Introduction to Animal Behavior and Veterinary Behavioral Medicine

Introduction to Animal Behavior and Veterinary Behavioral Medicine

Edited by

Meghan E. Herron
Gigi's (Shelter for Dogs), Ohio
US

WILEY Blackwell

Published by John Wiley & Sons, Inc., Hoboken, New Jersey.
Published simultaneously in Canada.

Library of Congress Cataloging-in-Publication Data
Names: Herron, Meghan E., editor.
Title: Introduction to animal behavior and veterinary behavioral medicine / edited by Meghan E. Herron.
Description: Hoboken, New Jersey : Wiley-Blackwell, [2024] | Includes bibliographical references and index.
Identifiers: LCCN 2024000377 (print) | LCCN 2024000378 (ebook) | ISBN 9781119824480 (paperback) | ISBN 9781119824503 (adobe pdf) | ISBN 9781119824497 (epub)
Subjects: MESH: Behavior, Animal–physiology | Veterinary Medicine–methods | Human-Animal Interaction. | Dogs | Cats | Horses
Classification: LCC SF756.7 (print) | LCC SF756.7 (ebook) | NLM SF 756.7 | DDC 636.089–dc23/eng/20240206
LC record available at https://lccn.loc.gov/2024000377
LC ebook record available at https://lccn.loc.gov/2024000378

Cover Design: Wiley
Cover Images: Calf - © Emily Miller-Cushon, University of Florida, Horse - © Jill E. Sackman, Dog - © Ryan Hughes, Cat - © Aditi Czarnomski

Set in 9.5/12.5pt STIXTwoText by Straive, Pondicherry, India
SKY10074521_070324

Dedication

I dedicate this book to the late Linda Lord. I had the pleasure of knowing Linda for over three decades. My formative years were spent in awe and mild annoyance, listening to my mother go on and on about Linda's pure perfection. She was the smart, natural beauty who excelled in sports while still getting straight A's – every mother's dream. As such, I idolized Linda like an eager grasshopper for years. Given my interest in science and animal behavior, she was the first person to suggest that I consider veterinary school. She told it to me straight and helped me set practical and realistic expectations.

Something I admired most about Linda was her never-ending desire to better the community around her. If there was an issue with students, she enacted a plan to fix it and prevent it from recurring. When a friend was in need, she dropped everything, hopped on a plane, and was there and present. When elderly and disabled pet owners needed a way to get care for themselves and their pets, she created a program and funding to provide it. She did not complain about the woes of the world as most of us do; she made plans, acted to create change, and, more importantly, motivated others to do the same.

Linda chose veterinary medicine as a second career. This late start did not stop her from quickly ascending into leadership roles and becoming a strong public advocate for the profession. While Linda earned numerous awards throughout her career, what she found most important was not just helping animals but also helping and guiding people. She understood and valued the importance that pets brought to people's lives. Her advocacy and dedication for proper care and protection of animals have been valuable and appreciated. Her publications on pet identification and the importance of microchipping set a course for drastic improvement in owner-pet reunification, and her findings set today's standard for pet identification and recovery. Much of her early work focused on the human–animal bond, animal welfare, and shelter medicine, thus improving the lives of pets and their people around the world.

Linda had a professional and personal maturity beyond her years, and her unique combination of values and skills led to her eventually becoming the Associate Dean for Professional Programs at the College, President of the Ohio Veterinary Medical Association, and the Ohio delegate to the American Veterinary Medical Association. I could not possibly list the many programs and initiatives she either started or enhanced, but all of them were to help others. Linda blazed a trail in every role she served. She positively impacted the people around her and beyond through her vision, commitment, and actions to promote diversity and inclusion, health and wellbeing, shelter medicine, outreach and engagement, professional development, leadership, and much more.

She was a gifted teacher, role model, advisor, and administrator. The contributions she made to our profession have been remarkable, and her legacy will live on through programs and people who have grown through her initiatives. Although we can no longer ask Linda for her advice and counsel, what we can do, and what I have already done, is ask ourselves in certain situations, "What would Linda do"? And this will serve us all well.

Contents

List of Contributors *xiii*
Acknowledgments *xv*
About the Companion Website *xvii*

Part I Introduction to Animal Behavior and Handling Concepts *1*

1 **Introduction** *3*
Meghan E. Herron
Why We Study Behavior *3*
How We Study Behavior *4*
What Comes Next *5*

2 **The Process of Domestication** *7*
Carlos A. Driscoll
Introduction *7*
Animal Domestication *8*
Dogs *14*
Cats *15*
Farm Animals *17*
Horses *19*
Entrained Beasts *22*
Domestication in Fast- Forward: The Farm- Fox Experiment *22*
References *24*

3 **Social Behavior** *31*
R. Julia Kilgour, Traci Shreyer, and Candace Croney
Introduction *31*
Evolutionary and Environmental Constraints on Social Behavior *32*
The Costs and Benefits of Group Living *32*
Types of Social Groupings *36*
Conflict in Social Groups *39*
Social Structures and Dominance Hierarchies *44*
Affiliative Behaviors *47*
Parent–Offspring Relationships *50*
Conclusion *54*
References *55*

4 **Sensory and Perception** *65*
Shana Gilbert-Gregory
Introduction *65*
Vision *66*
Audition *73*
Olfaction *77*
Gustation (Taste) *81*
Conclusion *82*
References *82*

5 **Animal Learning** *91*
Lisa Radosta
Introduction *91*
Factors Affecting Learning *91*
Types of Learning *96*
Choosing the Right Training Method *101*
Techniques for Changing Behavior *103*
Reinforcement Schedules *104*
Conclusion *107*
References *107*

6 **The Development of Behavior and the Shaping of the Human–Animal Bond: Dogs** *111*
Marie Hopfensperger and Jacquelyn Jacobs
Introduction *111*
Developmental Stages in Dogs *111*
Veterinary Care *119*
Behavior Support for Clients *121*
Managing Typical Puppy Behaviors *123*
Conclusion *128*
References *128*

7 **The Development of Behavior and the Shaping of the Human–Animal Bond: Cats** *135*
Kersti Seksel
Introduction *135*
Developmental Periods *136*
Setting Up for Success *143*
Veterinary Experiences *150*
Conclusion *151*
References *151*

8 **The Development of Behavior and the Shaping of the Human–Animal Bond: Horses** *153*
Katherine A. Houpt and Sharon Madere
Introduction *153*
The Neonatal Period *153*
Mare–Foal Communication *156*
Early Training *157*
Play *158*
Sick Foals *159*

Foal Rejection *160*
The Orphan Foal *160*
Weaning *160*
Predicting Adult Behavior *162*
Additional Problem Prevention Tips *162*
References *162*

9 **Bovine Communication, Handling, and Restraint** *165*
Kathryn L. Proudfoot
Introduction *165*
How Cattle Perceive Their World *165*
How Cattle Communicate Their Emotions *167*
Impact of Human Handlers on Cattle Affective States *170*
Cattle Handling and Restraint *172*
Cattle Handling in the Real World *175*
Conclusion *176*
References *176*

10 **Equine Communication, Handling, and Restraint** *181*
Jeannine Berger and Kathryn Holcomb
Introduction *181*
Body Language and Emotional States *181*
Tools, Handling Skills, and Procedures *186*
Medications to Aide in Handling *200*
References *203*

11 **Canine and Feline Communication, Restraint, and Handling** *205*
Meghan E. Herron, Allison Shull, Traci Shreyer, and Susan Barrett
Introduction *206*
Step 1: Assess the Environment *207*
Step 2: Assess the Patient's Comfort Level and Indicators of Intent *214*
Step 3: Assess Yourself *215*
Step 4: Make a Handling Plan *220*
Conclusion *238*
References *238*

Part II Clinical Concepts in Animal Behavior *241*

12 **Addressing Canine and Feline Behavior Problems in Clinical Practice: The Art of Behavior Triage** *243*
Traci Shreyer, Susan Barrett, and Allison Shull
Introduction *244*
The Importance of Communication *245*
The Five Steps of Behavior Triage *246*
Setting Up the Behavior-focused Visit *262*
Other Important Certifying Organizations *265*
References *265*

13 Feline Elimination Disorders *269*
Amy L. Pike
Introduction *269*
Normal Elimination Behavior *269*
History Taking for Elimination Disorders *272*
Ruling Out Medical Disorders *275*
Behavior Diagnoses for Undesirable Elimination *276*
Approach to Treatment *278*
Conclusion *284*
References *284*

14 Feline Aggression *289*
Carlo Siracusa
Introduction *289*
Neurophysiology of Aggression *289*
Aggression As a Normal Social Behavior of Cats *290*
When Cat Aggression Becomes a Behavior Problem *292*
Physical Disease and Aggression *293*
Classification of Cat Aggression *294*
General Guidelines for the Treatment of Aggression *296*
Using Psychoactive Medication to Treat Affective Aggression *299*
Cat Aggression Directed to People *300*
Aggression Between Cats *303*
References *306*

15 Canine Aggression *311*
Gabrielle Carter
Introduction *311*
The Body Language of Aggression *313*
Factors that Influence Aggression *315*
Making an Aggression Diagnosis *320*
General Principles of Treating Aggression Cases in Dogs *326*
Prognosis *331*
Considerations for Rehoming/Relinquishing/Euthanasia *333*
Conclusion *334*
References *334*

16 Separation-Related Disorders in Dogs *337*
Niwako Ogata
Introduction *337*
Definitions and Variations on Separation-Related Disorders *338*
Risk Factors *340*
Common Signs *340*
Making a Definitive Diagnosis *343*
Approach to Treatment *345*
Concluding Remarks *348*
References *349*

17 **Equine Aggression** *351*
Jeannine Berger and Kathy Holcomb
Introduction *351*
Categories of Aggression *353*
Diagnosis and Treatment Summary *361*
What to Avoid When Addressing Aggression *363*
Medication *363*
References *364*
Further Reading *365*

18 **Repetitive Behaviors in Companion Animals** *367*
Melissa Bain
Introduction *367*
Definitions and Motivating Factors *367*
Specific Repetitive Behaviors *370*
Physiological Differentials *373*
Gathering a History *375*
Treatment *376*
Conclusion *380*
References *380*

19 **Repetitive and Other Abnormal Behaviors in Wild Animals Under Human Care** *385*
Mark Flint and Randall E. Junge
Introduction *385*
Behavior and Other Domains as a Welfare Indicator *386*
Common Abnormal Repetitive Behaviors *388*
Applying What We have Learned in Zoos and Wildlife Sanctuaries *391*
Prevention, Management, and Treatment *395*
Conclusion *399*
References *399*

20 **Repetitive and Other Abnormal Behaviors in Livestock and Horses** *403*
Emily Miller-Cushon and Carissa Wickens
Introduction *403*
Behavioral Indicators of Sickness *403*
Behavioral Indicators of Pain *404*
Cognitive Approaches to Understanding Emotional States *407*
Importance of Meeting Behavioral Needs *407*
Common Abnormal Behaviors in Horses, Pigs, Cattle, and Poultry *408*
Medical Considerations *410*
Prevention, Management, and Treatment Concepts *412*
References *416*

21 **Approach to Psychopharmacology in Companion Animals** *419*
M. Leanne Lilly
Introduction *419*
Daily Medications *420*
Specific Medications *422*

Selecting a Daily Medication *425*
Event Medications *426*
Polytherapy *430*
Administering Medications *431*
Weaning *432*
References *434*

22 Chemical Restraint and Sedation in Small Animals *443*
M. Leanne Lilly
Introduction *443*
Medications and Routes *444*
Protocols, Combinations, and Decision-Making *450*
Safely Getting Injections into Your Patients *451*
Achieving and Maintaining Sedation *451*
Record Keeping and Communication *455*
References *457*

23 Behavior Considerations for Aging Dogs and Cats *461*
Margaret O'Brian
Introduction *461*
Sensory Changes *461*
Brain Changes *463*
Cognitive Dysfunction Syndrome *464*
References *469*

Appendix A: Books to Keep in Practice – Clinical Textbook Recommendations *471*
Appendix B: Teaching Your Cat to Like the Carrier *473*
Lisa Radosta

Glossary *475*
Index *483*

List of Contributors

Melissa Bain
School of Veterinary Medicine, University of California, Davis, Davis, CA, USA

Susan Barrett
VCA Morris Animal Hospital, Small Animal Clinical Private Practice, Lancaster, OH, USA

Jeannine Berger
Sacramento Veterinary Behavior Services, Vacaville, CA, USA

Gabrielle Carter
Royal Society for the Prevention of Cruelty to Animals Victoria, Burwood East VIC, Australia

Candace Croney
Department of Comparative Pathobiology, Department of Animal Sciences, Purdue University, West Lafayette, IN, USA

Carlos A. Driscoll
InnerCat, Frederick, MD, USA

Mark Flint
One Welfare and Sustainability Center, College of Veterinary Medicine, The Ohio State University, Columbus, OH, USA

Shana Gilbert-Gregory
Behavioral Medicine Service, Mount Laurel Animal Hospital, Mount Laurel, NJ, USA

Meghan E. Herron
Gigi's, (Shelter for Dogs) Canal Winchester, OH, USA

Kathryn Holcomb
School of Veterinary Medicine, University of California, Davis, Davis, CA, USA

Marie Hopfensperger
College of Veterinary Medicine, Michigan State University, East Lansing, MI, USA

Katherine A. Houpt
College of Veterinary Medicine, Cornell University, Ithaca, NY, USA

Jacquelyn Jacobs
Department of Animal Science, College of Agriculture and Natural Resources, Michigan State University, East Lansing, MI, USA

Randall E. Junge
Columbus Zoo and Aquarium, Powell, OH, USA

R. Julia Kilgour
Department of Integrative Biology, University of Guelph, Guelph, ON, Canada

M. Leanne Lilly
Veterinary Medical Center, The Ohio State University, Columbus, OH, USA

Sharon Madere
International Association of Animal Behavior Consultants (IAABC), Cranberry Township, PA, USA

Emily Miller-Cushon
Department of Animal Sciences, University of Florida, Gainesville, FL, USA

Margaret O'Brian
Southeast Animal Behavior and Training, Charlotte, NC, USA

Niwako Ogata
Department of Veterinary Clinical Sciences, College of Veterinary Medicine, Purdue University, West Lafayette, IN, USA

Amy L. Pike
Animal Behavior Wellness Center, Fairfax, VA, USA

Kathryn L. Proudfoot
Sir James Dunn Animal Welfare Centre, Atlantic Veterinary College, University of Prince Edward Island, Charlottetown, PEI, Canada

Lisa Radosta
Florida Veterinary Behavior Service, West Palm Beach, FL, USA

Kersti Seksel
Adjunct Professor in Veterinary Behaviour, University of Queensland, Australia

Traci Shreyer
The Croney Research Group, Purdue University, West Lafayette, IN, USA

Allison Shull
ASPCA Cruelty and Recovery Center, Columbus, OH, USA

Carlo Siracusa
Department of Clinical Sciences and Advanced Medicine, School of Veterinary Medicine, University of Pennsylvania, Philadelphia, PA, USA

Carissa Wickens
Department of Animal Sciences, University of Florida, Gainesville, FL, USA

Acknowledgments

This book is the realization of a long-held dream, and I have many to thank for its remarkable content and organization. I first want to thank each one of the authors for their incredible contributions. With unwavering dedication, they poured countless hours into crafting their manuscripts, ensuring that content was not only well-researched but also presented in a clear, captivating manner. I am ever appreciative for their patience and understanding as they unbegrudgingly navigated my repeated edits and numerous requests for photos, figures, and permissions. I found myself continually learning and gaining new insights from each chapter, and I am beyond thrilled at last to share this knowledge with our readers.

The photo content in this book was no small feat. I am indebted to my colleagues at Gigi's for tolerating my following them around, butting into exam rooms, and asking them to repeat what they just did so I could get it on camera, as they enriched the lives of shelter dogs daily and practiced animal handling in the most graceful and patient of ways. Thank you also to my clients, friends, and coworkers – both from Gigi's and The Ohio State University Behavioral Medicine Service for sharing their photos – revealing all sorts of cuteness and quirks to the world. My biggest thanks go to my partner-in-crime, Aditi Czarnomski, for her prolific contributions to the photos in this book and for dropping everything just to capture a photo of her cat, Steve, pooping outside of the litterbox.

Thank you to my early mentors in animal behavior, Traci Shreyer and Candace Croney, for illuniating the path that led to my career and that of many other students you inspired.

Thank you to my residency mentor, Dr. Ilana Reisner, the goddess of editing, for teaching me the difference between "lay" and "lie" and giving me a true appreciation for the written word in veterinary medicine. I owe all my writing successes to you, just as much as my clinical skills in veterinary behavior.

A book has no future without a publisher that believes in it. Wiley has supported this idea since my early days at The Ohio State University College of Veterinary Medicine. Without their patience and persistence with my years of delay, Introduction to Animal Behavior and Veterinary Behavioral Medicine may not have ever seen a bookshelf.

Thank you, Josh Black, for your unrelenting support and patience as I read, re-read, edited, and re-edited page after page, month after month. I am so grateful to share this life's journey with you and our smart, strong, and beautiful girls, Rowan and Amelia. Girls, mommy can finally read books at bedtime again. And with that, a special thanks goes to the furry friends in my life who have helped give this book its personal perspective (and several photos): Junebug, Willett, Ranger, and Junior.

Meghan E. Herron

About the Companion Website

This book is accompanied by a companion website.

www.wiley.com/go/introductiontoanimalbehavior

This website includes:

- Videos
- Handouts
- Weblinks

Part I

Introduction to Animal Behavior and Handling Concepts

1

Introduction

Meghan E. Herron

Gigi's, Canal Winchester, OH, USA

Why We Study Behavior

You have either picked up this book as a requirement for an introductory course, or you have chosen to seek knowledge on behavior because there is an absence in your veterinary school's curriculum. Perhaps you are a freshly minted veterinarian eager to acquire information that wasn't covered during your studies, or you are a seasoned practitioner seeking a refresher now that behavior seems more pertinent in practice. Whatever brought you to this page, you are welcome here, and I hope you find this journey to be insightful, interesting, and, most of all, fun.

Some of you may be wondering why behavior is even part of your veterinary curriculum. How does it tie into the crucial task of saving lives and the thrilling career that lies ahead of you? While behavior may not have been at the forefront of your mind when you decided to pursue veterinary medicine, I am here to tell you it will inevitably become a fundamental aspect of your daily lives, regardless of what field or specialty lands in your path.

To begin, let's talk about how behavioral medicine IS medicine. The brain is an organ, and it oversees the entirety of the body's functions and actions. It is the grand central station for emotions, movements, and actions, all of which shape behavior, whether voluntary or reflexive. While the brain may have anatomical or biochemical abnormalities directly affecting the behavior of an animal, as veterinarians, we must also recognize that behavior problems are not solely the result of brain-related abnormalities. Metabolic diseases, hormonal imbalances, pain, and discomfort can also exert significant influence on behavior, even if the physical abnormality is not overtly severe. The question we should ask ourselves is not "Is this a behavior problem or a medical problem," but rather "What medical problem might be causing or influencing this behavior" before ever reaching for a behavior modification plan. In many cases, behavior is merely a symptom of what is going on beneath the surface.

Understanding animal behavior and how to apply it will help you practice better medicine in many ways. Behavior recognition plays a central role in livestock rearing and handling. Many of these animals are bigger and/or stronger than we humans and have the potential to be dangerous if they feel threatened. The ability to recognize and respond to animals' emotional states, and when they might be feeling threatened, will keep you, your staff, and your clients safer. Furthermore, reproductive

Introduction to Animal Behavior and Veterinary Behavioral Medicine, First Edition. Edited by Meghan E. Herron.

Companion website: www.wiley.com/go/introductiontoanimalbehavior

medicine is heavily dependent on behavioral signs of estrus, and a successful breeding program requires a solid understanding of animal behavior. Each species of livestock has unique social behavior, which will dictate how and where animals should be housed, fed, and handled. Poor understanding of social behavior leads to injury, fighting, poor welfare, and loss of product. In dairy cows, posture, movement, and time spent in recumbency are all primary indicators of foot pain. A veterinarian must rely on these behaviors to accurately assess individual and herd health.

In wild animal sanctuaries and zoos, knowledge of natural behavior is crucial for survival in captivity. Attempts to breed endangered species in captivity have only been successful thanks to insight from their behavior in the wild and the ability to adapt habitats that allow them to engage in as many normal behaviors as possible. Since frequent physical examination of wild animals has its challenges, careful monitoring of behavior allows for early detection of underlying medical problems. Understanding learning theory, and how emotions are conditioned, allows for animal caretakers and healthcare providers to perform physical assessments without sedation. Animals that would otherwise be extremely dangerous to handle are readily complying with venipuncture and medication administration as a result of training and the establishment of trust.

How companion animals behave and interact with their caretakers forms the core of the human–animal bond. With that, problematic behaviors are a top reason this bond may weaken or break. Veterinarians have the advantage of meeting many pets at a young age, presenting an opportunity for problem prevention and early intervention when problems do arise. We have not always been viewed as a person of expertise in this subject matter, but as veterinary curriculums and continuing education programs expand to include behavioral medicine, our collective confidence is changing for the better.

The Bayer veterinary care usage study revealed that a large percentage of feline patients do not receive annual wellness care. Clients reported that the stress their pet experiences both at and on the way to the veterinary clinic was a bigger barrier to obtaining care for their cat than was the cost of that care. We must make this experience better for both clients and cats if we want to make a dent in this alarming statistic. Knowledge of behavioral stress signals and how to mitigate them is the first step. This book will give you those tools, which will serve as a foundation for additional learning through programs aimed at improving the veterinary experience for small animals, such as Fear Free®, Low Stress Handling®, and Cat Friendly Practice® certifications.

How We Study Behavior

There are three main approaches to the study of behavior – ethological, experiential, and physiological. The ethological approach examines an animal's natural behavior in the wild and specifically considers how their behavior has an adaptive, evolutionary value. For domesticated species, humans have artificially selected behavior traits that work well for companionship and/or group housing. Wild animals, on the other hand, have been naturally selected based on traits that have allowed them to survive and evolve without human influence. The early chapters of this book will walk you through the process of domestication and how behavior has influenced it, social behavior and its influence on the husbandry of animals, and how the evolution of various sensory and perception systems has shaped animal behavior.

The experiential approach attempts to understand an animal's behavior based on what they learned during early life experiences. Each species has early developmental stages where experiences gained have dramatic effects on adult behavior. How, when, and to what extent that occurs differs between species, with domesticated species having the most prolonged periods of susceptibility to human influence. We will delve into early influences on the behavioral development of companion animals as we move toward the central portion of this book.

Lastly, the physiological approach delves into how the biology and physiology of animals intricately shape their individual behaviors. Take, for instance, the endocrine system, which governs the onset and cessation of numerous behaviors, ranging from reproductive activities to food and water intake, parental care, and sleep patterns. Any deviations from these behavioral norms may indicate an underlying physiological issue. As veterinarians, we hold both a moral and professional responsibility to comprehend and grasp these behavioral changes, understanding the diverse physiological processes that can influence them.

In the latter part of this book, we introduce concepts of clinical behavioral medicine, taking a physiological approach to understand various abnormal behaviors observed across multiple species. Through this journey, we seek to deepen our insights and begin to gain the expertise needed to address behavioral issues in a comprehensive manner, rooted in the interplay between biology, physiology, and behavior. This knowledge equips us to provide the best care possible for our animal patients and fulfill our commitment to their health and well-being.

After reading this book, you should be able to:

- Understand how different factors (e.g. genetics, physiology, learning, the environment) impact normal and abnormal animal behavioral development and expression.
- Reliably read and interpret the body language and behaviors of various domesticated species.
- Apply knowledge about animal behavior to safely handle animals and promote positive welfare.
- Anticipate situations in which animal behavior and/or well-being may be problematic and develop an appropriate plan of action.
- Examine fundamental principles related to the development of behavior in domesticated animals.
- Demonstrate how knowledge of animal behavior is relevant to clinical practice and how it can be applied to facilitate safe and humane animal handling, care and management, behavioral wellness, and positive human–animal interactions.
- Feel prepared for advanced coursework in applied animal behavior such as clinical treatment of problem behaviors.

What Comes Next

Those of you seeking to expand your knowledge and abilities are encouraged to seek out clinical experiences with veterinary behaviorists. This may include signing up for a clinical rotation while in school or spending time shadowing a behavior practice as a veterinarian. Several formal externships exist if your institution does not offer clinical behavioral medicine opportunities. Additionally, most of the major veterinary conferences, including the Midwest Veterinary Conference, Western Veterinary Conference, VMX, and the AVMA Annual Convention routinely offer continuing education on behavior topics.

Whether you are triaging a behavior case as elaborated in Chapter 11, conducting a full appointment within your practice, or preparing patients for referral to a behavior specialist, you can confidently approach these situations. This book can serve as an invaluable future reference, providing you with essential insights and strategies. Moreover, it would be beneficial to have clinically focused textbooks readily available, especially those specific to the species you commonly encounter in your practice. Appendix A contains a comprehensive list of books that can be of great interest to you as a veterinarian. By building a library with these resources, you enhance your ability to address behavior-related challenges and further elevate the level of care you provide to your patients.

If you discover a passion for behavioral medicine and want to learn more about specializing in this amazing field, visit www.DACVB.org for information on residency programs and how to find a veterinary behaviorist in your area. After veterinary school, Diplomates of the American College of Veterinary Behaviorists (DACVBs) have completed at least one year of clinical veterinary practice or a rotating internship, a three-year (on average) residency program, published a clinical case report and a scientific paper, and passed an exam to achieve board certification. If you think this may be your intended career path, I encourage you to reach out to DACVBs for shadowing opportunities and network with them at annual Veterinary Behavior Symposiums.

Regardless of where your path takes you, remember, with the right knowledge and resources at hand, you have the potential to make a significant difference in the lives of the animals you serve. So embrace these opportunities, stay curious, and keep learning for the well-being of your patients and the fulfillment of your practice.

2

The Process of Domestication

Carlos A. Driscoll

InnerCat, Frederick, MD, USA

Introduction

Domestication is the most important thing humans have ever done. The clever use of raw materials to make tools and the mastery of fire separated our hominid forefathers from most of the natural world, but domesticating animals and plants brought surpluses of materials, energy, and food, which drove a human population explosion still continuing to this day (Harris 1996a). Today, at the dawn of the latest geological era, the Anthropocene, 96% of all land mammals are livestock or humans, and only 4% of animals are wild; of birds, only 30% are wild, and the remaining 70% are poultry (Bar-On et al. 2018). 12% of the world's land surface is used for agriculture; 70% of fresh water consumed is used to water it; and the food produced has allowed the human population to grow from an estimated 5 million in the Neolithic to 7.9 billion, and growing, today (Groube 1996; World Resources Institute 2000). Naturally evolved "wild" species are going extinct at a rate 100–1,000 times faster than the "background" rate, primarily as a result of habitat loss, itself overwhelmingly driven by conversion of natural habitats to raising domestic animals and plants. Yet no domesticated animal has ever gone extinct (Zeder 2008).

What does this have to do with animal behavior and veterinary medicine? Behavioral disorders are increasingly common in companion and farm animals and constitute a large and growing fraction of veterinary expenses. Behavior is the driving factor in the domestication process, and so the study of domestication is really the study of heritably modified behavior. Although domesticates have been structurally refashioned by processes of selection (Natural and Artificial), domestic animals today are nevertheless reflections of the wild ancestors from which they descend. Behaviors observed today are not elementally different from the behaviors expressed by those ancestors, but the environmental context is unimaginably different than that which shaped life in the wild (Tinbergen 1951). We, as humans, have pulled these animals out of their naturally evolved contexts and exposed them to challenges for which they were not originally adapted to cope. Studying how domesticates came to be and what they came from will enlighten practitioners regarding the genetic etiology of behavioral disorders, thereby improving the health and welfare of their patients (Boissey and Erhard 2014; Grandin and Deesing 2014).

This approach to understanding is not in itself new but has recently been re-addressed as Evolutionary Medicine (Perry 2021). This is

Introduction to Animal Behavior and Veterinary Behavioral Medicine, First Edition. Edited by Meghan E. Herron.

Companion website: www.wiley.com/go/introductiontoanimalbehavior

a way of thinking about medicine – human and animal – that seeks to inform practitioners about medically significant genetic variation, mismatches to modernity, reproductive medicine, degenerative disease, pathogen evolution, and comparative medicine by explicitly incorporating an evolutionary perspective (Benton et al. 2021; Stearns 2012).

One avenue to understanding behavioral disorders (in both animals and humans) is to discover the genetic underpinnings of behavior. This is challenging because it is difficult to define a behavior in question accurately and precisely, and it is difficult to discover and parse contributions of individual genes to behavior. Moreover, there is high ecophenotypic variability in behavior, that is, the expression of gene products is greatly influenced by the environment. Students of behavioral genetics seek to understand the combined role of genetics and the environment in forming individual behavioral variation. And perhaps the most profitable approach to an understanding of behavior is the study of domestication in animals.

Animal Domestication

In the Beginning

Six centers of independent animal domestication are shown in Figure 2.1 along with some of the more important locally derived domesticates. Their ancestral origins and relationships are listed in Table 2.1. Looking at this list, there are several obvious questions: why were some species domesticated and not others? Why, out of some 2 million wild animals, are there only about 30 domestic animal species worldwide? Why are there only these few homelands of domestication?

These few places had certain characteristics that encouraged domestication to develop (Bellwood 2007; Harris 1969; Sauer 1952). From an early age, these locations hosted human societies that were stable, sedentary, had social complexity, and were relatively long-lasting. Not incidentally, these areas each also had wild animals that were ecologically suitable for human use. These locales are

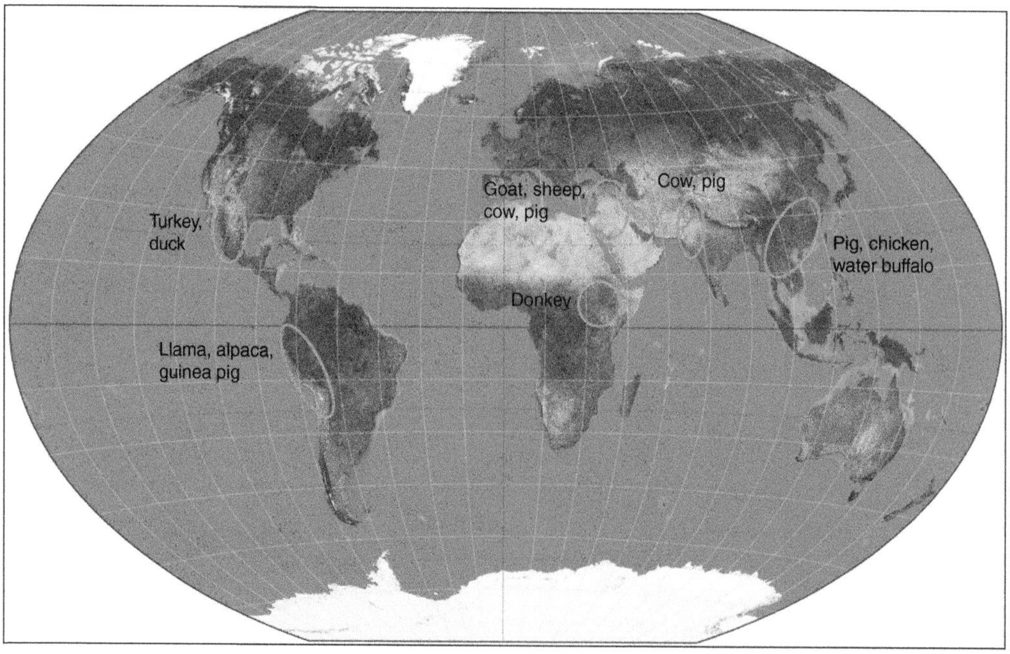

Figure 2.1 A map of the world showing the six centers where the domestication of animals occurred independently. *Source:* Background photo credit: WikiMediaCommons/Daniel R. Strebe.

Table 2.1 Origin of eight common domesticated animals inferred by mitochondrial DNA.

	Domesticated species		Wild ancestor			
Clade	Name	Latin	Name	Latin	Location	References
Mammals	Dog	*Canis lupus familiaris*	Gray wolf	*Canis lupus*	Beringia	Ni Leathlobhair et al. 2018 Perri et al. 2021 Bergstrom et al. 2020 Loog et al. 2020
	Cat	*Felis sylvestris catus*	African wildcat	*Felis silvestris lybica*	Near East	Driscoll et al. 2007
	Donkey	*Equus asinus*	African wild ass	*Equus africanus*	Northeast Africa	Beja-Pereira et al. 2004 Orlando 2015
	Pig	*Sus scrofa domesticus*	Wild boar	*Sus scrofa*	East Asia South Asia Southeast Asia West Asia Europe	Larson et al. 2005 Wu et al. 2007
	Cattle	*Bos taurus*	Aurochs	*Bos primigenius*	West Asia North Africa Europe?	Troy et al. 2001 Achilli et al. 2008 Achilli et al. 2009 Bonfiglio et al. 2010 Bonfiglio et al. 2012
	Horse	*Equus caballus*	Wild horse	*Equus ferus*	Lower Volga-Don	Librado et al. 2021
	Sheep	*Ovis aries*	Asian mouflon	*Ovis orientalis*	West Asia	Hiendleder et al. 2002 Meadows et al. 2007 Pedrosa et al. 2005 Tapio et al. 2006
	Goat	*Capra aegagrus hircus*	Bezoar	*Capra aegagrus*	West Asia; East Asia	Naderi et al. 2008 Chen et al. 2005 Luikart et al. 2001
Birds	Chicken	*Gallus gallus domesticus*	Red junglefowl	*Gallus gallus*	Southern East Asia South Asia	Liu et al. 2006 Miao et al. 2013

Source: Adapted from Wang et al. 2014, with permission from Annual Reviews.

recognized as centers of domestication today because they were the first to develop in their region. This is significant because the process of domestication can take several thousands of years, and once an animal has come to be domesticated, it is easier for that animal to spread to new cultural centers than for each civilization to develop its own variant (Zeder 2008). We can extend that reasoning to believe that if today's familiar domesticates had not spread and preempted autochthonous development elsewhere, there would have been other different centers of domestication, with other different domestic animals, if other places had developed stable, sedentary, complex human societies earlier than those recognized today.

Although domestication and agriculture originated independently in several spots around the world, accumulated archaeological, cultural, and genetic evidence suggests it happened first in a region of the Near East called the Fertile Crescent beginning between 15,000 and 12,000 years ago (Bellwood 2007; Breasted 1916; Harris 1996b; Uerpmann 1989), and it makes a good example for the sequence of events that happened worldwide. It is in the Fertile Crescent during the Protoneolithic that nomadic hunter-gatherers, supported with ample wild game and wild cereals, first began to live in settled communities; first developed agriculture, both agronomy and animal husbandry; and first developed the more advanced sociopolitical organizations that we continue to this day (Bar-Yosef 1998; Breasted 1916; Uerpmann 1996).

Up to this point in human history, for over 250,000 years, humans had been nomadic hunter/gatherers, moving as they hunted an area out and building no permanent structure. But the Fertile Crescent was so bountiful it was possible to hunt and gather all that was needed without being nomadic (Ucko et al. 1969; Uerpmann 1996). This set the stage for sedentism where, between 12,500 and 10,800 BC, the movable base camps of this hunting/gathering elite, called Natufians by archaeologists, evolved into permanent, semi-subterranean pit houses, where they stored wild grains for use throughout the year (Uerpmann 1989). Note that sedentism, living in one place all year around, proceeds plant and animal domestication by at least several thousand years.

Traits that Favor Domestication

It has long been argued that only certain wild animals are suitable for domestication. Francis Galton was the first to publish thoughts on what makes a good candidate (Galton 1865). Although varying criteria have been set forth since, such lists usually include components similar to his in spirit, if not name (Driscoll et al. 2009). The following traits of a species favor domestication:

1) Proclivity to form large social groups with modifiable social hierarchies – Group living animals are naturally calmer when in groups (when grouped appropriately), thus reducing the drive to flee, and also increasing the efficiency of husbandry since they do not have to be housed individually.
2) Promiscuous mating – The ability to breed in captivity is an absolute mandate for success. Propagating the stock is important for obvious reasons, but captive breeding also opens the door to intensive artificial selection.
3) Sexual signals are behavioral – having obvious signals for optimal fertility windows allows humans to maximize success of mating strategies.
4) Parental-offspring bonding – A prolonged window of opportunity for humans to insert themselves as familiar and safe caretakers leads to less fear early in life and promotes longer-lasting tameness.
5) Short flight distance – This involves a heightened fear threshold, the outcome being an overall relatively lessened drive to flee from humans (be it a human's sight, sound, or smell).
6) Flexible diets – A flexible diet is important since animals in captivity are unlikely to be fed the same spread of foods that they

would source themselves in the wild. Finicky animals would have been eliminated quickly.

7) Limited agility – A limited ability to escape confinement and/or containment allows for greater ease of housing/penning.
8) Climate adaptability – Animals that are "hardy" and can thrive in changing climates are better suited for populating a variety of geographic locations.
9) Fast growth rates – A fast growth rate ensures that the harvest – of milk, meat, wool, or even antler – is attained within a reasonable time and with reasonable effort, while consuming a reasonable number of resources.
10) **Docility** – Perhaps one of the most important traits to favor domestication. This encompasses a native openness to tameness, if not outright human interaction. These animals have a fair temperament and do not panic.

Not all traits are required for candidacy and there are traits not listed that might be useful. Most important among the traits of domestication, and the only one common to all domesticates, is docility – a lack of fear of people, an important consequence of which is the inborn ability to live in proximity to people.

These aspects of personality are strongly genetically influenced, and individual personality is highly variable (Koolhaas et al. 2007; Korte et al. 2005). It is this individual variation that is subject to selection (Sloan Wilson et al. 1994; Houslay et al. 2022; Oswald et al. 2013). Individual variability in personality is the key to making a domestic animal because that individual variability is the grist on which Darwinian selection works.

Evolution and Selection

Darwin grouped selection into *natural*, including **sexual selection**, and *artificial*, which is effected either methodically or unconsciously, intent being the heart of the difference (Darwin 1991; Darwin 1890; Darwin 1972; Reznick 2010). **Natural selection** predominates in "the wild" where the survival of individuals long enough to breed and raise offspring to maturity is the sole criterion for selection. No less mechanistic, **artificial selection** is effected by humans, who are possessed of rational thought. By Darwin's reckoning, unconscious selection implies no wish or expectation to alter a population, whereas methodical selection is guided by some predetermined standard as to what is best. The distinction between methodical or unconscious is important when considering domestication and its origins because that intent might tell us something about the people who are husbanding those animals. Unconscious selection might, for example, be the preferential elimination of aggressive captive goats in a pen simply because they are unpleasant to deal with. Methodical selection includes a forward-looking criterion, such as a desire for cattle with shorter, less dangerous horns.

Darwinian evolution requires four things: that animal produces more offspring than are required for generational replacement; that individuals are genetically/phenotypically variable; that the phenotypes are heritable; and that those differences influence reproduction and survival. This is as true of instinctive behaviors as it is of sharp claws, and strong bones, and appropriate beaks. Regardless, whether Natural or Artificial or any subtype of those, those four requirements are indispensable to evolution by selection. In the structure of a managed environment, humans unwittingly used the mechanistic power of Evolution by Selection to evolve animals faster than might occur in the wild, and by deciding which animals lived and died based on their tractability and utility to those people, humans became the driving force in the evolution of those populations.

Domestication Syndrome

The term **Domestication Syndrome** has been applied to a suite of modified characteristic traits involving physiology, morphology, and behavior that consistently occur across species of domestic animals (Price 1984; Price 2002). Physical and physiological characteristics common among domesticated mammals are described in Table 2.2 and include: dwarfs and giants, piebald coat color, wavy or curly hair, fewer vertebrae, shorter tails, rolled tails, floppy ears, and manifestations of **neoteny** (the retention of juvenile features into sexual maturity) such as a foreshortening of the skull and jaw, deposits of fat under the skin, and playfulness and purring (Clutton-Brock 1992b; Hemmer 1990; Zeuner 1963; Trut 1999; Zeder et al. 2006). Additional changes to the reproductive cycle, such as polyestrousness, and adaptations to a new, often poorer, diet are common.

Behaviorally too, domestication is not a single trait but a suite of traits comprising elements affecting mood, emotion, agnostic and affiliative behavior, and social communication, all modified in some way from their wild antecedents. Domesticates show reductions in adrenal development, fear of humans, and inter- and intra-species aggression, but increases in activity levels and explorative tendencies (Wright 2015). Changes mostly imply a tolerance of humans – human control of daily activity and reproduction; control of food supply; and utility to humans. But note that domesticates do not have to be "nice"; Miura toro bravo, for instance, or fighting cocks (in fact, chickens were domesticated for cockfighting, not for food (Zeuner 1963) are good examples.

Learn the Lingo

What exactly is **domestication,** and when is an animal domesticated? Domestication, as with all of evolution, is an ongoing process and not an endpoint (Albarella et al. 2006). No species, wild or domestic, is ever "perfectly adapted."

It is becoming commonly understood that behavioral adaptation is prerequisite to domestication and that the characteristic morphological cues of the Domestication Syndrome follow (Zeder et al. 2006). The outward morphological phenotypes are not individually defining characters – they are just symptoms of domestication. Thus, the nidus of domestication is the behavioral modification that allows humans to interact with a population. At its most elemental, domestication is a heritable docility (propensity for tameness). This allows humans to craft tame temperaments in individual animals more quickly and effectively.

Tame and domestic are blanket terms colloquially (and unevenly) applied to many animals habitually used by humans or habituated

Table 2.2 Domestication Syndrome includes a suite of modified characteristics that consistently occur across species of domesticated animals (Based on: Price 1984; Price 2002; Dobney and Larson 2006; Trut 1999).

Characteristic	Species
Dwarfs and giant varieties	All domesticated mammals
Piebald coat color	All domesticated mammals
Wavy or curly hair	Sheep, dogs, cats, donkeys, horses, pigs, goats, mice, and guinea pigs
Rolled tails	Dogs and pigs
Shortened tails, fewer vertebrae	Dogs, cats, and sheep
Floppy ears	Dogs, cats, pigs, horses, sheep, goats, cattle, and rabbits
Changes in reproductive cycle	All except sheep

to human places. But to the behavioral specialist looking through an evolutionary lens, taming and domestication are related but not identical and should not be conflated. Taming is conditioned behavioral modification of an individual animal at some point in its natural life and is not passed down from parent to offspring; domestication is genetic modification of populations which leads to an intergenerational predisposition toward human association: a *heritable* tameness (docility).

An ideal **wild** population is one unmodified by adaptation to a post-Neolithic human environment. In their niche, wild animals are subject to natural selection (which may include predation by humans) but not, except incidentally, to artificial (unconscious) selection. This idealization has caveats of course, the primary one being the occasional genetic exchange between wild and captive camps, as has been detected in pigs, goats, sheep, wolves, and wildcats, among others (Barbato et al. 2017; Daly et al. 2018; Driscoll et al. 2007; Frantz et al. 2019; Pilot et al. 2018).

Wild and **feral** are also often confused. A feral animal is an individual which has gone fully down the genetic path to domestication, perhaps having sustained selective breeding or even line breeding, but which has become reacquainted to some degree of independent living. "Wild" horses captured by Native Americans in the 1800s and mustangs in the contemporary American west, for example, and the ponies of Assateague, Chincoteague, and the Outer Banks, are decedents of *domesticated* European horses either liberated or escaped at the time of European settlement and are not at all wild in a genetic sense. *Feral* mustangs and *feral* ponies would be the more accurate terminology to describe these equids. A domesticated population experiencing sustained independence from humans is subject to heightened natural selection in a "natural" habitat, whatever form that might take, and adaptation proceeds according to those lines (Mangan et al. 2021). Much like the "wild" (feral) hogs plaguing farmlands, feral horses have adapted to predators, forage, and weather and live totally independent of humans. One might find it helpful to note that domesticated and wild refer to species and reflect genome changes as a result mostly of artificial selection over thousands of years. This is in contrast to terms like tame and feral, which refer to individual animals who have either lost their fear of humans (tame) or were born outside of and are living independently of human care (feral).

Peri-domestic animals are those that have ventured to exploit human environments, often settlements, and have become adapted to that environment through natural selection. These animals provide no human utility, in fact peri-domestic describes mice, rats, and sparrows often considered pests (i.e. parasitic).

Semi-domestic describes animals as a stage closer to human dependence and utility. These animals are part of, and are derived from, a human landscape, though they have not been subjected to conscious selective breeding. Due to their long association with humans and our environment, they are effectively reproductively isolated from their ancestors. The dingo and New Guinea singing dog have arrived, apparently chiefly by natural selection, at a stage where they are adapted to living in close quarters with people when the situation suits, even engaging in mutually beneficial tandem hunting parties, yet they are still capable of living altogether independent of humans.

Pathways to Domestication

All living things have personalities, that is, individual variations in behavior. Humans unwittingly mined this genetic variation when selecting those animals more readily amenable to human association, so producing domestic animals. Selection on behavior is thus the driving factor in domestication. But how did this selection come about? Here, we explore domestication pathways for: the dog (a special case), the cat (as a commensal), farm animals, and entrained beasts. Critically, all domesticates, relative to their ancestral "wild" state, manifest an inborn and lifelong tolerance of proximity to, or outright lack of fear of, people, brought about by selection and adaptation.

Dogs

Wolves were the first animals domesticated (Freedman et al. 2014; Hemmer 1990), with evidence of morphologically identifiable dogs dating to 14,500 ya (Janssens et al. 2018), but mitochondrial coalescent data suggests dog domestication by around 23,000 ya (Ameen et al. 2019). Phylogenetic inference indicates that all modern dogs have common a ancestry and are derived from one or more populations (concluded to be now extinct) of Eurasian grey wolf, *Canis lupus* (Bergstrom et al. 2020; Freedman et al. 2014; Freedman et al. 2016; Ni Leathlobhair et al. 2018). It is likely this population of wolves, and their domestic derivatives, originated in Siberia (Loog et al. 2020; Ni Leathlobhair et al. 2018). Subsequent to domestication, but most likely prior to 11,600 ya, several ancestral Eurasian lineages diverged (Bergstrom et al. 2020). This divergence is indicative of restricted gene flow between sub-populations attributed to population growth and spread across both distance and landform barriers.

Interestingly, modern grey wolves themselves have a genetic and temporal origin in northeast Siberia (Beringia) at roughly the same time (~25 kya) as domestication – a happenstance that may have clouded earlier genetic analysis (Loog et al. 2020). As the climate moderated and habitats opened, modern grey wolves spread out across Eurasia and later North America, entirely replacing earlier and distinct Pleistocene wolves (Fan et al. 2016; Freedman et al. 2014; Loog et al. 2020; Sinding et al. 2018).

Human Cultural Aspects of Wolf Domestication

While the genetic origin story of dogs has recently become less ambiguous, the human cultural context of just how wolves came to be domesticated is less clear, with explanations relying to a greater extent on untestable hypotheses (Clutton-Brock 1995; Driscoll et al. 2009; Driscoll and Macdonald 2010; Morey 1994; vonHoldt and Driscoll 2017; Zeuner 1963). In part because the ancestral population of wolves cannot yet be identified, there is no definitive evidence of the precise location of domestication (Bergstrom et al. 2020), limiting the inferences that can be made regarding the specific lifeways of the human groups that were involved. Also, the dramatically expository archaeological finds that make the reconstruction of farm animal domestication so clear are unlikely to survive for dogs up to the present day. Frustratingly, the most likely area of domestication includes Beringia, now largely under the Chukchi and Bering seas. In any event, because the Late Pleistocene humans domesticating wolves were at least semi-nomadic, there are few fixed sites where artifactual evidence would have accumulated in a time series, and any evidence that exists is likely spread over a geographic area the size of Australia.

That said, given the known climatic and ecological contexts and combined with genomic data, it seems most plausible that grey wolves and a lineage of Pleistocene hunter-gatherers, the Ancient North Siberians, became isolated in glacial refugia during the Late Glacial Maximum (~26,500–19,000 ya), where they would have relied on the same prey species and habitats and been forced to closely coexist (Perri et al. 2021). Wolves and humans are both social hunters/scavengers of large, herding, prey animals (e.g. mammoths, wapiti, bison, camels, and horses), and both rely on visual and auditory communication. The nature of earliest wolf – human interaction can only be conjectured, but it is possible that wolves followed human encampments, scavenging kills, or, indeed, humans and wolves scavenged the same kills. Over time, as wolves and humans became accustomed to a mutual presence, those wolves more bold and less fearful moved into a closer human orbit and benefited from an increased availability of scraps unsuitable or undesirable for human consumption.

Through a process of assortative mating, those wolves less fearful of humans bred with other wolves sharing similar personalities, bounded by their proximity to, and comfort in, anthropogenic environments. At this point, genetic differentiation between human-associated proto-dogs and the larger population of wild wolves would have become evident (to a time-traveling geneticist), and traits relating to heritable tameness may have appeared. Once introduced to the human niche, such proto-dogs may have manifested utility as barking nighttime sentinels, leveraging their enhanced faculties of smell and hearing (Lindsay 2000). A cultural aspect of domestication (let us say found pups are raised for a time by humans) would accelerate selection (unconscious and conscious) for increasingly sociable and approachable animals. It is notable that communication between wolves and humans is intrinsically intuitive, with aggression, fear, submission, and joy being mutually understood (Darwin and Lorenz 1965; Uerpmann 1996). As the relationship between early dogs and humans developed, connections between dogs and wolves dissolved. Once dogs were reliant on humans, dogs and wolves increasingly defined separate ecological niches, and barriers to interbreeding became higher. And while an early dog might survive amongst wolves, wolves were no longer welcome amongst dogs and their humans. This is detectable in dog and wolf genomes, where gene flow is substantial from dog to wolf but less so from wolves to dogs (Bergstrom et al. 2020; Pilot et al. 2018).

With the melting of the glaciers in the terminal Pleistocene, tundra yielded to forest, and new habitats opened up where a mobile, active companion with superior senses of hearing and smell and an inborn taste for the hunt would have a chance to shine. Dogs eventually spread from Beringia west throughout central Eurasia, India, the Near East, and into Africa, and east across Beringia into the Americas; south through Indo-China to Austronesia; and to the Pacific Islands and New Zealand. It is not known whether early dogs dispersed independently of humans. Other than the dingo, modern dogs do not live independently of settlements.

Dogs in Europe are of particular interest. Dogs accompanied Neolithic agriculturalists from the Near East as they migrated to Europe (Ollivier et al. 2018), and, again mirroring human demography, Neolithic Near Eastern dogs interbred with resident Mesolithic European hunter-gatherer dogs to produce a genetically variegated population. However, under circumstances not yet clear, dogs in Europe became genetically homogenized at 7,000 years old, completely overwriting the prior population diversity. This new, blended ancestry has dispersed worldwide and is now a ubiquitous and dominant component of all dog populations (Bergstrom et al. 2020).

Cats

In contrast to dog origins amongst the nomadic hunter-gatherers of the late Mesolithic, animals following the commensal pathway, including the mouse, house sparrow, pigeon, and cat, originate in settled communities of the early Neolithic. It was the very existence of year-round settlements that made their domestication possible. The short story is that in establishing permanent settlements, humans created a new ecological niche that was exploited by several species to their own benefit.

The first finds of house mouse remains have been identified from Israel and are dated to around 12,000 years ago, shortly after the first evidence of stores of wild grain (Auffray et al. 1988; Boursot et al. 1996). Stockpiles of grain would have supported a resident peri-domestic rodent population, which in turn provided an additional food source for local Near Eastern wildcats, which then became adapted to an "urban" environment as peri-domestic human commensals themselves. But a greater draw than the grain stores, at least initially, for both wildcats and mice, were discarded food wastes, which would have provided rich grounds for scavenging with no fear of human persecution while being close enough to people that larger predators are denied access. This rich new urban habitat, rather than the people living there, was the attraction for wildcats.

Initially, there would be little if any genetic or behavioral distance between a habituated urban-wildcat and a wild-wildcat, and they could move freely from one environment to another. Through a process of assortative mating, whereby animals with similar genetic backgrounds mate more frequently with each other than expected by chance (Via 2001), those wildcats more tolerant of living in human-dominated environments would meet and mate with other wildcats so disposed. In this model, cats (and other commensals) are not actively selected from the wild, but are simply allowed to persist, and over time and perhaps space, they gradually diverge from their "wild" relatives (Driscoll et al. 2007; Driscoll et al. 2009; Todd 1978). Cat domestication is a surety by 3,600 ya when house cats are clearly depicted in tomb paintings of the Egyptian New Kingdom, but the oldest archaeological evidence of cat *taming* dates to ~9,500 ya in Crete (Vigne et al. 2004). Thus, the window for cat domestication ranges between ~9,500 ya and 3,600 ya.

Unlike other domesticates that were used for meat, traction, milk, or wool, it is difficult to suppose cats had much utility to Neolithic people. Thus, selection was effectively only for habituation to human environments (docility), and only natural selection was responsible for the differential reproduction and survival of those wildcats better adapted to a human environment. Darwin recognized the unique phenomenon of cat domestication when he noted, "But man, owing to the difficulty of paring cats, has done nothing by methodical selection; and probably very little by unintentional selection. . ." (Darwin 1890). Because cats were uncared for, there was no abatement of natural selection pressure on hunting skill, and so their ability to feed themselves remained undiminished. The result today is that house cats retain the ability to hunt and can survive independently of humans (Passanisi et al. 1991; Sarmento et al. 2009; Say et al. 2002).

Although domestic cats have their origins in the Fertile Crescent at the dawn of sedentism, prior to the development of agriculture proper, it appears that cat husbandry was invented in Egypt after the introduction of Near Eastern farm animals, crops, and the cat as a package around 3100 BC (Butzer 1959; Harris 1996b; Ottoni et al. 2017; Wenke 2009). Egyptian worship of cats eventually led to captive rearing. Bastet is so well known as to be iconic, and Bubastis, the necropolis built in her honor, is famous for the vast catacombs of cat mummies found there.

Domestic cats spread to China during the Tang dynasty (618–907) via Mesopotamia and India in a combination of land (on the Silk Road) and sea routes (Clutterbuck 2004; Zeuner 1963; Baldwin 1975; Baldwin 1979; Haruda et al. 2020). Oriental domestic cats developed a distinct evolutionary trajectory early on because there are no *Felis silvestris* native to the Far East with which house cats might mix. Isolation from the parent stock, in combination with restricted population sizes, allowed a greater probability of fixing coat color mutations by genetic drift. This led to the eventual development of the first breeds – "natural breeds" Darwin called them – such as the Korat, Siamese, and Birman (Clutterbuck 2004; Darwin 1890). Darwin and others of his day noted a distinction between the so-called "natural" breeds and more "ordinary" breeds depending on the intentional influence of human selection for desired traits. The natural breeds from the Orient developed with only limited human guidance, probably no earlier than the thirteenth century (Clutterbuck 2004). Modern genetic analysis detects a shallow but noteworthy rift between today's European and Oriental domestic cat breeds (Lipinski et al. 2008; Menotti-Raymond et al. 2008) reflecting the 2,000 year divergence in their development from a common Near Eastern ancestor (Driscoll et al. 2007).

The first cat breeds, besides the natural breeds noted by Darwin, were developed beginning in England in the nineteenth century, with the first cat show taking place at the

Crystal Palace in London in 1871 (Weir 1889). Today, there are around a hundred recognized breeds, but superficial coat color variation aside, cats are remarkably uniform. The huge variance in size, shape, and behavior seen in dogs, cows, horses, pigeons, and chickens is nowhere to be seen in cats. Why? Several factors of biology and history come into play. First, unlike dogs and farm animals that had value for meat or fur or tasks like hunting or herding, cats have no such utility. As a result, there was never any selection pressure on them to fill such roles. Tameness was the only selective criterion; once cats adapted to living with people they were sufficiently adapted. Second, even if one wanted to select for a particular trait, maintaining reproductive isolation of a cat is difficult in a world before routine spaying and neutering. Containing a queen in heat is notoriously difficult, making control over her mate selection near impossible.

Are Cats Domesticated?

Today, there are 36 species of cats yet only one, *F. silvestris*, was domesticated (Driscoll et al. 2007). Though other felines have been tamed for hunting, like the cheetah and caracal, or for circuses, like lions and leopards, or for prestige pets, like tigers, members of *F. silvestris* are the only ones who live and breed in our homes. There are five subspecies of wildcat, *F. silvestris*, and all domestic cats descend from one of those, *Felis silvestris lybica*, which is native to the broad Near East and North Africa (Driscoll et al. 2007). As candidates for domestication, wildcats are contraindicated on every count. Felids are obligate carnivores, meaning they have a limited metabolic ability to digest anything but proteins (Bradshaw et al. 1996), with even blood sugar derived from meat (Li et al. 2005). Moreover, wildcats have exclusive territories and are solitary, following no pack or group leader (Daniels et al. 2001; Macdonald et al. 2004). Domestic cats are singular in being the only animal that is social under domestication despite having been solitary in the wild. Domestics retain their territoriality, and it is still the case today that cats are more attached to places than people. Morphologically, the average domestic varies little from the wild body plan (Daniels et al. 1998), with a slightly reduced cranial volume (Hemmer 1972; Lesch et al. 2022; Yamaguchi et al. 2004a; Yamaguchi et al. 2004b) and, as Darwin noted, longer intestines than wildcats due to a "less strictly carnivorous" diet than any wild feline, an adaptation he attributed to scavenging kitchen scraps (Darwin 1890). They also have become **polyestrous**, and of course their coat colors now vary wildly from the wild-type stripped mackerel tabby. But since the majority of the world's domestic cats live feral (Legay 1986), only a small fraction of a percent of domestic cats, mostly those in registered breeds, have mates chosen for them (i.e. pre-zygotic artificial selection), and people have little control over what and when they eat. So, by far the overwhelming majority of domestic cats, whether house cats or feral, choose their own mates and most source their own food. Also particularly notable is the cat's lack of utility and pathway to domestication, as cats alone among domesticates can be said to have avoided artificial selection entirely (Ritvo 1998). Given all this, cats seem unlikely domesticates. However, they do overwhelmingly satisfy the one key criterion for domestication: tolerance of humans. See Figure 2.2a,b for an illustration of how similar today's domestic housecat and its wild ancestor are in physical appearance.

Farm Animals

Dogs and cats began their journey to domestication as commensals, not prey or captives, on the outskirts of human influence when bold individuals sought to exploit whatever human niche was available to them at the time. Those individuals more amenable to life around humans began to predominate as a result of assortative mating over time. Thus, selection had begun at the first sight of humans. In contradistinction, farm animals were gathered

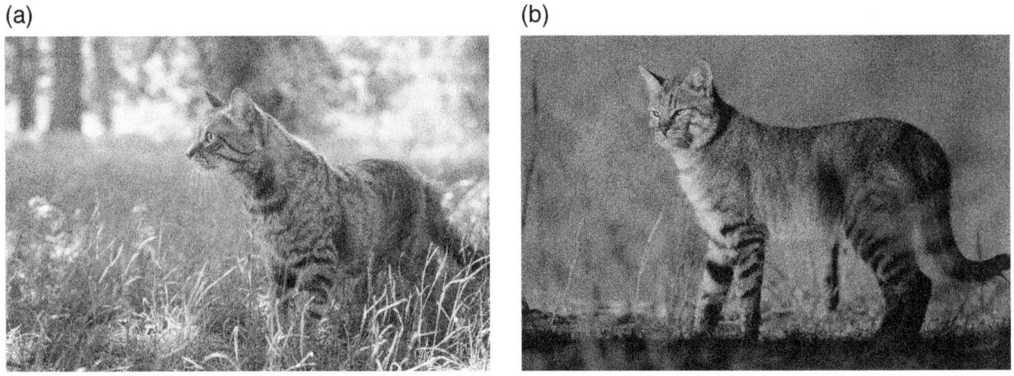

Figure 2.2 The physical appearance of today's domestic housecat, *Felis sylvestris* (a), is remarkably similar to that of the African wild cat, *Felis sylvestris lybica* (b), putting into question the true extent of domestication our housecats have undergone. *Source:* Photo credit: Africa Studio/AdobeStock (a) and EcoView/Adobe Stock (b).

randomly from their wild populations and only selected for domestication once under human dominion. For them, capture and captivity were the first steps toward domestication. Capture myopathy, the trauma of being captured, can cause serious stress injuries, damage to internal organs, or even death. Further selection was imposed by a substandard diet and diseases resulting from corralling in the same area for generations in what today must be considered appalling hygiene.

Goats, sheep, pigs, and cattle were sources of meat for Neolithic hunter-gatherers 12,000 years ago, before the emergence of permanent settlements. It seems likely that as sedentism emerged, orphaned young, unable and unwilling to flee, were husbanded for a time before themselves were being led to slaughter (Galton 1865; Serpell 1989). This approach to live storage – a "walking larder" – would have provided easy meat over winter and around seasonal herd migration patterns, as well as for ritual offerings and feasts (Clutton-Brock 1989). Eventually time and chance led to breeding in captivity and enrollment in the domestication train. Estimated dates for these events range from 10,350 ya for the goat to 8,000 ya for cattle.

Archaeological time-series reconstruction from excavations in the south-central Anatolian site of Asikli Hoyuk shows just this pattern in the remains of sheep and goats (Stiner et al. 2022), where three stages are described; in the first, from ~8,350 BC, hunting and live storage, or "Catch-and-Grow," live spring kids and lambs are captured and raised for a short time in captivity. There is no reproduction and significant selection from capture myopathy. Miscarriages are absent from animal collections from hunting. In the second stage, by 8,000 BC, incidental captive reproduction begins as evidenced by an increase in preterm remains, aborted due to stressful conditions and poor care. There is evidence of sex-based culling, where males are preferentially slaughtered young, at around seven months old, as they are disruptive and not limiting to population growth. In the last stage, there are fewer preterm individuals indicating better conditions and perhaps more resilient animals. Both males and females reach adulthood, indicating an appreciation of non-meat products (milk and hair), and production of goat milk is also notable, indicating active breeding.

Stiner et al. (2022) estimate this archaeological sequence entails roughly 250 generations, corresponding to about one thousand years. Over the entire sequence from Catch-and-Grow to full domestication, there would be lateral admixture from the wild as wild lambs and kids were introduced to a growing flock. This introgression is important, as it will maintain genetic diversity, counteracting the high selection pressures for tolerance to captivity and poor diet that may otherwise result in inbreeding depression.

It cannot at present be known with absolute certainty whether cattle and pigs followed paths similar to that described for goats and sheep, and in the same timescale, but the circumstantial evidence suggests they did (Baig et al. 2005; Bradley 2006; Bradley and Magee 2006; Larson et al. 2005; Price and Evin 2019; Smyser et al. 2020).

Horses

Equids have an importance in human history on par with the dog, enabling transportation of people, ideas, and goods over distances, habitats, languages, religions, and lifeways. Until the sailing ship, nothing moved as fast over great distances, and, even so, the horse remained a land-bound complement to seafaring through the age of steam locomotives, until finally being made obsolete by the automobile ecosystem (Breen et al. 1994; Clutton-Brock 1992a). Equids, along with their associated technologies (bit, bridle, saddle, chariot, pants), have an unparalleled importance in warfare and the spread of complex societies, laying the foundations of the socio-political landscape of modern times (Turchin et al. 2021; Wagner et al. 2022). It has been frustrating then, that their domestication has been so challenging to reconstruct (Jansen et al. 2002; Warmuth et al. 2012).

The family Equidae has an almost ideal fossil representation spanning 55 million years, making it a textbook exemplar of macroevolution and diversification. By 5 million years ago, the family represented more than 20 genera, all except one that is now extinct (Orlando et al. 2009). The sole surviving genus, *Equus*, originated in North America ~23 million years ago; the lineage surviving today has a most recent common ancestor (MRCA) about 4 million years ago (Orlando 2015; Orlando et al. 2008).

It was not until 700,000 years ago that a second exodus from North America saw caballine equids (including the MRCA of domestic horses (*Equus caballus ferus*) and Przewalski's horses (*Equus przewalskii*)) cross to Eurasia. More recently, between 10,000 and 12,000 years ago, all equids in the Americas went extinct, victims of the same climate-driven Pleistocene mass extinctions that wiped out most other medium and large mammals, leaving all remaining equids in the Old World (Orlando 2015).

As known today, the equid cast of characters is comprised of caballine and non-caballine equids (Groves and Ryder 2000; Vilstrup et al. 2013). There are four known lineages of caballine, or true, horses: Siberian, Iberian, Przewalski's, and domestic. The largest basal population is identified in Siberia and was extinct by the fourth millennium BC. A European population (called the Iberian) extended from Scandinavia to Iberia, Britain to Poland, and was bridled and harnessed by people until the third millennium BC. Przewalski's horses ranged from the Urals to the Altai and were exploited by Central Asian cultures such as the Botai. The Western Eurasian steppes that are the home of modern horses include southeastern Ukraine around the Dnieper River, southern Russia north of the Caucasus through the Volga River drainage, and into Eastern Kazakhstan. Negligible genetic input from Iberian or Przewalski's lineages has been detected in modern horses, indicating a total genetic replacement (Librado et al. 2021).

Extant non-caballines include zebras (plains, *Equus quagga/burchelli*; mountain, *Equus zebra*; Grevy's, *Equus grevi*), half-asses (also called hemionids) (Asiatic wild ass, *Equus hemionus*), and ass (African wild ass, *Equus africanus*) (Vilstrup et al. 2013).

As in the dog, advances in ancient DNA extraction have made possible comprehensive phylogenetic assessments of equids, with startling effect (Librado and Orlando 2021).

At least four events and taxa should be recognized in equid domestication: donkey, Botai, Przewalski's, Kungas, and the true domestic horse.

Donkey. The first, estimated to between 5,000 and 6,000 years ago, is the domestication of African asses in northeast Africa to create the donkey, *Equus africanus asinus* (Orlando 2015). It is likely this occurred twice, once certainly from the Nubian wild ass, *Equus africanus africanus,* and once, perhaps from a taxon not yet identified and now extinct, but not from the extant Somali wild ass, *Equus africanus somaliensis,* nor the extinct Atlas wild ass, *Equus africanus atlanticus* (Kimura et al. 2011). As these subspecific taxa are interfertile, the distinct parental genomes have become blended in the resulting domestic donkey, *Equus africanus asinus*, but two mitochondrial clades remain distinct (Beja-Pereira et al. 2004). Evidence of genetic bottlenecking by the third millennium BC is interpreted as the result of translocation out of their native range and captive breeding.

Botai. The earliest evidence of horse management is from 5,500 years ago in Kazakhstan, where the Botai culture was highly dependent on them. Excavations at Botai sites revealed tons of animal bones, almost entirely of horses. Horses of all ages had been butchered, suggesting hunting wild animals, but some had teeth worn in characteristic ways, suggesting harnessing with a bit. A protein analysis of pottery shards indicated fatty acid deposits consistent with horse milk, put forward as further evidence of domestication (Outram et al. 2009). These findings of milking and bits were taken as *prima facia* evidence of domestication, erroneously it seems, as, in a surprising twist revealed by DNA analysis, these early bridled horses were shown to be Przewalski's horses (*Equus przewalskii*) (Gaunitz et al. 2018) and not the caballine horses from which all modern horses descend. Categorization of these horses regarding domestication status is awkwardly unsettled. Though integrated into settled life, the demographic structure of the found remains gives no impression of selection or captive breeding, and it is thus difficult to hypothesize any genetic deviation from the wild genetic structure of the horses, making them essentially captive, though highly managed, tame wild animals.

Kungas. The third event, dated between 4,550 and 4,300 years ago, is the product of hybridization between a female of the aforementioned domestic donkey (*Equus africanus asinus*) and a male Syrian wild ass, or hemippe (*Equus hemionus hemippus*) (Bennett et al. 2022), making this interesting phenomenon a domesticate along a unique pathway.

Known only from cuneiform tablets and carved stone panels, kungas were strong and fast and of indisputably high value, given as gifts to political elites and as dowries in royal marriages. Archaeological and written evidence indicates that they were harnessed to the plow, and they are pictured pulling four-wheel war-wagons. Kungas were more valued than donkeys, given their greater size and strength. They retained their high value status until displaced by the introduction of the horse to the region at the end of the third millennium BC.

Analyzing 25 equids buried over a 250-year period at the Mesopotamian site of Umm el-Marra in present-day Syria, Bennett et al. report on animals found in a vast complex of tombs. These animals show dental evidence of cribbing, typical of corralled animals, as well as wear on the anterior of the upper incisors, evidence of a lip ring used for control. Further evidence of care includes heavily worn cheek teeth relative to their incisors, suggesting they were foddered as may be expected given that a lip ring prevents effective grazing. Also, leg bones show evidence of draft work, as opposed to loading, indicative of their use pulling chariots. Genetic analysis based on Y-chromosome and mitochondrial DNA presents clear evidence of the Kunga being first generation hybrids between donkey and hemippe (Bennett et al. 2022), confirming longstanding speculation (Clutton-Brock 1981; Zarins 1976).

Such interspecies crosses are usually sterile, particularly here, where the parental species have differing chromosome numbers (Graphodatsky et al. 2020). The import of that fact is that kungas have to be hybridized each generation since there is no line propagation possible, as is also true of today's horse/ass mules. Doing this involves considerably more effort than simply breeding kunga stock at hand since hemippes must be sourced from the wild. It seems that as a result of hunting pressure, these wild hemippes became scarce, further belaboring the process. When true domestic horses were introduced toward the end of the third millennium BC their temperament, ease of breeding and care, and their notable speed and strength, led to total replacement, to the point that knowledge of kungas themselves was completely lost.

Modern horse. Fourth, is the domestication of the caballine horse, *Equus cabalus*, which evolved into the domestic horse of today. The progression is complex, with evidence of multiple taming events. While it has become clear that localized horse management and herding practices were widespread in Eurasia, not all populations so managed resulted in stable domestic populations, as illustrated by Botai. Early archaeology pointed variously to Iberia, Anatolia, Kazakhstan, and southern Ukraine/Russia as the cradle of horse culture, technology, and domestication. These putative centers were each backed by early genetic studies, without finding a consensus. Horses are uniquely mobile, resulting in high spatial genetic connectivity across the Eurasian continent, exacerbating the sparce sampling that hamstrung these genetic surveys, and there is no living ancestor against which to compare in order to genetically define "wild." However, recent comprehensive genetic reconstructions of wild and kept equids, both prehistoric and contemporary, from all candidate regions, have made it clear that although four lineages of caballine horse (Iberian, Siberian, Przewalski's, and domestic) were alive at the time of domestication – and there is evidence for all lineages except Siberian having been captive and used extensively by humans – it is only *E. cabalus* horses that survived to the present as domestics (Fages et al. 2019; Gaunitz et al. 2018; Librado et al. 2021; Orlando et al. 2009; Vilstrup et al. 2013).

Mules. Mules in the sense that exist today, as infertile hybrids of a male domestic donkey and a female domestic horse, are known from at least 2,200 years ago (Fages et al. 2019). In modern times, crosses of each zebra species with horses and wild asses have been accomplished for research or in hopes of conferring a zebra's innate disease resistance. Such zebra mules are sterile, as are most other equine hybrids. Crosses between Przewalski's horse and domestic horse are viable however (Ryder 1978). Przewalski's and domestic horses still maintain distinct genetic profiles; modern Przewalski's horses do not descend from the same ancestral population as modern domestic horses.

While genetic inferences have succeeded in identifying the lineages of wild horses that ultimately became domestic, these analyses do not shed as much light on the various human cultural conditions and lifeways that led to their entrainment and domestication in the first place. Whether the people who domesticated the ancestors of the modern horse, or those involved in any of the alternate incipient domestication trials, were settled or transhumant pastoralists, semi-nomadic hunters, cultivators, or agriculturalists is not on the whole clearly known. It is too soon to say whether all, some, one, or none of these equid management events followed the same series of steps as did goats and sheep, though that is the supposition. Regardless, it is now clear that "horse culture" developed numerous times in human history, linked to both caballine and non-caballine equids. In the end, one taxon superseded and genetically over-wrote the rest, but the culture and technologies developed from north-eastern Africa to Iberia, eastern Europe, and central Asia combined synergistically over millennia to advance equestrianism.

Entrained Beasts

Sometimes referred to as "exploited captives," these are a hodgepodge bestiary of animals in captivity (Clutton-Brock 1981; Clutton-Brock 1989; Clutton-Brock 1992b; Zeuner 1963). The only unifying feature is a symbiosis according to its most basic definition of two species, human and animal, living together. Excluding most animals taken from the wild and kept solely as modern pets (e.g. aquarium fishes, and reptiles), and focusing on those whose salient feature is their past or present history of utility in their native, unadulterated state, we are still left with too long a list, including deer of many species, caracal, cheetah, fox, elephant, otter, cormorant, falcon, vicuna, guanaco, and still many others.

Populations range from captive bred to entirely wild-caught. Asian elephants from southwest to southeast Asia used for timbering are turned out into the forest to breed before being collected for the next term of service. Otters used for herding fish into nets are collected from the wild but also breed in captivity. Parrots in the pet trade are both bred and poached from the wild. Cheetahs were once collected by the thousands from the wild for use in hunting, but only once were they recorded breeding in captivity.

Through extended association with, and management by humans, some have become undisputed domesticates. Yet, even this group of animals will get along just fine without humans. Reindeer of the Sami, perhaps the most "domesticated" of the exploited captives, would migrate, foal, and feed according to their natural script if left to do so. While others are, in all senses, wild animals. Among these, some are tractable and can be trained to task (Asian elephants); others are simply exploited as they are for their natural abilities (e.g. cormorants). Breeding takes place in their natural environment; mate choice is determined by the animals; and individuals are collected from the wild for work. These are tamed wild animals, not domesticated in the genetic sense of differing from their ancestral population due to selection. Asian elephants, when "retired" to liberty in the forest, are *wild* animals, not *feral*.

Many such populations are managed, but fewer are selectively bred. Vicuna and guanaco are wild but have a well-documented history of demographic interventions by pre-Columbian civilizations. Yearly round-ups of wild herds were held so that old, weak, and unsuitable animals could be culled before returning the remainder to the wild (Clutton-Brock 1981; Darwin 1890). It seems likely that the Przewalski's horses of the Botai culture were similarly wild, albeit occasionally captive, herds. Whether they were similarly subjected to differential culling is unknown. This system of food procurement is somewhat beyond a simple predator–prey relationship but still does not rise to the level of food production (Clutton-Brock 1981).

Entrained beasts go to show that, in fact, there is tremendous flexibility in the behavior of wild animals. Many of the behaviors that are considered reserved for domesticates are present in the wild and become obvious when human interaction is pressed upon them. As the following farmed fox experiment shows, all of the alleles for tame behavior/docility are already in the unselected population, and what selection did was aggregate those alleles for tameness into individual genotypes.

Domestication in Fast-Forward: The Farm-Fox Experiment

Seeking to explore the genetics behind domestication, Dr. Dimitry Belyaev and his assistant Lyudmilla Trut began an experimental domestication of the silver fox, a coat color variant of the red fox, raised industrially on commercial fur farms in Siberia (Trut 1999; Trut et al. 2009). Selective breeding began with 100 females and 30 males. The two primary axes of personality are the shy/bold axis and the aggressive/tame axis. Belyaev describes the initial fox population as being around 30% extremely aggressive,

20% fearful, 40% aggressively fearful, and 10% displayed neither fear nor aggression, but only a quiet, exploratory behavior (what we might consider docile).

The standard phenotyping assessment included five simple steps, where an observer: (1) approaches the fox cage (2) stands near cage (3) opens cage but stands motionless and does not initiate contact (4) attempts physical contact (5) stays near the closed cage. Each of these steps is timed to one minute. Using this rather course test of mansuetude, he selected the top 5% of males and 20% of females for each successive generation, while keeping the population roughly the same size. To avoid conditioning the animals to human contact, that is, taming them, the foxes were never handled prior to evaluating their phenotype, and selection of breeders was determined by that phenotyping. Within a few generations, demonstrable changes in behavior toward people were evident in the foxes' vocalizations, position in their cages on approach, the attitude of ears and tails, and their willingness to be touched. Within 10 generations, they had succeeded in breeding a reasonably domestic fox. With additional generations of selection, again solely for nonaggression, morphological changes like coat color variation, floppy ears, and curled tails became increasingly common. Note that these morphological and physiological changes correspond to the domestication syndrome described earlier as being common among domestic animals of all kinds. Changes in estrus cycle and mating behavior were also noted, and the animal became increasingly social, not just with humans, but with other foxes as well (Belyaev 1978; Belyaev et al. 1981).

In a parallel experiment, Belyaev and Trut selected foxes at the bottom of the tameness scale. This resulted in aggressive animals that were never handleable, regardless of history of human encounters. Aggressive kits cross-fostered to more docile, tame mothers, who likewise grew into aggressive, un-handleable adults. Hormonal assays indicate the aggressive foxes show signs of stress during test encounters with humans, but that tame foxes do not and seem to genuinely enjoy these encounters. Tame and aggressive foxes even differ in the words they use to communicate with humans. Tame foxes cackle and pant, but never cough or snort, while aggressive foxes do the opposite.

The farm-fox experiment continues to the present. After more than 40 generations of selection and more than 45,000 foxes, the fox is completely tame. Affiliative displays intended to solicit attention from humans are clear, such as holding mouths ajar, wagging, rolling onto their sides and exposing their bellies, and generally adopting submissive poses.

Conclusions drawn from this experiment are important. Foremost, domestication, by even the strictest definition, is in fact heritable. Selecting docile behavior led the resulting progeny to interpret their environment differently than the preceding generations. Thus, individual differences in personality are the selectable unit. Also, the entire repertoire of commonly recognized morphological domestication syndrome traits can be recapitulated by artificial selection on nonaggression only – that is, on behavior and behavior alone. It is significant too that recognizable domestication occurred in so few generations (<10) because this indicates that the alleles for domestication are present in the unselected population, as there simply had not been enough time for mutation to give rise to any new allelic variation. The short timeframe also indicates that the number of genes involved in domestication cannot be exceedingly large. Belyaev estimated perhaps 5–10 genes of major effect, while current estimates range from 10 to 20, but the magnitude is the same.

This brilliant experiment unambiguously reveals how artificial selection can take advantage of a population's standing genetic diversity and assemble heritable behaviors consistent with our recognized ideas of domestication, and how this can arise simply by selecting against aggression toward humans. These foxes are now acknowledged as the gold-standard model of domestication.

References

Achilli, A., Bonfiglio, S., Olivieri, A. et al. (2009). The multifaceted origin of taurine cattle reflected by the mitochondrial genome. *PLoS ONE* 4 (6): e5753.

Achilli, A., Olivieri, A., Pellecchia, M. et al. (2008). Mitochondrial genomes of extinct aurochs survive in domestic cattle. *Curr. Biol.* 18 (4): R157–R158.

Albarella, U., Dobney, K., and Rowley-conwy, P. (2006). The domesticatin of the pig (*Sus scrofia*): new challenges and approaches. In: *Documenting Domestication: New Genetic and Archaeological Paradigms* (ed. M.A. Zeder, D.G. Bradley, E. Emshwiller, and B.D. Smith), 209–227. Berkely, CA: University of California Press.

Ameen, C., Feuerborn, T.R., Brown, S.K. et al. (2019). Specialized sledge dogs accompanied Inuit dispersal across the North American Arctic. *Proc. Biol. Sci.* 286 (1916): 20191929.

Auffray, J.-C., Tchernov, E., and Nevo, E. (1988). Origine du commensalisme de la souris domestique (Mus musculus domesticus) vis-a-vis de l'homme. *C.R. Acad. Sci. Paris* 307: 517–522.

Baig, M., Beja-Pereira, A., Mohammad, R. et al. (2005). Phylogeography and origin of Indian domestic cattle. *Curr. Sci.* 89: 38–40.

Baldwin, J.A. (1975). Notes and speculations on the domestication of the cat in Egypt. *Anthropos* 70 (3/4): 428–448.

Baldwin, J.A. (1979). Ships and the early diffusion of the domestic cat. *Carnivore Genet. Newsl.* 4: 32–33.

Bar-On, Y.M., Phillips, R., and Milo, R. (2018). The biomass distribution on Earth. *Proc. Natl. Acad. Sci. USA* 115 (25): 6506–6511.

Bar-Yosef, O. (1998). The natufian culture in the levant, threshold to the origins of agriculture. *Evol. Anthropol.* 6: 159–177.

Barbato, M., Hailer, F., Orozco-Terwengel, P. et al. (2017). Genomic signatures of adaptive introgression from European mouflon into domestic sheep. *Sci. Rep.* 7 (1): 7623.

Beja-Pereira, A., England, P.R., Ferrand, N. et al. (2004). African origins of the domestic donkey. *Science* 304 (5678): 1781.

Bellwood, P. (2007). *First Farmers, the Origins of Agricultural Societies*. New York, NY: Wiley.

Belyaev, D.K. (1978). Destabilizing selection as a factor in domestication. *J. Hered.* 70 (5): 301–308.

Belyaev, D.K., Ruvinsky, A.O., and Trut, L.N. (1981). Inherited activation–inactivation of the star gene in foxes: its bearing on the problem of domestication. *J. Hered.* 72 (4): 267–274.

Bennett, E.A., Weber, J., Bendhafer, W. et al. (2022). The genetic identity of the earliest human-made hybrid animals, the kungas of Syro-Mesopotamia. *Sci. Adv.* 8: eabm0218.

Benton, M.L., Abraham, A., Labella, A.L. et al. (2021). The influence of evolutionary history on human health and disease. *Nat. Rev. Genet.* 22: 269–283.

Bergstrom, A., Frantz, L., Schmidt, R. et al. (2020). Origins and genetic legacy of prehistoric dogs. *Science* 370: 557–564.

Boissey, A. and Erhard, H.W. (2014). How studying interactions between animal emotions, cognition, and personality can contribute to improve farm animal welfare. In: *Genetics and the Behavior of Domestic Animals* (ed. T. Grandin and M. Deesing), 95–129. London, UK: Academic Press.

Bonfiglio, S., Achilli, A., Olivieri, A. et al. (2010). The enigmatic origin of bovine mtDNA haplogroup R: Sporadic interbreeding or an independent event of *Bos primigenius* domestication in Italy? *PLoS ONE* 5: e15760.

Bonfiglio, S., Ginja, C., De Gaetano, A. et al. (2012). Origin and spread of *Bos taurus*: new clues from mitochondrial genomes belonging to haplogroup T1. *PLoS ONE* 7: e38601.

Boursot, P., Din, W., Anand, R. et al. (1996). Origin and radiation of the house mouse: mitochondrial DNA phylogeny. *J. Evol. Biol.* 9: 391–415.

Bradley, D.G. (2006). Documenting domestication: reading animal genetic texts. In: *Documenting Domestication: New Genetic and Archaeological Paradigms* (ed. M.A. Zeder, D.G. Bradley, E. Emshwiller, and B.D. Smith), 273–278. Los Angeles, CA: Univeristy of California Press.

Bradley, D.G. and Magee, D.A. (2006). Genetics and origins of domestic cattle. In: *Documenting Domestication: New Genetic and Archaeological Paradigms* (ed. M.A. Zeder, D.G. Bradley, E. Emshwiller, and B.D. Smith), 317–328. Los Angeles: University of California Press.

Bradshaw, J.W.S., Goodwin, D., Legrand-Defretin, V., and Nott, H.M.R. (1996). Food selection by the domestic cat, an obligate carnivore. *Comp. Biochem. Physiol. A comp. Physiol.* 114: 205–209.

Breasted, J.H. (1916). *Ancient Times, a History of the Early World*. Chicago: Ginn and Co.

Breen, M., Downs, P., Irvin, Z., and Bell, K. (1994). Intrageneric amplification of horse microsatellite markers with emphasis on the Przewalski's horse (*E. przewalskii*). *Anim. Genet.* 25: 401–405.

Butzer, K.W. (1959). Environment and human ecology in Egypt during predynastic and early dynastic times. *Bulletin de la Societe de Geographie d'Egypte* 32: 43–87.

Chen, S.Y., Su, Y.H., Wu, S.F. et al. (2005). Mitochondrial diversity and phylogeographic structure of Chinese domestic goats. *Mol. Phylogenet. Evol.* 37: 804–814.

Clutterbuck, M.R. (2004). *Siamese Cats : Legends and Reality*. Bangkok, Thailand: White Lotus.

Clutton-Brock, J. (1981). *Domesticated Animals from Early Times*. Austin and London: University of Texas Press; British Museum (Natural History).

Clutton-Brock, J. (1989). *The Walking Larder : Patterns of Domestication, Pastoralism, and Predation*. London: Unwin Hyman.

Clutton-Brock, J. (1992a). *Horse Power : A History of the Horse and the Donkey in Human Societies*. Cambridge, MA: Harvard University Press.

Clutton-Brock, J. (1992b). The process of domestication. *Mammal Rev.* 22: 79–85.

Clutton-Brock, J. (1995). Origins of the domestic dog: domestication and early history. In: *The Domestic Dog: It's Evolution, Behaviour, and Interactions with People* (ed. J. Serpell), 7–20. Cambridge University Press.

Daly, K.G., Maisano Delser, P., Mullin, V.E. et al. (2018). Ancient goat genomes reveal mosaic domestication in the Fertile Crescent. *Science* 361: 85–88.

Daniels, M.J., Balharry, D., Hirst, D. et al. (1998). Morphological and pelage characteristics of wild living cats in Scotland: implications for defining the "wildcat". *J. Zool.* 244: 231–247.

Daniels, M.J., Beaumont, M.A., Johnson, P.J. et al. (2001). Ecology and genetics of wild-living cats in the north-east of Scotland and the implications for the conservation of the wildcat. *J. Appl. Ecol.* 38: 146–161.

Darwin, C. (1991). *On the Origin of Species by Means of Natural Selection*. Norwalk, Connecticut: The Easton Press.

Darwin, C. (1890). *The Variation of Animals and Plants Under Domestication*. New York: D. Appleton and company.

Darwin, C. (1972). *The Descent of Man, and Selection in Relation to Sex*. New York: Heritage Press.

Darwin, C. and Lorenz, K. (1965). *The Expression of the Emotions in Man and Animals*. Chicago: University of Chicago Press.

Dobney, K. and Larson, G. (2006). Gentics and animal domestication: new windows on an elusive process. *J. Zoology* 269: 261–271.

Driscoll, C.A. and Macdonald, D.W. (2010). Top dogs: wolf domestication and wealth. *J. Biol.* 9: 10.

Driscoll, C.A., Macdonald, D.W., and O'brien, S.J. (2009). From wild animals to domestic pets, an evolutionary view of domestication. *Proc. Natl. Acad. Sci. USA* 106 (Suppl 1): 9971–9978.

Driscoll, C.A., Menotti-Raymond, M., Roca, A.L. et al. (2007). The near Eastern origin of cat domestication. *Science* 317: 519–523.

Fages, A., Hanghoj, K., Khan, N. et al. (2019). Tracking five millennia of horse management with extensive ancient genome time series. *Cell* 177: 1419, e31–1435.

Fan, Z., Silva, P., Gronau, I. et al. (2016). Worldwide patterns of genomic variation and admixture in gray wolves. *Genome Res.* 26: 163–173.

Frantz, L.A.F., Haile, J., Lin, A.T. et al. (2019). Ancient pigs reveal a near-complete genomic turnover following their introduction to Europe. *Proc. Natl. Acad. Sci. USA* 116: 17231–17238.

Freedman, A.H., Gronau, I., Schweizer, R.M. et al. (2014). Genome sequencing highlights the dynamic early history of dogs. *PLoS Genet.* 10: e1004016.

Freedman, A.H., Schweizer, R.M., Ortega-Del Vecchyo, D. et al. (2016). Demographically-based evaluation of genomic regions under selection in domestic dogs. *PLoS Genet.* 12: e1005851.

Galton, F. (1865). The first steps towards the domestication of animals. *Trans. Ethnol. Soc. London* 3: 122–138.

Gaunitz, C., Fages, A., Hanghoj, K. et al. (2018). Ancient genomes revisit the ancestry of domestic and Przewalski's horses. *Science* 360: 111–114.

Grandin, T. and Deesing, M. (2014). Genetics and animal welfare. In: *Genetics and the Behavior of Domestic Animals*, 2e (ed. T. Grandin and M. Deesing). London, UK: Academic Press.

Graphodatsky, A., Perelman, P., and Obrien, S.J. (2020). *Atlas of Mammalian Chromosomes*. Hoboken, NJ: Wiley.

Groube, L. (1996). The impact of diseases upon the emergence of agriculture. In: *The Origins and Spread of Agriculture and Pastoralism in Eurasia* (ed. D.R. Harris), 101–129. London: University College London.

Groves, C.P. and Ryder, O.A. (2000). Systematics and phylogeny of the horse. In: *The Genetics of the Horse* (ed. A.T. Bowling and A. Ruvinsky), 1–24. Wallingford, UK: CABI Publishing.

Harris, D.R. (1969). Agricultural systems, ecosystems and the origins of agriculture. In: *The Domestication and Exploitation of Plants and Animals* (ed. P.J. Ucko and G.W. Dimbleby), 3–16. Chicago: Aldine Publishing Company.

Harris, D.R. (ed.) (1996a). *The Origins and Spread of Agriculture and Pastoralism in Eurasia*. London: UCL Press.

Harris, D.R. (1996b). The origins and spread of agriculture and pastoralism in Eurasia: an overview. In: *The Origins and Spread of Agriculture and Pastoralism in Eurasia* (ed. D.R. Harris), 552–573. London: UCL Press.

Haruda, A.F., Miller, A.R.V., Paijmans, J.L.A. et al. (2020). The earliest domestic cat on the Silk Road. *Sci. Rep.* 10: 11241.

Hiendleder, S., Kaupe, B., Wassmuth, R., and Janke, A. (2002). Molecular analysis of wild and domestic sheep questions current nomenclature and provides evidence for domestication from two different subspecies. *Proc. Biol. Sci.* 269: 893–904.

Hemmer, H. (1972). Variations in brain size in the species *Felis silvestris*. *Experientia* 28: 271–272.

Hemmer, H. (1990). *Domestication : The Decline of Environmental Appreciation*, 2e. Cambridge England ; New York: Cambridge University Press Publisher description http://www.loc.gov/catdir/description/cam023/89009993.html.

Houslay, T.M., Earley, R.L., White, S.J. et al. (2022). Genetic integration of behavioural and endocrine components of the stress response. *eLife* 11: e67126.

Jansen, T., Forster, P., Levine, M.A. et al. (2002). Mitochondrial DNA and the origins of the domestic horse. *Proc. Natl. Acad. Sci. USA* 99 (16): 10905–10910.

Janssens, L., Giemsch, L., Schmitz, R. et al. (2018). A new look at an old dog: Bonn-Oberkassel reconsidered. *J. Archaeol. Sci.* 92: 126–138.

Kimura, B., Marshall, F.B., Chen, S. et al. (2011). Ancient DNA from Nubian and Somali wild ass provides insights into donkey ancestry and domestication. *Proc. Biol. Sci.* 278: 50–57.

Koolhaas, J.M., De Boer, S.F., Buwalda, B., and Van Reenen, K. (2007). Individual variation in coping with stress: a multidimensional approach of ultimate and proximate mechanisms. *Brain Behav. Evol.* 70: 218–226.

Korte, S.M., Koolhaas, J.M., Wingfield, J.C., and Mcewen, B.S. (2005). The Darwinian concept of stress: benefits of allostasis and costs of allostatic load and the trade-offs in health and disease. *Neurosci. Biobehav. Rev.* 29: 3–38.

Larson, G., Dobney, K., Albarella, U. et al. (2005). Worldwide phylogeography of wild boar reveals multiple centers of pig domestication. *Science* 307: 1618–1621.

Legay, J.M. (1986). Tentative estimation of the total number of domestic cats in the world. *C. R. Acad. Sci. III* 303: 709–712.

Lesch, R., Kitchener, A.C., Hantke, G. et al. (2022). Cranial volume and palate length of cats, *Felis* spp., under domestication, hybridization and in wild populations. *R. Soc. Open Sci.* 9: 210477.

Li, X., Li, W., Wang, H. et al. (2005). Pseudogenization of a sweet-receptor gene accounts for cats' indifference toward sugar. *PLoS Genet.* 1: 27–35.

Librado, P., Khan, N., Fages, A. et al. (2021). The origins and spread of domestic horses from the Western Eurasian steppes. *Nature* 598: 634–640.

Librado, P. and Orlando, L. (2021). Genomics and the evolutionary history of equids. *Annu. Rev. Anim. Biosci.* 9: 81–101.

Lindsay, S.R. (2000). *Handbook of Applied Dog Behavior and Training*. Iowa: Iowa State Press, Blackwell Publishing Company.

Lipinski, M.J., Froenicke, L., Baysac, K.C. et al. (2008). The ascent of cat breeds: genetic evaluations of breeds and worldwide random-bred populations. *Genomics* 91: 12–21.

Liu, Y.P., Wu, G.S., Yao, Y.G. et al. (2006). Multiple maternal origins of chickens: out of the Asian jungles. *Mol. Phylogenet. Evol.* 38: 12–19.

Loog, L., Thalmann, O., Sinding, M.S. et al. (2020). Ancient DNA suggests modern wolves trace their origin to a Late Pleistocene expansion from Beringia. *Mol. Ecol.* 29: 1596–1610.

Luikart, G., Gielly, L., Excoffier, L. et al. (2001). Multiple maternal origins and weak phylogeographic structure in domestic goats. *Proc. Natl. Acad. Sci. USA* 98: 5927–5932.

Macdonald, D.W., Daniels, M.J., Driscoll, C. et al. (2004). *The Scottish Wildcat Analyses for Conservation and an Action Plan*. Oxford: Wildlife Conservation Research Unit.

Mangan, A., Piaggio, A.J., Bodenchuck, M.J. et al. (2021). Rooting out genetic structure of invasive wild pigs in Texas. *J. Wildl. Manage.* 85 (8): 1563–1573.

Meadows, J.R., Cemal, I., Karaca, O. et al. (2007). Five ovine mitochondrial lineages identified from sheep breeds of the near East. *Genetics* 175: 1371–1379.

Menotti-Raymond, M., David, V.A., Pflueger, S.M. et al. (2008). Patterns of molecualr genetic variation among cat breeds. *Genomics* 91: 1–11.

Miao, Y.W., Peng, M.S., Wu, G.S. et al. (2013). Chicken domestication: an updated perspective based on mitochondrial genomes. *Heredity* 110: 277–282.

Morey, D.F. (1994). The early evolution of the domestic dog. *Amer. Sci.* 82: 336–347.

Naderi, S., Rezaei, H.R., Pompanon, F. et al. (2008). The goat domestication process inferred from large-scale mitochondrial DNA analysis of wild and domestic individuals. *Proc. Natl. Acad. Sci. USA* 105: 17659–17664.

Ni Leathlobhair, M., Perri, A.R., Irving-Pease, E.K. et al. (2018). The evolutionary history of dogs in the Americas. *Science* 361: 81–85.

Ollivier, M., Tresset, A., Frantz, L.A.F. et al. (2018). Dogs accompanied humans during the neolithic expansion into Europe. *Biol. Lett.* 14: 0286.

Orlando, L. (2015). Equids. *Curr. Biol.* 25: R973–R978.

Orlando, L., Male, D., Alberdi, M.T. et al. (2008). Ancient DNA clarifies the evolutionary history of American late pleistocene equids. *J. Mol. Evol.* 66: 533–538.

Orlando, L., Metcalf, J.L., Alberdi, M.T. et al. (2009). Revising the recent evolutionary history of equids using ancient DNA. *Proc. Natl. Acad. Sci. USA* 106: 21754–21759.

Oswald, M.E., Singer, M., and Robison, B.D. (2013). The quantitative genetic architecture of the bold-shy continuum in zebrafish, *Danio rerio*. *PLoS One* 8: e68828.

Ottoni, C., Van Neer, W., De Cupere, B. et al. (2017). The palaeogenetics of cat dispersal in the ancient world. *Nat. Ecol. Evol.* 1: 0139.

Outram, A.K., Stear, N.A., Bendrey, R. et al. (2009). The earliest horse harnessing and milking. *Science* 323: 1332–1335.

Passanisi, W.C., Macdonald, D.W., and Kerby, G. (1991). *Wild Cats and Feral Cats*. McMahons Point: Weldon Owen.

Pedrosa, S., Uzun, M., Arranz, J.J. et al. (2005). Evidence of three maternal lineages in Near Eastern sheep supporting multiple domestication events. *Proc. Biol. Sci.* 272: 2211–2217.

Perri, A.R., Feuerborn, T.R., Frantz, L.A.F. et al. (2021). Dog domestication and the dual dispersal of people and dogs into the Americas. *Proc. Natl. Acad. Sci. USA* 118 (6): e2010083118.

Perry, G.H. (2021). Evolutionary medicine. *eLife* 10: e69398.

Pilot, M., Greco, C., Vonholdt, B.M. et al. (2018). Widespread, long-term admixture between grey wolves and domestic dogs across Eurasia and its implications for the conservation status of hybrids. *Evol. Appl.* 11: 662–680.

Price, E.O. (1984). Behavioral aspects of animal domestication. *Q. Rev. Biol.* 59: 1–32.

Price, E.O. (2002). *Animal Domestication and Behavior*. New York: CABI Pub.

Price, M.D. and Evin, A. (2019). Long-term morphological changes and evolving human-pig relations in the northern fertile crescent from 11,000 to 2,000 cal BC. *Archaeol. Anthropol. Sci.* 11: 237–251.

Reznick, D.N. (2010). *The Origin Then and Now : An Interpretive Guide to the Origin of Species*. Princeton: Princeton University Press.

Ritvo, H. (1998). *Forward. The Variation of Animals and Plants Under Domestication*, Johns Hopkins paperbackse. Baltimore, Maryland: The Johns Hopkins University Press.

Ryder, O.A. (1978). Chromosomal polymorphism in *Equus hemionus*. *Cytogenet. Cell Genet.* 21: 177–183.

Sarmento, P., Cruz, J., Eira, C., and Fonseca, C. (2009). Spatial colonization by feral domestic cats *Felis catus* of former wildcat *Felis silvestris silvestris* home ranges. *Acta. Theriologica.* 54: 31–38.

Sauer, C.O. (1952). *Agricultural Origins and Dispersals; the Domestication of Animals and Foodstuffs*. Cambridge, MA: MIT Press.

Say, L., Devillard, S., Natoli, E., and Pontier, D. (2002). The mating system of feral cats (*Felis catus* L.) in a sub-Antarctic environment. *Polar Biol.* 25: 838–842.

Serpell, J. (1989). Pet-keeping and animal domestication: a reappraisal. In: *The Walking Larder: Patterns of Domestication, Pastoralism, and Predation* (ed. J. Clutton-Brock). London: Unwin.

Sinding, M.S., Gopalakrishan, S., Vieira, F.G. et al. (2018). Population genomics of grey wolves and wolf-like canids in North America. *PLoS Genet.* 14: e1007745.

Smyser, T.J., Tabak, M.A., Slootmaker, C. et al. (2020). Mixed ancestry from wild and domestic lineages contributes to the rapid expansion of invasive feral swine. *Mol. Ecol.* 29: 1103–1119.

Stearns, S.C. (2012). Evolutionary medicine: its scope, interest and potential. *Proc. Biol. Sci.* 279: 4305–4321.

Stiner, M.C., Munro, N.D., Buitenhuis, H. et al. (2022). An endemic pathway to sheep and goat domestication at Asikli Hoyuk (Central Anatolia, Turkey). *Proc. Natl. Acad. Sci. USA* 119: e2110930119.

Tapio, M., Marzanov, N., Ozerov, M. et al. (2006). Sheep mitochondrial DNA variation in European, Caucasian, and Central Asian areas. *Mol. Biol. Evol.* 23: 1776–1783.

Tinbergen, N. (1951). *The Study of Instinct*. Oxford, England: Clarendon Press.

Todd, N.B. (1978). An ecological, behavioral genetic model for the domestication of the cat. *Carnivore Genet. Newsl.* 1: 52–60.

Troy, C.S., MacHugh, D.E., Bailey, J.F. et al. (2001). Genetic evidence for Near-Eastern origins of European cattle. *Nature* 410: 1088–1091.

Trut, L., Oskina, I., and Kharlamova, A. (2009). Animal evolution during domestication: the domesticated fox as a model. *BioEssays* 31: 349–360.

Trut, L.N. (1999). Early canid domestication: the farm-fox experiment. *Am. Sci.* 87: 160–169.

Turchin, P., Hoyer, D., Korotayev, A. et al. (2021). Rise of the war machines: charting the evolution of military technologies from the neolithic to the industrial revolution. *PLoS One* 16: e0258161.

Ucko, P.J., Dimbleby, G.W., and University of London. Institute of Archaeology (1969). *The Domestication and Exploitation of Plants and Animals*. Chicago: Aldine Pub. Co.

Uerpmann, H.-P. (1996). Animal domestication - accident or intention? In: *The Origins and Spread of Agriculture and Pastoralism in Eurasia* (ed. D.R. Harris). London: UCL Press.

Uerpmann, H.P. (1989). Animal exploitation and the phasing of the transition from the paleolithic to the neolithic. In: *The Walking Larder : Patterns of Domestication, Pastoralism, and Predation* (ed. J. Clutton-Brock). London, Boston: Unwin Hyman.

Via, S. (2001). Sympatric speciation in animals: the ugly duckling grows up. *Trends Ecol. Evol.* 16: 381–390.

Vigne, J.D., Guilaine, J., Debue, K. et al. (2004). Early Taming of the Cat in Cyprus. *Science* 304 (5668): 259.

Vilstrup, J.T., Seguin-Orlando, A., Stiller, M. et al. (2013). Mitochondrial phylogenomics of modern and ancient equids. *PLoS One* 8: e55950.

Vonholdt, B. and Driscoll, C. (2017). Origins of the dog: genetic insights into dog domestication. In: *The Domestic Dog*, 2e (ed. J. Serpell). Cambridge, England: Cambridge University Press.

Wagner, M., Hallgren-Brekenkamp, M., Xu, D. et al. (2022). The invention of twill tapestry points to Central Asia: archaeological record of multiple textile techniques used to make the woollen outfit of a ca. 3000-year-old horse rider from Turfan, China. *Archaeological Research in Asia* 29: 100344.

Wang, G.D., Xie, H.B., Peng, M.S. et al. (2014). Domestication genomics: evidence from animals. *Annu. Rev. Anim. Biosci. 2* (1): 65–84.

Warmuth, V., Eriksson, A., Bower, M.A. et al. (2012). Reconstructing the origin and spread of horse domestication in the Eurasian steppe. *Proc. Natl. Acad. Sci. USA* 109: 8202–8206.

Weir, H. (1889). *Our Cats and All About Them : Their Varieties, Habits, and Management, and for Show, the Standard of Excellence and Beauty*. Tunbridge Wells (England): R. Clements and Co.

Wenke, R.J. (2009). *The Ancient Egyptian State : The Origins of Egyptian Culture (c. 8000-2000 BC)*. Cambridge, UK ; New York: Cambridge University Press.

Wilson, D.S., Clark, A.B., Coleman, K., and Dearstyne, T. (1994). Shyness and boldness in humans and other animals. *Trends Ecol. Evol.* 9: 442–446.

World Resources Institute (2000). *People and Ecosystems: The Fraying Web of Life*, 389. Washington DC: World Resources Institute.

Wright, D. (2015). The genetic architecture of domestication in animals. *Bioinform. Biol. Insights* 9 (S4): 11–20.

Wu, G.S., Yao, Y.G., Qu, K.X. et al. (2007). Population phylogenomic analysis of mitochondrial DNA in wild boars and domestic pigs revealed multiple domestication events in East Asia. *Genome Biol.* 8: R245.

Yamaguchi, N., Driscoll, C.A., Kitchener, A.C. et al. (2004a). Craniological differentiation between European wildcats (*Felis silvestris silvestris*), African wildcats (*F. s. lybica*) and Asian wildcats (*F. s. ornata*): implications for their evolution and conservation. *Biol. J. Linnean Soc.* 83: 47–63.

Yamaguchi, N., Kitchener, A.C., Ward, J.M. et al. (2004b). Craniological differentation amongst wild-living cats in Britain and southern Africa: natural variation or the effects of hybridization? *Anim. Conserv.* 7: 339–351.

Zarins, J. (1976). *The Domestication of Equidae in Third Millennium BC Mesopotamia*. Chicago: University of Chicago.

Zeder, M.A. (2008). Domestication and early agriculture in the Mediterranean Basin: origins, diffusion, and impact. *Proc. Natl. Acad. Sci. USA* 105: 11597–11604.

Zeder, M.A., Bradley, D.G., Emshiwiller, E., and Smith, B.D. (2006). Documenting domestication: bringing together plants, animals, archaeology, and genetics. In: *Documenting Domestication: New Genetic and Archaeological Paradigms* (ed. M.A. ZEDER, D.G. Bradley, E. Emshiwiller, and B.D. Smith). London: University of California Press.

Zeder, M.A., Emshwiller, E., Smith, B.D., and Bradley, D.G. (2006). Documenting domestication: the intersection of genetics and archaeology. *Trends Genet.* 22: 139–155.

Zeuner, F.E. (1963). *A History of Domesticated Animals*. New York: Harper & Row.

3

Social Behavior

R. Julia Kilgour[1], Traci Shreyer[2], and Candace Croney[3]

[1] University of Guelph, Department of Integrative Biology, Guelph, ON, Canada
[2] Purdue University, The Croney Research Group, West Lafayette, IN, USA
[3] Purdue University, Department of Comparative Pathobiology, Department of Animal Sciences, West Lafayette, IN, USA

Introduction

Social behavior occurs whenever two or more individuals interact. It encompasses a broad scope of behaviors, including whether and how animals form groups, the ways in which they maintain their social status within them, how, what, and when they communicate, and the types of behaviors they exhibit that support or undermine group cohesion. Additionally, sociality includes animals' preferences and tolerance for **conspecifics** (others of their own species), how they select mates, care for their offspring, and otherwise engage with each other.

For those working or interacting with animals regularly, understanding social behavior is critical to supporting the welfare of animals in virtually all situations in which they are kept and cared for by people. Certainly, those charged with the husbandry, care, and management of wild animals in captivity must be keenly aware of whether animals are more solitary or gregarious in nature to ensure that their housing environments and social groups permit biologically relevant behaviors. However, a solid understanding of animal sociality is just as important for veterinary practitioners focused on domesticated animal species. For example, knowledge about the sociality of the domesticated cat is necessary to support decision-making about housing cats singly or in groups in catteries, shelters, or laboratories. For veterinarians needing to counsel prospective or current cat households about whether and how to introduce and manage cats living together in households, incorporating knowledge of cat social behavior is essential to ensure positive outcomes. Likewise, the social behaviors of livestock and poultry dictate numerous aspects of their husbandry, care, and environmental management. These include housing designs, space allocations, feeding, and social groupings that are species appropriate. Incorporating such knowledge into decision-making affords farmers the opportunity to maximize agricultural animals' ability to access key resources (e.g. food, water, shelter, and resting areas) while minimizing unnecessary competition and aggressive encounters between them.

In this chapter, we provide an overview of different types of social behaviors domesticated animals display, an introduction to the advantages and costs of sociality, and the implications for animal care, management, and welfare in clinical and other applied settings.

Introduction to Animal Behavior and Veterinary Behavioral Medicine, First Edition. Edited by Meghan E. Herron.

Companion website: www.wiley.com/go/introductiontoanimalbehavior

Evolutionary and Environmental Constraints on Social Behavior

Almost all animals are social, at least some of the time. Some species have strong social bonds and live in large, complex groups for their entire lives, like humans. Others may live closely in complex associations with conspecifics for a portion of their lives, at predictable times of the year. Some may only interact briefly with conspecifics, such as for mating and reproduction. The degree of sociality varies across all animal groups, including mammals, birds, reptiles and amphibians, fishes, insects, and many other species of invertebrates. Furthermore, sociality encompasses a wide variety of behaviors, including mating and reproduction, parental care of offspring, and agonistic or **affiliative** interactions. Social behaviors can include cooperative defense from predators, as is often seen with ungulates, or cooperative hunting, as displayed by wolves. Given the ubiquity of sociality across the animal kingdom, these behaviors are certainly advantageous for animals to engage in, and therefore are adaptive.

Just as with any other trait, like scales, thick fur, hooves, or opposable thumbs, behaviors can evolve and be shaped by natural selection. Natural selection is the process by which traits that are more advantageous to individuals (i.e. those that enhance survival and reproduction rates) are passed on to future generations more often than less advantageous traits. The ability of an organism to survive and reproduce, thus propagating its traits, describes that individual's "fitness." Fitness refers to how much an individual contributes genetically to the next generation.

Social behaviors evolve when individuals who engage in them have higher fitness (survival and reproduction) than those who do not. Understanding the origins of animal behavior in wild species can provide important insights into our understanding of the behavior of domesticated species. As discussed in Chapter 2, domesticated animals have undergone generations of artificial selection, whereby humans have deliberately selected which animals will survive and reproduce based on desirable traits. Despite this, there are often strong legacy effects of wild ancestors in the behaviors that result from both intentional and inadvertent selection. Unsurprisingly, multiple domesticated animal species, such as pigs, cattle, and horses, show evidence that they have retained ancient behavioral traits that likely benefited their evolutionary ancestors (Koolhass and Van Reenen 2016).

A common misperception is that farmed livestock and poultry species may not need accommodations that allow expression of certain behaviors because these have been selectively eliminated through the process of domestication. For instance, some may believe that hens reared for commercial egg production have little need to perch or dustbathe. This notion is not supported by science. Although wild and domesticated members of a species may vary greatly in many aspects of their behavior, domestication does not appear to eliminate behaviors from the repertoire of a species. Rather, *quantitative* differences in behavioral expression are more common than qualitative changes (Price 1984). For example, in sheep, selection of birth sites away from the herd prior to parturition may vary as a function of domestication. Prior to parturition, wild and feral breeds of sheep will isolate either by distancing themselves from their herds, or by seeking out areas that are rocky and secluded to give birth. Some may choose to do both.

The Costs and Benefits of Group Living

As with any other trait or characteristic, social behavior can be shaped by natural selection when the fitness benefits are greater than the

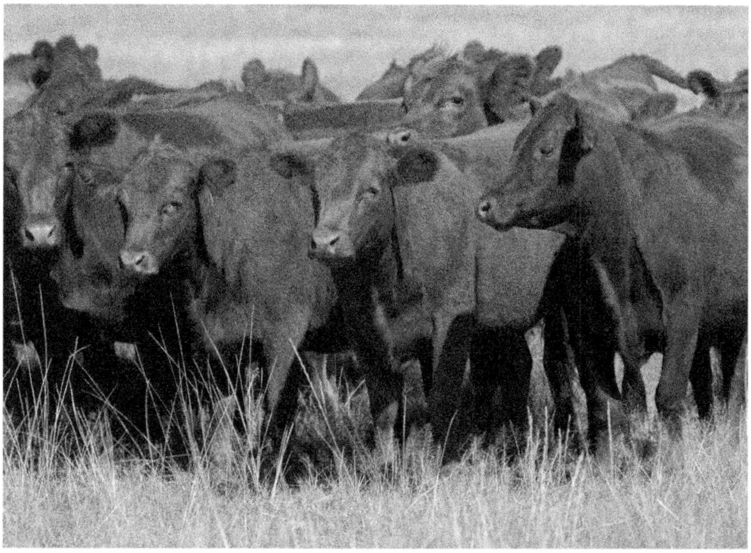

Figure 3.1 An example of the dilution effect – Cattle huddle together to create fewer opportunities for predators to single out one individual. *Source:* Photo credit: EcoView/Adobe Stock

fitness costs. Given the ubiquity of sociality in animals, it is fair to expect there to be a great many benefits of life in groups, but proximity to conspecifics can also have downsides. Therefore, many animals have evolved mechanisms to maximize the benefits while simultaneously reducing the costs of group life (Alexander 1974). Several studies have documented how fitness costs increase as group sizes swell beyond a certain number (Avilés and Tufino 1998; Stokes and Boersma 2000), demonstrating the trade-offs of sociality, and how individuals must minimize costs in order to maximize benefits of group living. In this section, we will describe the benefits and the costs of sociality.

Benefits of Sociality

Predator Defense

Among the most important benefits of living in groups is the potential for improved defense from predators. Solitary prey animals will certainly become targets if they encounter predators. Thus, living in groups offers individuals protection via the **dilution effect**, similar to the idea that there is "safety in numbers." Additionally, congregating in large, closely packed groups can result in increased protection from predators through predator confusion (Figure 3.1). For example, animals like fish that aggregate very closely and move synchronously can cause visual confusion for predators.

There are other benefits based on position within the group, such as being on its periphery. Many social ungulates, such as muskox and domestic cattle, will deliberately place the most vulnerable members of their social group, such as young, in the center of a defense ring. Animals on the exterior of the ring provide a protective shield, defending attacks by predators using horns and other weaponry.

Other species will use collective predator detection, sharing the responsibility for "standing watch," called the "Many Eyes hypothesis" (Powell 1974). If solitary, these animals would spend far more time engaged in vigilance behaviors, thereby interrupting other important behaviors, like foraging or resting, whereas vigilance can be shared amongst group members. **Mobbing**, another example of active defense, occurs when multiple individuals work together to attack or harass an approaching predator. This behavior is commonly observed in songbirds, where multiple species will dive bomb a threatening hawk or other predator in mid-air. Mobbing is also an example of cooperation, as individuals work together to harass and deter the incoming predator.

Information Transfer

Seasonal differences in environmental resource availability may make it difficult to find quality food at certain times of the year, such as during colder months. When this is the case, many animals use social information to locate resources. A form of passive information transfer is **local enhancement**, when an observer is drawn to a location or item simply by the presence of other individuals (Shettleworth 1998). Through **social facilitation** (described in detail later), vultures soaring in search of food are more likely to land in areas as a result of seeing conspecifics foraging on the ground (Buckley 1996), just as hens from a backyard flock rush over to areas where others are pecking in the grass. Animals also deliberately share information with each other on finding resources (any material necessary for survival and reproduction, such as food, water, or shelter), and social learning plays a critical role in the survival and reproduction of individuals from countless animal species.

Foraging Efficiency

For many species, locating and acquiring food can be challenging. For predators, survival is contingent on their ability to hunt successfully. Taking down a prey animal often depends on the relative size of the predator and its prey. Group hunting evolves if individuals can acquire more calories without increasing their energy expenditure. Indeed, cooperative hunting has evolved in many predator species, particularly in canids. Examination of cooperative hunting in African wild dogs has demonstrated that per capita food intake per kilometer chased was optimized by hunting in groups (Creel and Creel 1995).

Reproductive Benefits

There are reproductive benefits to life in groups, such as the ability to find a mate. Unlike those who live solitarily, animals who live in large flocks or herds can spend less energy searching for a mate and have more choices in their selection. Many species of birds, including wild turkeys and other species of fowl, use leks, wherein males congregate in a specific area and females arrive to choose a mate. The males use visual and vocal displays to attract the observing females, who subsequently select a male.

Other reproductive benefits relate to the rearing of offspring. Cooperative rearing of young occurs when individuals other than the parents (such as siblings or aunts) assist in the care of offspring. The decision to help rear their siblings or relatives, instead of dispersing and seeking a mate of their own, is often related to the availability of suitable nest sites or other features of the environment (Arnold and Owens 1999; Hatchwell 2007). Cooperative rearing of young is found in many species of social insects (Wilson 1975), crustaceans (Emmett and Macdonald 2010), and mammals (Jarvis 1981).

Costs of Sociality

Predation Risk

While gregarious species may benefit from reduced risks of predation, living in groups can also result in increased detection by predators. For example, Hebblewhite and Pletscher (2002) found that large groups of elk were more likely to be detected and hunted when they were in groups of 30 than when solitary or in groups of 5 individuals or less. However, the individual risk of mortality was low in large groups, likely due to the dilution effect, showing the net positive effect of sociality in this group. The increased encounter rates by predators also apply to farming, when livestock are at greater risk of predation where they are more abundant or more closely congregated (Kuiper et al. 2021).

Parasites and Disease

Transmission of pathogens and parasites is often related to proximity between individuals. Sociality increases the risk of illness and parasite infestation through increased transmission rates (Altizer et al. 2003), resulting in considerable fitness declines in both wild and domesticated species. In contemporary livestock and poultry production, disease transmission is a major welfare concern, requiring significant deliberation about how to house animals in groups while protecting their health, behavioral needs, and productivity. Animals living in larger groups may interact more with conspecifics and have less opportunity to disengage, resulting in more opportunities for parasite and pathogen transmission. Under such circumstances, highly virulent pathogens such as avian influenza or Porcine Reproductive and Respiratory Syndrome (PRRS) may be more easily transmitted between animals (Alizon et al. 2009). Thus, attention must be paid to avoid stocking at densities that may exacerbate these risks. Similar concerns exist for dogs kept in groups in various forms and sizes of kennels, where confinement near others may increase their chances of transmitting parasites and pathogens, such as fleas, ticks, influenza, distemper, parvovirus, and *Giardia* (Capelli et al. 2003) to each other.

Resource Competition

When animals congregate in areas where resources such as food and water are plentiful, there is no concern as to whether or which individuals will be able to access them. However, as group size increases and resources become more limited, individuals must compete to gain and maintain access to them. Indeed, competition for resources is considered to be one of the major forces limiting the evolution of sociality (Alexander 1974; Bourke 2011; Korb and Heinze 2016). Groups of animals can only be sustained if individuals can overcome the costs of competition or reduce them sufficiently to be outweighed by the fitness benefits.

Management of problematic levels of aggression in domestic animals can be at least in part a function of high animal density, low perceived resources, or space restrictions that constrain or prevent animals from leaving the group. When boarding facilities offer limited pasture time to horses, this creates both a limited resource (the pasture) and an inability to flee from conflict (fenced-in pasture). In such cases, horses may aggressively attack one another, causing injuries, because though they may want to control the pasture resource, the constrained environment prevents individuals from escaping or signaling submission. Similar challenges may arise in group-housed swine where food is typically restricted, and animals are kept at relatively high densities. Under these conditions, it is essential for farmers to attend carefully to the type and number of feeding stations the animals can access simultaneously to avoid unnecessary competition and fighting.

Reproductive Competition

While there are reproductive advantages to sociality, as highlighted above, there are also reproductive costs. These can come in aggressive forms of reproductive interference. For example, in many mammalian (Hoogland 1985; Lukas and Clutton-Brock 2012) and fish species (Heg 2008), a dominant female may actively suppress reproduction in other females, effectively coercing them to assist her in the rearing of her young. In acorn woodpeckers, a female will occupy the same nest and remove the eggs of her sister, destroying them (Mumme et al. 1983). Competition for mates can also increase the costs of sociality and result in competitive dynamics, as with any form of resource competition (West-Eberhard 1979).

Pros/cons of group-living	Feature	Examples
Benefits of group-living	Predator defense	Cattle grazing on rangeland attacked by a bear arrange themselves so that young are protected in the center of the group while adult animals on the periphery of the group simultaneously charge at and ultimately deter the bear.
	Information transfer	Kittens learn to hunt the same prey as their mothers through observation.
	Foraging efficiency	Chickens vocalize when feed is scattered, indicating to groupmates where food can be found.
	Reproductive efficiency	In large flocks of sheep, cross-fostering of lambs is possible when one ewe has twins or triplets and might otherwise not be able to provide nutrition and maternal care for all offspring.
Costs of group-living	Predation risk	A group of cows grazing in a field with their newborn calves draws the attention of coyotes in the area.
	Parasites and disease	Horses living in barns with large numbers and open access contract diseases such as Strangles or Equine Influenza.
	Resource competition	In a kennel housing multiple dogs, the largest dog housed in the run quickly eats most of their food and then displaces a smaller dog, leaving the other hungry.
	Reproductive competition	Roosters in a large flock initiate fights with each other for access to hens.

Types of Social Groupings

Both wild and domesticated animal species vary widely in their social groupings. These groupings may impact reproduction by influencing access to mates and parental care in its many forms, thus contributing to an individual's fitness (Gans 1996). The type of social grouping a species forms also has significant implications at the individual and group levels, in terms of territorial defense and coping with conflict over limited resources (Wolff 1997; Lopez-Sepulcre and Kokko 2005). For species categorized as **territorial**, social behaviors associated with conflict are central to their fitness. Though definitions of territoriality vary, generally, they refer to a strategy that enables individuals to gain and/or maintain exclusive access to the resources in a fixed area (Davies and Houston 1981; Kaufmann 1983; Stamps 1994). Territoriality therefore involves social interactions between individuals and their neighbors (Siracusa et al. 2017), requiring understanding of behaviors related to conflict management and cooperation. The type of species determines the territory size and the frequency at which interactions between conspecifics occur. Domesticated cats, for example, often occupy and share a relatively large territorial range but they do not generally interact frequently, unless to share "kills" or other resources (Turner 2014).

The tendency of different species to form groups, and the types of social groups formed have implications for their housing and management under human care. For example, many species live in **solitary-territorial** social groupings. Here, adults occupy and defend their own territories – males typically solitarily, and females with young. Males approach females around the reproductive period, when they are receptive and therefore more tolerant of their presence. Most carnivores, including bears, most wild felids (except lions and cheetahs), and domestic cats (when dependent on small prey for food), demonstrate solitary-territorial living. For these animals, the costs of group living, including competition between conspecifics, do not outweigh the benefits, especially since most of these species do not cooperatively hunt, parent, or defend resources (Bekoff et al. 1984; Caro 1989; Sandell 1989; Elbroch and Quigley 2017). The domestic cat is unique in that high individual variability exists for social tolerance, making it difficult to predict which cats may cope well with group living. In fact, the cat's ability to do well when kept in colonies depends on the availability and abundance of resources, such as shelter, food, and space to establish a territory (Flockhart et al. 2016). Colonies with an abundance of these resources are most conducive to large group living.

While the social needs of species differ, in both wild and domesticated animals, very few species are "asocial." Although some animals may appear to rely on and seek out companions more than others, some degree of social contact is normal and important to most species. For example, when in zoos, solitary-territorial cats such as tigers experience less stress when in the presence of a social companion. Veterinarians managing cats and those practicing zoo or exotic animal medicine should be cognizant of the fact that while these animals' social groupings are unique, their evolutionary history dictates dynamic social interactions with members of their own kind as well as other species. Care must be taken when determining whether and how to group solitary-territorial species, as individuals may be highly selective about which social companions they will tolerate. Their related behavioral needs must be appropriately incorporated into their housing, care, and husbandry in both the home and hospital environments to ensure their welfare.

Another common social organization is the **pairing-territorial** grouping, characterized by a male and female pair occupying and defending a territory, as is commonly observed in many songbird species. In these groups, the pair will also participate in the rearing of offspring – another benefit of sociality for these species. Both the solitary-territorial and pairing-territorial groupings present significant challenges for efficient management and reproduction of a species, making it unsurprising that few domesticated species group in this way.

Female groupings (often **matriarchal**) consist of multiple females and their dependent offspring. Such groups may occupy a specific **home range**, or they may range freely. Adult males live singly or in **bachelor herds** (all-male groups), joining the females during the breeding season. This is among the most common social groups formed by wild pigs, though another grouping may consist of a peri-parturient sow and her litter, which remain temporarily isolated from the herd until around 10 days post-parturition (Gonyou 2001). Similarly, wild elephants live in herds of related adult females of overlapping generations, creating extended, multigenerational family units (Douglas-Hamilton 1972). Cattle likewise form matrilineal groups of adult females and their calves. This form of social grouping is often reflected in contemporary cow–calf operations that are foundational to beef production. In such groupings, selection for maternal behavior is critical to the survival and behavioral development of young, particularly when the animals are raised under extensive conditions, where risk of encountering predators exists. In managed groups of feral cats where resources are provided in abundance by humans, social groups called "colonies" form that are based on a matrilineal composition. Here, females live together and cooperate in rearing each other's offspring and defending the colony from intruders (Bradshaw 2012; Turner 2014).

Some readers may wonder why group housing of sows presents a challenge for commercial pork production given that wild pigs naturally form groups that can resemble some of those used in industry management (large groups of females, sows and offspring, and juveniles of both sexes). However, Gonyou (2001) notes that it is not the grouping of sows that is problematic, but rather the *mixing* of sows (as commonly occurs in modern swine production management) that creates challenges. In nature, sows usually are closely-related and they group together for most of their lives, making them very familiar with one another. Thus, fighting is rare. Commercial production, however, requires that new groups of sows be formed with each breeding cycle, and it is the lack of familiarity between newly mixed animals that triggers potentially injurious aggression (Stookey and Gonyou 1998). These interactions can create enough distress to disrupt embryo implantation or cause loss of pregnancies. Unfortunately, in commercial production, where groups are at least somewhat dynamic, it is not feasible for sows and gilts to be completely familiar with each other, and it may take weeks for newly introduced animals to become fully integrated (Gonyou 2001). In the interim, the social disruption that occurs may jeopardize behavioral and physical welfare of the animals, adversely impacting performance and productivity.

Single male-multiple female groupings (**natal bands**) are commonly observed in equids such as zebras, the domesticated horse, lions, sea-lions and seals, and others. Typically, males will either defend the females and their young, or the territory where they are located, from other adult males. Male elephant seals, for example, will remain close to and defend the breeding females (Le Boeuf and Peterson 1969). Though uncommon, in some species, infanticide may occur when a new male takes over the breeding group (Lukas and Huchard 2014). Such behavior has been observed in lions as well as in horses. This clearly favors the fitness of the male, as females will quickly re-enter estrus and males do not provide care for the young of other males (Vitet et al. 2021). However, females have also evolved counter-strategies involving mating with multiple males so as to confuse the paternity of their offspring and reduce infanticide (Agrell et al. 1998).

Multi-male and multi-female groups are common in dogs, rodents, non-human primate species, and many other species. In this type of grouping, males and females co-exist with juvenile offspring, often organized into dominance hierarchies (detailed later in this chapter). This type of social grouping is difficult to replicate in captive settings, particularly those such as farms, or companion animal colonies where breeding must be synchronized to facilitate management and production, and decisions about which animals are bred must be tightly controlled to achieve desirable characteristics.

Maintaining animals in social groups to which they are not well adapted or acclimated may result in undesirable behavior and welfare outcomes. For example, learning and other aspects of animal cognition are impaired when animals that normally form social groups are kept in isolation. Learning deficits have been demonstrated in socially isolated rodents (Jones et al. 1992) and calves (Gaillard et al. 2014) and behavioral development was significantly impaired in socially isolated infant monkeys (Harlow et al. 1965). Dogs housed individually in shelters displayed more behavioral problems, including stereotypical behaviors, than those housed in groups (Mertens and Unshelm 1996). Further, in keeping with the idea that even solitary species have social needs, paired tigers had more diverse behavioral repertoires than those who were singly housed (De Rouck et al. 2005).

Conflict in Social Groups

Conflict within a social group is typically unavoidable. Whenever two or more individuals want access to the same limited and/or "unshareable" resource, a conflict arises. As a result, animals are forced to compete, which is a major cost of group living. Conflicts are worsened when the resource in question is easily defendable, is temporally and spatially clumped and predictable, or if population density is high (Grant 1993) (see Figure 3.2a,b). To avoid these conditions, clinicians and applied behaviorists often advise owners and animal caretakers to provide multiples of the resources animals living in groups need and want, especially those that are of high value to them (e.g. chew bones for dogs and litter pans for cats). They also may advise dispersing them throughout the environment in a manner that makes it difficult for one animal to monopolize or prevent others from accessing them.

When a conflict does arise, animals may use multiple strategies to resolve it in relatively quick and non-injurious ways. This can occur through threat displays, ritualized behaviors, or overt aggression. The term **agonistic behavior** refers to all of the behaviors involved in a competitive interaction, including threat, attack (fighting behavior), submission, and retreat (fleeing).

Competitive Agonistic Interactions

Agonistic interactions include a wide range of behaviors that vary in their level of intensity. Logically, animals should avoid engaging in fights as the risk of injury (or even death) increases as fights become more intense. Indeed, competitive interactions between two

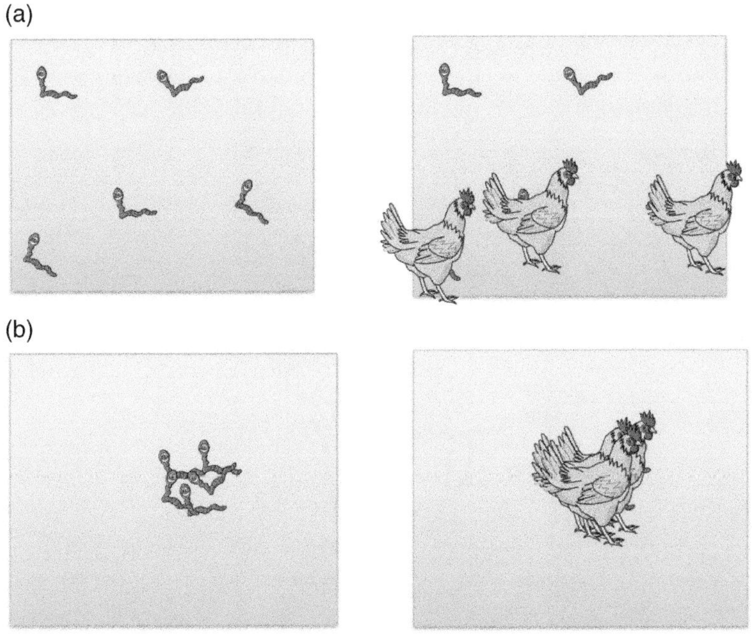

Figure 3.2 (a) In this example of a food (worms) resource, the resource is spatially dispersed, making it difficult for one animal to hoard and defend. Each individual animal also has space to access the resource without coming into conflict with another. (b) In this scenario of a food (worms) resource, the resource is clumped into one location, making it easy for one animal to access and defend from others. Clumped resources can lead to social tension, conflict, and injury. *Source:* Image credit: Katy Proudfoot.

or more individuals typically begin with displays, without any physical contact. These threats often take the form of auditory or visual signals, which inform potential competitors of an animal's presence and indicate the potential for a physical fight. Growling in dogs, piloerection (raised hackles), and specific physical postures serve as auditory and visual signals of intent. Physical postures during these displays can indicate what behaviors are likely to follow, depending on the response shown by the recipient of the communication. Cattle engage in a broad side threat as an offensive signal of their intent to move forward aggressively if the approaching animal does not retreat (Figure 3.3). Displays may also indicate an individual's willingness to progress further along the sequence of agonistic behaviors, though most competitive interactions cease at this stage, with one individual disengaging or retreating (Figure 3.4).

If neither animal retreats following threat signalment, animals will engage in physical contests, which may include **ritualized** behaviors. These behaviors allow the animals to test each other's competitive ability and determine if they want to continue in the contest. While these "tests" may appear risky to an outside observer, the intention is not to cause physical harm but instead to show off one's fighting ability. Ungulates will lock horns, a display of their relative strength (Clutton-Brock et al. 1979). Animals have evolved traits to minimize the impact of these displays. For example, rams have very thick skulls and extra cushioning around the brain as protection when they run at each other head-on (Geist 1966). There may be minor injuries incurred during these interactions, but typically one individual will show **submissive** behaviors and retreat or flee, signaling the end of the interaction.

On occasion, though rarely in wild animals, neither competitor will submit, and the level of aggression will escalate, with the intention of causing each other physical harm. Animals will use any part of their bodies, such as teeth, claws, horns, or body size, to injure the opponent. Predator species, such as cats, will shift from using claws to also using canine teeth – weaponry more often reserved for hunting prey (Hart 1985). It is important to note that if an animal is unable to flee following the ritualized displays, this will also result in

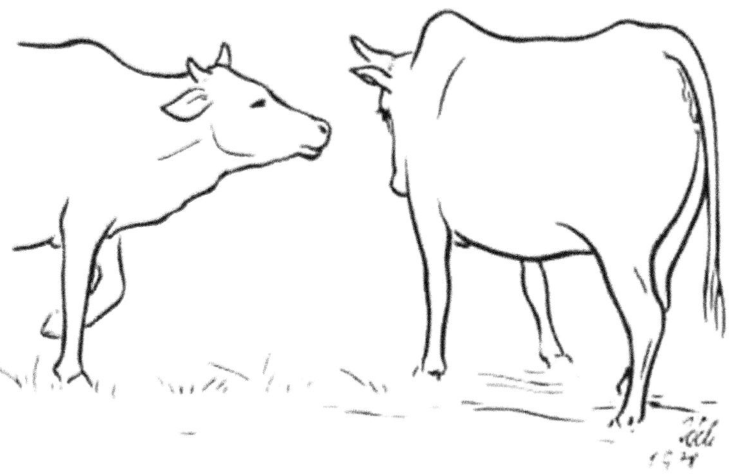

Figure 3.3 A strange cow (left) submissively approaches another herd and is blocked from proceeding by a cow who displays the broadside-threat gesture. *Source:* Image reproduced with permission from Comfortable Quarters for Laboratory Animals (2002), Reinhardt V, Reinhardt A (eds), page 90, Animal Welfare Institute, Washington, DC 2000; Drawing by Ingrid Schaumburg.

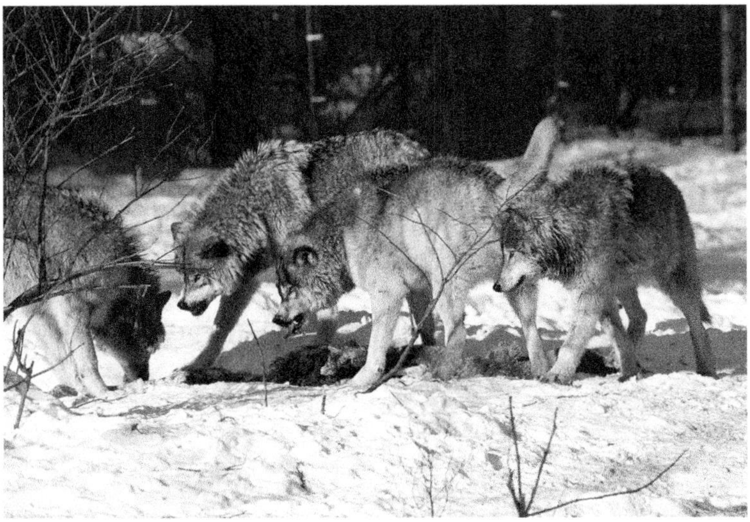

Figure 3.4 The two center wolves are moving forward with a direct stare, front teeth showing, which are both indications they are willing to move forward if the wolf on the left does not retreat. The wolf on the left is cowering slightly and if he does not back away a fight may ensue. *Source:* Photo credit: Martin Cathrae / Wikimedia Commons / CC BY-SA 2.0.

high-intensity fights. This is one reason why injurious fights are common in farm animals, such as pigs, that are socially housed in contained areas (Arey and Edwards 1998).

Determining Contest Outcomes

During competitive interactions, animals will make decisions about whether to continue or to retreat. Animals must be able to gauge the likelihood of winning or the extent of the potential costs, and then alter their behaviors. There are several factors that can predispose one individual to "win" more so than another and these may work in concert. Below, we outline prominent determinants of contest outcomes.

Resource Holding Potential

What determines the outcome of a contest is the relative competitive abilities of the animals involved. The ability of an individual to successfully win a competition can be influenced by animal's body size, endurance capacity, and weapon size. In combination, these factors describe an individual's **resource holding potential**, or RHP (Briffa and Sneddon 2010). Competitive interactions are rooted in the desire to acquire and/or maintain access to a limited resource, or an individual's potential to *hold* a resource. Strategic fight decisions are made based on relative RHP. If competitors differ in their RHP (for example, they are very different sizes), then the contest is unlikely to escalate into high-intensity aggression because the likely outcome is obvious from the beginning. However, if individuals are more closely matched in RHP, then the fight is more likely to escalate, (Dehnen et al. 2022; Maynard and Parker 1976). Competitive abilities can reflect the dynamics and structure of a social group, as dominance ranks are determined based on RHP differences between individuals (Feltes et al. 2020).

Perceived Resource Value

An animal is more likely to engage in a contest if it highly values the resource for which it is competing, regardless of its own RHP (Figure 3.5). Keep in mind the perceived value

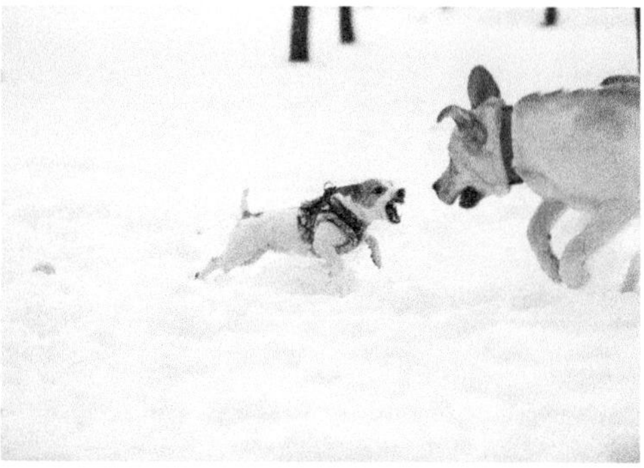

Figure 3.5 A small dog clearly has a lower resource holding potential in comparison to the larger dog on the right. The value of the blue toy on the ground is of great value to this dog, though, prompting her to engage in resource guarding behavior. *Source:* Photo credit: alexei_tm / Adobe Stock

of a resource may vary significantly between individuals. For example, a hungry lion is more likely to value a low-quality prey item, and thus fight over access to its carcass, than one who is well nourished. If the availability of a resource is restricted, then it will be of higher value and individuals will be more likely to compete aggressively. It is important to note that items that are highly valued by one individual may be of low value to another. This is often observed in dogs, where one individual might be more likely to compete for access to food, while another is more likely to compete for a resting space or a specific toy (Bradshaw et al. 2009).

Winner–Loser Effects

In the previous section, we described how aggressiveness is influenced by prior social experiences. This trend is reflected in competitive contests and is called the **winner–loser effect**, where the outcome of a contest is influenced by the individual's previous contest result. That is, when an individual "wins" a competition, it is more likely to win a subsequent competition (Chase et al. 1994). Similarly, if an animal "loses" a competition, it is more likely to lose the following contest. These effects can subsequently influence the rank structure within the group (Dugatkin 1997). Interestingly, winner and loser effects occur regardless of the relative RHP of the opponent and are likely due to psychological and physiological consequences of contest outcomes (Earley et al. 2013). In domestic pigs, winner–loser effects are stronger predictors of contest escalation than the level of aggressiveness of the pigs themselves (Oldham et al. 2020).

The sequence of agonistic behaviors between two dogs competing over a resource such as a favorite toy or chew might include growling, barking, lip lifting, or hard, sustained staring at each other, combined with rigid, forward body language (threat). If such displays were ineffective in causing one individual to yield, attack (fighting) behavior that might ensue would likely include any or all of the following: lunging, biting, or pinning the other dog. Eventually, one of the dogs would likely yield by retreating or by signaling submission by lowering their body, tail tucking, averting their head or eyes, or by rolling over and exposing their belly. Clear indication of submission or retreat should act as an inhibitory stimulus that discontinues threat or aggression from an opponent. It is therefore concerning when, in situations like this, one dog has clearly yielded or retreated, but the winner continues to attack. Bite placement on recipient dogs that indicate retreat (rump, anogenital, hind legs) or performance submissive signaling/postures (entire ventrum, particularly the inguinal area), or injury that punctures the skin should serve as a prompt for immediate intervention by the clinician, including referral to an academically trained animal behaviorist. It is also abnormal for adult dogs to display injurious aggressive behavior toward young puppies. Veterinarians should counsel owners about early intervention and monitoring of dogs showing such behavior patterns to ensure safe interactions with others. These risk factors, along with aggression triggered by the sight of the recipient, same-sex pairs (particularly female-female), and owner use of aversive training techniques, were found by Feltes et al. (2020) to be associated with poor outcomes (e.g. permanent separation, rehoming, or euthanasia).

Owner versus Intruder

When animals compete for resources in nature, it is often the case that one individual will already have access to the resource which the opponent wants. For example, animals will fight for access to a high-quality territory, resulting in a competition with the individual currently occupying the territory. Although RHP factors into the likelihood of engaging in the competition to begin with, the initial ownership status is also relevant. Similar to a "home team advantage," animals who are current resource "owners" are more likely to win a contest than the opponent, or "intruder" (Krebs 1982). This premise is relevant to understanding aggression among livestock, such as pigs, whose social groups are regularly shuffled (Gonyou 2001).

Aggression

Aggression is expressed in a range of contexts, not only competitive interactions, and involves species-specific behaviors which indicate an intention to do harm (Hinde 1970). Aggression may be triggered by multiple motivational states and may serve different functions. For example, there are competitive, protective, and parental types of aggression (Archer 1988). Take, for instance, a self-defensive situation such as when a hen is attacked by a coyote. This might elicit self-protective, fear-based aggression from the hen. If her chicks were nearby, the hen would likely also display parental aggression to protect her young from danger. In this case, aggression from her would be highly adaptive, as hens who appropriately exhibit aggression under such circumstances would likely experience greater fitness benefits (via survival of self and/or offspring) than those who did not.

Animals may also display aggressive behaviors in contexts where they may not serve an obvious function to the outside observer. For example, while protective aggression may be motivated by and displayed in response to a real or perceived threat, animals may also display fear-based aggression that is not necessarily adaptive in the moment but may instead reflect previous learning based on past experiences. Similarly, the expression of pain-induced aggression, which is all too familiar to veterinary practitioners, while still a form of self-protection, may not reflect any actual risk to an animal. Nonetheless, intense pain or chronic stress may cause an animal to behave aggressively in response to relatively inert or typically non-threatening stimuli.

Aggression is therefore a complex behavioral response that is influenced by both innate qualities of the individual and their environment. It has a genetic component, and can thus be shaped by natural and artificial selection (McClearn 1970). Due to the consistency in behavior across contexts, aggressiveness is considered a personality trait in both domestic and wild animals (Briffa et al. 2015). As with any personality trait, inheriting alleles that code for aggression does not mean that individuals will behave aggressively all the time, but may indicate a predisposition toward acting aggressively. For example, livestock guardian dogs such as the Great Pyrenees were selectively bred to readily guard flocks from predators, and Bullmastiffs were bred to guard hunting grounds from poachers. While these breeds are predisposed to behaving aggressively, this is not an indicator that they will be aggressive in all contexts. Further, when assessing animals showing aggression, clinicians should be aware of the specific motivations for aggressive behavior. It is crucial to understand the difference between context-dependent aggression and animals who are aggressive in most or all contexts, as the latter almost never exists. For example, the Great Pyrenees may show levels of intense aggression directed toward a wolf approaching a flock but not human visitors. Similarly, the fearfully aggressive Bullmastiff may direct aggression toward a stranger entering the yard, but not to a trusted family member. Unfortunately, misunderstanding motivation and context-specific aggression can result in efforts to punish aggression and the associated agonistic behavioral displays that predict it and that precede fighting. This may result in diminished threat behavior, thus reducing warning before attack or fighting ensures, or create the paradoxical effect of inadvertently eliciting aggression in individuals, thus reducing safety for all.

Most animals are heavily influenced by their social surroundings, both past and present. Aggressiveness as an adult can be a reflection of early life experiences, either through learned behavior or physiological changes (Haller et al. 2014; Holekamp and Strauss 2016; Spencer 2017). For example, the social environments of piglets, relating to litter size and nutrition, influence the aggressiveness of pigs later in life (D'eath and Lawrence 2004). The expression of aggression can also be influenced by an animal's recent social experience. For example, when green swordtail fish witness a competitive interaction between familiar individuals, they are more likely to subsequently behave aggressively in future competitive interactions (Earley and Dugatkin 2002). In this way, we can say that individuals are "primed" to behave aggressively. Lastly, the present social environment influences whether an animal decides to behave aggressively. That is, an animal may be less aggressive (or not aggressive) in the presence of an individual with higher RHP but may be highly aggressive toward one with a lower RHP.

Social Structures and Dominance Hierarchies

In many social groups, individuals develop relationships with each other, which assist in navigating conflict and minimizing the costs of competition. The nature of structured social groups was first described in groups of domestic chickens (Schjelderup-Ebbe 1922), where it was noted that individuals who "won" in competitive interactions also had priority access to food and roosting locations. It was from these observations that the term "pecking order" was coined, as competitive interactions were identified based on pecking behaviors between hens. In social groups structured into dominance ranks, individuals with the highest ranks have priority access to resources, such as food, mates, or resting areas, and others are organized in descending or overlapping rank orders.

If individuals were to engage in competitive contests with escalating levels of risk each time they encountered one another, they would expend considerable time and energy at every meeting. Instead, establishing social hierarchies provides information about likely outcomes ahead of time, enabling animals to avoid such aggressive interactions. Indeed, once the hierarchical order has been established within a group, there is a reduction in overall aggression among group members (Bernstein 1981; Drews 1993; Chase et al. 1994; Gonyou 2001). Therefore, although dominance relationships result in unequal distribution of resources, they can be advantageous to both higher and lower ranking individuals. Additionally, social groups which develop strong hierarchical structures have improved stability over time, as ranks can be maintained using less costly behaviors, such as non-physical cues or even affiliative behaviors (Tibbetts et al. 2022).

The relative ranks of individuals are established through either a series of competitive contests (as described earlier in this chapter) or through demographic factors. Ranks can also be established through coalitions, or alliances, of subordinate individuals, who work together to challenge the top-ranking individual (Smith et al. 2010). Alliances are usually established between siblings (Parsons et al. 2003; Smith et al. 2010), though not always (Chapais et al. 1991). In multi-male and multi-female groups, individuals of one sex will be dominant over all members of the other sex. For example, in spotted hyenas, females outrank males (Frank 1986), a trend also observed in many species of primates, although often depending on the male to female ratio (Hemelrijk et al. 2008). In some groups, ranks are inherited, where the young of high-ranking females are inherently also high-ranking, (Holekamp and Smale 1991).

Despite the stability that dominance ranks can create within a group, social ranks change over time as group members die, disperse, or lose their competitive ability. Resource availability may change, inducing new series of competitive interactions. Sudden changes in group membership, particularly among high-ranking individuals, can function as a "re-set" button, where remaining group members challenge one another for higher-ranking positions.

Hierarchical ranks can also vary across contexts. For example, some individuals may be more likely to compete for resources which are unvalued by others, resulting in different sets of competitors and thus dominance ranks may be relative to the resources in question. The influence of perceived resource value in relative ranks, particularly compared to RHP, may be strong determinants of social structure in domestic dogs (Bradshaw et al. 2009).

Types of Dominance Hierarchies

Because animals must coexist in environments where resources are constrained, and some conflict is inevitable, different types of dominance hierarchies emerge as animals attempt to maintain preferential access to resources. One of the most common hierarchical arrangements is unidirectional or linear, as with the pecking order. In a **linear dominance hierarchy**, the animal at the top of the pecking order outranks all others. The next highest-ranking animal in the group outranks all members but the one above it and this pattern continues through to the lowest ranked member of the group. This pattern is very common, and has been observed in swine (Mauget 1981) chickens, captive giraffes (Horová et al. 2015), and free-ranging dogs (Cafazzo et al. 2010).

A **parallel hierarchy** may be seen in groups where animals of different ages coexist. In such groups, it is not uncommon to find a linear hierarchy among the adults and a similar linear hierarchy among the juveniles within the group. Such patterns have been observed in several domestic species, such as turkeys, pigs, cattle, and sheep. For example, Mauget (1981) noted that in groups consisting of sows and their offspring, the sows will outrank all other individuals and maintain a linear hierarchy relative to each other, whereas the juveniles will mirror a linear hierarchy within their age group (Gonyou 2001).

In contrast, in a **despotic hierarchy**, one individual is clearly dominant while the other individuals in the group share relatively equal subordinate status. Domesticated cats kept in laboratory colonies at higher densities than are usually seen in homes or in feral groups have been shown to exhibit despotic hierarchies (Voith and Borchelt 1986).

Triangular or multi-angular (**complex**) arrangements (see Figure 3.6a,b) may be observed in many species where large groups are formed, including those that form linear or parallel hierarchies. In this arrangement, the relationships between three individuals may vary relative to each other (thus forming a triangle). These animals might outrank all others in the group, who might then fall into a relatively linear hierarchy or multiple triangles

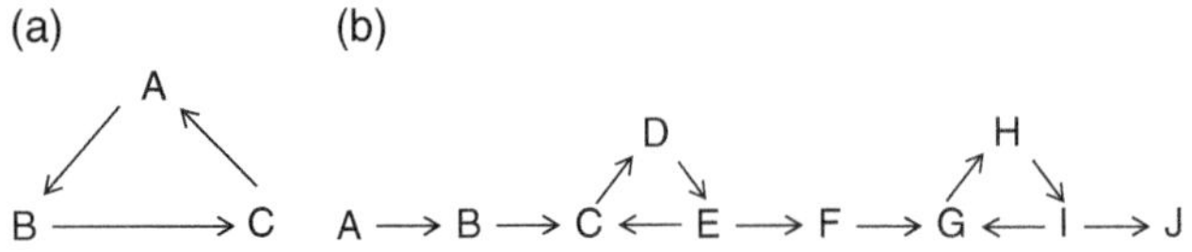

Figure 3.6 Triangular (a) and complex (b) hierarchies: The first figure (a) illustrates a triangular hierarchy whereby animal A has a higher social ranking (preferential access to resources) over animal B; animal B outranks animal C; and C outranks animal A, thus forming a "triangle." The second figure (b) shows a complex social hierarchy with multiple triangles. Here, animal A is the top-ranking animal and J is the lowest-ranking animal; animals C, D, and E, as well as G, H, and I, form their own triangles within the hierarchy.

might be formed at different levels within an otherwise linear hierarchy.

While discussions about animal social organizations and networks may seem esoteric, it can be valuable for veterinarians and all animal caretakers to understand the kinds of dominance hierarchies that may occur in different social groupings for several reasons. For example, understanding that pigs quickly and naturally form hierarchies that protect them from injurious aggressive interactions should inform or underscore advice against mixing of unknown individuals and repeated remixing of pigs once stable groups are formed. Furthermore, having knowledge of companion animal social hierarchies (or, in some cases, lack thereof) helps dispel popular misconceptions, such as those common in the domestic dog training world (see Box 3.1).

The Role of Aggressiveness in Contest Outcome and Dominance Rank

There is a common misconception that aggressiveness is equated with RHP or dominance rank. That is, individuals with a high dominance rank and a high RHP are inherently the most aggressive. This is not the case. Research has repeatedly demonstrated that the most aggressive animals in a group are often not the highest ranking (Kim and Zuk 2000; Kralj-Fišer et al. 2010; McGhee and Travis 2010), and multiple factors can determine relative ranks (Lewis 2022). As previously described, aggression is often classified as an animal personality trait, predisposing certain individuals to behave more aggressively than others. Research on pigs has shown that the escalation in the intensity of fights is often due to the aggressive personality

Box 3.1 The Pack

A pack is a well-organized social structure, adopted by grey wolves, African wild dogs, and a few other wild canid species. Members of this social group follow a strict linear hierarchy, led by a breeding male and female pair – **breeders**. Key characteristics of a pack structure include communal rearing of young and cooperative hunting. This system allows large groups of mostly related individuals to cover large territories, protect their young, minimize conflict, and take down large prey. A common misconception is that domestic dogs inherited this social structure, despite evidence to the contrary (Bradshaw et al. 2009; Majumder et al. 2014). Studies of *Canis familiaris* both in feral and in-home settings fail to demonstrate strict linear hierarchies, cooperative rearing or hunting, or any establishment of large family groups. Dogs living with people and other dogs do form bonds and social groups – just not the pack-like structure that has been popularized over the past two decades.

of the individual and not its RHP or dominance rank (Camerlink et al. 2016). This is likely because there are many costs to obtaining and maintaining a high dominance rank, as individuals with higher ranks often experience chronic stress (Creel 2001). Individuals with a higher RHP may be able to gauge competitive situations more appropriately, thereby only engaging in high-intensity aggression when necessary. Due to the high physiological costs of maintaining a high dominance rank, it is logical that higher-ranking individuals are not those who are simply the most aggressive, but those who are selective when they behave aggressively.

Aggression certainly plays a role in the establishment of dominance ranks; however, the terms *cannot and should not be used interchangeably*. Indeed, the definition of dominance does not rely on the use of aggression, simply because social **dominance** refers to a relationship between multiple individuals. In contrast, **aggression** is a behavior expressed by a single individual. To infer a high dominance rank, the aggressive behavior must be followed by submission from the opponent, not just by the aggressive behaviors themselves (East and Hofer 2010). For example, wolves do not force others onto their backs to gain dominance rank. A submissive animal voluntarily performs that behavior as a signal of deference. It should also be emphasized that the term, "dominance" refers to a relationship established after many interactions, and is not a characteristic of an individual (e.g. "he is a dominant dog"). Most of the companion animal behaviors that clients struggle with are not related to preferential access to resources but are those that are inadvertently rewarded, never trained in the first place, or rooted in fear. The use of "**dominance theory**" in attempts to change pet behavior is not evidence-based, encourages adversarial interactions and physical punishment, and decreases empathy from people toward their pets. Confrontational techniques, such as "alpha rolls," "dominance downs," "staring the dog down," as well as hitting, kicking, and yelling used in an attempt to reduce unwanted behaviors frequently elicit aggressive responses in dogs (Herron et al. 2009).

The American Veterinary Society of Animal Behavior (AVSAB) recommends that veterinarians not refer clients to trainers or behavior consultants who coach and advocate dominance theory and the subsequent confrontational training that follows. The AVSAB emphasizes that the standard of care for veterinarians specializing in behavior is that dominance theory should not be used as a general guide for behavior modification. Instead, they emphasize that behavior modification and training should focus on reinforcing desirable behaviors, avoiding the reinforcement of undesirable behaviors, and striving to address the underlying emotional state and motivations, including medical and genetic factors, that are driving the undesirable behavior (AVSAB 2008).

Affiliative Behaviors

In contrast to agonistic behavior, affiliative behaviors, such as cooperation, help to reinforce bonds within members of a social group, thereby facilitating group cohesion as well as individual and group success (Pellegrini 2008). Pro-social behaviors are those performed by one individual that helps another meet their needs and, in so doing, contributes to the other's improved welfare (Cronin 2017). Animals exhibit a wide range of pro-social behaviors, through parental care, socially-facilitated learning, and cooperative and altruistic behaviors. For example, rats have been shown to free cage-mates trapped in a restrainer in response to conspecific distress signals. When given the opportunity to free a cage-mate or open another restrainer containing chocolate, they chose to open both restrainers and share the chocolate

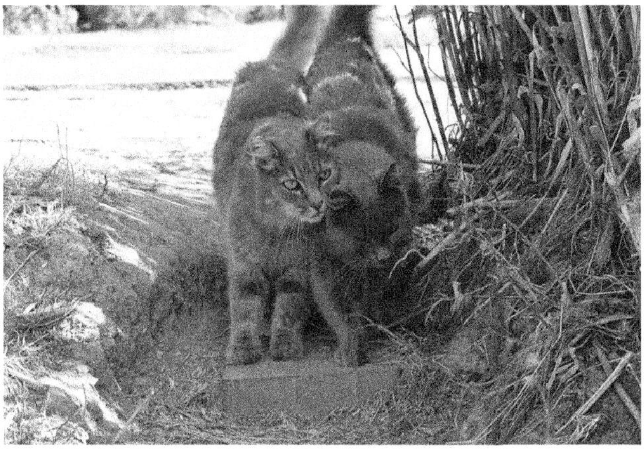

Figure 3.7 Two cats rub against each other to exchange scents and show affiliative intentions – an activity known as allorubbing. *Source:* Photo credit: Rhonda Van.

(Bartal et al. 2011), suggesting they may be capable of empathy-driven, cooperative prosocial behavior.

Multiple factors may elicit pro-sociality in animals, with some consensus emerging that pro-social behaviors are tied to their effects on social relationships. For instance, the possibility of reciprocal altruism may explain such behaviors (Trivers 1971) and it is plausible that individual animals may preferentially aid those with whom they have close social bonds (Preston and de Waal 2002). Other factors, such as social status, the context in which the behavior is occurring (including adequacy of available resources), and experience may influence pro-sociality (Rault 2019).

Allogrooming and Allorubbing

Other examples of prosocial behaviors include allogrooming and allorubbing (grooming and rubbing of others). Allogrooming, where one individual grooms another, has clear benefits in reducing parasite loads on groupmates. The social benefits are also well known. Cats frequently direct grooming behavior toward **preferred associates**, typically resulting in purring, postural changes, and other behaviors wherein the recipient indicates that such interactions are welcomed (Crowell-Davis et al. 2004). Allogrooming may serve to strengthen social bonds in cats and in many other species, including cattle and non-human primates (Dunbar 1991), and may be particularly beneficial to subordinate animals, as with meerkats who use allogrooming to placate more dominant females (Kutsukake and Clutton-Brock 2006). Cats also allorub (Figure 3.7), using their heads, sides, and tails to rub against a familiar group member (including humans). This behavior may allow them to exchange scents with each other (aiding in mutual recognition) as well as engage in positive tactile contact with those with whom they interact (Crowell-Davis et al. 2004).

Social Buffering

A major way in which sociality may help animals adapt to environmental demands is through social buffering. During distressful circumstances, the presence of familiar conspecifics with whom social bonds are shared can help to mitigate fear and other unpleasant emotional states animals may experience. Therefore, animals may seek contact with each other on such occasions. Heifers, for instance, showed less avoidance of strange noises when penmates were present (Boissy and Le Neindre 1990), and they were less fearful in a novel environment when they had a social partner versus when they were alone (Veissier and Le Neindre 1992). Likewise, chicks subjected to restraint stress rapidly sought contact with conspecifics when given the opportunity to do so (Marin et al. 2001). Chicks also showed reduced stress responses in the presence of their mothers (Edgar et al. 2015), illustrating the effects of maternal bonds and care. Given these findings, clinicians and others working with farm animals in novel environments, maintaining them temporarily for treatment purposes, or subjecting them to procedures that are likely to elicit distress, may facilitate easier handling and positive welfare states simply by ensuring they are handled in the presence of familiar conspecifics.

Studies conducted with dogs reveal similar patterns while illustrating that, in addition to familiar dogs being able to provide stress-buffering effects for each other, having an affiliative relationship with a human may also alleviate stress (Bauer et al. 2017; Cimarelli et al. 2019). Facilitating the presence of familiar caretakers when providing veterinary care is advised whenever possible for this reason. "Owner" presence has been shown to reduce both physiological (e.g. heart rate) and behavioral (e.g. low posture escape) indicators of fear in dogs during routine exams (Stellato et al. 2020). Incorporating a calm, affiliative canine housemate into stressful situations that may be difficult for more timid or fearful dogs can be helpful advice for pet families, as well as shelters and rescue groups rehabilitating extremely fearful dogs (Schultz 2016). Interestingly, findings suggest that the strong social bonds dogs and humans share can permit dogs to reciprocate as substitute sources of support and stress-buffering for socially isolated people (Bowen et al. 2021).

Social Facilitation

It is not uncommon to see animals in groups engaged in behaviors that appear to elicit the same behaviors in others. This phenomenon, termed social facilitation (Zajonc 1965), is also referred to as "contagion" (Miller et al. 2009). Yawning in humans is a classic example of socially facilitated behavior. Chickens demonstrate social facilitation when they are drawn to peck in areas where others are seen pecking. Some have been shown to drink more quickly if they observe another hen drinking quickly (Hoppitt and Laland 2008). Similarly, mice have shown contagious itching when they observe others scratching themselves (Yu et al. 2017). Many examples of social facilitation are highly beneficial.

Pigs exhibit emotional contagion, a foundation for empathy, wherein their emotional states may be impacted by their groupmates (Reimert et al. 2013). This finding has implications for their welfare when housed socially, particularly where distress by one individual may elicit a similar unpleasant state in another. Likewise, dogs can be emotionally contagious to each other (Palagi et al. 2015), resulting in behaviors that are problematic to manage in housing and hospital situations, including barking in kennels, and fearful behaviors that make handling and the provision of medical care difficult or dangerous. Because dogs also show emotional contagion to humans (Yong and Ruffman 2014; Van Bourg et al. 2020) clinicians may be able to facilitate positive emotional states in dogs during ambiguous or distressful circumstances by treating them in the presence of owners who are calm, positive, and encouraging. Conversely, two animals that are fearful may be intentionally separated during behavior modification work so that one does not escalate the fear responses in the other from avoidance to aggression (Bowen et al. 2021).

Play

Play behavior in animals often involves exaggerated, uncoordinated, and unpredictable movement (Spinka et al. 2001). While it is most often seen in juvenile animals, many domesticated species, such as cats and dogs, play as adults, although play may occur with less frequency with age. Play may be solitary or social, with social play involving at least two animals

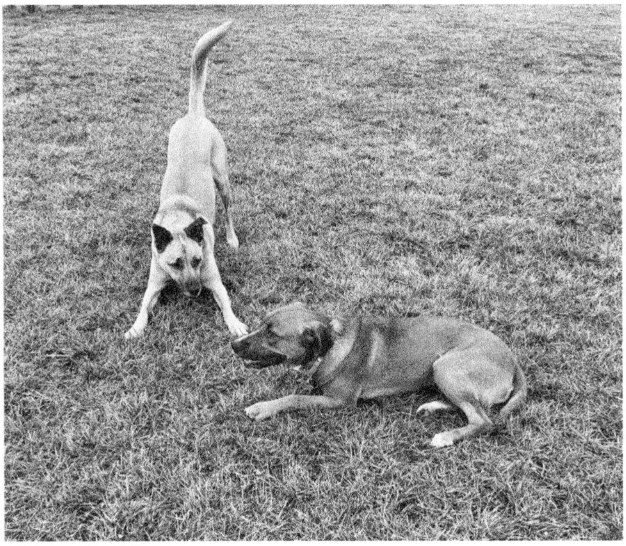

Figure 3.8 The play bow. Dogs will engage in this position when soliciting play as a signal to the other dog that they mean no harm. The tail and rump are held high with the tail broadly wagging, the front end is lowered with bent forearms, and the mouth is open. Dogs will typically bow for only a few seconds before bouncing forward in a playful manner or running in another direction. *Source:* Photo credit: Aditi Czarnomski.

that are often similar in size and age (Spinka et al. 2001). Animals may initiate play using species-typical behaviors and postures. The play bow demonstrated in dogs is easily recognized by other dogs and humans as a solicitation to engage in play (Figure 3.8).

Burghardt (2005) describes play as behavior that is not fully functional in that it does not contribute to the animal's survival in the moment; is self-rewarding; different in form and timing from the adult version of the behaviors displayed; is performed in a repeated but not stereotypic manner; and is initiated when the animal is relaxed. Many benefits of play have been suggested (Fagen 1982). Social play may encourage and aid the formation of the bonds and social skills required to cooperate or compete successfully in groups. It may help animals train cognitively and physically for unexpected future situations, such as predation or avoidance of predators, while also aiding in skeletal muscle fiber differentiation (Weller et al. 2020). During play fighting, which may closely simulate actual fighting behavior, animals do not typically injure each other (Beckel 1991). Instead, this kind of play may give animals a frame of reference by which to gauge their fighting ability and that of their playmates. In other words, play may help animals to accurately assess their RHP (Weller et al. 2020).

Play is connected to the experience of positive emotional states in animals (Fraser and Duncan 1998; Spinka et al. 2001) and therefore can be useful to clinicians trying to assess the welfare of patients. The presence or absence of play might be used diagnostically to identify animals in need of supportive interventions, or it might provide supporting evidence of whether they are responding positively to treatment. For example, the newly adopted young cat not engaging in solitary play (e.g. with toys) or social play (e.g. people or other animals) should be screened for distress, and their caretakers should be advised of stress-reduction strategies. It is often a positive prognosticator when play behaviors return between dogs experiencing intrahousehold inter-dog aggression.

Parent–Offspring Relationships

For many animals, interactions with one or both of their parents are their first social experiences. As a result, the relationship between parents and offspring can have a profound influence on later physical and behavioral development. Early life experiences play a critical role in brain development, somatic health, and an individual's ability to navigate its environment, including its social environment (Rilling and Young 2014).

Across different taxa, both parents have the potential to provide some kind of care for offspring. However, the type of care can vary between no parental care, bi-parental care, and only paternal or maternal care. There are often biological explanations that indicate who can provide sufficient care of young. In fish, amphibians, reptiles, and birds (as well as many invertebrates) where embryos develop external to the body, both parents are equally equipped to provide care for the eggs and hatched young, and biparental care is common in these taxa (Cockburn 2006; Reynolds et al. 2002). In contrast, among mammals, only females can provide certain care for young through lactation. Therefore, many species of mammals have only maternal care, where the fathering male spends minimal or no time caring for offspring, depending on the social structure of the species (Woodroffe and Vincent 1994). Although they cannot provide nutrition for neonates, mammalian fathers are able to protect young from predators and conspecifics, protect their mates, and help secure food for their mates and young after weaning.

The level of development of young when born or hatched influences the amount of care provided by parents. Some animals, such as ducks, geese, and many species of ungulates, including horses, are precocial, meaning they are born or hatch at a later stage of development, typically with mostly functioning sensory systems, and the ability to quickly rise and demonstrate mobility, which allows them to feed or nurse while standing and staying close to their mothers. Other animals, such as cats and dogs, are altricial, in that offspring are born or hatch at an earlier stage of development, often with undeveloped sensory systems, lack of capacity to move on their own. They are therefore heavily dependent on parental care for survival. Altricial young require considerably more support upon birth or hatching, and this, in turn, influences the intensity and duration of the parent–offspring relationship.

A vital component of the care and proper development of young is the bond that is established between them and their parents. In mammals, interactions between mother and infant that begin almost immediately following birth or hatching result in increased offspring recognition and facilitate parental care. Maternal care is motivated by both external and internal cues. Maternal behavior in mammals may be elicited by a combination of olfactory and other chemical cues emitted directly from neonates, and from the placenta or amniotic fluid (Edwards 1983; Jones and Wynne-Edwards 2001; Lévy and Keller 2009; Okabe et al. 2012). Maternal and paternal behaviors may also be driven by neurochemical and hormonal changes (Angelier and Chastel 2009; Broad et al. 2006; Wynne-Edwards and Timonin 2007; Ziegler 2000). For example, in mammals, the release of oxytocin, which occurs during parturition and nursing in mammals is important in establishing mother–offspring bonds (Nagasawa et al. 2012), whereas vasopressin is important in creating father-offspring bonds (McGraw et al. 2010). Circulating prolactin results in similar prosocial and parental behaviors in birds (Boos et al. 2007; Spée et al. 2010). These external and internal motivators result in the initiation of behaviors that assist in the development of the parental-offspring bond. Research on rats, for instance, has illustrated that tactile contact, such as grooming, results in the release of oxytocin in both mother and young (Nagasawa et al. 2012; Uvnas-Moberg 1998). Further, in cows, the mother begins to lick her newborn calf within hours, stimulated by the presence of amniotic fluid (Edwards 1983). This behavior engages tactile, gustatory, odor, and pheromonal cues that aid in both recognition of and bonding with the calf. In short, these kinds of early, repeated, positive social interactions between animals and their parents shortly after birth or

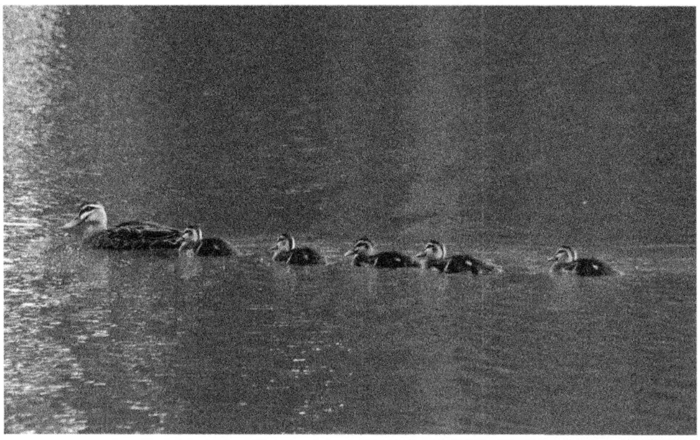

Figure 3.9 Ducklings imprint on their mother, as she is the first moving object they see after hatching. They will then follow her movements throughout their neonatal period. *Source:* Ross, CC BY-SA 2.0, via Wikimedia Commons.

hatching may strongly influence the young animal's social and behavioral development. In this regard, the effects of early social interactions, exposures, and related social bond formation may somewhat resemble those that might result from socialization of juvenile animals (to be detailed later). However, the processes that influence behavioral changes in young animals (early social interactions with parents versus intentional early exposures to social and other stimuli that result in socialization) and the time periods during which they occur differ significantly.

A second form of parent–offspring bond formation occurs through a process called filial **imprinting**, wherein animals develop social preferences for objects they encounter at a specific age. In the natural world, that object is usually a parent. One should be aware that imprinting is not equivalent to socialization. Most mammalian young do not imprint, but rather have a sensitive period in early life when social bonds and social capacity are established. This gives them the ability to interact with conspecifics, humans, and other species with whom they might interact later in life without intense fear. In companion animals (i.e. dogs, cats, horses), adequate exposure to people, animals, and various environments is essential during the socialization periods to prevent fear and/or aggression problems from developing (see Chapters 6–8 for more detailed information on socialization of companion animals). Because of imprinting, young will subsequently follow their parent(s) as they move around the environment, as well as mimic their motions and feeding habits (Bateson 1990) (Figure 3.9). Imprinting enables young to distinguish their own parents from other conspecifics and to distinguish conspecifics from members of other species (Bateson 1990). Indeed, proper imprinting affects an offspring's ability to survive into adulthood. It influences their preferences for food, habitats, and mates, and it affects their ability to reproduce as adults and to navigate long distances, such as during migration (Immelmann 1975). This type of bond formation is commonly observed in precocial birds and is well studied in ducks and chickens (Bateson 1966), although it is also found in altricial birds and mammals (Junco 1988; Lynn et al. 2010), including humans (Di Giorgio et al. 2017). Precocial young are often highly exploratory in their first few days of life, and during this critical period they develop preferences for familiar objects. Here again, the outcomes may appear to resemble those that occur as a result of socialization. Although this imprinting is generally considered adaptive in terms of the development of social bonds and anti-predator behavior, definitions use the term "object" as research has shown that imprinting can occur not only on conspecifics, such as parents, but also on heterospecifics, artificial animal models, or objects with no biological significance (reviewed in Bateson 1966, 1990). Both visual stimuli (including motion), as well as olfactory and auditory cues are important for imprinting (Bolhuis 1991; Immelmann 1975). It should be noted that socialization and imprinting are not mutually exclusive processes. Instead, imprinting represents a learning mechanism wherein young are predisposed to attend to specific stimuli early in life and thus develop specific preferences and biases for those stimuli, resulting in the formation of strong bonds with parents (Di Giorgio et al. 2017).

Parents can often, though not always, distinguish their own offspring from other similarly aged young. Among highly social species, where a parent may be interacting with many other young, it is adaptive for the parent to recognize its own offspring over non-related individuals (Mateo 2004). In some social groups, young may risk injury or death by other conspecific adults, such as through cannibalism or infanticide. Therefore, it is also advantageous for young to distinguish their own parents from other adults (Lefevre et al. 1998; Leonard et al. 1997). Individual recognition occurs through familiarity of phenotypes, either developed through imprinting or associative learning of individual specific calls, odors, or cues (Mateo 2004). Parental behavior can also be triggered by a generic cue not specific to the relatedness of young, such as a specific auditory or visual signal from young. For example, young Nile crocodiles elicit acoustic cues before and after hatching, which initiate a strong maternal response; however, mothers cannot distinguish between the calls of individual young (Vergne et al. 2007). Similarly, provisioning behavior in birds is highly motivated by the behavioral or chemical cues emitted by young (Kölliker et al. 2005; Mas et al. 2009; Whittingham et al. 2003), regardless of who is emitting the cues.

Predation of young is much more common than predation of adults due to their overall vulnerability, and therefore protection from predators (or conspecifics) is an essential role of parents. One antipredator strategy is based on the level of integration of young into the social group. This distinction, where some are "hiders" and others are "followers" is observed in ungulates as an antipredator strategy (Caro 2005). Hiders are animals who break away from their social group to give birth, often concealing their offspring in vegetation for weeks before re-joining the group (Figure 3.10). In contrast, among follower species, offspring join mothers and the social group shortly after birth and rely on maternal and group defense to avoid predation. Additionally, follower offspring will remain physically close to their mothers and will interact with them frequently. Interestingly, differences in hider/follower antipredator strategies differ in parent–offspring recognition. For example, among follower species such as sheep, parents and young

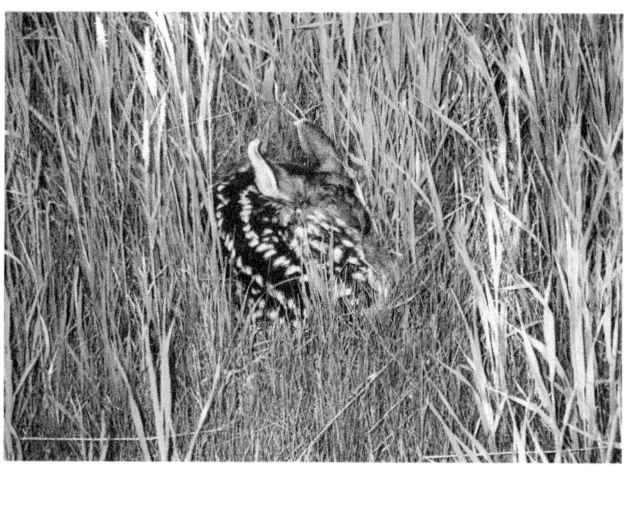

Figure 3.10 A newborn fawn sets tucked away in tall grass for safe hiding from predators during its first few days of life while the doe forages. She will return that evening to feed and care for the fawn. *Source:* Photo credit: Wikimedia Commons/runt35.

can often identify one another through contact calls (Searby and Jouventin 2003), whereas hiders, such as fallow deer, show asymmetrical recognition, where young can distinguish between vocalizations of adults, but not the other way around (Torriani et al. 2006). A second antipredator strategy is through parental aggression, a form of protective aggression that is used against any predator or conspecific who puts the lives of young at risk (Archer 1988). The intensity of parental aggression may vary depending on context. For example, the parent may be less likely to engage in protective behaviors if the survival risk to them is high or if the parent can reproduce shortly thereafter.

In addition to these essential needs for growth, parents serve as models to demonstrate or teach their young necessary skills, such as selection of appropriate food items or how to handle more complex food items or prey (Caro and Hauser 1992; Mikeliban et al. 2021; Shettleworth 1998; Thornton and Raihani 2008). In many species of carnivores, parents go through extensive training periods with their young to teach them how to hunt successfully (Caro and Hauser 1992; Shettleworth 1998). For instance, wild meerkats will actively teach young prey-handling skills of risky items like scorpions, deliberately providing increased predation opportunities to young as they get older (Thornton and McAuliffe 2006). Similar teaching can be observed in domestic cats, as mothers bring dead prey back to their young, switching to live prey as offspring age, thereby allowing the development of hunting skills (Caro and Hauser 1992). In addition to hunting, young can rely on parents for geographic learning, as with the Caspian tern, where young will follow their fathers to learn about migration routes (Byholm et al. 2022). These examples emphasize just some of the critical roles parents play in the social development of their offspring.

Two other important social components of parenting are rejection or abandonment of one's own offspring and the adoption or **alloparenting** of other offspring. In nature, parents may decide to abandon their young if it compromises their own survival and potentially future reproduction (Webb et al. 2002). For example, this may occur when surrounding conditions result in high stress (Ciminelli et al. 2021). This behavior may be mediated by high levels of circulating stress hormones in combination with other endocrine levels, as is observed in terms of nest abandonment in birds (Groscolas et al. 2008; Ouyang et al. 2012; Spée et al. 2011) and mammals (Berlin et al. 2018; Maestripieri et al. 2009). Further, rejection or abandonment of young is more common among first-time parents (Dwyer and Lawrence 2000; Pittet et al. 2012). In the common eider, a species of duck, parents with poor body condition are more likely to abandon their brood (Bustnes and Erikstad 1991). In the same species, "foreign" young will often join the groups (called creches) of other females, thereby receiving alloparental care (Bustnes and Erikstad 1991). Providing parental care for unrelated offspring may seem "maladaptive," however, it is prevalent across the animal kingdom and can result in increased fitness for the alloparents (Riedman 1982). There may be advantages to caring for the young of others if they are related (e.g. nieces and nephews) or provide "practice" for future parenting efforts (Finton et al. 2022; Riedman 1982). In domestic and wild mammals, allonursing or allosuckling is not uncommon (Mota-Rojas et al. 2021) and as noted previously, animal caretakers may take advantage of these behaviors to help offset or avoid animal welfare issues resulting from insufficient or poor maternal behavior (Kent 2020).

Conclusion

In this chapter, we have described the ways in which animals socially interact with each other. We have explored the pros and cons of sociality, and how it can evolve in different animal groups. We have highlighted the nature of competitive interactions, as well as the use of aggression. Further, we have shown how aggression and dominance status are not synonymous, emphasizing how aggression can be adaptive, but is also expressed under periods of distress where it may not be advantageous. Understanding these concepts may help veterinarians make evidence-based recommendations for housing, grouping, and managing animals in biologically relevant ways. This may facilitate safe interactions between animals and with those who provide care for them, and in so doing, support animal welfare.

References

Agrell, J., Wolff, J., and Yinen, H. (1998). Counter-strategies to infanticide in mammals : costs and consequences. *Oikos* 83 (3): 507–517.

Alexander, R.D. (1974). The evolution of social behavior. *Annu. Rev. Ecol. Syst.* 5: 325–383.

Alizon, S., Hurford, A., Mideo, N., and Van Baalen, M. (2009). Virulence evolution and the trade-off hypothesis: history, current state of affairs and the future. *J. Evol. Biol. 22* (2): 245–259.

Altizer, S. et al. (2003). Social organization and parasite risk in mammals: integrating theory and empirical studies. *Annu. Rev. Ecol., Evol. Syst.* 34: 517–547. https://doi.org/10.1146/annurev.ecolsys.34.030102.151725.

American Veterinary Society of Animal Behavior (2008). Dominance position statement. https://avsab.org/resources/position-statements/ (accessed 14 December, 2023).

Angelier, F. and Chastel, O. (2009). Stress, prolactin and parental investment in birds: a review. *General and Comparative Endocrinology* 163 (1–2): 142–148. https://doi.org/10.1016/j.ygcen.2009.03.028.

Archer, J. (1988). *The Behavioural Biology of Aggression*. Cambridge, UK: Cambridge University Press.

Arey, D.S. and Edwards, S.A. (1998). Factors influencing aggression between sows after mixing and the consequences for welfare and production. *Livest. Prod. Sci.* 56 (1): 61–70. https://doi.org/10.1016/S0301-6226(98)00144-4.

Arnold, K.E. and Owens, I.P.F. (1999). Cooperative breeding in birds: the role of ecology. *Behav. Ecol.* 10: 465–471.

Avilés, L. and Tufino, P. (1998). Colony size and individual fitness in the social spider *Anelosimus eximius. Am. Nat.* 152 (3): 403–418. https://doi.org/10.1086/286178.

Bartal, I.B.A., Decety, J., and Mason, P. (2011). Empathy and pro-social behavior in rats. *Science 334* (6061): 1427–1430.

Bateson, P. (1990). Is imprinting such a special case? *Phil. Trans. – R. Soc., B* 329 (1253): 125–131. https://doi.org/10.1098/rstb.1990.0157.

Bateson, P.P. (1966). The characteristics and context of imprinting. *Biol. Rev. Cambridge Phil. Soc.* 41 (2): 177–211. https://doi.org/10.1111/j.1469-185x.1966.tb01489.x.

Bauer, A.E., Jordan, M., Colon, M. et al. (2017). Evaluating FIDO: developing and pilot testing the field instantaneous dog observation tool. *Pet Behav. Sci.* 4: 1–16.

Beckel, A.L. (1991). Wrestling play in adult river otters, Lutra canadensis. *J. mammalogy 72* (2): 386–390.

Bekoff, M., Daniels, T.J., and Gittleman, J.L. (1984). Life history patterns and the comparative social ecology of carnivores. *Annu. Rev. Ecol. Syst. 15* (1): 191–232.

Berlin, D., Steinman, A., and Raz, T. (2018). Post-partum concentrations of serum progesterone, oestradiol and prolactin in Arabian mares demonstrating normal maternal behaviour and Arabian mares demonstrating foal rejection behaviour. *Vet. J.* 232: 40–45. https://doi.org/10.1016/j.tvjl.2017.12.007.

Bernstein, I.S. (1981). Dominance : the baby and the bathwater. *Behav. Brain Sci.* 4: 419–457.

Boissy, A. and Le Neindre, P. (1990). Social influences on the reactivity of heifers: implications for learning abilities in operant conditioning. *Appl. Anim. Behav. Sci. 25* (1–2): 149–165.

Bolhuis, J.J. (1991). Mechanisms of avian imprinting: a review. *Biol. Rev.* 66: 303–345.

Boos, M., Robin, J., and Petit, O. (2007). *Post-hatching parental care behaviour and hormonal status in a precocial bird* 76: 206–214. https://doi.org/10.1016/j.beproc.2007.05.003.

Bourke, A.F. (2011). *Principles of Social Evolution.* New York, NY: Oxford University Press.

Bowen, J., Bulbena, A., and Fatjó, J. (2021). The value of companion dogs as a source of social support for their owners: Findings from a pre-pandemic representative sample and a convenience sample obtained during the COVID-19 lockdown in Spain. *Front. Psych. 12*: 622060.

Bradshaw, J.W. (2012). *The Behaviour of the Domestic Cat.* Cabi.

Bradshaw, J.W.S., Blackwell, E.J., and Casey, R.A. (2009). Dominance in domestic dogs - useful construct or bad habit ? *Journal of Veterinary Behavior: Clinical Applications and Research* 4 (3): 135–144. https://doi.org/10.1016/j.jveb.2008.08.004.

Briffa, M. and Sneddon, L.U. (2010). Contest behavior. In: *Evolutionary Behavioral Ecology* (ed. D.F. Westneat and C.W. Fox), 246–265. New York, NY: Oxford University Press.

Briffa, M., Sneddon, L.U., and Wilson, A.J. (2015). Animal personality as a cause and consequence of contest behaviour. *Biol. Lett.* 11 (3): 20141007. https://doi.org/10.1098/rsbl.2014.1007.

Broad, K.D., Curley, J.P., and Keverne, E.B. (2006). Mother-infant bonding and the evolution of mammalian social relationships. *Phil. Trans. R. Soc. B: Biol. Sci.* 361 (1476): 2199–2214. https://doi.org/10.1098/rstb.2006.1940.

Buckley, N.J. (1996). Food finding and the influence of information, local enhancement, and communal roosting on foraging success of North American vultures. *Auk* 113 (2): 473–488. https://doi.org/10.2307/4088913.

Burghardt, G.M. (2005). *The Genesis of Animal Play: Testing the Limits.* MIT press.

Bustnes, J.A.N. and Erikstad, E. (1991). Factors affecting abandonment and adoption of young. *Can. J. Zoo.* 69 (1991): 1538–1545.

Byholm, P. et al. (2022). Paternal transmission of migration knowledge in a long-distance bird migrant. *Nat. Commun.* 13 (1): 1–7. https://doi.org/10.1038/s41467-022-29300-w.

Cafazzo, S., Valsecchi, P., Bonanni, R., Natoli, E., 2010. Dominance in relation to age, sex, and competitive contexts in a group of free-ranging domestic dogs. *Behav. Ecol.* 21, 443–455. https://doi.org/10.1093/beheco/arq001

Camerlink, I., Arnott, G., Farish, M., and Turner, S.P. (2016). Complex contests and the influence of aggressiveness in pigs. *Anim. Behav.* 121: 71–78. https://doi.org/10.1016/j.anbehav.2016.08.021.

Capelli, G., Paoletti, B., Iorio, R. et al. (2003). Prevalence of *Giardia* spp. in dogs and humans in Northern and Central Italy. *Parasitol Res.* 90: S154–S155.

Caro, T.M. (1989). The brotherhood of cheetahs. *Nat. History 6*: 50–59.

Caro, T.M. (2005). *Antipredator Defenses in Birds and Mammals.* Chicago: University of Chicago Press.

Caro, T.M. and Hauser, M.D. (1992). Is there teaching in nonhuman animals? *Q. Rev. Biol.* 67 (2): 151–174.

Chapais, B., Girard, M., and Primi, G. (1991). Non-kin alliances, and the stability of matrilineal dominance relations in Japanese macaques. *Anim. Behav.* 41: 481–491.

Chase, I.D., Bartolomeo, C., and Dugatkin, L.A. (1994). Aggressive interaction and inter-contest interval: how long do winners keep winning? *Anim. Behav.* 48: 393–400.

Cimarelli, G., Marshall-Pescini, S., Range, F., and Virányi, Z. (2019). Pet dogs' relationships vary rather individually than according to partner's species. *Sci. Rep. 9* (1): 3437.

Ciminelli, G. et al. (2021). Social distancing: high population density increases cub rejection and decreases maternal care in the giant panda. *Appl. Anim. Behav. Sci.* 243: 105457. https://doi.org/10.1016/j.applanim.2021.105457.

Clutton-Brock, T.H., Albon, S.D., Gibson, R.M., and Guinness, F.E. (1979). The logistical stag: adaptive aspects of fighting in red deer. *Anim. Behav.* 27: 211–225.

Cockburn, A. (2006). Prevalence of different modes of parental care in birds. *Proc. R. Soc. B: Biol. Sci.* 273 (1592): 1375–1383. https://doi.org/10.1098/rspb.2005.3458.

Creel, S. (2001). Social dominance and stress hormones. *Trends Ecol. Evol.* 16 (9): 491–497. https://doi.org/10.1016/S0169-5347(01)02227-3.

Creel, S., Creel, N.M., 1995. Communal hunting and pack size in African wild dogs, Lycaon pictus. *Anim. Behav.* 50, 1325–1339. https://doi.org/10.1016/0003-3472(95)80048-4.

Cronin, K.A. (2017). *Comparative Studies of Cooperation: Collaboration and Prosocial Behavior in Animals.* American Psychological Association.

Crowell-davis, S.L., Curtis, T.M., Knowles, R.J., 2004. Social organization in the cat : a modern understanding 19–28. *J. Feline Med. Surg.* 6(1): 19–28. https://doi.org/10.1016/j.jfms.2003.09.013.

Davies, N.B. and Houston, A.I. (1981). Owners and satellites: the economics of territory defence in the pied wagtail, Motacilla alba. *J. Anim. Ecol.* 157–180.

D'eath, R.B. and Lawrence, A.B. (2004). Early life predictors of the development of aggressive behaviour in the domestic pig. *Anim. Behav.* 67 (3): 501–509. https://doi.org/10.1016/j.anbehav.2003.06.010.

Dehnen, T. et al. (2022). Costs dictate strategic investment in dominance interactions. *Phil. Trans. R. Soc. B – Biol. Sci.* 377: 20200450.

De Rouck, M., Kitchener, A.C., Law, G., and Nelissen, M. (2005). A comparative study of the influence of social housing conditions on the behaviour of captive tigers (*Panthera tigris*). *Anim. Welf. 14* (3): 229–238.

Douglas-Hamilton, I. (1972). On the ecology and behaviour of the African elephant. PhD thesis. University of Oxford.

Drews, C. (1993). The concept and definition of dominance in animal behaviour. *Behaviour* 125 (3–4): 283–313.

Dugatkin, L.A. (1997). Winner and loser effects and the structure of dominance hierarchies. *Behav. Ecol.* 8: 583–587.

Dunbar, R.I.M. (1991). Functional significance of social grooming in primates. *Folia Primatologica* 57 (3): 121–131. https://doi.org/10.1159/000156574.

Dwyer, C. M. and Lawrence, A. B. (2000) 'Maternal behaviour in domestic sheep (Ovis aries): Constancy and change with maternal experience. *Behaviour* 37 (10): 1391–1413.

Earley, R.L. et al. (2013). Winner and loser effects are modulated by hormonal states. *Front. Zoo.* 10 (1): 1–13. https://doi.org/10.1186/1742-9994-10-6.

Earley, R.L. and Dugatkin, L.A. (2002). Eavesdropping on visual cues in green swordtail (*Xiphophorus helleri*) fights: a case for networking. *Proc. R. Soc. B: Biol. Sci.* 269 (1494): 943–952. https://doi.org/10.1098/rspb.2002.1973.

East, M.L. and Hofer, H. (2010). Social environments, social tactics, and their fitness consequences in complex mammalian societies. In: *Social Behaviour: Genes, Ecology and Evolution* (ed. T. Szekely, A.J. Moore, and J. Komdeur), 360–394. Cambridge, UK: Cambridge University Press.

Edgar, J., Kelland, I., Held, S. et al. (2015). Effects of maternal vocalisations on the domestic chick stress response. *Appl. Anim. Behav. Sci. 171*: 121–127.

Edwards, S.A. (1983). The behaviour of dairy cows and their newborn calves in individual or group housing. *Appl. Anim. Ethol.* 10 (3): 191–198. https://doi.org/10.1016/0304-3762(83)90140-2.

Elbroch, L.M. and Quigley, H. (2017). Social interactions in a solitary carnivore. *Curr. Zool. 63* (4): 357–362.

Emmett, D.J. and Macdonald, K.S. (2010). Kin structure, ecology and the evolution of social organization in shrimp: a comparative analysis. *Proc. R. Soc. B: Biol. Sci.* 277 (1681): 575–584. https://doi.org/10.1098/rspb.2009.1483.

Fagen, R. (1982). Skill and flexibility in animal play behavior. *Behav. Brain Sci. 5* (1): 162.

Feltes, E.S., Stull, J.W., Herron, M.E., and Haug, L.I. (2020). Characteristics of intrahousehold interdog aggression and dog and pair factors associated with a poor outcome. *J. Am. Vet. Med. Assoc.* 256: 12–17.

Finton, C.J., Kelly, A.M., and Ophir, A.G. (2022). Support for the parental practice hypothesis: subadult prairie voles exhibit similar behavioral and neural profiles when alloparenting kin and non-kin. *Behav. Brain Res.* 417: 113571. https://doi.org/10.1016/j.bbr.2021.113571.

Flockhart, D.T.T., Norris, D.R., Coe, J.B., 2016. Predicting free-roaming cat population densities in urban areas. *Anim. Conserv.* 19, 472–483. https://doi.org/10.1111/acv.12264

Frank, L.G. (1986). Social organization of the spotted hyaena *Crocuta crocuta*. II. Dominance and reproduction. *Anim. Behav.* 34 (5): 1510–1527. https://doi.org/10.1016/S0003-3472(86)80221-4.

Fraser, D. and Duncan, I.J. (1998). Pleasures', 'pains' and animal welfare: toward a natural history of affect. *Anim. Welf. 7* (4): 383–396.

Gaillard, C., Meagher, R.K., von Keyserlingk, M.A., and Weary, D.M. (2014). Social housing improves dairy calves' performance in two cognitive tests. *PloS One 9* (2): e90205.

Gans, C. (1996). An overview of parental care among the reptilia. In: *Advances in the Study of Behavior* (ed. J. Rosenblatt and C. Snowdon), 145–157. Academic Press Ltd.

Geist, V. (1966). The evolutionary significance of mountain sheep horns. *Evolution* 20 (4): 558–566.

Di Giorgio, E. et al. (2017). Filial responses as predisposed and learned preferences: early attachment in chicks and babies. *Behav. Brain Res.* 325: 90–104. https://doi.org/10.1016/j.bbr.2016.09.018.

Gonyou, H.W. (2001). The social behaviour of pigs. In: *The Social Behaviour of Farm Animals* (ed. L.J. Keeling and H.W. Gonyou). CABI Publishing.

Grant, J.W. (1993). Whether or not to defend? The influence of resource distribution. *Mar. Behav. Physiol.* 23: 137–153.

Groscolas, R., Lacroix, A., and Robin, J.P. (2008). Spontaneous egg or chick abandonment in energy-depleted king penguins: a role for corticosterone and prolactin? *Horm. Behav.* 53 (1): 51–60. https://doi.org/10.1016/j.yhbeh.2007.08.010.

Haller, J., Harold, G., Sandi, C., and Neumann, I.D. (2014). Effects of adverse early-life events on aggression and anti-social behaviours in animals and humans neuroendocrinology. *J. Neuroendocrinol.* 26: 724–738. https://doi.org/10.1111/jne.12182.

Harlow, H.F., Dodsworth, R.O., and Harlow, M.K. (1965). Total social isolation in monkeys. *Proc. Nat. Acad. Sci. 54* (1): 90–97.

Hart, B.L. (1985). *The Behavior of Domestic Animals*. New York, NY: W. H. Freeman and Company.

Hatchwell, B.J. (2007). Avian reproduction: role of ecology in the evolution of cooperative breeding. *Curr. Biol.* 17 (19): 845–847. https://doi.org/10.1016/j.cub.2007.08.002.

Hebblewhite, M. and Pletscher, D.H. (2002). Effects of elk group size on predation by wolves. *Can. J. Zoo.* 80 (5): 800–809. https://doi.org/10.1139/z02-059.

Heg, D. (2008). Reproductive suppression in female cooperatively breeding cichlids. *Biol. Lett.* 4 (6): 606–609. https://doi.org/10.1098/rsbl.2008.0365.

Hemelrijk, C.K., Wantia, J., and Isler, K. (2008). Female dominance over males in primates: self-organisation and sexual dimorphism. *PLoS ONE* 3 (7): https://doi.org/10.1371/journal.pone.0002678.

Herron, M.E., Shofer, F.S., and Reisner, I.R. (2009). Survey of the use and outcome of confrontational and non-confrontational training methods in client-owned dogs showing undesired behaviors. *Appl. Anim. Behav. Sci. 117* (1-2): 47–54.

Hinde, R.A. (1970). *Animal Behaviour*. New York, NY: McGraw-Hill.

Holekamp, K.E. and Smale, L. (1991). Dominance acquisition during mammalian social development: the "inheritance" of maternal rank. *Am. Zool.* 317: 306–317.

Holekamp, K.E. and Strauss, E.D. (2016). Aggression and dominance: an interdisciplinary overview. *Current Opinion in Behavioral Sciences* 12: 44–51. https://doi.org/10.1016/j.cobeha.2016.08.005.

Hoogland, J.L. (1985). Infanticide in prairie dogs: lactating females kill offspring of close kin. *Science* 230 (4729): 1037–1040. https://doi.org/10.1126/science.230.4729.1037.

Hoppitt, W. and Laland, K. (2008). Social processes affecting feeding and drinking in the domestic fowl. *Anim. Behav.* 76: 1529–1543. https://doi.org/10.1016/j.anbehav.2008.07.011.

Horova, E., Brandlova, K., and Glonekova, M. (2015). The first description of dominance hierarchy in captive giraffe: not loose and egalitarian, but clear and linear. *PLoS One 10* (5): e0124570.

Immelmann, K. (1975). Ecological significance of imprinting and early learning. *Annu. Rev. Ecol. Syst.* 6 (1975): 15–37.

Jarvis, J.U.M. (1981). Eusociality in a mammal: cooperative breeding in naked mole-rat colonies. *Science* 212 (4494): 571–573. https://doi.org/10.1126/science.7209555.

Jones, G.H., Hernandez, T.D., Kendall, D.A. et al. (1992). Dopaminergic and serotonergic function following isolation rearing in rats: study of behavioural responses and postmortem and in vivo neurochemistry. *Pharmacol. Biochem. Behav. 43* (1): 17–35.

Jones, J.S. and Wynne-Edwards, K.E. (2001). Paternal behaviour in biparental hamsters, *Phodopus campbelli*, does not require contact with the pregnant female. *Anim. Behav.* 62 (3): 453–464. https://doi.org/10.1006/anbe.2001.1765.

Junco, F. (1988). Filial imprinting in an altricial bird. *Behaviour* 106 (1): 25–42.

Kaufmann, J.H. (1983). On the definitions and functions of dominance and territoriality. *Biol. Rev.* 58: 1–20.

Kent, J.P. (2020). The cow-calf relationship: from maternal responsiveness to the maternal bond and the possibilities for fostering. *J. Dairy Res.* 87 (S1): 101–107. https://doi.org/10.1017/S0022029920000436.

Kim, T. and Zuk, M. (2000). The effects of age and previous experience on social rank in female red junglefowl, *Gallus gallus* spadiceus. *Anim. Behav.* 60: 239–244. https://doi.org/10.1006/anbe.2000.1469.

Kölliker, M., Chuckalovcak, J.P., and Brodie, E.D. (2005). Offspring chemical cues affect maternal food provisioning in burrower bugs, *Sehirus cinctus. Anim. Behav.* 69 (4): 959–966. https://doi.org/10.1016/j.anbehav.2004.06.031.

Koolhaas, J.M., Reenen, C.G. Van, 2016. Animal behavior and well-being symposium: interaction between coping style/personality, stress, and welfare: relevance for domestic farm animals. *J. Anim. Sci.* 94, 2284–2296. https://doi.org/10.2527/jas2015-0125.

Korb, J. and Heinze, J. (2016). Major hurdles for the evolution of sociality. *Annu. Rev. Entomol.* 61: 297–316. https://doi.org/10.1146/annurev-ento-010715-023711.

Kralj-Fišer, S., Weiß, B.M., and Kotrschal, K. (2010). Behavioural and physiological correlates of personality in *greylag geese* (Anser anser). *J. Ethol.* 28: 363–370. https://doi.org/10.1007/s10164-009-0197-1.

Krebs, J.R. (1982). Territorial defence in the great tit (Parus major): do residents always win? *Behav. Ecol. Sociobiol.* 11 (3): 185–194. https://doi.org/10.1007/BF00300061.

Kuiper, T., Loveridge, A.J., and Macdonald, D.W. (2021). Robust mapping of human – wildlife conflict : controlling for livestock distribution in carnivore depredation models. *Anim. Conser.* 1–13. https://doi.org/10.1111/acv.12730.

Kutsukake, N. and Clutton-Brock, T.H. (2006). Social functions of allogrooming in cooperatively breeding meerkats. *Anim. Behav.* 72 (5): 1059–1068. https://doi.org/10.1016/j.anbehav.2006.02.016.

Le Boeuf, B.J. and Peterson, R.S. (1969). Social status and mating activity in elephant seals. *Science 163* (3862): 91–93.

Lefevre, K., Montgomerie, R., and Gaston, A.J. (1998). Parent – offspring recognition in thick-billed murres (Aves : Alcidae). *Anim. Behav.* 55 (4): 925–938.

Leonard, M.L., Horn, A.G., Brown, C.R., and Fernandez, N.J. (1997). Parent–offspring recognition in tree swallows, *Tachycineta bicolor*. *Anim. Behav.* 54 (5): 1107–1116.

Lévy, F. and Keller, M. (2009). Olfactory mediation of maternal behavior in selected mammalian species. *Behav. Brain Res.* 200 (2): 336–345. https://doi.org/10.1016/j.bbr.2008.12.017.

Lewis, R.J. (2022). Aggression, rank and power: why hens (and other animals) do not always peck according to their strength. *Phil. Trans. R. Soc. B – Biol. Sci.* 377: 20200450.

Lopez-Sepulcre, A. and Kokko, H. (2005). Territorial defence, territory size, and population regulation. *The American Naturalist* 166: 317–329.

Lukas, D. and Clutton-Brock, T. (2012). Cooperative breeding and monogamy in mammalian societies. *Proc. R. Soc. B: Biol. Sci.* 279 (1736): 2151–2156. https://doi.org/10.1098/rspb.2011.2468.

Lukas, D. and Huchard, E. (2014). The evolution of infanticide by males in mammalian societies. *Science 346* (6211): 841–844.

Lynn, B.L., Reichmuth, C., Schusterman, R.J., and Gulland, F. (2010). Filial imprinting in a steller sea lion (*Eumetopias jubatus*). *Aquat. Mamm.* 36 (1): 79–83. https://doi.org/10.1578/AM.36.1.2010.79.

Maestripieri, D. et al. (2009). Mother-infant interactions in free-ranging rhesus macaques: relationships between physiological and behavioral variables. *Physiol. Behav.* 96 (4–5): 613–619. https://doi.org/10.1016/j.physbeh.2008.12.016.

Majumder, S.S., Bhadra, A., Ghosh, A. et al. (2014). To be or not to be social: foraging associations of free-ranging dogs in an urban ecosystem. *Acta Ethologica* **17**: 1–8.

Marin, R.H., Freytes, P., Guzman, D., and Jones, R.B. (2001). Effects of an acute stressor on fear and on the social reinstatement responses of domestic chicks to cagemates and strangers. *App. Anim. Behav. Science 71* (1): 57–66.

Mas, F., Haynes, K.F., and Kölliker, M. (2009). A chemical signal of offspring quality affects maternal care in a social insect. *Proc. R. Soc. B: Biol. Sci.* 276 (1668): 2847–2853. https://doi.org/10.1098/rspb.2009.0498.

Mateo, J.M. (2004). Recognition systems and biological organization: the perception component of social recognition. *Ann. Zool. Fenn.* 41 (6): 729–745.

Mauget, R. (1981). Behavioural and reproductive strategies in wild forms of Sus scrofa (European wild boar and feral pigs). In: *The Welfare of Pigs: A Seminar in the EEC Programme of Coordination of Research on Animal Welfare held in Brussels*, 3–15. Dordrecht: Springer Netherlands.

Maynard, S.J. and Parker, G.A. (1976). The logic of asymmetric contests. *Anim. Behav.* 24 (1): 159–175. https://doi.org/10.1016/S0003-3472(76)80110-8.

McClearn, G.E. (1970). Behavioral genetics. *Annu. Rev. Genet.* 4: 437–468.

McGhee, K.E. and Travis, J. (2010). Repeatable behavioural type and stable dominance rank in the bluefin killifish. *Anim. Behav.* 79: 497–507. https://doi.org/10.1016/j.anbehav.2009.11.037.

McGraw, L., Szekely, T., and Young, L. (2010). Pair bonds and parental behaviour. In: *Social Behaviour: Genes, Ecology and Evolution* (ed. T. Szekely, A. Moorse, and J. Komdeur), 271–305. Cambridge: Cambridge University Press.

Mertens, P.A. and Unshelm, J. (1996). Effects of group and individual housing on the behavior of kennelled dogs in animal shelters. *Anthrozoös 9* (1): 40–51.

Mikeliban, M. et al. (2021). Orangutan mothers adjust their behaviour during food solicitations in a way that likely facilitates feeding skill acquisition in their offspring. *Sci. Rep.* 11 (1): 1–14. https://doi.org/10.1038/s41598-021-02901-z.

Miller, H.C., Rayburn-Reeves, R., and Zentall, T.R. (2009). Imitation and emulation by dogs using a bidirectional control procedure. *Behav. Process. 80* (2): 109–114.

Mota-Rojas, D. et al. (2021). Physiological foundations and explanatory hypotheses. *Animals* 11 (3092): 1–25.

Mumme, R.L., Koenig, W.D., and Pitelka, F.A. (1983). Reproductive competition in the communal acorn woodpecker: sisters destroy each other's eggs. *Nature* 306 (5943): 583–584. https://doi.org/10.1038/306583a0.

Nagasawa, M., Okabe, S., Mogi, K., and Kikusui, T. (2012). Oxytocin and mutual communication in mother-infant bonding. *Front. Hum. Neurosci.* 6 (February): 1–10. https://doi.org/10.3389/fnhum.2012.00031.

Okabe, S., Nagasawa, M., Mogi, K., and Kikusui, T. (2012). The importance of mother-infant communication for social bond formation in mammals. *Anim. Sci. J.* 83 (6): 446–452. https://doi.org/10.1111/j.1740-0929.2012.01014.x.

Oldham, L. et al. (2020). Winner – loser effects overrule aggressiveness during the early stages of contests between pigs. *Sci. Rep.* 1–13. https://doi.org/10.1038/s41598-020-69664-x.

Ouyang, J.Q., Quetting, M., and Hau, M. (2012). Corticosterone and brood abandonment in a passerine bird. *Anim. Behav.* 84 (1): 261–268. https://doi.org/10.1016/j.anbehav.2012.05.006.

Palagi, E., Nicotra, V., and Cordoni, G. (2015). Rapid mimicry and emotional contagion in domestic dogs. *Royal Soc. Open Sci. 2* (12): 150505.

Parsons, K.M. et al. (2003). Kinship as a basis for alliance formation among male bottlenose dolphins (*Tursiops truncatus*) in the Bahamas. *Anim. Behav.* 66: 185–194. https://doi.org/10.1006/anbe.2003.2186.

Pellegrini, A.D. (2008). The roles of aggressive and affiliative behaviors in resource control: A behavioral ecological perspective. *Development. Rev. 28* (4): 461–487.

Pittet, F. et al. (2012). Age affects the expression of maternal care and subsequent behavioural development of offspring in a precocial bird. *PLoS ONE* 7 (5): e36835. https://doi.org/10.1371/journal.pone.0036835.

Powell, G.V.N. (1974). Experimental analysis of the social value of flocking by starlings (*Sturnus vulgaris*) in relation to predation and foraging. *Anim. Behav.* 22 (2): 501–505. https://doi.org/10.1016/S0003-3472(74)80049-7.

Preston, S.D. and De Waal, F.B. (2002). Empathy: its ultimate and proximate bases. *Behav. Brain Sci. 25* (1): 1–20.

Price, E.O. (1984). Behavioral aspects of animal domestication. *Quarterly Rev. Biol. 59* (1): 1–32.

Rault, J.L. (2019). Be kind to others: prosocial behaviours and their implications for animal welfare. *Appl. Anim. Behav. Sci. 210*: 113–123.

Reimert, I., Bolhuis, J.E., Kemp, B., and Rodenburg, T.B. (2013). Indicators of positive and negative emotions and emotional contagion in pigs. *Physiol. Behav. 109*: 42–50.

Reynolds, J.D., Goodwin, N.B., and Freckleton, R.P. (2002). Evolutionary transitions in parental care and live bearing in vertebrates. *Phil. Trans. R. Soc. B: Biol. Sci.* 357 (1419): 269–281. https://doi.org/10.1098/rstb.2001.0930.

Riedman, M.L. (1982). The evolution of alloparental care and adoption in mammals and birds. *The Quarterly Review of Biology* 57 (4): 405–435.

Rilling, J.K. and Young, L.J. (2014). The biology of mammalian parenting and its effect on offspring social development. *Science* 345 (6198): 771–776. https://doi.org/10.1126/science.1252723.

Sandell, M. (1989). The mating tactics and spacing patterns of solitary carnivores. In: *Carnivore Behavior, Ecology, and Evolution*, 164–182. Boston, MA: Springer US.

Schjelderup-Ebbe, T. (1922). Beitrage zum Sozialpsychologie des Haushuhns. *Zeitschrift für Psychologie* 88: 225–252.

Schultz, B. (2016). The Effects of Conspecifics on Dog (Canis lupus familiaris) Behavior during Behavioral Rehabilitation Treatments. PhD thesis. *Academic Works. Hunter College.* https://academicworks.cuny.edu/hc_sas_etds/84.

Searby, A. and Jouventin, P. (2003). Mother-lamb acoustic recognition in sheep: a frequency coding. *Proc. R. Soc. B: Biol. Sci.* 270 (1526): 1765–1771. https://doi.org/10.1098/rspb.2003.2442.

Shettleworth, S.J. (1998). *Cognition, Evolution, and Behavior*. New York, NY: Oxford University Press.

Siracusa, E., Boutin, S., Humphries, M.M., Gorrell, J.C., Coltman, D.W., Dantzer, B., Lane, J.E., Mcadam, A.G., 2017. Familiarity with neighbours affects intrusion risk in territorial red squirrels. *Anim. Behav.* 133, 11–20. https://doi.org/10.1016/j.anbehav.2017.08.024

Smith, J.E. et al. (2010). Evolutionary forces favoring intragroup coalitions among spotted hyenas and other animals. *Behav. Ecol.* 21: 284–303. https://doi.org/10.1093/beheco/arp181.

Spée, M. et al. (2010). Should I stay or should I go? hormonal control of nest abandonment in a long-lived bird, the adélie penguin. *Horm. Behav.* 58 (5): 762–768. https://doi.org/10.1016/j.yhbeh.2010.07.011.

Spée, M. et al. (2011). Exogenous corticosterone and nest abandonment: A study in a long-lived bird, the adélie penguin. *Hormones and Behavior* 60 (4): 362–370. https://doi.org/10.1016/j.yhbeh.2011.07.003.

Spencer, K.A. (2017). Developmental stress and social phenotypes: integrating neuroendocrine, behavioural and evolutionary perspectives. *Phil. Trans. R. Soc. B: Biol. Sci.* 372 (1727): https://doi.org/10.1098/rstb.2016.0242.

Spinka, M., Newberry, R.C., and Bekoff, M. (2001). Mammalian play: training for the unexpected. *Quarterly Rev. Biology 76* (2): 141–168.

Stamps, J.A. (1994). Territorial behavior: testing the assumptions. *Adv. Study of Behav. 23* (173): 232.

Stellato, A.C., Dewey, C.E., Widowski, T.M., and Niel, L. (2020). Evaluation of associations between owner presence and indicators of fear in dogs during routine veterinary examinations. *J. Am. Vet. Med. Assoc. 257* (10): 1031–1040.

Stokes, D.L. and Boersma, P.D. (2000). Nesting density and reproductive success in a colonial seabird, the magellanic penguin. *Ecology* 81 (10): 2878–2891. https://doi.org/10.1890/0012-9658(2000)081[2878:NDARSI]2.0.CO;2.

Stookey, J.M. and Gonyou, H.W. (1998). Recognition in swine: recognition through familiarity or genetic relatedness? *Appl. Anim. Behav. Sci. 55* (3-4): 291–305.

Thornton, A. and McAuliffe, K. (2006). Teaching in wild meerkats. *Science* 313 (5784): 227–229. https://doi.org/10.1126/science.1128727.

Thornton, A. and Raihani, N.J. (2008). The evolution of teaching. *Anim. Behav.* 75 (6): 1823–1836. https://doi.org/10.1016/j.anbehav.2007.12.014.

Tibbetts, E.A., Pardo-Sanchez, J., and Weise, C. (2022). The establishment and maintenance of dominance hierarchies. *Phil. Trans. R. Soc. B-Biol. Sci.* 377: 20200450.

Torriani, M.V.G., Vannoni, E., and Mcelligott, A.G. (2006). Mother-young recognition in an ungulate hider species: a unidirectional process. *Am. Nat.* 168 (3): 412–420.

Trivers, R.L. (1971). The Evolution of reciprocal altruism. *Q. Rev. Biol.* 46: 35–57.

Turner, D.C. (2014). Social organisation and behavioural ecology of free-ranging domestic cats. In: *The Domestic Cat: The Biology of its Behaviour*, 3e (ed. D.C. Turner and P.P.G. Bateson), 63–80. Cambridge University Press.

Uvnas-Moberg, K. (1998). Oxytocin may mediate the benefits of positive social interaction and emotions. *Psychoneuroendocrinology* 23 (8): 819–835.

Van Bourg, J., Patterson, J.E., and Wynne, C.D. (2020). Pet dogs (Canis lupus familiaris) release their trapped and distressed owners: individual variation and evidence of emotional contagion. *PLoS One 15* (4): e0231742.

Veissier, I. and le Neindre, P. (1992). Reactivity of Aubrac heifers exposed to a novel environment alone or in groups of four. *Appl. Anim. Behav. Sci. 33* (1): 11–15.

Vergne, A.L., Avril, A., and Martin, S. (2007). Parent-offspring communication in the Nile crocodile *Crocodylus niloticus*: do newborns' calls show an individual signature? *Naturwissenschaften* 94: 49–54. https://doi.org/10.1007/s00114-006-0156-4.

Vitet, C., Duncan, P., Ganswindt, A. et al. (2021). Do infanticides occur in harem-forming equids? A test with long-term sociodemographic data in wild plains zebras. *Anim. Behav. 177*: 9–18.

Voith, V.L. and Borchelt, P.L. (1986). Social behavior of domestic cats. *Compendium Small Anim. 8* (9): 637–646.

Webb, J. N., Székely, T., Houston, A.I., & Mcnamara, J.M. (2002) 'A theoretical analysis of the energetic costs and consequences of parental care decisions', *Phil. Trans. R. Soc. B: Biol. Sci.*, 357(1419), pp. 331–340. doi: https://doi.org/10.1098/rstb.2001.0934.

Weller, J.E., Turner, S.P., Farish, M. et al. (2020). The association between play fighting and information gathering during subsequent contests. *Sci. Rep. 10* (1): 1133.

West-Eberhard, M.J. (1979). Sexual selection, social competition, and evolution. *Proc. Am. Phil. Soc.* 123 (4): 222–234.

Whittingham, L.A., Dunn, P.O., and Clotfelter, E.D. (2003). Parental allocation of food to nestling tree swallows: the influence of nestling behaviour, sex and paternity. *Anim. Behav.* 65 (6): 1203–1210. https://doi.org/10.1006/anbe.2003.2178.

Wilson, E.O. (1975). *Sociobiology: The New Synthesis*. Cambridge, Massachusetts: Harvard University Press.

Wolff, J.O. (1997). Population regulation in mammals : an evolutionary perspective. *J. Anim. Ecol.* 66: 1–13.

Woodroffe, R. and Vincent, A. (1994). Mother' s little helpers: patterns of male care in mammals. *Trends Ecol. Evol.* 9 (8): 294–297.

Wynne-Edwards, K.E. and Timonin, M.E. (2007). Paternal care in rodents: weakening support for hormonal regulation of the transition to behavioral fatherhood in rodent animal models of biparental care. *Horm. Behav.* 52 (1): 114–121. https://doi.org/10.1016/j.yhbeh.2007.03.018.

Yong, M.H. and Ruffman, T. (2014). Emotional contagion: dogs and humans show a similar physiological response to human infant crying. *Behav. Process. 108*: 155–165.

Yu, Y.Q., Barry, D.M., Hao, Y. et al. (2017). Molecular and neural basis of contagious itch behavior in mice. *Science 355* (6329): 1072–1076.

Zajonc, R.B. (1965). Social facilitation. *Science* 149 (July): 269–274.

Ziegler, T.E. (2000). Hormones associated with non-maternal infant care: a review of mammalian and avian studies. *Folia Primatologica* 71 (1–2): 6–21. https://doi.org/10.1159/000021726.

4

Sensory and Perception

Shana Gilbert-Gregory

Behavioral Medicine Service, Mount Laurel Animal Hospital, Mount Laurel, NJ, USA

Introduction

Animals communicate through visual, auditory, and olfactory signals. Understanding how animals send and perceive these signals allows for more humane and efficient management and is essential to better interpret and respond to communication between animals of the same species, as well as between humans and animals. This chapter will describe visual, auditory, olfactory, and gustatory senses as they pertain to domesticated animals, giving insight into their adaptive advantages and how each system relates to inter- and intraspecies communication.

Social species depend on the recognition of individuals, utilizing single or multiple sensory modalities to aid in that recognition. Humans and several non-human species use faces and voices as the most relevant cues for individual identity (Campanella and Belin 2007; Sliwa et al. 2011; Saito and Shinozuka 2013; Sankey et al. 2011; Huber et al. 2013). Cattle, horses, and dogs have efficient visual (Coulon et al. 2009; Wathan et al. 2016; Racca et al. 2010) and auditory (Watts and Stookey 2000; Lemasson et al. 2009; Andics et al. 2014) recognition of conspecifics. Sheep utilize visual (Kendrick et al. 1996) recognition, while pigs (Düpjan et al. 2011) and cats (Siniscalchi et al. 2016) utilize auditory recognition. Several species are also able to discriminate between familiar and unfamiliar humans (Taylor and Davis 1998; Casey and Bradshaw 2008) and some can even form a memory of an individual that influences their reactions in subsequent interactions with that individual (Tallet et al. 2016; d'Ingeo et al. 2019). Additionally, a growing number of species have been shown to recognize human faces and/or voices, including sheep (Knolle et al. 2017; Kendrick et al. 1995; Tallet et al. 2016; Bensoussan et al. 2019), horses (Stone 2010), cats (Saito and Shinozuka 2013) and dogs (Huber et al. 2013; Adachi et al. 2007). Animals not only identify **conspecifics** and humans through separate sensory modalities, but they are also capable of integrating identity cues from multiple sensory modalities for recognition (Pitcher et al. 2017; Proops and McComb 2012; Lampe and Andre 2012; Takagi et al. 2019; Gergely et al. 2019). Species living in close contact with humans are also capable of integrating visual and auditory cues to identify a familiar human, as recently demonstrated in horses (Proops and McComb 2012; Lampe and Andre 2012), and dogs (Adachi et al. 2007), who also generalize this ability to unfamiliar people (Gergely et al. 2019).

Introduction to Animal Behavior and Veterinary Behavioral Medicine, First Edition. Edited by Meghan E. Herron.

Companion website: www.wiley.com/go/introductiontoanimalbehavior

Vision

Visual information is key to interactions with the environment. Animals respond to both color and brightness when processing visual information. All domestic animals have color vision; however, there are species variations in this color vision. The spectrum of visual light ranges in frequency from approximately 380—750 nm in most mammals, including humans. Birds, fish, and many insects can see into the ultraviolet range, which may aid in reproductive success and pollination. Snakes have been known to see infrared frequencies, allowing them to see radiant heat from potential prey. Figure 4.1 illustrates wavelength frequencies and the visual spectrum for most mammals.

Humans are trichromats (three color processing cones), while most other mammals are dichromats (two color processing cones). Figure 4.2 compares trichromatic and dichromatic color vision perceptions. Birds and fish are often tetrachromatic (four color processing cones). Color vision is processed by the retina, which contains three classes of light-sensitive cells: rod photoreceptors (low light vision), multiple types of cone photoreceptors (color vision), and ganglion cells (which are intrinsically photosensitive as they contain the photopigment melanopsin).

The visual field of animals varies based on their eye placement. Species with eyes set close together on the front of the face will have predominantly **binocular vision**, utilizing both eyes together to see the world around them. Binocular vision allows an animal to have better depth perception but little to no perception of what is behind them. Binocular vision provides sharp acuity for better tracking, hunting, climbing, and picking out food, making it a common trait in predator species. Species with more laterally placed eyes have predominantly monocular vision, with the ability to use each eye separately when observing their environment. **Monocular vision** provides for greater peripheral vision, with the extent of the visual field dependent on how laterally placed the eyes are in that specific species. Monocular vision provides poor depth perception, and often animals with predominantly monocular vision may not see what is directly in front of their faces. One can appreciate the adaptive value of sharp frontal visual acuity for predator species, as well as the ability to see what may be sneaking up behind you in prey species. See Figure 4.3 for a comparison of binocular and monocular visual fields based on eye placement.

Horses

The equine eye is amongst the largest in land mammals and produces an image magnification that is 50% larger than the human eye (Roberts 1992). The equine retina is composed

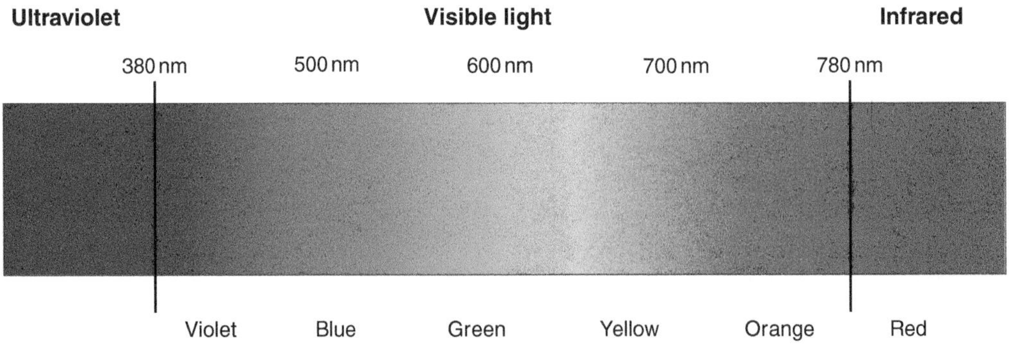

Figure 4.1 The electromagnetic spectrum of visible light for humans and most mammals includes violet, blue, green, yellow, orange, and red color gradients. Other species can see into higher and lower frequencies. *Source:* Image credit: Meghan E. Herron.

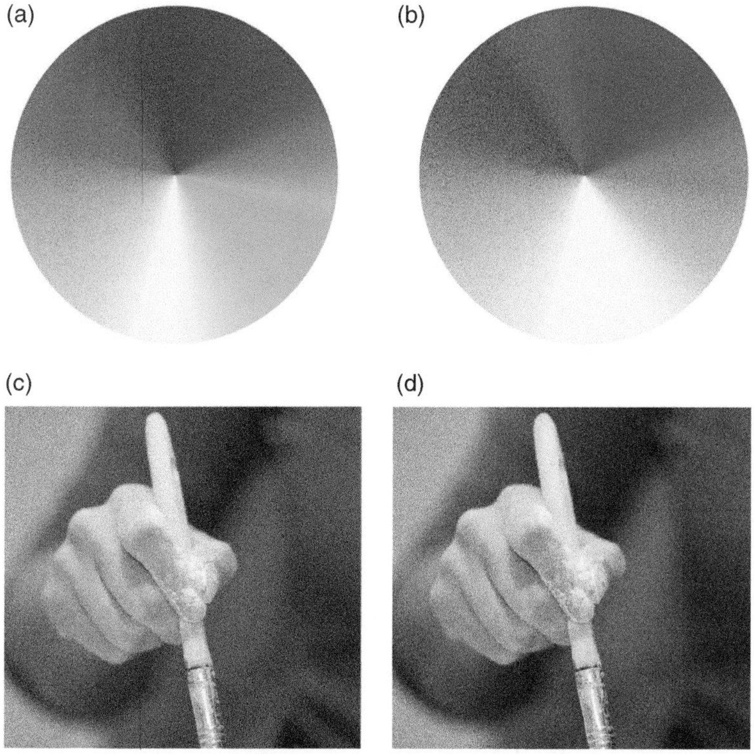

Figure 4.2 Humans have trichromatic vision, with three types of color cones that detect and process color, allowing them to perceive color along a red, yellow, and blue gradient (a and c), while most other mammals are dichromats with cones that only process two colors. Dogs, cats, horses, and pigs see a range of blue and yellow (b and d), with some variation between each species. *Source:* Bocskai István / AdobeStock.

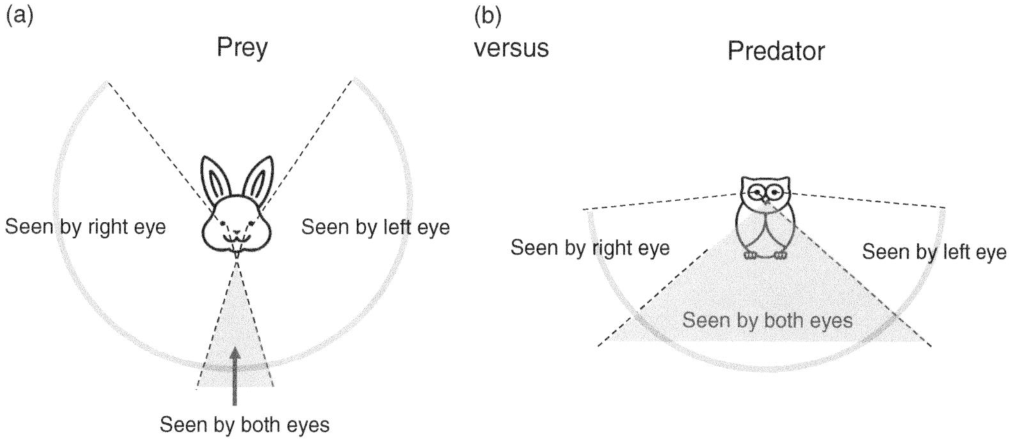

Figure 4.3 Monocular versus binocular visual fields. Note how the laterally placed eyes of prey species (a) allow for large peripheral visual fields, but poor frontal acuity, and the close set, frontally placed eyes of predator species (b) allow for precise vision of what is directly in front of them, yet their peripheral vision is limited. *Source:* Image credit: Meghan E. Herron.

of predominantly rods, with cones that are evenly distributed throughout the retina, and ganglion cells that concentrate in a narrow, but distinct, **horizontal streak** located just above the optic disc (Hebel 1976; Harman et al. 1999). This streak provides a narrow but panoramic area of visual acuity for the horse's surroundings (Figure 4.4). Horses have dichromatic color vision, predominantly facilitated by two cone types, sensitive to short (428 nm peak) and medium wavelengths (539 nm peak) (Carroll et al. 2001). When compared to human color vision, horses see colors along a continuous range from blue to yellow (Macuda and Timney 1999; Roth et al. 2008; Roth et al. 2007; Smith and Goldman 1999). Horses are unlikely to be able to distinguish between many of the colors that humans see as red, orange, and green, unless they also differ in brightness (Murphy et al. 2009).

The difference in color vision between humans and animals contributes to altered perceptions of visual cues in interactions that require teamwork between them, such as in animal sports. This is especially consequential for horses, where sport associated traditions commonly pre-date a broad knowledge and understanding of animal vision (DeMello 2012). Differences between human vision and that of animals used in competitions can result in important features of the sporting, training, and housing environments not being well-designed for visibility to the focal animal itself (Figure 4.5). Recent advances in the animal

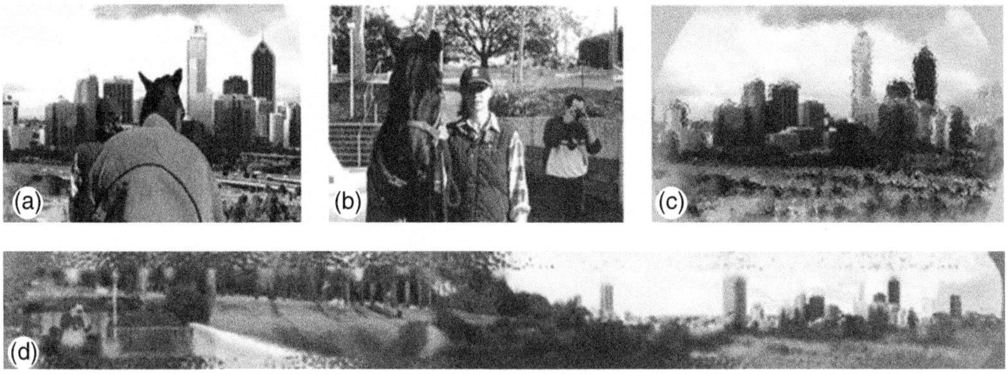

Figure 4.4 The view seen by the left eye of a horse and a human facing the same direction. In (a) is the front view of the city, in (b) is the rear view behind the horse and human. In (c) is the view seen by the human with a small high acuity central region surrounded by a lower acuity region. In (d) is shown the view seen by the horse, running from city almost all the way to the rear as a horizontal streak with much lower acuity above and below. *Source:* With permission from Alison Harman.

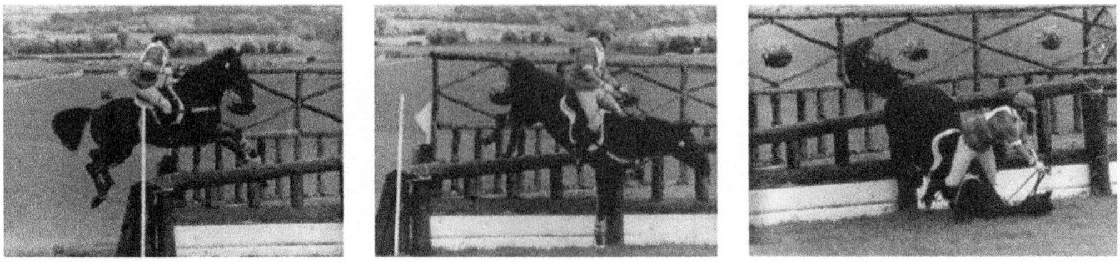

Figure 4.5 Some fence designs may challenge not only the athletic prowess of the performance horse but also the visual capability of the animal, which may have safety implications for both horse and rider. *Source:* Reproduced with permission from Murphy et al. 2009/Hindawi Publishing Corporation.

visual sciences mean that there has been the opportunity to re-assess these environments using approaches designed to quantify and predict how animals see and respond to visual information (Kelber et al. 2003; Kelber and Osorio 2010).

In a study performed by Paul and Stevens (2020) examining horse vision and obstacle visibility in horse racing (predominantly jump sports), they found that standard fence coloring, specifically the orange takeoff board and midrail, is not optimal for horse vision. They found poor contrast between the base of the fence (orange takeoff board) and the foreground, and the orange midrail with the mid-fence for the current fence colors and materials used. Additionally, they noted that weather and light conditions should be taken into account when considering alternative colors, but that blues, whites, and yellows generally had better contrast than current fence materials. The colors they found to have the most contrast against the foreground were blue and fluorescent yellow. Fluorescent yellow and light green were also several times more contrasting across all fence backgrounds than natural brush and had considerably higher contrast to the main fence than the orange midrail. They found that overall, the use of white, yellow, or blue would significantly improve the visibility of the takeoff board, midrail, and top of the fence/hurdle to horses, and the colors that were most contrasting against the foreground, in comparison to the orange takeoff board, were blue and fluorescent yellow (Paul and Stevens 2020).

Horses have laterally positioned eyes, which provide a broad field of vision. They use monocular and binocular visual cues. Their estimated horizontal field of vision for the uniocular field is 215° and 228°, with a mean of 190° to 195°. The vertical extent of the visual field in horses has been reported as approximately 178° (Roberts 1992). Their horizontal visual circumference has been reported as 330°–375° (when the head is held high). The amount of binocular overlap is expected to be between 55° and 65° (Hughes 1977; Duke-Elder 1958). Horses also have a region of binocular overlap below their heads, extending down approximately 75° (Duke-Elder 1958). The overlap of visual fields for horses results in them having an almost spherical field of view when holding their heads level. There is a narrow blind region directly to their rear as well as in the region of space extending forward perpendicular to the forehead and directly below the nose (Figure 4.6). There are practical consequences for the shape of the equine visual field, predominantly associated with the field of binocular vision being directed to the ground where the horse will feed (Timney and Macuda 2001).

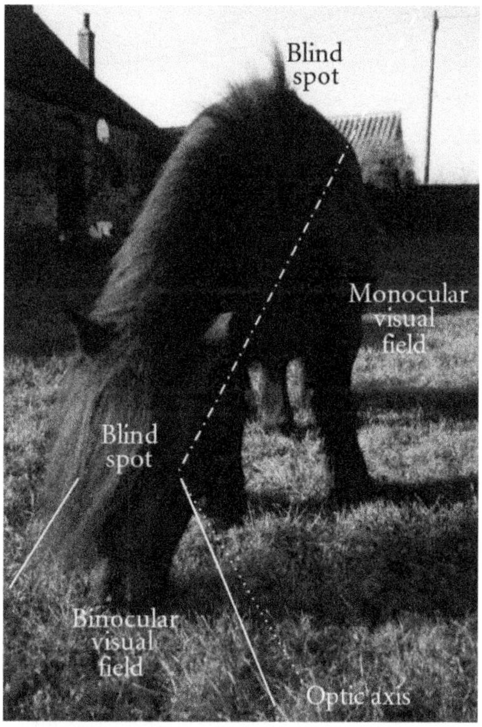

Figure 4.6 The position and extent of the binocular overlap in the region of the inferior visual field of the horse (approx. 65°). The extent of the monocular visual field, blind spots, and angle of the optic axis (approximately 40° from the midline) are also shown. *Source:* Reproduced with permission from Murphy et al. 2009/Hindawi Publishing Corporation.

Dogs and Cats

Dogs have functional vision during the day and night (Hughes 1977; Walls 1944) and have developed several mechanisms of visual function to adapt to dim light. The canine retina is predominantly composed of rod photoreceptors, which function in less intense light conditions (Kemp and Jacobson 1992), with only 3% of retinal cells composed of cone photoreceptors, which are responsible for color vision (Peichl 1992). In dogs, the area centralis, a region typically centrally located in the retina, contains the maximal density of rod and cone photoreceptor cells.

The **tapetum lucidum** is a biologic reflector system commonly found in vertebrates (Ollivier et al. 2004) but not humans and is responsible for the yellow/green reflection when direct light hits the eye (Figure 4.7a,b). This layer of tissue reflects light back through the retina a second time, allowing for additional photon/photoreceptor stimulation, enhancing visual sensitivity in dim light but reducing image detail due to light scatter (Walls 1944). There is variation in the tapetum lucidum (Lesiuk and Braekevelt 1983). The size varies with breed and body size, and variations can also exist within a breed. In fact, in a sample of 539 dogs, a tapetal area was completely present in only 70.3 % of them, being completely absent in 1.9% (Kasparson et al. 2013). Generally, smaller sized breeds, like Papillons, Shetland Sheepdogs, Dachshunds, American Cocker Spaniels, Miniature Schnauzers, Miniature Poodles, Bichon Frisé/Havanais, and Cavalier King Charles Spaniels, have a smaller tapetal area, while larger dogs, like Border Collies, Leonbergers, Samoyeds, Golden Retrievers, and English Springer Spaniels, typically have a full-sized tapetal area (Kasparson et al. 2013). Labrador Retrievers appear to have increased variation compared to other breeds, with a large portion appearing to lack a tapetal area (Kasparson et al. 2013).

Dogs have two classes of cones that provide them with dichromatic color vision, allowing

(a) (b)

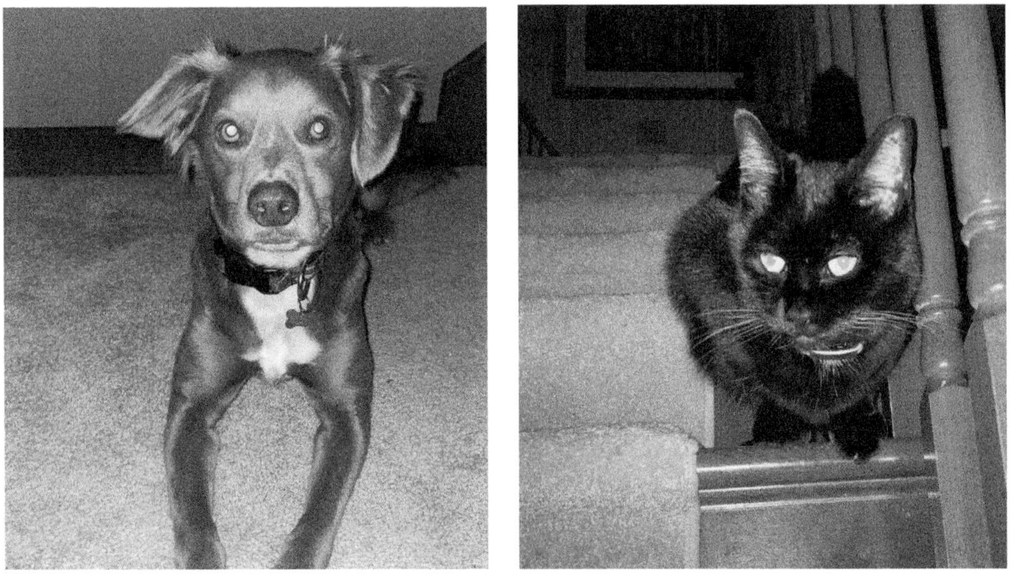

Figure 4.7 The tapetum lucidum is a reflective area of the retina present in most vertebrates besides humans. It reflects light within the globe of the eye, allowing enhanced vision in low-light environments. The eyes appear to "glow" when direct light illuminates them in dark settings. The tapetum lucidum of a dog (a) and cat (b) appear as a bright yellow/green color in most direct light. *Source:* Meghan E. Herron.

them to see shades of blue and yellow, but not red. There is evidence that dogs may use color over brightness cues when presented with a discrimination task between yellow and blue stimuli (Kasparson et al. 2013). Eight dogs were observed to use color over brightness when recognizing and discriminating visual objects (Kasparson et al. 2013), which suggests that color may be a fundamental feature of visual object perception in dogs. Additionally, in a study by Tanaka et al. (2000), two dogs (Shiba Inu) were able to appropriately identify a positive stimulus (red, blue, or green compared to grey) when given the choice between the two.

Cats also have two classes of cones that provide them with dichromatic color vision, similar to dogs, seeing violet, blue, and yellow, but not red (Pearlman and Daw 1971). There have been several studies detecting a third photopic receptor in cats that could allow trichromatic vision (Ringo et al. 1977); however, more recent studies have not found a third class of cones in the feline retina. Additionally, the behavioral study that indicates cats demonstrated trichromatic vision has a flaw in the experimental design that could allow achromatic intensity cues to allow accurate identification of medium wavelength cues (Clark and Clark 2016). Cats also have a tapetum lucidum (Figure 4.7b) that functions similarly to this structure in dogs, reflecting light that has not stimulated the retina back into the receptor cells for a second chance of absorption by the visual pigments. In cats nutritionally deprived of taurine, there is a severe disorganization of the lattice arrangement of tapetal rods in addition to photoreceptor degeneration, indicating taurine plays a vital role in maintaining the structural integrity of multiple structures in the feline eye. Visual evoked potentials and electroretinogram responses are severely reduced in taurine-depleted cats, indicating that they are deficient in light processing in addition to exhibiting structural changes. Normal vision in cats relies on dietary taurine for the maintenance of normal structure and function of the feline eye (Wen et al. 1979).

Ruminants/Cattle

Ruminants have two classes of cones, similar to horses, that provide them with dichromatic color vision. Evidence of these two classes of cones has been found in the family Suidae – the domestic pig (Sus scrofa) (Neitz and Jacobs 1989), the family Cervidae – white-tailed (Odocoileus virginiana) and fallow deer (Dama dama) (Jacobs et al. 1994), and the family Bovidae – domestic cattle (Bos taurus), sheep (Ovis aries), and goats (Capra hircus) (Jacobs et al. 1998). Ungulates see medium to long wavelengths better (yellow, orange, and red). Behavioral studies to establish visual capacities in ungulates can be difficult; however, cattle have been shown to visually discriminate between patches of green and dead forages, and this visual discrimination is most likely to occur when a distance away from the forages (Hirata and Kusatake 2020).

Visual perception of livestock is a significant factor in the design of handling facilities. Cattle and sheep have relatively poor depth perception, while pigs are better equipped to judge distances. Cattle, sheep, and pigs have wide-angle vision; therefore, it is recommended that there should be high sides to single-file lead-up chutes, crowing pens, and the curved holding lane to obscure moving objects and people outside the facility (Grandin 1980b) (Figure 4.8).

The effects of white, yellow, and blue light emitting diodes (LEDs) on milk production and composition in comparison to natural daylight were studied in Holstein cows. It was found that in the blue LED group, milk fat, protein, and lactose contents were the lowest and milk-urea-nitrogen levels were the highest, although high milk-urea-nitrogen was also found in the yellow LED group. Extended exposure to blue LED light lowered antioxidant enzyme activity and insulin-like growth factor-1 levels. Prolactin concentrations were higher in the white and blue LED groups than in the natural daylight control. Cortisol level was the highest in the blue LED group.

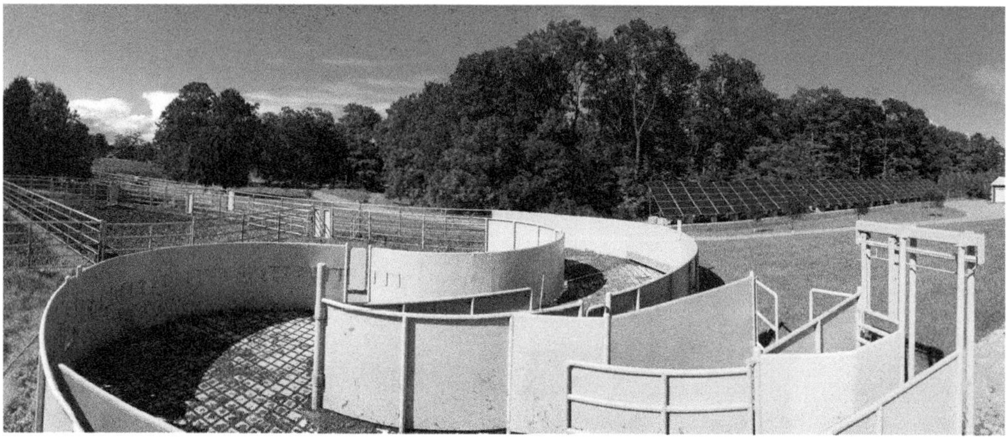

Figure 4.8 This lead-up chute has high, solid sides and follows a curved path, all of which prevent balking and should promote forward movement. *Source:* With permission from Jeff Lutzey / Waseda Farms.

Nonesterified fatty acid levels in the yellow and blue LED groups decreased to the greatest extent compared to the start point. The results suggest that blue LED lights can decrease milk production and generate more stress than white and yellow LED lights (Son et al. 2020).

Birds

In birds, color vision plays a role in behaviors such as finding food and choosing between mating partners (Bennett and Cuthill 1994; Bennett et al. 1997; Church et al. 1998; Hunt et al. 2001; Maddocks et al. 2001). Four types of single cone photoreceptors sensitive to red light (long wavelengths, L), green light (medium wavelengths, M), blue light (short wavelengths, S), and violet or ultraviolet light (very short wavelengths, VS/UVS) mediate color vision in birds (Hart 2001; Osorio et al. 1999; Vorobyev et al. 1998). These cone photoreceptors are equipped with colored oil droplets, which act as filters, narrowing cone spectral sensitivities. This potentially improves color discrimination and color constancy (Vorobyev et al. 1998; Govardovskiĭ 1983; Vorobyev 2003).

Visual fields vary extensively among avian species (Martin 2017). This variability has been attributed to foraging, predator detection, parental care, and gathering of social information (Martin 2014). A wider binocular field has been observed in birds that are visually guided compared with a narrower binocular field in birds that are more tactile-guided (Martin and Portugal 2011; Guillemain et al. 2002). The extent of blind area above the head also varies (Martin and Shaw 2010). Differences in visual field configuration have been linked to visual acuity differences, with a higher visual acuity in species with broader visual fields (Moore et al. 2015). Birds are believed to forage primarily utilizing visual cues, especially raptors. Due to the blind spot above the head, when scanning below for sources of food, raptors and other visually guided birds may not detect hazards directly in front of them, such as power lines or wind turbines. Potier et al. (2018) found that in raptors, binocular field shape is associated with bill and suborbital ridge shape and, ultimately, foraging strategies. Tyrrell and Fernández-Juricic (2017) found that the anterior blind area (the blind area in front of the head that is proximal to the binocular visual field) and beak visibility play a role in shaping avian binocular fields. They found that in visually guided foragers, the ability to see the beak (and how much of the beak can be seen) varies predictably with foraging habits: fish- and insect-eating birds see more of

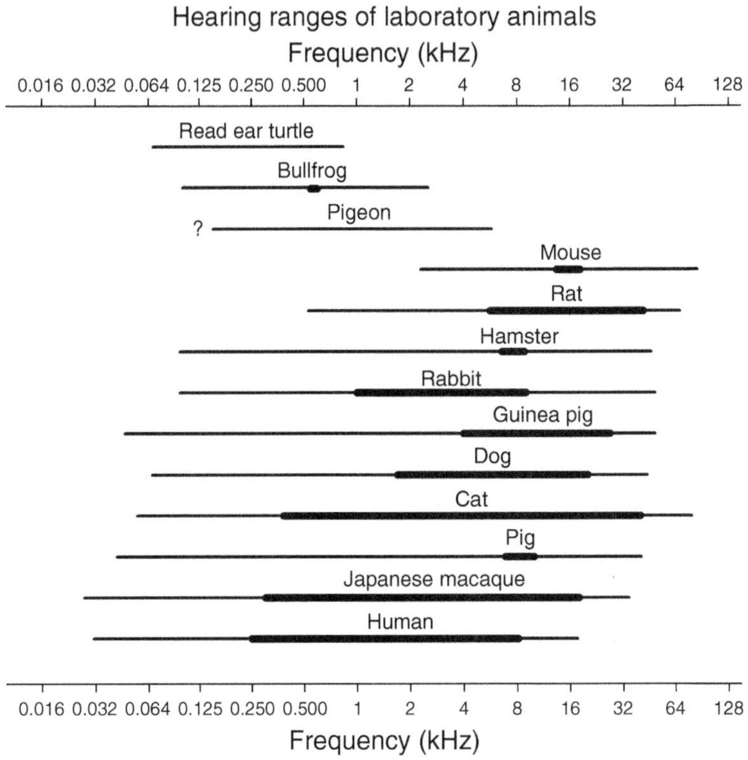

Figure 4.9 The hearing range of common laboratory animals compared to those of humans. The thin lines indicate the range of frequencies that can be detected at 60 dB sound pressure level (SPL). The thick lines indicate the range of frequencies that can be detected at 10 dB SPL. *Source:* Heffner and Heffner 2007, reproduced with permission from the Journal of the American Association for Laboratory Animal Science.

their own beak than birds eating immobile food. Additionally, in non-visually guided foragers, there is no consistent relationship between the beak and anterior blind area (Tyrrell and Fernández-Juricic 2017).

Audition

Auditory interactions with the environment are the result of three primary functions that hearing provides in all animals: sound detection, localization of the sound source, and sensory information for recognition of the source identity. The ability of animals to hear is dependent on a means of capturing sound waves from the environment (the pinnae), a means of converting sound waves into a signal (tympanic membrane and ossicles), and a means of sending signal to the brain (optic nerve and associated receptors) for processing. The ability to perceive high frequency versus low frequency sound waves varies between species (Figure 4.9). Generally, there is an inverse relationship between the mass of a mammal and its hearing frequency threshold (Fletcher 1985). Laterality of auditory processing has been demonstrated in a variety of species and has been shown to depend on factors such as sound structure, species specificity, and types of stimuli.

There are two physical characteristics of the auditory signal that affect localization of sound: the delay in time between the arrival of the signal at each pinna (Δt) and the frequency-intensity spectrum of the sounds reaching the ear (Δfi). For a sound source that is directly ahead or behind the head, the signal arrives simultaneously to both ears. For a sound source located at 90° azimuth, the delay would be maximal. Intermediate azimuthal angles would cause intermediate delays in the detection of the sound source. The ability of the nervous system to interpret (Δt) depends on its ability to resolve small temporal difference in time of arrival of the signal. Animals with large **pinnal distances** may have better sound localization capacities; their larger heads will generate a longer time delay between pinnal inputs (see Figure 4.10). The frequency-intensity spectrum results from the animal's head creating a sound-shadow that decreases intensity of the sound arriving at the ear on the side of the head opposite the sound source. This effect is frequency dependent, with high frequency sounds inducing maximal attenuation and low frequency sounds scarcely being affected. The ability to localize sound depends on the extent to which an animal can integrate information from (Δt) and (Δfi) (Timney and Macuda 2001).

Horses

Horses show visible reactions to sounds, with one or both ears typically moving toward the direction of the sound source. The funnel-shape of the equine ear provides an acoustic pressure gain of 10–20 dB (Fletcher 1985) improving the acuity of equine hearing. Horses hear from 55 to 33,500 Hz, but are only able to locate a sound accurately within 27°. In other words, they have sensitive hearing, but lack the ability to detect a precise location of a sound's source. The horse represents an outlier to the inverse relationship between the mass of a mammal and its hearing frequency threshold, exhibiting limited low frequency hearing but good acuity in the higher frequency ranges. Sensitive, high frequency hearing is likely adaptive in horses, providing important information for horses as prey species regarding, among other things, the stealthy advance of predators (Rørvang et al. 2020). Heffner and Heffner (Heffner and Heffner 1984; Heffner and Heffner 1986; Heffner and Heffner 1983)

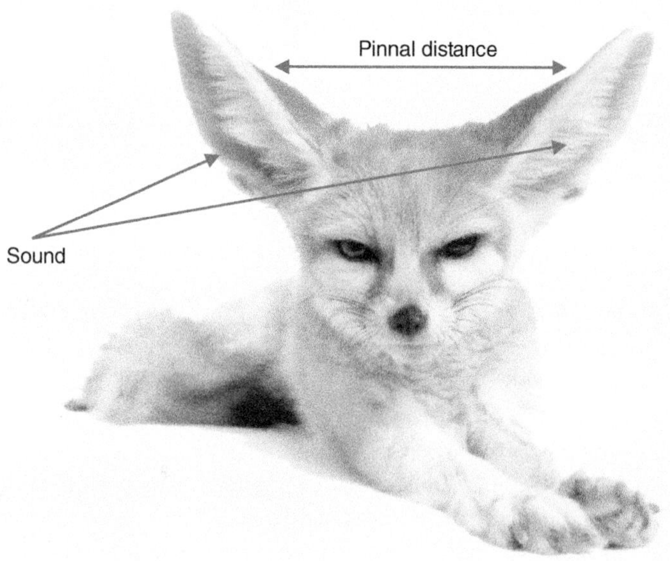

Figure 4.10 Animals with more distance between pinnae will have better sound localization as the time delay between sound hitting each pinna will be greater than it would be for animals with narrower heads/smaller pinnae. *Background image source:* Eastman Arts/AdobeStock.

mapped the range of frequencies horses can detect and demonstrated that while larger animals tend to be adept at hearing lower frequencies, horses are an exception. The lowest frequency detectable by horses is 50 Hz, which is higher than the lowest human detection threshold of 20 Hz. Conversely, equine hearing exceeds the highest frequencies that can be heard by humans (33 kHz compared to 20 kHz for humans). Horses have been found to demonstrate auditory laterality that is influenced by familiarity of the sound. Whinny calls from group members, neighbors, and strangers were played, and clear left hemispheric preference (the horse turns its right ear more toward to source) was found for familiar neighbor calls, whereas there was no preference for group member or strangers calls (Basile et al. 2009).

The effects of music on stress in horses have been examined in limited capacity. Classical music was demonstrated to reduce the intensity of stress responses in horses subjected to either a short transportation or a farrier treatment, suggesting that background music can have practical implications (Neveux et al. 2016). Another study investigated the potentially calming effects of music on ponies, but found no effects of either classical, jazz, country, or rock music (Houpt et al. 2000). Instrumental guitar music was shown to have a positive emotional influence on Arabian racehorses when played for 5 h per day for a period of between 1 and 3 months, after which the positive effect diminished (Stachurska et al. 2015). The same type of music was tested in a study that showed that the positive emotional effects of playing the music were greater when played for three hours per day than for one hour per day (Kedzierski et al. 2017), confirming the positive emotional effects of instrumental guitar music.

Horses have been shown to discriminate emotions in nonverbal vocalization from humans. When presented with positively and negatively valanced human vocalizations (laughter and growling, respectively) in the absence of all other emotional cues, horses adopted a freeze posture longer, held their ears forward for longer, and performed fewer ear movements in response to negative vocalizations, suggesting increased vigilance. In addition, horses exhibited a right-ear/left-hemisphere bias when attending to positive compared with negative vocalization, suggesting that laughter was perceived as more positive than growling (Smith et al. 2018).

Dogs and Cats

Dogs hear in the range of 40–60,000 Hz and their ability to rotate and erect their pinnae can enhance their auditory processing. Auditory lateralization in dogs shows the right ear (left hemisphere) is primarily utilized for intraspecific communication and the left ear (right hemisphere) is primarily used for intense emotions (Siniscalchi et al. 2008; Reinholz-Trojan et al. 2012). Canine congenital deafness has been reported in 80 different breeds of dogs (Strain 2004). The breeds with the highest observed prevalence of deafness include Dalmatian, Bull Terrier, English Cocker Spaniel, English Setter, and Australian Cattle Dog. Most deafness in dogs is congenital sensorineural hereditary deafness, associated with the genes for white pigment: piebald or merle. Dogs with blue eyes have a greater likelihood of hereditary deafness than brown-eyed dogs. Other common forms of sensorineural deafness include presbycusis, ototoxicity, noise-induced hearing loss, otitis interna, and anesthesia (Strain 2012).

Dog responses to classical music have been studied in multiple settings with variable results. In studies done within rescue/shelter/rehoming centers, classical music was found to promote relaxation, while heavy metal was found to increase behaviors associated with stress (Bowman et al. 2015; Wells et al. 2002; Kogan et al. 2012; Brayley and Montrose 2016). In one study at an animal rescue and rehoming center in Scotland, canine residents were divided into groups that were exposed to soft rock, Motown, pop music, reggae music, classical music, and control (before and after). Dogs were exposed to a different music treatment each day for five consecutive days. Music exposure (all genres) induced changes in behavior (less time standing) and altered heart rate variability, both indicative of reduced stress. Urinary cortisol levels were higher during soft rock exposure. Physiological and behavioral changes were maintained over the five days of auditory stimulation, suggesting that providing a variety of different genres may minimize habituation (Bowman et al. 2017). In studies done within a veterinary teaching hospital, no difference in behavior (aggression, anxiety) or physiology (body temperature and heart rate) of dogs was observed in one study, although classical music had a positive effect upon owner and employee satisfaction in that study (Engler and Bain 2017), while in the second study auditory stimulation reduced respiratory rate variability, suggesting the novel music exposure had an excitatory rather than a calming effect (Koster et al. 2019).

Cats hear in the range of ~30–64,000 Hz, which is a range that extends wider and higher than both humans and dogs. As obligate carnivores, the ability to detect the high frequency sounds emitted by their prey is advantageous. Cats also have excellent mobility in their pinnae that allows for precision sound localization (within a few degrees). Auditory lateralization in response to both conspecific and heterospecific (dog) vocalizations shows that cats turn their heads with the right ear leading (left hemisphere activation) in response to their typical-species vocalizations and have a distinct bias in the use of the left ear (right hemisphere activation) in response to dogs' vocalizations of "disturbance" and "isolation". This suggests that the auditory sensory domain seems to be lateralized with the left hemisphere for intraspecific communication and with the right hemisphere for processing threatening and alarming stimuli (Siniscalchi et al. 2016).

Snowdon et al. (2015) hypothesized that for music to be effective with other species, it must be in the frequency range and with similar tempos to those used in natural communication by each species. They utilized a theoretical framework to compose "species-appropriate music" for domestic cats and tested this music in comparison with music with similar affective content composed for humans. Cats showed a significant preference for, and interest in, "species-appropriate music" compared with human music. Additionally, they found younger and older cats were more responsive to cat music than middle-aged cats (Snowdon et al. 2015). In a study evaluating the ability of cat-specific music and classical music compared with no music to reduce stress in cats during hospitalization, there was no difference in the mean cat stress scoring (CSS) between cats listening to cat-specific music, classical music, and control throughout the five evaluations observed. Cat-specific music had a higher percentage of positive social interactions than the other groups during one of the five evaluations, and the average respiratory rate was significantly lower in the classical music group versus control at one of the five evaluations, although both findings were statistically insignificant (Paz et al. 2022). In another study, it was found that cats listening to cat-specific music prior to, and during, physical examination were associated with lower CSSs and lower mean handling scores (HS) in cats but had no effect on the physiological stress responses measured by neutrophil:lymphocyte ratios (NLR) (Hampton et al. 2020).

Ruminants

Cattle hear in the range of 23–40,000 Hz, while goats hear 78–37,000 Hz, and pigs hear in the range of 40–35,000 Hz. Best sensitivity in cattle and goats has a well-defined point of 8,000 Hz (Heffner and Heffner 1990) and 2,000 Hz (Heffner and Heffner 1992) (respectively) while pigs have a region of best sensitivity from 250 to 16,000 kHz (Heffner and Heffner 1992). Cattle and goats have relatively poor sound localization acuity compared with most mammals, 30° and 18° (respectively). Although both have large pinnal distances and large binaural locus cues available to them, it is not unexpected when other factors are considered. Like other poor localizers (both domesticated and nondomesticated), cattle and goats are prey species with their best vision directed throughout nearly the entire horizon. In contrast to mammals with very narrow foveal fields, they may not need very accurate locus information from their auditory systems to direct their gaze to a sound source (Heffner and Heffner 1992). Pigs, on the other hand, have significantly more accurate sound localization, 4.5°. The ability of pigs to localize low-frequency tones indicates that they can use the binaural phase-difference cue. However, they are unable to localize tones of 4 kHz and higher, indicating that, like other hoofed mammals; their ability to use binaural intensity cues is greatly restricted if not completely absent (Heffner and Heffner 1989).

Vocalization in cattle is potentially a useful indicator of their physiological and psychological functioning. Vocalizations provide information on the age, sex, social status, and reproductive status of the caller. Calves can recognize their mothers using vocal cues, but it is not clear whether cows recognize their offspring in this way. Vocal behavior may play a role in estrus advertisement and competitive display by bulls. Under experimental conditions involving pain or social isolation, vocal response is useful as an indicator of welfare, and unlike commonly used physiological measures, it can be recorded non-invasively and varies on a number of quantitative and qualitative dimensions (Watts and Stookey 2000).

Classical or slow instrumental music has been found to increase milk yield in dairy cows (Kenison 2016). Country music can facilitate dairy cows' voluntary approach and entry into the automatic milking system (AMS) (Uetake et al. 1997). Lullaby music reduces stress most significantly in dairy cattle when compared to country, jazz, reggae, pop, classical, opera, rap, hip hop and heavy metal (Kemp 2019). Additionally, in dairy cattle, auditory stimulation (classical and country music and an audiobook) may reduce abnormal behaviors (tongue rolling) and enhance behavioral diversity (increased locomotive behavior and positive social interactions), as periods of no auditory stimulation seem to increase resting and rumination, indicating auditory enrichment that incorporates periods of no auditory stimulation should be considered (Crouch et al. 2019). Soft background music is recommended for livestock in the stockyards, with a higher volume being played in the stunning area (due to the equipment sounds). Research finds that cattle are calm when music is played but become nervous if the music system is not functioning. Additionally, employees are more likely to handle the cattle humanely if music plays at the plant (Grandin 1980a).

Classical music promotes a significant increase in tail-wagging, playing, and exploring behaviors of growing pigs. Short-term (8d), pigs exposed to classical music had a reduced stress response (lower cortisol level) compared to those in the noise and control groups, while long-term (60d) music stimulus enhanced immune response (increased immunoglobulin G [IgG], interleukin-2 [IL-2], and interferon-gamma [IFN-γ] levels), indicating use of music can have both short- and long-term benefits (Li et al. 2021). In pregnant sows, Vivaldi's "Four Seasons" (played at 71.13 dB) promotes lower respiratory rate, fewer stereotypies, and better interactions with humans (Silva et al. 2017). Piglets, however, seem distressed by this same piece of music, and it disrupts their rest (Sartor et al. 2018). Rock and roll music played to pigs at 80–85 dB (twice daily during feeding) seems to have a negative effect on the daily growth rate (DGR) and feed conversion ratio (Talling et al. 1996).

Olfaction

> "Olfaction is to animals what writing is to humans"
>
> – Katherine Houpt.

Olfaction enables most mammalian species to detect and discriminate vast numbers of chemical structures, odorants, and pheromones. The perception of such chemical compounds is mediated via two major olfactory systems: the main olfactory system and the vomeronasal system, as well as minor systems, such as the septal organ and the Grueneberg ganglion. Distinct differences exist not only among species but also among individuals in terms of their olfactory sensitivity. The olfactory apparatus is composed of olfactory epithelium (which lines the nasal cavity), olfactory nerve axons that enter the skull via the cribiform plate and synapse at the olfactory bulb, and olfactory tracts that carry information to other parts of the brain, including the limbic system (amygdala, hippocampus, and hypothalamus) and olfactory cortex. The **vomeronasal organ** (VNO) detects nonvolatile compounds (pheromones) found in urine, feces, saliva, and other substances, which provide information such as sex, reproduction status, and stress of other animals. This organ is a group of sensory receptors located in the soft tissue of the nasal septum, in the nasal cavity just above the hard palate (roof of mouth) (Figure 4.11). Dogs, cats, and pigs have small ducts behind the canine teeth, connecting to the VNO, while horses and ruminants have ducts leading directly from the nasal passage. The VNO sends axons to the accessory olfactory bulb (AOB) (Wackermannová et al. 2016).

Scents/odors are volatile molecules. Deposited scents/odors are messages that can be transmitted in the absence of the sender, as they can persist for minutes to days after they have been deposited. To ensure these molecules make contact with the olfactory epithelium, animals must "sniff", increasing the

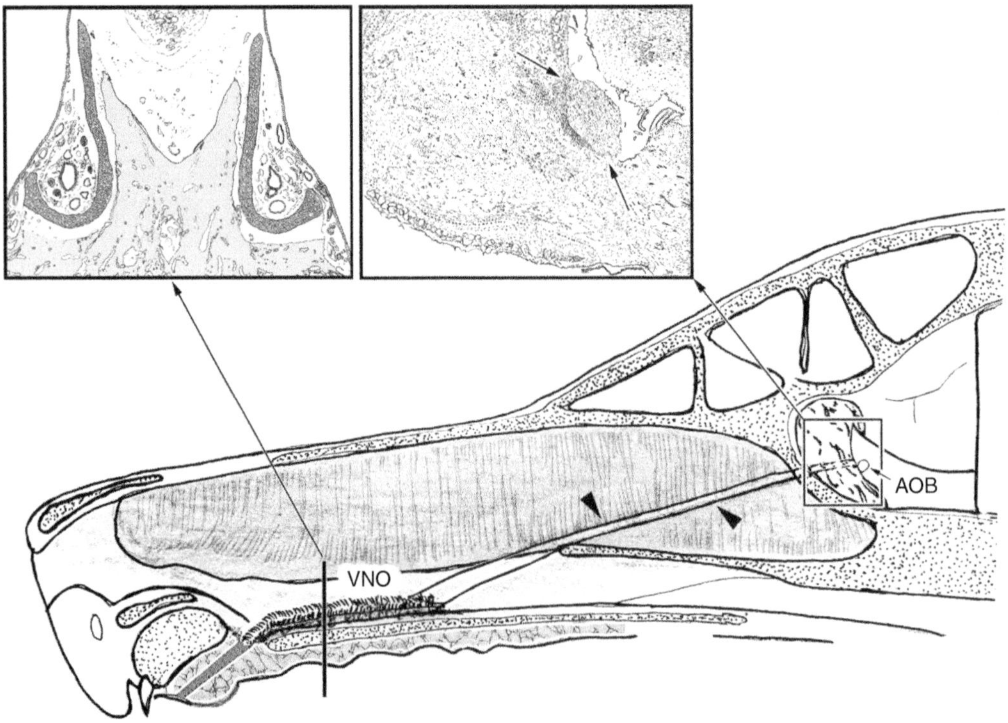

Figure 4.11 Diagram of a sagittal section through the head of a dog, showing the projection areas of the VNO and the AOB and the trajectory of the vomeronasal nerves (arrowheads) between them. Left box: transverse section of the pair of VNOs; right box: partial parasagittal section of the olfactory bulb, showing the location of the AOB (arrows). *Source:* Salazar et al. 2013; Reproduced with permission from John Wiley and Sons.

likelihood the scent is able to be processed. Scents can be deposited/detected in urine, feces, secretions (anal gland, ear, and vaginal), foot pads, skin glands, and saliva. There are two types of odors deposited/detected: identifier odors and emotional odors. Identifier odors are produced by normal metabolic processes and stable for long periods of time. These include sex-, age-, species-, colony-, and individual-specific odors. Emotional odors are produced or released in special circumstances, such as when an animal becomes stressed, is in estrus, starts lactating, or changes their social structure within the group (Brown 1979).

Pheromones are non-volatile molecules that carry messages between conspecifics. Pheromones persist in the environment longer than odors. Some examples of better characterized pheromones include the facial pheromone in cats, 5α-androstenone in boars, salivary pheromones in bulls, appeasing pheromones (dogs, cats, horses, and rabbits), estrus pheromones and stress pheromones. Pheromone detection relies on moving non-volatile substances across specialized olfactory epithelium – the action to do this is more than a "sniff" and may involve oral and nasal movements (flehmen, gaping, and tongue flicking).

Horses

Horses' olfactory organs consist of olfactory epithelium, olfactory neurons, and the olfactory bulb in the brain and respond to volatile molecules (scents). They also have a well-developed vomeronasal organ, which is receptive to non-volatile and poorly volatile molecules (pheromones). Pheromone activation of the vomeronasal organ triggers a flehmen response in which the horse curls its upper lip back and inhales, often with closed nostrils, which reduces the escape of air and increases the air pressure in the nasal cavity (see Figure 4.12). Flehmen enables the horse to analyze poorly volatile compounds with far greater accuracy.

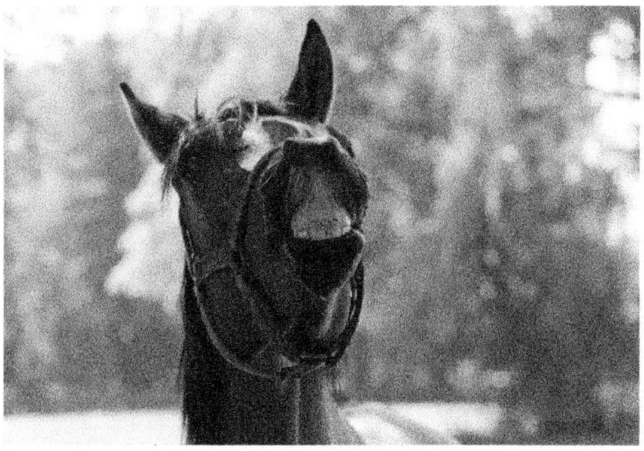

Figure 4.12 Flehmen response in a horse. *Source:* Dorota/AdobeStock.

In mammals, an important innate (non-learned) response to odors is the avoidance of/flight from predators. Horses show vigilance behavior when exposed to an unknown odor (eucalyptus oil; [Christensen et al. 2005]) and to a predator odor (wolf urine; [Christensen et al. 2005]). Additionally, if a predator odor is paired with a loud noise, the combination elicits significantly higher heart rates than when horses are only exposed to one of the stimuli (Christensen and Rundgren 2008), indicating that the presence of a predator odor alone (without the animal itself) can amplify the response to fear-eliciting situations.

There is evidence that odors are used by horses for social recognition. Stallions will sniff mares' feces longer than stallions' feces, will also exhibit more flehmen when sniffing mares' feces when compared to stallions' feces, and will exclusively urinate on mares' feces (Jezierski et al. 2018). Horses are also able to distinguish their own feces from conspecifics; however, they cannot differentiate between the feces of familiar and unknown horses or mare feces compared to gelding feces (Krueger and Flauger 2011). Studies of feral and free-ranging horses indicate these animals recognize each other based on body odors (Hothersall et al. 2010; Péron et al. 2014), as well as odors from urine and feces (Krueger and Flauger 2011; Hothersall et al. 2010). Horses also exhibit more interest in the feces of horses from whom they received the highest amount of aggressive behavior (Krueger and Flauger 2011). Additionally, hair samples from different horse breeds differ in their profiles of volatile organic compounds, and odor profiles in cohorts of related horses are different than in those of non-related horses. Odor profiles can indicate a degree of kinship, indicating that each horse has its own odor profile, but there is similarity in those profiles between related individuals. The ability to recognize conspecifics based on odor can be used by the horse to guide its response to other horses in a social group based on previous experiences, allowing odor profiles to aid in determining the potential outcome of a given interaction (Deshpande et al. 2018).

A synthetic analogue of the Equine Appeasing Pheromone (EAP) has been studied for its effects on reducing fear and anxiety, with inconsistent results. In a study examining the effects of EAP in a controlled fear-inducing situation (walking the horse through a fringed curtain), horses who received EAP underwent fewer stress-related consequences associated with cardiac physiology (significant differences were observed between the treated and control groups for heart rate data, both during the test and during the whole measured period). Horses treated with EAP also showed fewer behavioral signs characteristic of fear than those in the control group (Falewee et al. 2006). Another study examining the effects of EAP on horses thought to be experiencing separation anxiety, the pheromone was observed to dampen extreme anxiety but had no significant effect when bonded pairs were separated (Collyer and Wilson 2016). A study examining the effects of EAP on behavioral and physiologic indicators of stress (serum cortisol) in response to abrupt weaning of foals found no significant effects of the pheromone treatment on neither behavioral measures nor cortisol concentration (Berger et al. 2013).

The role of odor in emotional recognition between members of different species remains somewhat of a mystery, although emotional recognition between species using visual and auditory cues has been demonstrated repeatedly. Horses were studied to assess whether they displayed differential behavior in response to human fear and non-fear odors, in conditions designed to elicit fear or happiness. Horses lifted their heads significantly more frequently and for longer in the fear and control conditions compared to the happiness condition. Similarly, horses tended to touch a familiar person that was present during the test more frequently and for longer in the fear condition compared to the happiness condition. Additionally, depending on odor condition, the horses differed in the time they spent keeping their ears back (Sabiniewicz et al. 2020). **Autonomic nervous system** activity of horses in response to human body odors produced under happy and fear states was also examined, and both sympathetic and parasympathetic changes were observed in response to these odors, as was emotional stimulation of the horses (Lanata et al. 2018).

Dogs

The canine olfactory system can recognize more smells than it has receptors for scent molecules. This is made possible because olfactory receptors can have specific cross-reactions, building unique systems of patterns connected to different smells. There are 339 different receptors, and each odorant binds differently with one or more of these receptors, which then sends a specific signal, and a "code" is created in the olfactory cortex. As with most mammals, dogs have two main parts of the olfactory system: the main olfactory epithelium (MOE) and the vomeronasal organ (VNO). The MOE is located in the caudo-dorsal region of the nasal cavity (which is frequently the pigmented part of the mucosa), and the VNO lies between the nasal and oral cavity, near the vomer bone, just above the roof of the mouth. The nasopalatine duct, which starts behind the upper incisors on the palate, connects the mouth with the VNO, which is a tubular, elongated organ, separated by the nasal septum (Dzieciol et al. 2020; Salazar, Cifuentes, and Sanchez-Quinteiro 2013; Jezierski et al. 2016).

Dogs have precise scent acuity – they can detect as little as 1/100 – 1/100,000 the concentration of odors that are detectable to humans. Dogs can differentiate identical twins based on scent. They can detect odors in human fingerprints up to six weeks after they are deposited. Dogs are used to detect cancer, explosives, narcotics, and most recently, SARS-CoV-2 (Hag-Ali et al. 2021). Dogs have also demonstrated that an odor can be linked to memory recall, being able to access a spatial memory based on the odor present at the time the memory was formed (Quaranta et al. 2020).

Cats

Like other mammals, cats have at least two olfactory systems to perceive and process the various chemicals existing in their environment (Shreve and Udell 2017). Small volatiles that reach the main olfactory epithelium are often inhaled during breathing and detected by the main olfactory system. The perception of chemical signals by the accessory olfactory system occurs through the vomeronasal organ (VNO). The olfactory system and scent communication play critical roles in many activities, especially marking and social interactions (Verberne and de Boer 1976; Pageat and Gaultier 2003). Cats use smell in the detection and selection of food. Hullár et al. (2001) found that if cats find the odor of a certain food substantially more attractive, they will consume that food exclusively, without tasting the less attractive foods.

Gustation (Taste)

There arc significant species variations in taste. Pigs prefer sweet flavors (almond, raspberry, and peach) and are less perturbed by bitter tastes. Dogs prefer meaty/savory, with some preference for sweet. Cats prefer meaty/savory tastes, seem to have no preference for sweet/may not taste sweet at all, and are very sensitive to bitter tastes, thanks primarily to lingual lipases that break down short-chain fatty acids. This sensitivity to bitter tastes can make compliance with accepting oral medications a challenge for many cats. Every effort should be made to make oral medications as palatable as possible for cats.

Animals will avoid foods that have been associated with gastrointestinal (GI) malaise or nausea. **Food aversion** (FA) can occur spontaneously but is also a utilized tool with pasture/free-range grazed horses and wild canids. There are plants that grow alongside common forage for horses that are quite toxic, among them locoweed (Figure 4.13). An induced food aversion to locoweed can be created for horses that would forage on this toxic plant. Horses can be averted from locoweed using lithium chloride as an aversive agent with minimal side effects/discomfort from the lithium chloride, and this may provide a management tool to reduce the risk of intoxication for horses grazing locoweed-infested rangeland (Pfister et al. 2002).

Although there are not necessarily naturally occurring reasons to induce a FA in dogs, native predators and scavengers are threatened through the incidence of illegal poisoning due to increasing human-wildlife conflicts, and the use of conditioned taste aversion (CTA) may mitigate such conflicts. To introduce a food aversion to wild canids, dogs are studied for a conditioned food aversion to determine substances that can then be used in wildlife. Thiabendazole, thiram, levamisole, fluconazole, and fluralaner were tested in CTA assays with dogs. Thiabendazole, thiram, and levamisole caused targeted food rejection by dogs and reduced the time spent eating during post-conditioning; however, levamisole appeared to be detectable by dogs, whereas thiram and thiabendazole were not. Fluconazole and fluralaner did not produce any CTA effects. Thiabendazole, thiram, and levamisole can therefore induce CTA, and thus are potential candidates as aversive compounds for wildlife management. Thiram is an undetectable, relatively safe, and accessible compound that can induce CTA in canids and opens new possibilities to develop methods of non-lethal predation control (Tobajas et al. 2019).

In companion animals, the concern with avoidance of foods that have been associated

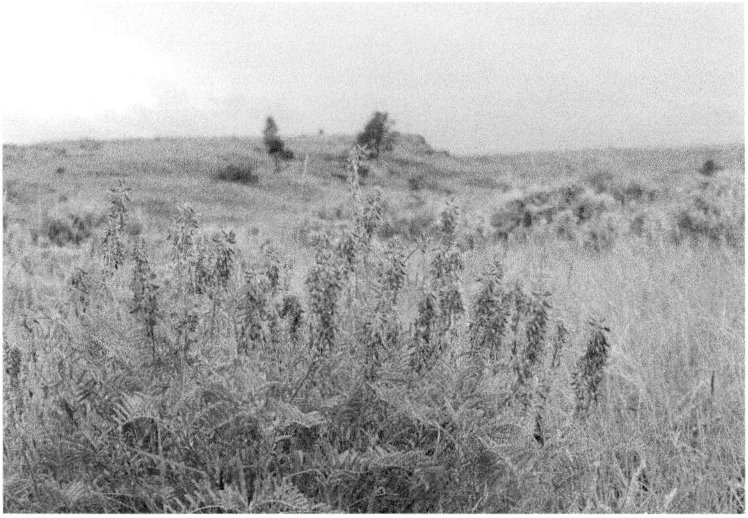

Figure 4.13 Locoweed contains toxins that, when consumed, lead to neurological damage in horses and cattle that is often irreversible. Caretakers can create an intentional food aversion to this plant by lacing a small amount of this plant with lithium chloride and feeding it to the animals. Due to the subsequent GI discomfort, the animals will avoid this plant and its toxins in the future. *Source:* aSculptor/AdobeStock.

with GI upset is that this avoidance can affect ability to treat physical health concerns that are diet responsive. In cats, controlling nausea and vomiting has clinical relevance in preventing the development of food aversion (Trepanier 2010). When considering a new prescription diet for a canine or feline patient, you should consider the GI status when introducing a new food and perhaps delay the start of it until the animal is home, settled, and no longer nauseated. Despite benefits of medium chain triglycerides (MCT) in some commercial pet foods, FA in dogs and cats has been detected when MCTs are included in diets (MacDonald et al. 1985), indicating palatability of food also plays a role in food aversion.

Conclusion

Perception of the environment by individual species and communication between and among species is unique but has similarities that can be utilized to better understand and manage companion animals and livestock under veterinary care. Making sure to consider all five senses when treating and managing patients is essential to success in ensuring appropriate inter- and intraspecies communication. Recognizing how companion animals and livestock will perceive the people around them, especially in a veterinary setting, allows for humane treatment and housing of the animals, not just successful treatment of their physical maladies.

References

Adachi, I., Kuwahata, H., and Fujita, K. (2007). Dogs recall their owner's face upon hearing the owner's voice. *Anim. Cogn.* 10: 17–21.

Andics, A., Gácsi, M., Faragó, T. et al. (2014). Voice-sensitive regions in the dog and human brain are revealed by comparative fMRI. *Curr. Biol.* 24: 574–578.

Basile, M., Boivin, S., Boutin, A. et al. (2009). Socially dependent auditory laterality in domestic horses (*Equus caballus*). *Anim Cogn.* 12 (4): 611–619. https://doi.org/10.1007/s10071-009-0220-5.

Bennett, A.T., Cuthill, I.C., Partridge, J.C., and Lunau, K. (1997). Ultraviolet plumage colors predict mate preferences in starlings. *Proc. Natl. Acad. Sci. U S A.* 94 (16): 8618–8621. https://doi.org/10.1073/pnas.94.16.8618.

Bennett, A.T. and Cuthill, I.C. (1994). Ultraviolet vision in birds: what is its function? *Vision Res.* 34 (11): 1471–1478. https://doi.org/10.1016/0042-6989(94)90149-x.

Bensoussan, S., Tigeot, R., Lemasson, A. et al. (2019). Domestic piglets (*Sus scrofa domestica*) are attentive to human voice and able to discriminate some prosodic features. *Appl. Anim. Behav. Sci.* 210: 38–45.

Berger, J.M., Spier, S.J., Davies, R. et al. (2013). Behavioral and physiological responses of weaned foals treated with equine appeasing pheromone: a double-blinded, placebo controlled, randomized trial. *J. Vet. Behav. Clin. Appl. Res.* 8: 265–277. https://doi.org/10.1016/j.jveb.2012.09.003.

Bowman, A., Dowell, F.J., Evans, N.P., and Scottish, S. (2015). Four Seasons in an animal rescue centre; classical music reduces environmental stress in kennelled dogs. *Physiol. Behav.* 143: 70–82.

Bowman, A., Dowell, F.J., Evans, N.P., and Scottish, S. (2017). The effect of different genres of music on the stress levels of kennelled dogs. *Physiol. Behav.* 171: 207–215.

Brayley, C. and Montrose, V.T. (2016). The effects of audiobooks on the behaviour of dogs at a rehoming kennels. *Appl. Anim. Behav. Sci.* 174: 111–115.

Brown, R.E. (1979). Mammalian social odors: a critical review. *Adv. Study of Behav.* 10: 103–162.

Campanella, S. and Belin, P. (2007). Integrating face and voice in person perception. *Trends. Cogn. Sci.* 11: 535–543.

Carroll, J., Murphy, C.J., Neitz, M. et al. (2001). Photopigment basis for dichromatic color vision in the horse. *J. Vis.* 1 (2): 80–87. https://doi.org/10.1167/1.2.2.

Casey, R.A. and Bradshaw, J.W.S. (2008). The effects of additional socialisation for kittens in a rescue centre on their behaviour and suitability as a pet. *Appl. Anim. Behav. Sci.* 114: 196–205.

Christensen, J.W., Keeling, L.J., and Nielsen, B.L. (2005). Responses of horses to novel visual, olfactory and auditory stimuli. *Appl. Anim. Behav. Sci.* 93: 53–65. https://doi.org/10.1016/j.applanim.2005.06.017.

Christensen, J.W. and Rundgren, M. (2008). Predator odour per se does not frighten domestic horses. *Appl. Anim. Behav. Sci.* 112: 136–145. https://doi.org/10.1016/j.applanim.2007.08.003.

Church, S.C., Bennett, A.T.D., Cuthill, I.C., and Partridge, J.C. (1998). Ultraviolet cues affect the foraging behaviour of blue tits. *Proc. Royal Society of London Series B* 265: 1509–1514.

Clark, D.L. and Clark, R.A. (2016). Neutral point testing of color vision in the domestic cat. *Exp. Eye Res.* 153: 23–26. https://doi.org/10.1016/j.exer.2016.10.002.

Collyer, P.B. and Wilson, H.S. (2016). Does a commercial pheromone application reduce separation anxiety in separated horse pairs? *J. Vet. Behav.* 15: 94. https://doi.org/10.1016/j.jveb.2016.08.064.

Coulon, M., Deputte, B.L., Heyman, Y., and Baudoin, C. (2009). Individual recognition in domestic cattle (*Bos taurus*): evidence from 2D-images of heads from different breeds. *PLoS ONE* 4: e4441.

Crouch, K.; Evans, B.; Montrose, V.T. (2019) The effects of auditory enrichment on the behaviour of dairy cows (*Bos taurus*). *Proceedings of the British Society of Animal Science Annual Conference 2019*, Edinburgh, UK: Hartpury University, (9–11 April 2019).

d'Ingeo, S., Quaranta, A., Siniscalchi, M. et al. (2019). Horses associate individual human voices with the valence of past interactions: a behavioural and electrophysiological study. *Sci. Rep.* 9: 11568.

DeMello, M. (2012). *Animals and Society: An Introduction to Human-Animal Studies.* Columbia University Press.

Deshpande, K., Furton, K.G., and Mills, D.E.K. (2018). The equine volatilome: volatile organic compounds as discriminatory markers. *J. Equine Vet. Sci.* 62: 47–53. https://doi.org/10.1016/j.jevs.2017.05.013.

Duke-Elder, S. (1958). *System of Ophthalmology* Vol. 1 The Eye in Evolution. Henry Kimpton.

Düpjan, S., Tuchscherer, A., Langbein, J. et al. (2011). Behavioural and cardiac responses towards conspecific distress calls in domestic pigs (*Sus scrofa*). *Physiol. Behav.* 103: 445–452.

Dziecioł, M., Podgórski, P., Stańczyk, E. et al. (2020). MRI Features of the vomeronasal organ in dogs (*Canis familiaris*). *Front. Veter. Sci.* 7: 159.

Engler, W.J. and Bain, M. (2017). Effect of different types of classical music played at a veterinary hospital on dog behavior and owner satisfaction. *J. Am. Vet. Med. Assoc.* 251: 195–200.

Falewee, C., Gaultier, E., Lafont, C. et al. (2006). Effect of a synthetic equine maternal pheromone during a controlled fear-eliciting situation. *Appl. Anim. Behav. Sci.* 101: 144–153. https://doi.org/10.1016/j.applanim.2006.01.008.

Fletcher, N.H. (1985). Sound production and hearing in diverse animals. *Acoustics Australia* 13: 49–53.

Gergely, A., Petró, E., Oláh, K., and Topál, J. (2019). Auditory–visual matching of conspecifics and non-conspecifics by dogs and human infants. *Animals* 9: 17.

Govardovskiĭ, V.I. (1983). On the role of oil drops in colour vision. *Vision Res.* 23 (12): 1739–1740. https://doi.org/10.1016/0042-6989(83)90192-x.

Grandin, T. (1980a). Livestock behavior as related to handling facilities design. *J. Study Anim. Probl.* 1: 33–52.

Grandin, T. (1980b). Observations of cattle behavior applied to the design of cattle handling facilities. *Appl. Anim. Ethol.* 6: 19–31.

Guillemain, M., Martin, G.R., and Fritz, H. (2002). Feeding methods, visual fields and vigilance in dabbling ducks (*Anatidae*). *Funct. Ecol.* 16: 522–529. https://doi.org/10.1046/j.1365-2435.2002.00652.x.

Hag-Ali, M., AlShamsi, A.S., Boeijen, L. et al. (2021). The detection dogs test is more sensitive than real-time PCR in screening for SARS-CoV-2. *Commun. Biol.* 4 (1): 686. https://doi.org/10.1038/s42003-021-02232-9.

Hampton, A., Ford, A., Cox, R.E. 3rd et al. (2020). Effects of music on behavior and physiological stress response of domestic cats in a veterinary clinic. *J. Feline Med. Surg.* 22 (2): 122–128. https://doi.org/10.1177/1098612X19828131.

Harman, A.M., Moore, S., Hoskins, R. et al. (1999). Horse vision and an explanation for the visual behaviour originally explained by the "ramp retina". *Equine Vet. J.* 31: 384–390.

Hart, N.S. (2001). The visual ecology of avian photoreceptors. *Prog. Retin. Eye Res.* 20 (5): 675–703. https://doi.org/10.1016/s1350-9462(01)00009-x.

Hebel, R. (1976). Distribution of retinal ganglion cells in five mammalian species: pig, sheep, ox, horse and dog. *Anat. Embryol.* 150: 45–51.

Heffner, H.E. and Heffner, R.S. (1984). Sound localization in large mammals: localization of complex sounds by horses. *Behav. Neurosci.* 98: 541–555. https://doi.org/10.1037/0735-7044.98.3.541.

Heffner, R.S. and Heffner, H.E. (1990). Hearing in domestic pigs (*Sus scrofa*) and goats (*Capra hircus*). *Hear Res.* 48 (3): 231–240. https://doi.org/10.1016/0378-5955(90)90063-u.

Heffner, R.S. and Heffner, H.E. (1983). Hearing in large mammals: horses (*Equus caballus*) and cattle (*Bos taurus*). *Behav. Neurosci.* 97: 299–309. https://doi.org/10.1037/0735-7044.97.2.299.

Heffner, R.S. and Heffner, H.E. (1992). Hearing in large mammals: sound-localization acuity in cattle (*Bos taurus*) and goats (*Capra hircus*). *J. Comp. Psychol.* 106 (2): 107–113. https://doi.org/10.1037/0735-7036.106.2.107.

Heffner, H.E. and Heffner, R.S. (2007). Hearing ranges of laboratory animals. *J. Am. Assoc. Lab. Anim. Sci. 46* (1): 20–22.

Heffner, R.S. and Heffner, H.E. (1986). Localization of tones by horses: use of binaural cues and the role of the superior olivary complex. *Behav. Neurosci.* 100: 93–103. https://doi.org/10.1037/0735-7044.100.1.93.

Heffner, R.S. and Heffner, H.E. (1989). Sound localization, use of binaural cues and the superior olivary complex in pigs. *Brain Behav. Evol.* 33 (4): 248–258. https://doi.org/10.1159/000115932.

Hirata, M. and Kusatake, N. (2020). How cattle discriminate between green and dead forages accessible by head and neck movements by means of senses: reliance on vision varies with the distance to the forages. *Anim. Cogn.* 23 (2): 405–414. https://doi.org/10.1007/s10071-019-01344-4.

Hothersall, B., Harris, P., Sörtoft, L., and Nicol, C.J. (2010). Discrimination between conspecific odour samples in the horse (*Equus caballus*). *Appl. Anim. Behav. Sci.* 126: 37–44. https://doi.org/10.1016/j.applanim.2010.05.002.

Houpt, K., Marrow, M., and Seeliger, M. (2000). A preliminary study of the effect of music on equine behavior. *J. Equine. Vet. Sci.* 20: 691–694. https://doi.org/10.1016/S0737-0806(00)80155-0.

Huber, L., Racca, A., Scaf, B. et al. (2013). Discrimination of familiar human faces in dogs (*Canis familiaris*). *Learn. Motiv.* 44: 258–269.

Hughes, A. (1977). The topography of vision in mammals of contrasting lifestyle: comparative optics and retinal organization. In: *Handbook of Sensory Physiology*. Vol VII/5. The visual system in vertebrates (ed. F. Crescitelli), 615–756. Berlin: Springer.

Hullár, I., Fekete, S., Andrásofszky, E. et al. (2001). Factors influencing the food preference of cats. *J. Anim. Physiol. Anim. Nutr. (Berl).* 85 (7-8): 205–211. https://doi.org/10.1046/j.1439-0396.2001.00333.x.

Hunt, S., Cuthill, I.C., Bennett, A.T. et al. (2001). Is the ultraviolet waveband a special communication channel in avian mate choice? *J. Exp. Biol.* 204 (Pt 14): 2499–2507. https://doi.org/10.1242/jeb.204.14.2499.

Jacobs, G.H., Deegan, J.F. 2nd, Neitz, J. et al. (1994). Electrophysiological measurements of spectral mechanisms in the retinas of two cervids: white-tailed deer (*Odocoileus virginianus*) and fallow deer (*Dama dama*). *J. Comp. Physiol. A* 174 (5): 551–557. https://doi.org/10.1007/BF00217375.

Jacobs, G.H., Deegan, J.F. 2nd, and Neitz, J. (1998). Photopigment basis for dichromatic color vision in cows, goats, and sheep. *Vis. Neurosci.* 15 (3): 581–584. https://doi.org/10.1017/s0952523898153154.

Jezierski, T., Jaworski, Z., Sobczynska, M. et al. (2018). Do ′ olfactory behaviour and marking responses of Konik polski stallions to faeces from conspecifics of either sex differ? *Behav. Processes.* 155: 38–42. https://doi.org/10.1016/j.beproc.2017.09.015.

Jezierski, T., Ensminger, J., and Papet, L.E. (2016). *Canine Olfaction Science and Law: Advances in Forensic Science, Medicine, Conservation, and Environmental Remediation*. Boca Raton, FL, USA: CRC Press/Taylor & Francis Group.

Kasparson, A.A., Badridze, J., and Maximov, V.V. (2013). Colour cues proved to be more informative for dogs than brightness. *Proc. Royal Society B: Biol. Sci.* 280 (1766): https://doi.org/10.1098/rspb.2013.1356.

Kedzierski, W., Janczarek, I., Stachurska, A., and Wilk, I. (2017). Comparison of effects of different relaxing massage frequencies and different music hours on reducing stress level in race horses. *J. Equine Vet. Sci.* 53: 100–107. https://doi.org/10.1016/j.jevs.2017.02.004.

Kelber, A. and Osorio, D. (2010). From spectral information to animal colour vision: experiments and concepts. *Proc. Biol. Sci.* 277 (1688): 1617–1625. https://doi.org/10.1098/rspb.2009.2118.

Kelber, A., Vorobyev, M., and Osorio, D. (2003). Animal colour vision--behavioural tests and physiological concepts. *Biol. Rev. Camb. Philos. Soc.* 78 (1): 81–118. https://doi.org/10.1017/s1464793102005985.

Kemp, A. (2019). *The Effects of Music on Dairy Production*. Murray, KY, USA: Murray State University Honors College Available online: https://digitalcommons.murraystate.edu/honorstheses/41.

Kemp, C. and Jacobson, S. (1992). Rhodopsin levels in the central retinas of normal miniature poodles and those with progressive rod-cone degeneration. *Exp. Eye Res.* 54 (6): 947–956.

Kendrick, K.M., Atkins, K., Hinton, M.R. et al. (1995). Facial and vocal discrimination in sheep. *Anim. Behav.* 49: 1665–1676.

Kendrick, K.M., Atkins, K., Hinton, M.R. et al. (1996). Are faces special for sheep? Evidence from facial and object discrimination learning tests showing effects of inversion and social familiarity. *Behav. Process.* 38: 19–35.

Kenison, L. (2016). *The effects of classical music on dairy cattle: a thesis presented to the faculty of alfred university*, 1–46. Fac Alfred Univ Available online at: http://hdl.handle.net/10829/7243.

Knolle, F., Goncalves, R.P., and Morton, A.J. (2017). Sheep recognize familiar and unfamiliar human faces from two-dimensional images. *Royal Soc. Open Sci.* 4: 171228.

Kogan, L.R., Schoenfeld-Tacher, R., and Simon, A.A. (2012). Behavioral effects of auditory stimulation on kenneled dogs. *J. Vet. Behav.* 7: 268–275.

Koster, L.S., Sithole, F., Gilbert, G.E., and Artemiou, E. (2019). The potential beneficial effect of classical music on heart rate variability in dogs used in veterinary training. *J. Vet. Behav.* 30: 103–109.

Krueger, K. and Flauger, B. (2011). Olfactory recognition of individual competitors by means of faeces in horse (*Equus caballus*). *Anim. Cogn.* 14: 245–257. https://doi.org/10.1007/s10071-010-0358-1.

Lampe, J.F. and Andre, J. (2012). Cross-modal recognition of human individuals in domestic horses (*Equus caballus*). *Anim. Cogn.* 15: 623–630.

Lanata, A., Nardelli, M., Valenza, G. et al. (2018). A case for the interspecies transfer of emotions: a preliminary investigation on how humans odors modify reactions of the autonomic nervous system in horses. *Annu. Int. Conf. IEEE Eng. Med. Biol. Soc.* 2018: 522–525. https://doi.org/10.1109/EMBC.2018.8512327.

Lemasson, A., Boutin, A., Boivin, S. et al. (2009). Horse (*Equus caballus*) whinnies: a source of social information. *Anim. Cogn.* 12: 693–704.

Lesiuk, T. and Braekevelt, C. (1983). Fine structure of the canine *tapetum lucidum*. *J. Anat.* 136 (Pt 1): 157.

Li, J., Li, X., Liu, H. et al. (2021). Effects of music stimulus on behavior response, cortisol level, and horizontal immunity of growing pigs. *J. Anim. Sci.* 99 (5): skab043. https://doi.org/10.1093/jas/skab043.

MacDonald, M.L., Rogers, Q.R., and Morris, J.G. (1985). Aversion of the cat to dietary medium-chain triglycerides and caprylic acid. *Physiol. Behav.* 35: 371–375.

Macuda, T. and Timney, B. (1999). Luminance and chromatic discrimination in the horse (*Equus caballus*). *Behav. Processes* 44: 301–307.

Maddocks, S.A., Church, S.C., and Cuthill, I.C. (2001). The effects of the light environment on prey choice by zebra finches. *J. Exp. Biol.* 204 (Pt 14): 2509–2515. https://doi.org/10.1242/jeb.204.14.2509.

Martin, G.R. (2014). The subtlety of simple eyes: the tuning of visual fields to perceptual challenges in birds. *Phil. Trans. R. Soc. B* 369: 20130040. https://doi.org/10.1098/rstb.2013.0040.

Martin, G.R. (2017). *The Sensory Ecology of Birds*. Oxford: Oxford University Press.

Martin, G.R. and Portugal, S.J. (2011). Differences in foraging ecology determine variation in visual fields in ibises and spoonbills (*Threskiornithidae*). *Ibis* 153: 662–671. https://doi.org/10.1111/j.1474-919X.2011.01151.x.

Martin, G.R. and Shaw, J.M. (2010). Bird collisions with power lines: failing to see the way ahead? *Biol. Conserv.* 143: 2695–2702.

Moore, B.A., Pita, D., Tyrrell, L.P., and Fernández-Juricic, E. (2015). Vision in avian emberizid foragers: maximizing both binocular vision and fronto-lateral visual acuity. *J. Exp. Biol.* 218: 1347–1358. https://doi.org/10.1242/jeb.108613.

Murphy, J., Hall, C., Arkins, S., 2009. What horses and humans see: a comparative review. *Int. J. Zool.* 2009 ID 721798 | https://doi.org/10.1155/2009/721798

Neitz, J. and Jacobs, G.H. (1989). Spectral sensitivity of cones in an ungulate. *Vis. Neurosci.* 2 (2): 97–100. https://doi.org/10.1017/s0952523800011949.

Neveux, C., Ferard, M., Dickel, L. et al. (2016). Classical music reduces acute stress of domestic horses. *J. Vet. Behav.* 15: 81. https://doi.org/10.1016/j.jveb.2016.08.019.

Ollivier, F., Samuelson, D., Brooks, D. et al. (2004). Comparative morphology of the *tapetum lucidum* (among selected species). *Vet. Ophthalmol.* 7 (1): 11–22.

Osorio, D., Vorobyev, M., and Jones, C.D. (1999). Colour vision of domestic chicks. *J. Exp. Biol.* 202 (Pt 21): 2951–2959. https://doi.org/10.1242/jeb.202.21.2951.

Pageat, P. and Gaultier, E. (2003). Current research in canine and feline pheromones. *Vet. Clin. North Am. Small Anim. Pract.* 33: 187–211. https://doi.org/10.1016/S0195-5616(02)00128-6.

Paul, S.C. and Stevens, M. (2020). Horse vision and obstacle visibility in horseracing. *Appl. Anim. Behav. Sci.* 222: 104882. https://doi.org/10.1016/j.applanim.2019.104882.

Paz, J.E., da Costa, F.V., Nunes, L.N. et al. (2022). Evaluation of music therapy to reduce stress in hospitalized cats. *J. Feline Med. Surg.* 20: 1098612X211066484. https://doi.org/10.1177/1098612X211066484.

Pearlman, A.L. and Daw, N.W. (1971). Behavioral and neurophysiological studies on cat color vision. *Int. J. Neurosci.* 1 (6): 357–360. https://doi.org/10.3109/00207457109146984.

Peichl, L. (1992). Topography of ganglion cells in the dog and wolf retina. *J. Comp. Neurol.* 324 (4): 603–620.

Péron, F., Ward, R., and Burman, O. (2014). Horses (*Equus caballus*) discriminate body odour cues from conspecifics. *Anim Cogn.* 17: 1007–1011. https://doi.org/10.1007/s10071-013-0717-9.

Pfister, J.A., Stegelmeier, B.L., Cheney, C.D. et al. (2002). Conditioning taste aversions to locoweed (*Oxytropis sericea*) in horses. *J. Anim. Sci.* 80 (1): 79–83. https://doi.org/10.2527/2002.80179x.

Pitcher, B.J., Briefer, E.F., Baciadonna, L., and McElligott, A.G. (2017). Cross-modal recognition of familiar conspecifics in goats. *Royal Soc. Open Sci.* 4: 160346.

Potier, S., Duriez, O., Cunningham, G.B. et al. (2018). Visual field shape and foraging ecology in diurnal raptors. *J. Exp. Biol.* 221 (Pt 14): jeb177295. https://doi.org/10.1242/jeb.177295.

Proops, L. and McComb, K. (2012). Cross-modal individual recognition in domestic horses (*Equus caballus*) extends to familiar humans. *Proc. R. Soc. B* 279: 3131–3138.

Quaranta, A., d'Ingeo, S., and Siniscalchi, M. (2020). Odour-evoked memory in dogs: do odours help to retrieve memories of food location? *Animals (Basel)* 10 (8): 1249. https://doi.org/10.3390/ani10081249.

Racca, A., Amadei, E., Ligout, S. et al. (2010). Discrimination of human and dog faces and inversion responses in domestic dogs (*Canis familiaris*). *Anim. Cogn.* 13: 525–533.

Reinholz-Trojan, A., Włodarczyk, E., Trojan, M. et al. (2012). Hemispheric specialization in domestic dogs (*Canis familiaris*) for processing different types of acoustic stimuli. *Behav. Processes.* 91 (2): 202–205. https://doi.org/10.1016/j.beproc.2012.07.001.

Ringo, J., Wolbarsht, M.L., Wagner, H.G. et al. (1977). Trichromatic vision in the cat. *Science* 198 (4318): 753–755. https://doi.org/10.1126/science.910161.

Roberts, S.M. (1992). Equine vision and optics. *Vet. Clin. North Am. Equine Pract.* 8: 451–457.

Rørvang, M.V., Nielsen, B.L., and McLean, A.N. (2020). Sensory abilities of horses and their importance for equitation science. *Front. Vet. Sci.* 9 (7): 633. https://doi.org/10.3389/fvets.2020.00633. eCollection 2020.

Roth, L.S.V., Balkenius, A., and Kelber, A. (2007). Colour perception in a dichromat. *J. Exp. Biol.* 210: 2795–2800.

Roth, L.S.V., Balkenius, A., and Kelber, A. (2008). The absolute threshold of colour vision in the horse. *PLoS One* 3: 1–6.

Sabiniewicz, A., Tarnowska, L.K., Świątek, R. et al. (2020). Olfactory-based interspecific recognition of human emotions: horses (*Equus ferus caballus*) can recognize fear and happiness body odour from humans (*Homo sapiens*). *A Anim. Behav. Sci.* 230: https://doi.org/10.1016/j.applanim.2020.105072.

Saito, A. and Shinozuka, K. (2013). Vocal recognition of owners by domestic cats (*Felis catus*). *Anim. Cogn.* 16: 685–690.

Salazar, I., Cifuentes, J.M., and Sanchez-Quinteiro, P. (2013). Morphological and immunohistochemical features of the vomeronasal system in dogs. *Anat. Rec. Adv. Integr. Anat. Evol. Biol.* 296: 146–155.

Sankey, C., Henry, S., André, N. et al. (2011). Do horses have a concept of person? *PLoS ONE* 6: e18331.

Sartor, K., de Freitas, B.F., de Souza Granja Barros, J., and Rossi, L.A. (2018). Environmental enrichment in piglet creeps: behavior and productive performance. *bioRxiv* 346023.

Shreve, K.R.V. and Udell, M.A. (2017). Stress, security, and scent: the influence of chemical signals on the social lives of domestic cats and implications for applied settings. *Appl. Anim. Behav. Sci.* 187: 69–76. https://doi.org/10.1016/j.applanim.2016.11.011.

Silva, F.R.S., da S. Miranda, K.O., de S. Piedade, S.M., and Salgado, MD.D.'a. (2017). Effect of auditory enrichment (music) in pregnant sows welfare. *Eng. Agric.* 37: 215–225.

Siniscalchi, M., Laddago, S., and Quaranta, A. (2016). Auditory lateralization of conspecific and heterospecific vocalizations in cats. *Laterality* 21 (3): 215–227. https://doi.org/10.1080/1357650X.2015.1116541.

Siniscalchi, M., Quaranta, A., and Rogers, L.J. (2008). Hemispheric specialization in dogs for processing different acoustic stimuli. *PLoS One* 3 (10): e3349. https://doi.org/10.1371/journal.pone.0003349.

Sliwa, J., Duhamel, J.R., Pascalis, O., and Wirth, S. (2011). Spontaneous voice face identity matching by rhesus monkeys for familiar conspecifics and humans. *Proc. Natl. Acad. Sci. USA* 108: 1735–1740.

Smith, A.V., Proops, L., Grounds, K. et al. (2018). Domestic horses (*Equus caballus*) discriminate between negative and positive human nonverbal vocalisations. *Sci. Rep.* 8 (1): 13052. https://doi.org/10.1038/s41598-018-30777-z.

Smith, S. and Goldman, L. (1999). Color discrimination in horses. *Appl. Anim. Behav. Sci.* 62: 13–25.

Snowdon, C.T., Teie, D., and Savage, M. (2015). Cats prefer species-appropriate music. *Appl. Anim. Behav. Sci.* 166: 106–111.

Son, J., Park, J., Kang, D. et al. (2020). Effects of white, yellow, and blue colored LEDs on milk production, milk composition, and physiological responses in dairy cattle. *Anim. Sci. J.* 91 (1): e13337. https://doi.org/10.1111/asj.13337.

Stachurska, A., Janczarek, I., Wilk, I., and Kedzierski, W. (2015). Does music influence emotional state in race horses? *J. Equine Vet. Sci.* 35: 650–656. https://doi.org/10.1016/j.jevs.2015.06.008.

Stone, S.M. (2010). Human facial discrimination in horses: can they tell us apart? *Anim. Cogn.* 13: 51–61.

Strain, G.M. (2012). Canine deafness. *Vet. Clin. North Am. Small Anim. Pract.* 42 (6): 1209–1224. https://doi.org/10.1016/j.cvsm.2012.08.010.

Strain, G.M. (2004). Deafness prevalence and pigmentation and gender associations in dog breeds at risk. *Vet. J.* 167 (1): 23–32. https://doi.org/10.1016/s1090-0233(03)00104-7.

Takagi, S., Arahori, M., Chijiiwa, H. et al. (2019). Cats match voice and face: cross-modal representation of humans in cats (*Felis catus*). *Anim. Cogn.* 22: 901–906.

Tallet, C., Rakotomahandry, M., Guérin, C. et al. (2016). Postnatal auditory preferences in piglets differ according to maternal emotional experience with the same sounds during gestation. *Sci. Rep.* 6: 37238.

Talling, J.C., Waran, N.K., Wathes, C.M., and Lines, J.A. (1996). Behavioural and physiological responses of pigs to sound. *Appl. Anim. Behav. Sci.* 48: 187–201.

Tanaka, T., Ikeuchi, E., Mitani, S. et al. (2000). Studies on the visual acuity of dogs using shape discrimination learning. *Nihon Chikusan Gakkaiho* 71 (6): 614–620.

Taylor, A.A. and Davis, H. (1998). Individual humans as discriminative stimuli for cattle (*Bos taurus*). *Appl. Anim. Behav. Sci.* 58: 13–21.

Timney, B. and Macuda, T. (2001). Vision and hearing in horses. *J. Am. Vet. Med. Assoc.* 218 (10): 1567–1574. https://doi.org/10.2460/javma.2001.218.1567.

Tobajas, J., Gómez-Ramírez, P., María-Mojica, P. et al. (2019). Selection of new chemicals to be used in conditioned aversion for non-lethal predation control. *Behav. Processes.* 166: 103905. https://doi.org/10.1016/j.beproc.2019.103905.

Trepanier, L. (2010). Acute vomiting in cats: rational treatment selection. *J. Feline Med. Surg.* 12 (3): 225–230. https://doi.org/10.1016/j.jfms.2010.01.005.

Tyrrell, L.P. and Fernández-Juricic, E. (2017). Avian binocular vision: it's not just about what birds can see, it's also about what they can't. *PLoS One* 12 (3): e0173235. https://doi.org/10.1371/journal.pone.0173235.

Uetake, K., Hurnik, J.F., and Johnson, L. (1997). Effect of music on voluntary approach of dairy cows to an automatic milking system. *Appl. Anim. Behav. Sci.* 53: 175–182. https://doi.org/10.1016/S0168-1591(96)01159-8.

Verberne, G. and de Boer, J. (1976). Chemo communication among domestic cats, mediated by the olfactory and vomeronasal senses. *Z Für Tierpsychol.* 42: 86–109.

Vorobyev, M., Osorio, D., Bennett, A.T. et al. (1998). Tetrachromacy, oil droplets and bird plumage colours. *J. Comp. Physiol. A.* 183 (5): 621–633. https://doi.org/10.1007/s003590050286.

Vorobyev, M. (2003). Coloured oil droplets enhance colour discrimination. *Proc. Biol. Sci.* 270 (1521): 1255–1261. https://doi.org/10.1098/rspb.2003.2381.

Wackermannová, M., Pinc, L., and Jebavý, L. (2016). Olfactory sensitivity in mammalian species. *Physiol. Res.* 65 (3): 369–390. https://doi.org/10.33549/physiolres.932955.

Walls, G. L. (1944). The Vertebrate Eye and Its Adaptive Radiation. *J. Nervous and Mental Disease.* 100(3):332.

Wathan, J., Proops, L., Grounds, K., and McComb, K. (2016). Horses discriminate between facial expressions of conspecifics. *Sci. Rep.* 6: 38322.

Watts, J.M. and Stookey, J.M. (2000). Vocal behaviour in cattle: the animal's commentary on its biological processes and welfare. *Appl. Anim. Behav. Sci.* 67 (1-2): 15–33. https://doi.org/10.1016/s0168-1591(99)00108-2.

Wells, D.L., Graham, L., and Hepper, P.G. (2002). The influence of auditory stimulation on the behaviour of dogs housed in a rescue shelter. *Anim. Welf.* 11: 385–393.

Wen, G.Y., Sturman, J.A., Wisniewski, H.M. et al. (1979). Tapetum disorganization in taurine-depleted cats. *Invest. Ophthalmol. Vis. Sci.* 18 (11): 1200–1206.

5

Animal Learning

Lisa Radosta

Florida Veterinary Behavior Service, West Palm Beach, FL, USA

Introduction

From the moment we are born, we are learning. We learn to walk, master (or just survive) biochemistry, and eventually diagnose all types of disorders in dogs and cats. Learning is so commonplace that it may be regarded as a conscious, non-physiologic process which is influenced only by the capacity to perform the behavior and material being learned. In fact, learning is so much more. It is a process occurring even on the cellular level, by which an animal's experiences alter the brain's neurochemistry and structure (creating or removing synaptic connections), causing an outward change in behavior (Eichenbaum 1996). From the outside, learning looks simple, but inside the brain, learning causes developmental changes, changes in electrical impulses, and the release of neurochemicals. Learning is powerful! As long as animals are awake, they are learning, associating events with consequences even when there is no formal teaching taking place (Marsick and Watkins 2001). These associations enable animals to set up contingencies which alter their perception of events, how they think, plan, and behave with an end goal of staying safe, healthy, and happy. The scientific laws of learning apply to every animal, from honeybees to humans.

Factors Affecting Learning

Learning does not occur in a vacuum, but instead is shaped continuously by extrinsic and intrinsic factors. Memories of lessons learned are stored in the brain as changes to the nervous system – a process called consolidation. Those memories can then be retrieved as the animal needs them.

Intrinsic Factors

Intrinsic factors include the overall health of the pet (e.g. systemic disease, and pain); age of the pet (e.g. puppy, kitten, and elderly); emotional state (e.g. fear, anxiety, stress, conflict, panic, calm, relaxed, and excited); previous learning (e.g. positive reinforcement, positive punishment, and trauma) and genetic makeup (e.g. predispositions).

Fear, Anxiety, Stress, Conflict, and Panic

The neurochemistry associated with fear, anxiety, stress, conflict, and panic (FAS-CP) affects what an animal learns and how those memories are stored. To fully appreciate how emotions and physiologic states affect learning, one must first understand the stress response. The stress

Introduction to Animal Behavior and Veterinary Behavioral Medicine, First Edition. Edited by Meghan E. Herron.

Companion website: www.wiley.com/go/introductiontoanimalbehavior

response is immediate – sometimes starting less than a second after the presentation of a threatening stimulus. It starts with input from the sensory organs sent to the limbic system's first stop – the thalamus. The thalamus then recruits the hypothalamus and pituitary gland, which together trigger cortisol secretion from the adrenal glands. This is known as the **hypothalamo-pituitary-adrenal (HPA) axis** (Figure 5.1). Norepinephrine and epinephrine are also released by the adrenal glands as a result of **sympathetic nervous system** (SNS) activation/arousal. Norepinephrine, epinephrine, and cortisol then act on the body and the brain to cause tachycardia, tachypnea, hyperglycemia, hypertension, immune response changes, and shunting of blood from vital organs to more engaged parts of the body (e.g. musculature) to prepare for fight, flight, freeze, or fidget. Meanwhile in the brain, the amygdala is busy processing emotions and connecting to the hippocampus, which assists in the retrieval of vital memories from the cerebral cortex to aid in decision-making. Finally, the locus coeruleus prepares for motor activity to begin. With so much of the brain and body's precious energy devoted to the stress response, allotting any extra energy strictly to emotional learning (strategies for staying safe) and motor activity, the animal is left with little bandwidth for non-emotional learning.

In fact, cortisol has been shown to interfere with the animal's cognitive abilities and learning when levels of stress are perceived as moderate to high (De Kloet et al. 1999). In other words, animals under moderate to high stress are less likely to learn, to pay attention, and to respond to non-survival-related stimuli (Bodnariu 2005; Walker et al. 1997; Mendl 1999). In addition, the stress response

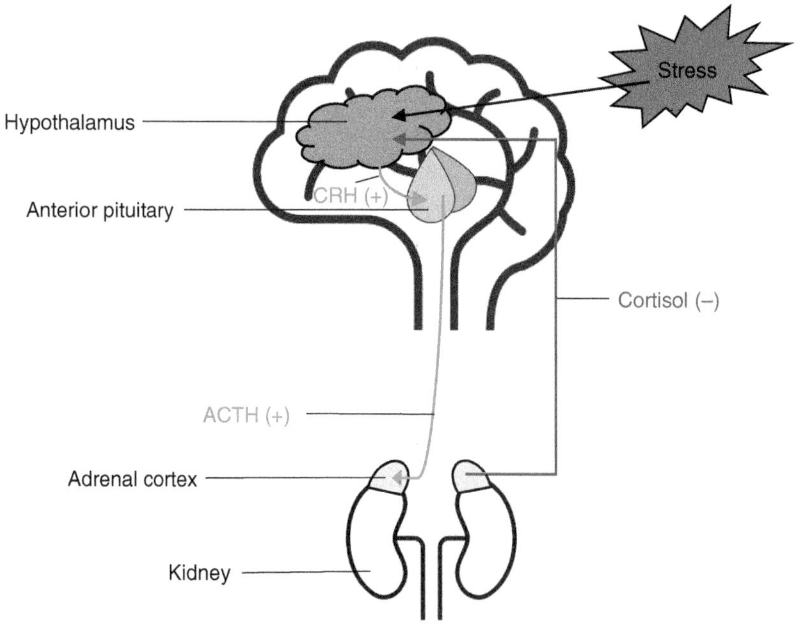

Figure 5.1 Simplified illustration of the hypothalamic-pituitary-adrenal (HPA) axis. Stress triggers the synthesis and release of corticotropin-releasing hormone (CRH) from the hypothalamus. Via the hypophyseal portal system, CRH travels to and acts at the anterior pituitary to stimulate the release of adrenocorticotropic hormone (ACTH), which in turn acts at the adrenal cortex to stimulate synthesis and release of cortisol. Cortisol regulates its own release from the hypothalamus via negative feedback control. Stimulation pathways represented in green; inhibitory pathways represented in red (negative feedback). *Source:* Image credit: Meghan E. Herron.

promotes vivid sensory memories of the environment, people, animals, and inanimate objects involved. Memories created when a dog or cat is suffering from FAS-CP are easily retrieved when the animal is in that situation again. These powerful memories lead to learned behavior patterns that are resistant to extinction (i.e. termination) and are more challenging to change than behaviors learned without the influence of SNS arousal (Johnson et al. 2012). This is one of the reasons why a single frightening visit to the veterinary clinic for a dog or cat can cause an instant and permanent change in behavior, but it may take 60–70 repetitions to teach a dog to lie down on cue. In addition, a fearful or stressed animal will have difficulty retrieving memories of learned behaviors outside of what is required to keep safe in that situation. In other words, a dog who is frightened at the veterinary clinic may learn quickly which efforts allow for escape, as well as what stimuli (e.g. scents, sounds, objects, and people) are associated with pain and stress; and may not be able to perform well-mastered behaviors such as sit or down when asked to do so in that situation (Roozendaal 2002). For all the reasons listed above, to maximize learning when teaching an animal, detrimental stress should be minimized or eliminated. Practically, that would entail teaching new behaviors in low stress situations until the animal is fluent (90% accurate) in performing the behavior, always choosing humane and low stress training methods, and avoiding pain and fear when teaching animals.

Pain

Pain is common in dogs and cats. In fact, up to 82% of dogs and cats presented to veterinary behaviorists have undiagnosed systemic disease or pain (Mills et al. 2020). Whether it comes in the form of orthopedic pain, gastrointestinal discomfort, or pruritus, each ailment has the potential to inhibit learning. In fact, in one study of school-aged children, those with pain had significantly lower reading scores than children without pain (Kosola et al. 2016). As veterinarians, we have an obligation to search out and alleviate animal pain and suffering while never intentionally causing unnecessary pain and suffering. When teaching animals, we should respect and adhere to those same tenets. Always, it should be ensured that the animal can physically perform the behavior being requested and that the performance of the behavior and/or the chosen training method does not cause pain or discomfort.

Extrinsic Factors

Extrinsic factors include type of **reinforcement** (e.g. food, play, freedom to run outside, treats, and toys); salience of the cue or stimulus (i.e. the likelihood that the stimulus will garner the pet's attention); salience or value of the reinforcement (e.g. fresh food versus commercial treats); the environment (e.g. veterinary clinic, home environment, and dog training facility); timing of the reinforcement (e.g. immediately following the behavior, delayed); and the behavior of the handler (e.g. skilled, unskilled, consistent, and inconsistent).

Timing of Reinforcement and Presentation of Cues (Contingency)

When stimuli are contingent on each other, one always predicts the other. For example, when a family member picks up the car keys, they almost always leave the house. The act of leaving the house is *contingent* on picking up the car keys from the dog's perspective. If the car keys are not picked up, the dog can feel comfortable that the family is not leaving. For dogs that have separation-related disorders, the aforementioned contingency can lead to panic behaviors when their human picks up the keys. In another example, from a cat's perspective each time that the caregiver tells the cat to get off the counter, she sprinkles silver vine on the cat's bed as a reward. The cat jumping off the counter on cue predicts the presentation of silver vine.

Lack of clear contingencies and deterioration of previously learned contingencies inhibit learning and contribute to the development of behavior disorders. In the example above of the cat who jumps off of the counter on cue, if the caregiver stops giving silver vine after the cat jumps off of the counter, the contingency is no longer valid, resulting in a lower likelihood that the cat will jump off of the counter. Many caregivers at this point scold the cat, not realizing that it was the change in their own behavior which caused the change in the cat's behavior. The scolding can cause confusion, frustration, and fear on the cat's part, affecting the relationship between the cat and the family in a negative way.

Consistency

Consistent interactions allow for efficient and effective learning. For example, if, when playing with the family dog, one member of the family allows the dog to mouth her during play and the other family member stops play immediately if the dog mouths her, the dog is likely to become confused as to whether or not mouthing is acceptable during play with people. The aforementioned example explains at least in part why animals behave differently with certain family members than others. In the example above, a lack of consistency causes a contingency: when playing with one family member, mouthing is acceptable; when playing with the other, it is not. If the dog understands that contingency and is without FAS-CP about those interactions, there may be few if any problems resulting from the family's inconsistency. When pets have FAS-CP, their behaviors have less plasticity, and inconsistencies lead to behavior problems.

Saliency

The factors which trigger, reinforce, and punish behaviors must be important to the animal and attract and keep the animal's attention long enough to facilitate learning. Saliency is often a factor when family members choose reinforcers for their pets. For example, if a cat gets petted frequently throughout the day on demand, that reinforcer most likely is not salient. Then, when the family uses petting as a reinforcer, it is not effective.

Reinforcement

The act of rewarding a behavior is termed reinforcement, and rewards are called reinforcers. Reinforcement increases the strength of a particular behavior and, as such, makes the behavior more likely to occur in the future. Behaviors that are not reinforced will eventually be extinguished (they will disappear). **Primary reinforcers** are those that the animal does not have to learn to like because they are inherently reinforcing (e.g. food, water, air, sex, control over situations/outcomes, and social companionship). **Secondary** (conditioned) **reinforcers** are previously neutral stimuli which are paired with primary reinforcers and, as such, gain value on their own. Grades, for example, are **conditioned reinforcers**. Grades themselves are not primary reinforcers and have no value, however they are paired with primary reinforcers such as recognition from peers, internal pride, access to additional opportunities, and love from family. Conditioned reinforcers such as clickers are especially helpful for fearful or aggressive patients who cannot be approached or handled. Clickers have been shown to increase the acquisition of new behaviors in many species under many conditions (Paredes-Ramos et al. 2020, Wood 2007). Any sound, word, or item can be a conditioned reinforcer. Some professionals use words such as "yes" or sounds such as the click of the tongue.

Reinforcement can be extrinsic, such as a toy offered by a caregiver, or intrinsic, such as relief from anxiety and fear after escape or pressure on the bladder after elimination. What is considered reinforcement will vary based on the individual animal and is affected by the extrinsic and intrinsic factors mentioned above (Killeen and Jacobs 2016; Schultz et al. 1997). The learner determines what is reinforcing, not the teacher. To that end, caregivers may not know what their pet likes. In fact, in one study on dogs, caregiver's predictions of what their dog valued as a reinforcer were significantly different than the dog's actual preference (Waite and Kodak 2021). Ideally, a functional analysis where the pet is offered several types of reinforcers in a systematic way, even if casually done, should be completed to assess the pet's reinforcement preference. If the caregiver is "reinforcing" with food or play, which is not considered rewarding by the pet, the behavior will not be effectively reinforced. This can lead to a mismatch in the caregiver's perception of the dog or cat's ability to learn or their opinion of their personality. They may call the pet stubborn or say that he failed obedience class, when in fact, the caregiver has yet to find a way to reinforce the pet for the behaviors which are desirable. In this case, the responsibility lies with the teacher (caregiver) to find the right reinforcement so that the learner (pet) can acquire new behaviors.

Different reinforcers may have different values for the same animal at different times of day or in different situations (Cook et al. 2016). For example, a caregiver may perceive that their dog loves petting, and that may be true when the pet is lying on the sofa with them; however, when the pet is asked to do something more challenging than lying on the sofa, such as looking over their paws, they may need the promise of more powerful reinforcement, such as food. In situations where the pet is stressed or distracted (those situations in which we want behavior to change), petting and praise are almost always ineffective reinforcers (Feuerbacher and Wynne 2014; Fukuzawa and Hayashi 2013; Feuerbacher and Wynne 2015) and high value food rewards have been shown to increase the speed of learning (Riemer et al. 2018). Thus, learning effectiveness is maximized when the reward value is adequate from the learner's perspective and matched to the difficulty of the task.

Scarcity of a certain reinforcer can make that reinforcer more valuable to the animal. It may seem logical, then, to withhold or restrict access to certain reinforcers to increase their salience. It follows then that withholding food in the way of delaying meals would increase the animal's drive to learn new behaviors. However, in some dogs, there is evidence that withholding food has the opposite effect on learning. One study found that dogs who were fed a meal 40 minutes prior to training were more successful than dogs who were fasted (Miller and Bender 2012). In addition, in a study of military working dogs, the ability to interact with a food-filled toy regularly increased the ability of the dogs to learn via reinforcement and did not negatively affect the likelihood of playing with a toy, acting playful, or motivation to possess or retain toys when compared to control dogs (Gaines et al. 2008). Because eating and playing decrease stress, the effect seen in this study could be a result of lowered stress in those dogs who had access to food toys. Dogs who are less stressed learn better. Finally, the welfare of the pet should be considered when withholding food for behavior modification. If the withholding of food increases FAS-CP, it will most likely decrease the learning of desirable behaviors. Withholding meals can be detrimental to the quality of life of the pet, and can negatively affect their ability to learn, and is not necessary to increase motivation to learn. Instead, rotating reinforcement types (Bremhorst et al. 2018), scheduling training sessions prior to meals, feeding a small meal before training, and increasing the value of reinforcement will suffice (Riemer et al. 2018).

Punishment

Punishment describes a consequence that, when applied correctly, causes a behavior to decrease or stop. Punishment can take many forms, from removing attention or a toy, to speaking a stern "no," squirting with water, or hitting a pet. For punishment to be effective, the animal receiving it must perceive it as punishing or aversive (salient) so that the target behavior decreases, but not aversive enough to cause FAS-CP; and it should be applied immediately (contiguous) in all circumstances (consistency) where the unwanted behavior is exhibited, but before the next behavior is exhibited (contingency). In most real-life situations, it is challenging to meet the criteria necessary to effectively use punishment as a learning tool. For that reason, certain types of punishment are rarely, if ever, recommended. Just as reinforcers can be conditioned, so can punishers. A conditioned or secondary punisher is a previously neutral stimulus that is associated with a punishing stimulus (unconditioned punisher) so that it acts as punishment. A cat carrier, which was neutral the first time that a cat was placed inside of it, soon becomes a predictor of unconditioned punishers such as car rides, nausea, and veterinary visits.

Timing of Reinforcement and Punishment (Contiguity)

Reinforcement and punishment must closely follow the behavior or be *contiguous* with it for desirable learning to occur. The reinforcement or punishment will have its effect on the behavior just preceding even if it is not the desired behavior. In the next two examples, consider for which behavior the puppy is being reinforced. A puppy who is being housetrained urinates outside. Immediately, the caregiver walks the puppy inside the house and gives the puppy a treat. The puppy was reinforced for coming into the house. In the next example, a puppy urinates outside, and the caregiver gives a treat outside as soon as the puppy finishes urinating. In this case, the behavior of urination in that spot outside was reinforced. Which puppy will be housetrained more quickly? The puppy in the second example, of course, because the reinforcement was timed perfectly and therefore, contiguous with outdoor elimination.

Types of Learning

Learning can be divided into two broad categories: **non-associative** and **associative**. Non-associative learning changes behavior without discrete antecedents and consequences. Habituation and sensitization are two such types. Associative learning (stimulus-response learning) involves discrete signals and consequences to aid in learning. **Classical** and **operant conditioning** are two types of associative learning. While the different types of learning have their own definitions distinct from one another, more often than not, several types of learning are acting on the same animal or on even the same behavior at the same time. There are also different types of responses: emotional, non-emotional, voluntary, and involuntary. Emotional responses might include fear, anxiety, stress, conflict, panic, aggression, joy, and SNS arousal. Non-emotional responses are those that involve cognition and rational reasoning, but not necessarily emotion (e.g. a dog moving his paw to engage in high-fives). Voluntary responses include behaviors which are under conscious control. Involuntary responses include emotions and reflexive responses beyond the animal's control (e.g. fear, joy, tachycardia, tachypnea, mydriasis, injected sclera, urination, defecation, and anal sac expression).

Non-associative Learning

Sensitization

Sensitization takes place when, through exposure, an animal has a more pronounced reaction to a stimulus. It is the opposite of habituation. For example, a dog who lives with a family in an apartment building with a buzzer at its entrance, may become sensitized to the noise of the buzzer. When the dog was adopted, the buzzer was a neutral sound. Then, over time, the buzzer became a more salient stimulus, to which the dog had a more pronounced reaction. The nature of the dog's reaction will depend on the extrinsic and intrinsic influences and classically or operantly conditioned behaviors.

Habituation

Habituation occurs when a stimulus which was previously salient becomes less salient due to exposure, resulting in a decreased response to that stimulus or event, without any positive or negative association. In other words, an animal habituates to something, adjusts to it, and learns to ignore it. For example, a cat hears for the first time a loud coffee grinder. There are no consequences which directly affect the cat when the coffee grinder is in use. In the weeks that follow, each day the coffee grinder is turned on as the caregiver makes their morning coffee. Over that time period, the cat habituates to the sound until the morning ritual of coffee grinding becomes meaningless. In the scenario described above with the apartment buzzer, another dog might learn to ignore the loud noise and habituate, rather sensitize to it. Whether an animal habituates or sensitizes to a previously neutral stimulus depends on the extrinsic and intrinsic factors noted above and conditioning.

Associative Learning

Classical (Pavlovian, Respondent) Conditioning

Classical conditioning (e.g. **Pavlovian conditioning**) occurs when a word, sound, smell, or sight of something, which was previously without meaning (neutral stimulus), comes to mean that a particular event is going to happen and results in an involuntary, emotional, and/or reflexive response. Emotional responses might run the gamut from fear or happiness, and reflex behaviors might include physiological changes such as tachypnea, tachycardia, and mydriasis. This type of learning does not necessarily require an active, conscious response by the participant and can be emotionally positive or negative. Classical conditioning is powerful and is difficult to change once it has occurred.

During classical conditioning, a previously **neutral stimulus** (NS) becomes a **conditioned stimulus** (CS) through pairing with an **unconditioned stimulus** (UCS) to then evoke the same response (UCR) as the unconditioned stimulus, deemed a **conditioned response** (CR). See Box 5.1 for definitions of these terms.

Conditioned Stimuli

Conditioned stimuli are those which were previously neutral and through pairing with a UCS when presented alone, will evoke the involuntary response. For example, a cat hears a can of cat food pop open for the first time. The first time that the cat hears the sound of the can popping open, it does not have any meaning and is, therefore, a neutral stimulus. However, soon after the pop of the can opening, the smell of cat food (UCS) reaches the cat and salivation occurs (UCR). Over the next two weeks, the sound of the can opening (CS) is associated with the smell and the taste of cat food until the cat salivates (CR) just by hearing the sound of the can popping open - before any smell is apparent. The UCS is the smell of food. The UCR is the cat salivating. The CS is the popping of the cat food can. The CR is the salivation before actually smelling the food.

Conditioned Emotional Response

When emotional states are conditioned in response to a previously neutral stimulus, they are called **conditioned emotional responses** (CER). A CER can be positive (e.g. happy, relaxed; Figure 5.2) or negative (e.g. unhappy, fear, and anxiety; Figure 5.3). Often, pets have conditioned negative emotional responses to stimuli in the veterinary office such as scrubs, stethoscopes, and thermometers.

Operant Conditioning (Instrumental Learning)

Operant conditioning (aka **instrumental learning**) includes voluntary actions (behaviors) which are cued or triggered by an antecedent and have positive or negative consequences affecting the likelihood of the response occurring in the future. This paradigm is abbreviated

Box 5.1 The Language of Learning

Stimulus: Anything in the environment (e.g. object, person, animal, or event) and any sensory factors (e.g. sight, smell, and taste) associated with that object or event that cause a sensory or behavioral response.

Neutral Stimulus (NS): A stimulus that does not elicit any emotional response.

Unconditioned stimulus (UCS): A stimulus that elicits an innate emotional response without previous training or learning.

Unconditioned response (UCR): An individual's automatic/reflexive/innate reaction to a stimulus. There is no training or learning needed to elicit this response.

Conditioned stimulus or reinforcer (CS or CR): A once neutral stimulus that now causes a specific response after a period of training where it has been paired repeatedly with an unconditioned stimulus (UCS).

Conditioned response (CR): The learned reaction to a conditioned stimulus (CS)

Classical conditioning: A kind of learning that occurs when a word, sound, smell, or sight of something, which was previously without meaning (NS), is paired with a stimulus (UCS) that evokes an involuntary response (UCR) until the NS becomes a conditioned stimulus (CS) evoking a conditioned response (CR) which is generally very close or identical to the UCR.

Classical conditioning: A kind of learning that occurs when neutral stimulus (NS) is paired with an unconditioned stimulus (UCS) which evokes an unconditioned, involuntary response (UCR) until the NS becomes a conditioned stimulus (CS), evoking a conditioned response (CR) which is generally very close or identical to the UCR.

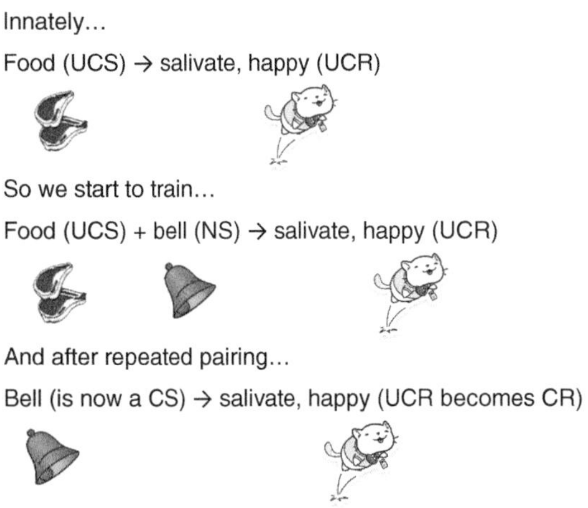

Innately...
Food (UCS) → salivate, happy (UCR)
So we start to train...
Food (UCS) + bell (NS) → salivate, happy (UCR)
And after repeated pairing...
Bell (is now a CS) → salivate, happy (UCR becomes CR)

Figure 5.2 Offering an unconditioned stimulus, in this case a piece of meat, triggers the innate (unconditioned) reflex of salivation and emotion of joy. A positive conditioned emotional response is created by introducing a neutral stimulus, in this case a bell, just prior to offering the unconditioned stimulus (meat). After several repetitions, the ringing of the bell triggers salivation and a positive emotion on its own. This is how the neutral stimulus (bell) becomes a conditioned stimulus and the cat's response becomes the conditioned emotional response.

as A (antecedent), B (behavior), and C (consequence). Antecedents can be intended, such as a client saying, "sit" or unintended such as a veterinarian entering the exam room. Please see Chapter 12 for a more in-depth description of the ABC's of behavior. As explained above, reinforcement increases the probability of the behavior recurring, and punishment decreases that probability. In other words, behaviors followed by pleasant consequences are likely to be repeated (reinforcement), and behaviors followed by unpleasant consequences are likely to be avoided (punishment).

Because operant conditioning depends so substantially on consequences, it is worth reiterating the basics of punishment and reinforcement. Delivery of consequences should follow the guidelines below.

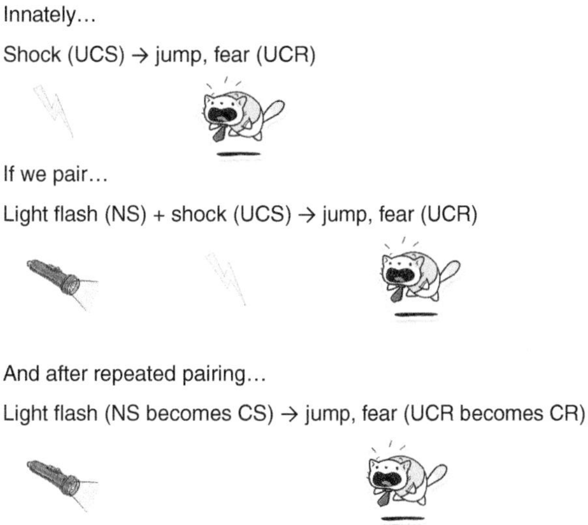

Innately...
Shock (UCS) → jump, fear (UCR)
If we pair...
Light flash (NS) + shock (UCS) → jump, fear (UCR)
And after repeated pairing...
Light flash (NS becomes CS) → jump, fear (UCR becomes CR)

Figure 5.3 Offering an unconditioned stimulus, in this case a shock, triggers the innate (unconditioned) reflex of jumping and emotion of fear. A negative conditioned emotional response is created by introducing a neutral stimulus, in this case a flash of light, just prior to delivering the unconditioned stimulus (shock). After several repetitions (sometimes just one for fear learning), the flashing of light triggers jumping and the negative emotion on its own. This is how the neutral stimulus (light flash) becomes a conditioned stimulus and the cat's response becomes the conditioned emotional response.

1) Reinforcement or punishment should be contiguous with the expression of the behavior on which they are acting, and delivered before any other behavior is exhibited.
2) Reinforcement or punishment should be salient enough to the animal to cause the desired effect without causing FAS-CP or pain.

In operant conditioning, there are four possible consequences which follow a behavior, and each consequence either decreases or increases the behavior to which it is applied (Table 5.1). Consequences that increase the likelihood of that behavior being repeated are known as reinforcers, and the method of delivering the consequence is known as reinforcement. Consequences that will decrease the likelihood of a behavior being repeated are known as punishers, and the method of delivering the consequence is known as punishment. It is also important to note that the term *negative* in regard to operant conditioning means something was *removed* or *taken away*, and the term *positive* means that something was *added*, *applied*, or *given*. Putting them together, we have the four quadrants of operant conditioning:

1) Positive reinforcement
2) Negative reinforcement

Table 5.1 Four consequences in operant conditioning.

	The pet's perspective	**Effect on target behavior**
Positive reinforcement	Something desirable is added/applied	Increases
Negative reinforcement	Something aversive is removed	Increases
Positive punishment	Something aversive is added/applied	Decreases
Negative punishment	Something desirable is removed	Decreases

3) Positive punishment
4) Negative punishment

Positive Reinforcement

Positive reinforcement is the addition of something the animal likes as a consequence of a specific or cued (requested) behavior, resulting in an increase in the likelihood of that behavior occurring in the future. The caregiver is adding something good after the behavior, which motivates the pet to perform that behavior again in the future. For example, a caregiver is training the new family cat to eliminate in the litterbox. When the cat eliminates in the box, the caregiver gives a tasty treat. Positive reinforcement sounds easy; just give animals something they like. However, as explained above, choosing the right reinforcement for the situation and the particular animal, while essential, is not always straightforward. This technique is recommended for training animals, is highly effective when implemented correctly, meets the standard of care, and has the least likelihood of doing harm.

Negative Reinforcement

Negative reinforcement is the removal of something aversive as a consequence of a cued (requested) behavior, which results in an increase in the likelihood of that behavior occurring in the future. The caregiver is subtracting something that the animal perceives as undesirable to motivate him to perform that behavior in the future. For example, the caregiver says "down" and steps on the dog's leash. When the dog lies down, the caregiver takes their foot off of the leash so that the pressure on the collar is released. In this case, the pressure on the leash was uncomfortable/painful and the dog moved away from the pressure when lying down. The movement of the caregiver's foot further released the pressure. In the future, when the dog hears "down," they will be more likely to lie down. When the previous example is examined more closely, it is easy to understand why the risk of injury, pain, and FAS-CP is higher with this technique. For that reason, negative reinforcement is typically avoided. Imagine if you were trying to learn the anatomy of the cat's forelimb for the first time. Would you be motivated to learn if, each time you attempted to memorize a structure, someone pulled on your hair and only let go when you gave the correct answer? Of course not! Just as we would not teach veterinary students in this way, nor should we teach animals with this method.

Positive Punishment

Positive punishment occurs when something that the animal does not like is applied immediately after the behavior which then decreases the likelihood of that behavior occurring in the future. By definition positive punishment is aversive. Methods may include hitting, yelling, grabbing, and holding animals down. They may also use tools, such as choke, shock, and pinch collars. Just as the learner decides what is reinforcing, they also determine what is punishing. For some animals, a raised voice might be punishing, while for others it may not. The risk of physical and emotional injury to the animal is high, and the use of positive punishment can cause intense, generalized fear in situations where the animal associates the pain or punishment with a neutral stimulus and then generalizes to other, similar stimuli. Positive punishment has been shown to be less effective, more stressful, and more likely to lead to serious behavior problems such as aggression toward family members, unfamiliar people, and veterinary healthcare team members than positive reinforcement methods (Hiby et al. 2004; Jones and Josephs 2005, de Castro et al. 2019, Blackwell et al. 2008; Herron et al. 2009; Hsu and Sun 2010; Rooney and Cowan 2011). In addition, dogs trained with positive reinforcement were more outgoing, playful, engaged with their handlers, and easily trained when compared to dogs who were trained with positive punishment who were more likely to be fearful, less likely to play, and were less trainable (Horváth et al. 2008).

Positive punishment is not a recommended method for teaching animals because negative emotional effects are inherent with aversive training, jeopardizing the animal's welfare and the human–animal bond.

Negative Punishment

In negative punishment, something that the dog likes is removed in order to decrease a behavior. Negative punishment can be a powerful yet humane way to decrease behaviors.

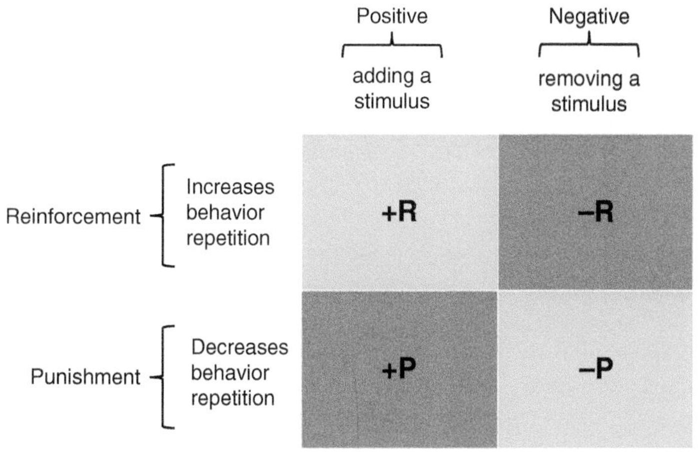

Figure 5.4 Operant conditioning can be broken down into four quadrants: Positive reinforcement (+R), negative reinforcement (–R), positive punishment (+P), and negative punishment (–P). Here the positive (+) indicates a stimulus was added or applied in order to achieve a specific behavior while negative (–) indicates a stimulus was removed in order to achieve a specific behavior. If the result of the application or removal of the stimulus is that the behavior is repeated, then the method is termed reinforcement. If the result of the application or removal of the stimulus is that the behavior decreases, then the term is punishment. Note the (+) and (–) refer to stimulus application and do not relate to emotional learning or whether something is "good" or "bad." The quadrants highlighted in green (+ R and –P) are conditioning methods that do not utilize aversive or unpleasant stimuli to teach behavior and are typically safer, more humane options for training in animals than those highlighted in red (–R and +P). *Source:* Image credit: Meghan E. Herron.

For example, a dog barks at the caregiver as she prepares his dinner. When he barks, the caregiver puts the bowl away and walks out of the room. In this case, the predictor of dinner (food being prepared) disappears, signaling that dinner will not be forthcoming, reducing the likelihood of the barking in the future.

The terminology of associative learning can be confusing at first. The terms *negative* and *positive* in relation to operant conditioning are, as described above, indicative of whether something was added or subtracted (think math equation). In classical conditioning, *positive* refers to a pleasant emotion and *negative* refers to an emotion associated with FAS-CP (think good versus bad). One way to remember the difference between the two forms of associative learning is that classical conditioning is the training (whether intentional or not) of involuntary emotions and their associated reflex behaviors, while operant conditioning is the training of voluntary behaviors, learned through consequences as an animal operates within its environment. Keep in mind that while operant conditioning strictly refers to voluntary behavior, there is an emotional association naturally established with various operant conditioning methods. Animals who experience pleasure during a training session, as they would with positive reinforcement, are likely to feel good about training. Animals experiencing fear, discomfort, or pain during training are likely to feel worried or stressed and, in some cases, respond with aggression as a result of training (Herron et al. 2009). See Figure 5.4 for an illustration and breakdown of the four quadrants of operant conditioning.

Choosing the Right Training Method

Whether recommending a training tool (e.g. collar, leash, and harness) or a training professional, the welfare of the pet being trained should be the top priority. Choose the most effective methods which do not cause fear, anxiety, stress, conflict, panic, or pain. Positive reinforcement and negative punishment are the recommended methods for changing behavior in most animals. They are highly effective and have the least likelihood of harm.

Shock collars, positive punishment, and negative reinforcement methods have a high likelihood of negative emotional and behavioral consequences (fear, aggression). In addition, there are no studies demonstrating quicker learning or improved retention of new behaviors when shock collars are compared to positive reinforcement training (Hiby et al. 2004). As explained above, the undesirable and detrimental consequences of negative reinforcement and positive punishment are many. Training professionals and tools which rely on those methods should be avoided. Unfortunately, too many families reach for punishment-based methods which cause detriment to their pets and make it more challenging to help the pet after the fact.

There are some tools which should never be used to teach animals. Shock is one of those tools. The use of shock, remote training, or electronic stimulation collars at any level of intensity for any length of time is not recommended as a part of a behavior modification plan for pets. The risk far outweighs any potential benefits. Shock collars are considered inhumane and are illegal to use in many countries and regions, including Scotland, Denmark, Norway, Sweden, Austria, Switzerland, Slovenia, Germany, Quebec, Wales, and parts of Australia. Organizations across the globe have published position statements recommending avoidance of the use of electronic collars, including but not limited to the European Society of Veterinary Clinical Ethology (ESVCE), American Veterinary Society of Animal Behavior (AVSAB), Association of Pet Dog Trainers (APDT), Pet Professionals Guild (PPG), Humane Society of the United States, and the United Kingdom Kennel Club. Considering that in the last decade, a dearth of peer reviewed literature has been published showing the risks of using shock collars to train animals, it is no wonder that so many have stepped forward to recommend against their use.

For any punishment to be effective, the intensity of the punishment must be controllable. Too high, and the animal is likely to suffer FAS-CP, and learning will be inhibited (Jacques and Myers 2007; Polsky 2000). Too low, and the punishment will not be salient, and learning will be slowed. Tissue impedance (the resistance electricity encounters to complete a circuit) varies indirectly with the intensity of the shock and is affected by degree of humidity, hair length, hydration of the pet, location of the electrodes on the tissue during the training session, position of the head, dirt and debris on the hair coat, and subcutaneous fat (Jacques and Myers 2007). Many of these variables are outside of the control of the person using the shock collar, resulting in varying levels of shock being delivered to the animal based on environmental conditions without the handler's knowledge. For those animals who wear shock collars much or all of the day, the threat of pain at any moment and at any intensity is constantly present. The lack of control over intensity not only makes using a shock collar less effective, but also inhumane.

Some people may feel that using electronic fencing is less risky than remote activated shock collars. However, electric fencing does not keep people or other animals off the property and may not keep the dog on the property. To that end, one study found that dogs on electric fences are more likely to have escaped (44%) than dogs who are confined by a physical fence (Starinksy et al. 2017).

Another characteristic of punishment which must be met for it to be effective is that it should not create FAS-CP, which inhibits non-emotional learning and affects the pet's quality of life. Studies in dogs have demonstrated the physiologic effects of shock, such as increases in salivary cortisol and heart rate (indicator of physiologic stress) (Beerda et al. 1998; Schalke et al. 2005), stress-related body language, (Cooper and Mills 2014; Schilder and van der Borg 2004) and development of lasting fear of the environment and the person doing the training (Schilder and van der Borg 2004). In fact, dogs trained by experienced handlers who used shock showed more stress behaviors than those trained in other ways, and positive reinforcement training was found to be more effective in teaching target behaviors without the risks to welfare and quality of life (Deldalle and Gaunet 2014; China et al. 2020).

Because shock causes pain and discomfort, it can lead to unintended associations (negative conditioned emotional response) between pain and any person, location, scent, auditory stimulus, object, or animal in the environment (Follette et al. 2019; Blackwell and Casey 2006; Polsky 1994), leading to aggression toward animals and people, refusal to walk outside, unexplained or "unpredictable" panic, and/or FAS-CP associated with previously neutral stimuli (Tortora 1982). Even the tone which precedes shock can cause physiologic changes. Dogs who are conditioned to the tone/shock sequence show increases in heart rate from 82 to 150 BPM after the presentation of the tone and before the shock (Lynch and McCarthy 1996).

Techniques for Changing Behavior

If changing behaviors, even normal ones, were easy, clients would not need help with their pets' behavior problems. In fact, changing behavior can take significant skill. The criteria for changing behavior include:

1) The animal understands the behavior being taught.
2) The animal understands the consequences of performing or not performing that behavior.
3) The animal is motivated to perform the behavior.
4) The animal is not too fearful, anxious, stressed, conflicted, panicked, or painful to perform the behavior.

When dealing with unwanted behaviors or behavior problems, very often there is an underlying emotional component. In these cases, the goal of learning is for the animal to be conditioned to exhibit a new emotional state in response to the stimulus.

Before you can change an animal's behavior, you need to know several things:

1) What is the specific behavior you want to change?
   a) This must be very specific. For example, if a cat meows during the night, jumps up on the caregiver while she is sleeping, and swats her in the face until she wakes up, there are three behaviors to change: meowing, jumping up on the bed, and swatting the caregiver.
2) What will the new behavior look like (e.g. what do you want the pet to do instead)?
   a) This too must be clear. Does the caregiver above object to meowing, jumping on the bed, and the swat in the face? She may choose to change only the swat to the face.
3) What is the underlying motivation/function?
   a) Finding the underlying motivation or function of the behavior allows treatment plans to be tailored to the behavior which is being altered and speeds the process of change. In the example above, the cat wakes up the caregiver in the hopes that she will feed him. His motivation is hunger. The function of the behavior pattern (meow, jump, swat) is to yield food and reduce uncomfortable hunger.
4) What is the reinforcement which perpetuates the behavior?
   a) This is sometimes related to the motivation/function and sometimes it is extraneous to what underlies the behavior. Returning to the previous example, when the pet parent gets up from the bed, she pets her cat, which he finds reinforcing, and she then feeds him. In this case, he is reinforced in two ways for the behaviors exhibited. The function of the behavior was not to receive petting; however, the behavior is further reinforced by the petting.

Reinforcement Schedules

A reinforcement schedule is a guideline which outlines how frequently a behavior will be reinforced. Reinforcement can be given for each correct attempt, a specific number of correct attempts, after a designated amount of time, or after varying amounts of time or correct attempts. The reinforcement schedule being used has a direct effect on the acquisition and retention of behaviors.

Continuous Reinforcement Schedule

A **continuous reinforcement schedule** is one in which the animal is given a reward for each correct attempt. When a pet is first learning a skill, a continuous reinforcement schedule is the most effective. Usually, when the pet is fluent in a behavior (accurate 9/10 times when cued), it is advantageous to move to a variable reinforcement schedule; however, there are some exceptions. First, most caregivers are not skilled dog training professionals and, as such, often do not time reinforcements (or punishments) as they should. For this reason, many pets are effectively on a variable reinforcement schedule, despite the family's efforts to reinforce each correct attempt. Second, most of the problems for which caregivers seek help from veterinarians are related to FAS-CP, such as aggression, separation-related disorders, generalized anxiety, noise phobia, and global fear. Continuous reinforcement is often necessary even after the animal is fluent in the behavior to overcome conditioned emotional responses.

Fixed Interval Reinforcement Schedule

When using a **fixed interval reinforcement** schedule, the pet is reinforced after a fixed amount of time has elapsed. For example, a dog who is fearful of sounds on a walk might be reinforced with food every 60 seconds while on the walk.

Fixed Ratio Reinforcement Schedule

In a **fixed ratio reinforcement schedule**, the reinforcer is given after a specified number of responses. For example, a dog who is fearful of sounds on a walk might be reinforced with food every two steps throughout the walk.

Variable Interval Reinforcement Schedule

When using a **variable interval reinforcement schedule**, the pet is reinforced based on interval of time, but the time varies between reinforcers. In the example above of the fearful dog on a walk, if using a variable interval reinforcement schedule, the dog would be reinforced after 1 minute, then 30 seconds, then 90 seconds, and so on.

Variable Ratio Reinforcement Schedule

A **variable ratio reinforcement schedule** means that the pet is reinforced after a varying number of correct attempts. Considering again the dog on a walk, if a variable ratio reinforcement schedule is used, the dog would be reinforced first for 2 steps, then 4 steps, then 2 steps, then 8 steps.

Extinction

Extinction occurs when a behavior that has been previously reinforced is no longer reinforced, thus eliminating the behavior. Behaviors on variable reinforcement schedules are more difficult to extinguish than behaviors on continuous reinforcement schedules. To be most effective, all possible reinforcers associated with the display of the behavior must be eliminated. When a previously rewarded behavior is no longer rewarded, there is an increase in the frequency of the behavior before the behavior is extinguished, which is called an extinction burst. In other words, when you start to ignore a behavior that has been previously reinforced, it will be offered more intensely before it fades away.

Flooding (Response Blocking, Response Prevention)

Imagine that you are afraid of spiders. Your friend, in an effort to cure you of your fear, locks you in a small room filled with thousands of spiders. Instead of feeling calmer and less scared of spiders, your heart races and you rush to escape the room. This technique is called **flooding**. Flooding (response blocking, response prevention) occurs when an animal is exposed to a fear-inducing stimulus at full intensity until the animal habituates (gets use to it) and no longer exhibits a fear response. For example, a dog is afraid of fireworks and exhibits that fear through trembling and pacing. The caregiver plays fireworks sounds at full volume on a computer to try to "cure" the dog of the noise phobia. For this to work the sound must play it at full volume until the dog habituates. It is easy to see why this method of changing behavior is rarely effective at making the change that we desire, but can be very effective at worsening behaviors which have an emotional component. If the treatment is performed incorrectly, it can result in learned helplessness and/or a worsened fear response. Learned helplessness is a state of emotional paralysis where the animal ceases to learn due to a lack of control over the outcomes of its behavior. In other words, because the animal does not understand how to escape a fear-inducing stimulus or a physical punishment, they cease to try to escape it. One of the first historical notes regarding this type of response was in 1976 (Maier and Seligman 1976), where dogs were placed in harnesses and shocked without a way to escape. Later, when those animals were given opportunities to escape, they did not attempt to do so. Animals can be changed behaviorally in a severe and sometimes irreversible way by **learned helplessness**. Learned helplessness is a sign of inhumane and/or ill-informed training techniques and should be avoided.

Redirection and Distraction

Redirection and distraction involve reorienting the animal to another behavior or stimulus to decrease the focus on the original stimulus. This can be a very effective method of keeping animals from escalating when they are in a negative emotional state. It requires little training prior to use and interrupts learning, which has been shown to decrease the likelihood of associating the stimulus with a negative emotional state. For example, if a cat stalks and pounces on the legs of a certain family member as they walk, the person being stalked can toss a toy when they see that the cat is focused on their feet, but before the cat has pounced. This will divert the attention and focus from feet to toy.

Differential Reinforcement (DRO, DRA, DRI)

Differential reinforcement (**response substitution**) involves reinforcing with a higher value reinforcer for the desired behavior when compared to the undesirable behavior. Alternative (DRA), other (DRO), and incompatible (DRO) behaviors can be reinforced. This is a highly effective way to change behavior when it is combined with extinction. Extinction (removal of reinforcement) for the undesirable behavior is contrasted with reinforcement for a desirable behavior. Continuing with the example of the cat who stalks the caregiver at night, when the caregiver moves around the house and the cat is not stalking them, they can toss a toy or mark the behavior with a conditioned reinforcer and follow with food. In this case, the alternate, incompatible behavior of not stalking her is being reinforced. If the cat is lying calmly, that is incompatible with stalking. In order to create the differential, the cat must never be reinforced for the undesirable play behavior. To do this, the caregiver must continue with redirection and distraction, as described in the previous paragraph.

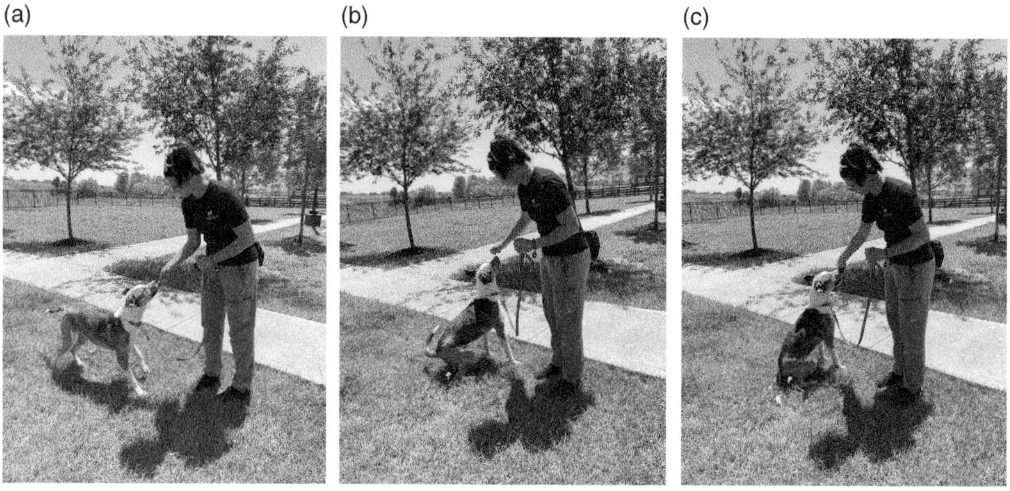

Figure 5.5 A trainer uses the luring method to teach a dog to sit. She allows the dog to sniff and investigate the food lure (a) and then moves her hand down and back in a 45° angle (b). As the dogs nose goes up and back the rear end naturally goes into a sit position (c) at which point she marks the behavior with a conditioned reinforcer and gives the treat. *Source:* Meghan E. Herron (Author).

Luring

Luring involves using a prompt (e.g. food, toy, and target stick) or physical gesture, usually in the form of food, to move the animal into position so that a behavior can be reinforced (Figure 5.5). This is a common way of teaching animals and can be highly effective. Dogs, and potentially cats, are better visual than auditory learners and tend to focus on lures. If the end criteria for the behavior are for the pet to respond to a verbal cue alone, the lure must eventually fade.

Shaping

When **shaping** a behavior, successive approximations of the final behavior are reinforced until the final behavior is achieved. This is one of most common ways that we learn. For example, if the end goal is to graduate from veterinary school, many smaller steps need to be reinforced, such as satisfactory grades on each test in each class in undergraduate and veterinary school. In the case of the cat who stalks the caregiver, shaping can be used to advance the cat from differential reinforcement and distraction to a behavior which is cued. The caregiver would start by using a conditioned reinforcer (clicker) and food to reinforce the behavior of not stalking. Then, they could increase the time required for the cat to remain in a calm state to achieve reinforcement until the cat can lie still for one minute as the caregiver moves around. Finally, the word "stay" can be added just prior to the shaped behavior. Then, when the caregiver moves around the house, they can ask the cat to "stay" and reinforce that behavior.

Systematic Desensitization

This technique is useful for behaviors which are classically conditioned and those for which the underlying motivation is fear or anxiety. The animal is exposed to the fear-inducing stimulus at an intensity low enough that it does not trigger fear (below threshold). The intensity of the stimulus is gradually increased over time in small enough increments to maintain a state of calm and not trigger fear. Eventually a high level of intensity is reached, but the animal remains in a calm state because they have habituated (gotten used to) each step. This method can take months to complete, and it is almost always combined with counterconditioning for the most lasting effect.

Counterconditioning

Counterconditioning is used to alter a conditioned fear response by pairing a frightening stimulus with a pleasurable stimulus, which then causes a strong, opposite emotional response. This technique is often used with systematic desensitization (see Desensitization and Counterconditioning). For best learning, the conditioned fear-inducing stimulus would be presented first, and then the unconditioned stimulus (food, play) would be presented immediately after. Sometimes, that is not possible because the situation does not allow for the intensity of the stimulus to be controlled or predicted. As a matter of fact, this is very common when teaching animals in real-life conditions. For example, during toenail trims in the hospital, food is used to distract the patient. While some counterconditioning does occur here, the learning is not nearly as effective as it would be were the stimulus (toenail handling, trimmers, restraint) systematically graded and the food presented immediately following each step.

Desensitization and Counterconditioning

Desensitization and counterconditioning (DS/CC) results from the combination of controlled exposures to the fear-inducing stimulus at a level below the animal's emotional response threshold with the presentation of a stimulus that evokes a pleasurable emotional response. The timing of the pleasurable stimulus must occur precisely after the presentation of the fear-inducing stimulus. Many caregivers and even dog training professionals express that they have tried this technique before coming to the veterinarian for assistance. Unfortunately, many times they were instead flooding the pet by not controlling the intensity, distance, or frequency of the fear-inducing stimulus, or they were introducing the pleasurable stimulus at the incorrect time. True DS/CC requires a good deal of skill and control over the environment.

Conclusion

Learning involves both emotions and voluntary behaviors and behavior is ever-changing in response to each experience an animal has. Understanding this opens the door to improving the quality of life of the animals that we treat. In turn, a strong foundation in animal learning concepts allows for endless possibilities, including setting up our patients for a lifetime of positive veterinary experiences, recommending appropriate training tools and training professionals, and creating treatment plans tailored to each behavior problem and patient.

References

Blackwell, E. and Casey, R. (2006). *The Use of Shock Collars and Their Impact on the Welfare of Dogs*. Bristol, England: University of Bristol.

Blackwell, E.J., Twells, C., Seawright, A. et al. (2008). The relationship between training methods and the occurrence of behaviour problems as reported by owners, in a population of domestic dogs. *J. Vet. Behav.* 3: 207–217.

Beerda, B., Schilder, M.B.H., van Hooff, J.A.R.A.M. et al. (1998). Behavioural, saliva cortisol and heart rate responses to different types of stimuli in dogs. *Appl. Anim. Behav. Sci.* 1998 (58): 365–381.

Bodnariu, A. (2005). The effects of stress on cognitive abilities in kennelled dogs. MSc thesis. The University of Edinburg, Royal School of Veterinary Studies, Division of Animal Health and Welfare, Easter Bush Veterinary Centre.

Bremhorst, A., Butler, S., Wurbel, H., and Riemer, S. (2018). Incentive motivation in pet dogs –preference for constant vs varied food rewards. *Sci. Rep.* 8: 9756. https://doi.org/10.1038/s41598-018-28079-5.

China, L., Mills, D.S., and Cooper, J.L. (2020). Efficacy of dog training with and without electronic collars vs. a focus on positive reinforcement. *Front. Vet. Sci.* 7: 508. https://doi.org/10.3389/fvets.2020.00508.

Cook, P.F., Prichard, A., Spivak, M. et al. (2016). Awake canine fMRI predicts dogs' preference for praise vs food. *Soc. Cogn. Affect. Neurosci.* 11: 1853–1862.

Cooper, J.J. and Mills, D. (2014). The welfare consequences and efficacy of training pet dogs with remote electronic training collars in comparison to reward based training. *Plos One* 9: e102722.

de Castro, A.C.V., Fuchs, D., Pastur, S. et al. (2019). Does training matter? Evidence for the negative impact of aversive-based methods on companion dog welfare. BioRixiv, https://www.biorxiv.org/content/10.1101/823427v1 (accessed 18 October 2023).

Deldalle, S. and Gaunet, F. (2014). Effects of two training methods on stress related behaviors of the dog (*Canis familiaris*) and on the dog – owner relationship. *J. Vet. Behav.* 9 (2): 58–65.

De Kloet, E.R., Oitzl, M.S., and Joels, M. (1999). Stress and cognition: are corticosteroids good or bad guys? *Trends Neurosci.* 22: 422–426.

Eichenbaum, H. (1996). Learning from LTP: a comment on recent attempts to identify cellular and molecular mechanisms of memory. *Learn Mem.* 3: 61–73.

Feuerbacher, E.N. and Wynne, C.D.L. (2014). Most domestic dogs (*Canis lupus familiaris*) prefer food to petting: population, context, and schedule effects in concurrent choice. *J. Exp. Anal. Behav.* 101: 385–405.

Feuerbacher, E.N. and Wynne, C.D.L. (2015). Shut up and pet me! Domestic dogs (*Canis lupus familiaris*) prefer petting to vocal praise in concurrent and single-alternative choice procedures. *Behav. Processes* 110: 47–59.

Follette, M.R., Rodriguez, K.E., Ogata, N. et al. (2019). Military veterans and their PTSD service dogs: associations between training methods, PTSD severity, dog behavior, and the human-animal bond. *Front. Vet. Sci.* 6: 23. https://doi.org/10.3389/fvets.2019.00023.

Fukuzawa, M. and Hayashi, N. (2013). Comparison of 3 different reinforcements of learning in dogs (*Canis familiaris*). *J. Vet. Behav. Clin. Appl. Res.* 8: 221–224.

Gaines, S.A., Rooney, N.J., and Bradshaw, J.W.S. (2008). The effect of feeding enrichment upon reported working ability and the behavior of kenneled working dogs. *J. Forensic Sci.* 53: 6. https://doi.org/10.1111/j.1556-4029.2008.00879.x.

Herron, F., Shofer, F., and Reisner, I. (2009). Survey of the use and outcome of confrontational and non-confrontational training methods in client-owned dogs showing undesirable behaviors. *Appl. Anim. Behav. Sci.* 117: 47–54.

Hiby, E.F., Rooney, N.J., and Bradshaw, J.W.S. (2004). Dog training method: their use, effectiveness and interaction with behaviour and welfare. *Anim. Welfare* 13: 63–69.

Horváth, Z., Dóka, A., and Miklósi, Á. (2008). Affiliative and disciplinary behaviour of human handlers during play with their dog affects cortisol concentrations in opposite directions. *Horm. Behav.* 54: 107–114.

Hsu, Y. and Sun, L. (2010). Factors associated with aggressive responses in pet dogs. *Appl. Anim. Behav. Sci.* 123: 108–123.

Jacques, J. and Myers, S. (2007). Electronic training devices: a review of current literature. *Anim. Behav. Consult.: Theor. Pract.* 3: 22–39.

Johnson, L.R., McGuire, J., Lazarus, R. et al. (2012). Pavlovian fear memory circuits and phenotype models of PTSD. *Neuropharmacology* 62 (2): 638–646. https://doi.org/10.1016/j.neuropharm.2011.07.004.

Jones, A.C. and Josephs, R.A. (2005). Predicting canine cortisol response from humane affiliative and punitive behaviors. Current issues and research in veterinary behavioral medicine. Papers presented at the 5th International Behavior Meeting, West Lafayette, IN: Purdue University Press, pp. 194–197.

Killeen, P.R. and Jacobs, K.W. (2016). Coal is not black, snow is not white, food is not a reinforcer: the roles of affordances and dispositions in the analysis of behavior. *Behav. Anal.* 40: 1–22.

Kosola, S K, Mundy L K, Sawyer, S, et al. 2016. Pain and learning in Australian primary school students. *Eur J Public Health*, 26(suppl_1), https://doi.org/10.1093/eurpub/ckw165.039.

Lynch, J.J. and McCarthy, J.F. (1996). The effects of petting on classically conditioned emotional response. *Behav. Res. Ther.* 5: 55–62.

Maier, S.F. and Seligman, M.E.P. (1976). Learned helplessness: theory and evidence. *J. Exp. Psychol.: General* 105: 3–46.

Marsick, V.J. and Watkins, K.E. (2001). Informal and incidental learning. In: *New Directions for Adult and Continuing Education*, 25–34. Wiley, 89,.

Mendl, M. (1999). Performing under pressure: stress and cognitive function. *Appl. Anim. Behav. Sci.* 65: 221–244.

Miller, H.C. and Bender, C. (2012). The breakfast effect: dogs (*Canis familiaris*) search more accurately when they are less hungry. *Behav. Processes* 91: 313–317.

Mills, D.S., Demontigny-Bedard, I., Gruen, M. et al. (2020). Pain and problem behavior in cats and dogs. *Animals* 10: 318. https://doi.org/10.3390/ani10020318.

Paredes-Ramos, P., Diaz-Morales, J.V., and Espinosa-Palencia, M. (2020). Clicker training accelerates learning of complex behaviors but reduces discriminative abilities of Yucatan Minature Pigs. *Animals* 10: 959. https://doi.org/10.3390/ani10060959.

Polsky, R.H. (1994). Electronic shock collars – are they worth the risks? *J Am. Anim. Hosp. Assoc.* 30 (5): 463–468.

Polsky, R.H. (2000). Can aggression in dogs be elicited through the use of electronic pet containment systems? *J. Appl. Anim. Welfare Sci.* 3: 345–357.

Riemer, S., Ellis, S.L.H., Thompson, H., and OHP, B. (2018). Reinforcer effectiveness in dogs–The influence of quantity and quality. *J. Appl. Anim. Behav. Sci.* https://doi.org/10.1016/j.applanim.2018.05.016.

Rooney, N.J. and Cowan, S. (2011). Training methods and owner-dog interactions: Links with dog behaviour and learning ability. *Appl. Anim. Behav. Sci.* 132: 169–177.

Roozendaal, B. (2002). Stress and memory: opposing effects of glucocorticoids on memory consolidation and memory retrieval. *Neurobiol. Learn. Mem.* 78: 578–595. https://doi.org/10.1006/nlme.2002.4080.

Schalke, E., Stichnoth, J. and Jones-Baade, R. (2005). Stress symptoms caused by the use of electric training collars on dogs (*Canis Familiaris*) in everyday life situations. Current issues and research in veterinary behavioural medicine. Papers presented at the 5th International Veterinary Behaviour meeting, West Lafayette, IN: Purdue University Press.

Schilder, M.B.H. and van der Borg, J.A.M. (2004). Training dogs with the help of the shock collar: short and long term behavioural effects. *Appl. Anim. Behav. Sci.* 85 (3–4): 319–334.

Schultz, W., Dayan, P., and Montague, P.R. (1997). A neural substrate of prediction and reward. *Science* 275: 1593–1599.

Starinsky, N.S., Lord, L.K., and Herron, M.E. (2017). Escape rates and biting histories of dogs confined to their owner's property through the use of various containment methods. *J. Am. Vet. Med. Assoc. 250* (3): 297–302.

Tortora, D.F. (1982). Understanding electronic dog training part 3. *Canine Practice* 9 (4): 8–17.

Waite, M.R. and Kodak, T.M. (2021). Simple food preference assessments for companion dogs. 2021 Veterinary Behavior Symposium Proceedings, p. 21, American College of Veterinary Behaviorists.

Walker, R., Fisher, J., and Neville, P. (1997). The treatment of phobias in the dog. *Appl. Anim. Behav. Sci.* 52: 275–289.

Wood, L. 2007. Clicker bridging stimulus efficacy. Unpublished thesis. Hunter College, New York.

6

The Development of Behavior and the Shaping of the Human–Animal Bond

Dogs

Marie Hopfensperger[1] *and Jacquelyn Jacobs*[2]

[1] *Michigan State University, College of Veterinary Medicine, East Lansing, MI, USA*
[2] *Michigan State University, Department of Animal Science, College of Agriculture and Natural Resources, East Lansing, MI, USA*

Introduction

When searching for the perfect dog, most people want a friendly personality as much as an adorable appearance. While physical features are largely informed by DNA, a wide variety of factors affect the development of behavior. These include genetics and epigenetics, prenatal experiences of both the fetus and dam, and experiences starting in the first few days to weeks of life, including maternal care, nutrition, and environment. Clients should be informed of the vast array of factors that influence behavioral development and expression, both prior to the acquisition of the dog and while in their care. This chapter will focus on periods of marked physical and behavioral development from in utero to young adulthood in the domestic dog (Table 6.1), with specific lenses for how this information applies to puppies in the home environment and in the veterinary setting.

Developmental Stages in Dogs

Early life experiences have profound and persistent effects on behavioral development (Battaglia 2009; Miklosi 2014; Dietz et al. 2018). A series of longitudinal experiments in the 1960s outlined developmental periods and how experiences in each stage can later affect adult behavior in domestic dogs (e.g. Elliot and Scott 1961; Freedman et al. 1961; Scott and Fuller 1965; Scott et al. 1968; Scott et al. 1974). It is important to be cognizant that this pioneering work was based on puppies who were not reared in typical home environments. It is also worthy to note that the upper and lower limits of each developmental period are soft edges within the process of behavioral development. This section will review the primary literature regarding canine developmental periods, examine recent research regarding experiences during these developmental periods, and consider how to apply the historic and current literature to the pet dog population.

Prenatal Period

The **prenatal period** encompasses the time a puppy spends in utero, essentially from conception to birth. In rodents, humans, and primates, experiences while in utero have been demonstrated to have significant effects on short- and long-term behavior. For example, pregnant female rats subjected to stressful stimuli of sufficient intensity and frequency release glucocorticoids (cortisol) from their

Introduction to Animal Behavior and Veterinary Behavioral Medicine, First Edition. Edited by Meghan E. Herron.

Companion website: www.wiley.com/go/introductiontoanimalbehavior

Table 6.1 Developmental periods in dogs by age – note that age ranges are approximate and may vary slightly in each breed and individual.

Developmental period	Age
Prenatal	Conception–birth
Neonatal	0–14 days
Transitional	14–20 days
Socialization	3 to 12–14 weeks
Juvenile	12–14 weeks to 5–9 months
Sexual maturity	Range 6–24 months, with smaller breeds averaging earlier than larger breeds
Social maturity	Reached around 18–36 months
Senior	7+ years (9+ for toy breeds)
Geriatric	10+ years (12+ for toy breeds)

adrenal glands into their bloodstream, which is also shared by their developing fetuses. When tested later in life, these offspring displayed higher levels of stress sensitivity and an altered **hypothalamo-pituitary-adrenal** (HPA) **axis** (Weinstock 2008).

The degree to which maternal stress and other hormones influence behavior in dogs has not yet been directly explored. One can infer, though, that prolonged cortisol exposure in utero might have similar effects on the developing canine HPA axis, leading to similarly altered stress sensitivities. This concept emphasizes the importance of comfortable, low-stress housing and handing for the pregnant dam. Retired breeding dogs from high-stress commercial breeding operations (CBO) often display persistent and increased behavioral and psychological changes, such as increased rates of social and non-social fear and physical health problems (McMillan 2017). Further, dogs obtained as puppies from pet stores and CBO's have increased incidences of aggression toward human family members, unfamiliar people, and other dogs; greater fear of other dogs and nonsocial stimuli; greater separation-related problems; and more house soiling problems as compared with dogs obtained as puppies from noncommercial breeders (Pirrone et al. 2016; McMillan 2017). While it is difficult to separate between the effects of prenatal and postnatal stressors on later stress sensitivity in puppies and dogs, it can be inferred that stressful breeding practices may have a prolonged influence, regardless of whether transferred during the prenatal period or directly after parturition.

Neonatal Period

The **neonatal period** includes the time between birth and approximately two weeks of age. Dogs are born blind and deaf with limited motor abilities, although they are sensitive to tactile stimuli (Scott and Fuller 1965) (Figure 6.1a). In this underdeveloped state, puppies are dependent on the dam for nourishment, warmth, and elimination. Despite their sensory limitations, neonates are capable of learning and forming associations (Bacon and Stanley 1970a; Bacon and Stanley 1970b; Stanley et al. 1970).

During the neonatal phase, interactions between the dam and pup are frequent, and maternal care plays a substantial role in the social development of the puppies (Figure 6.1b). The quantity and quality of interactions between the dam and pup may influence cognition and behavior at a later age (Bray et al. 2017; Foyer et al. 2016; Guardini et al. 2017). Pups experiencing more frequent maternal care behaviors (e.g. licking, sniffing, nursing, and mother-puppy contact) from birth to three weeks were better able to cope during exploratory and social isolation tests at eight weeks of age (Guardini et al. 2017). Further, pups that received more physical contact from dams were reported to have higher engagement with humans at 18 months of age (Foyer et al. 2016). However, contrary to these results, increased maternal behavior was associated with increased anxiety-related behaviors during a social isolation test and inferior performance during a problem-solving task in

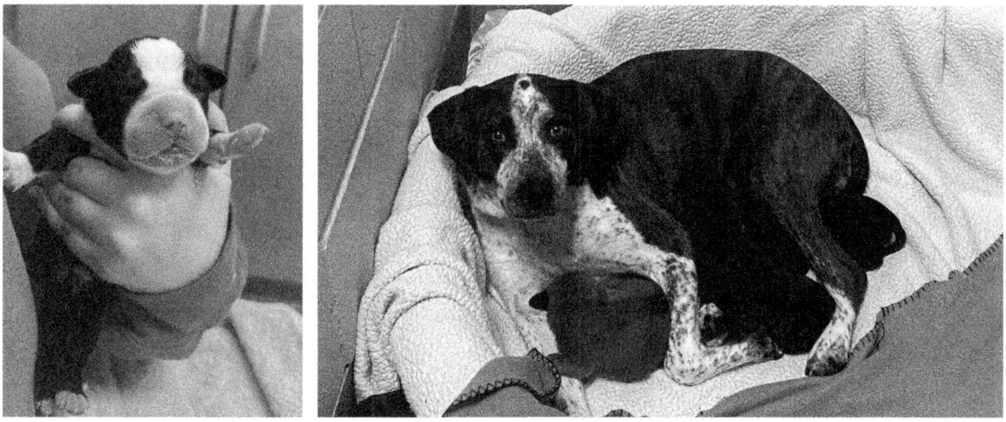

Figure 6.1 A neonatal puppy (a) is blind and deaf with limited locomotor abilities until two weeks of age. During this time, puppies require a great deal of maternal care (b) for warmth, nourishment, and elimination. *Source:* With permission from Hannah Henschen (a), Gigi's Shelter for Dogs (b).

another population (Bray et al. 2017). Rather than a linear relationship with greater maternal care equating to greater coping, it may be that the relationship is curved, as in primates (Parker and Maestripieri 2011), such that extremes on either end of attention are associated with poorer coping in offspring.

While the maternal-pup bond is the primary relationship, reports have also considered the impacts of human handling and stress during this timeframe. Fox and Stelzner (1966b) reported that pups experiencing an hour of sensory stimulation and handling from birth to five weeks were more explorative, performed better on a barrier task, and were more social with humans. In a more recent study, litters of puppies were evaluated, with half of each litter receiving five-minute sessions of tactile stimulation near the dam and littermates from days three to 21. At eight weeks of age, all pups were subjected to an isolation test. Those in the handling group had a longer latency to vocalize when isolated, spent more time exhibiting exploratory behavior, and were generally calmer (Gazzano et al. 2008b). Lyons et al. (2010) reported that brief periods of separation from the mother and littermates resulted in better motor and problem-solving skills. While excessive and chronic stress during periods of rapid neurological development has negative effects, minor, acute stress may improve coping with future stimuli.

Transitional Period

The **transitional period** is of short duration but marked by rapid motor and behavioral changes in the puppy. It begins around 12–16 days of age with the opening of the eyes (Figure 6.2) and ends at approximately 18–20 days (Serpell et al. 2017) with the

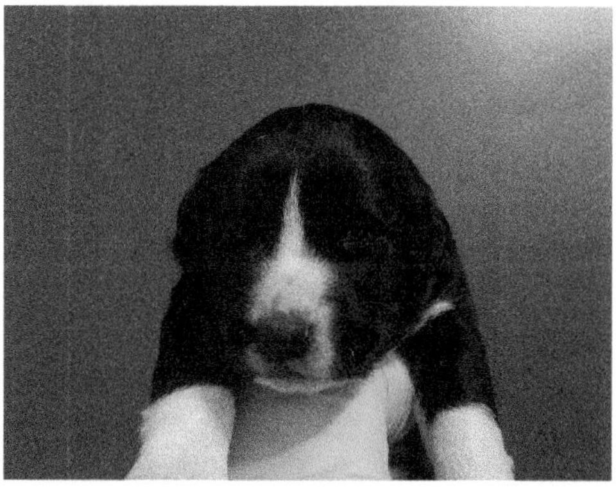

Figure 6.2 A two-week-old puppy opens his eyes for the first time as he moves from the neonatal to transitional period. *Source:* With permission from Gigi's.

opening of the ear canals (and an associated startle response), as well as the ability to stand, awkwardly locomote, and eliminate without stimulation from the dam. As the pups' sensory capabilities are expanding, they become more aware of their surroundings, and distress signaling, such as yelping, will occur if the pup is placed in an unfamiliar environment outside the nest, even if well-fed and warm (Fox 1971). Social interactions with littermates increase during this period, and behaviors such as tail wagging and growling are displayed during engagement in play. According to Scott and Fuller (1965), rates of learning and performance on operant conditioning tasks start to improve as compared to the neonatal phase. Given the increase in motor, social, and sensory capabilities, it is likely that this transitional period is also marked by increased cognitive function.

Socialization Period

Once termed a critical period in the dog's life, it is now understood that the **socialization period,** between three weeks and approximately three months of age, is a notably sensitive phase. The socialization period is a time during which puppies may be especially vulnerable and responsive to social encounters, and social experiences during this time may have a greater and longer-lasting impact in comparison to similar or more extensive social experiences later in life (Fox 1971). Thus, small amounts of experience are very meaningful, and total absence of experience has profound, negative impacts. See the online materials for Chapter 6 for a case example of a puppy presenting with inadequate socialization.

It is important to note that the age ranges that define the socialization period may not be precisely fixed. The lower age range (three weeks) of the socialization period was defined based on the average age at which puppies exhibit a startle response to auditory stimuli (Scott and Fuller 1965). The upper limit (12–14 weeks) is based upon a small group of puppies (n = 9) raised without human contact or exposure to other dogs (Freedman et al. 1961). The puppies reared without human contact were persistently avoidant and fearful of human investigators, while those reared without dog exposure were attacked when reunited with their littermates. When the socially isolated puppies were housed together, they were able to cohabitate without aggression; however, they tended to ignore one another and only exhibited independent play (Scott and Fuller 1965). Despite the limited of evidence to support an exact timeframe of the socialization period, there is general consensus that lack of exposure to social and non-social stimuli during this period has a substantial contribution to the development of problem behaviors later in life (Miklosi 2014; Serpell et al. 2017) and, therefore, should be a priority for clients with puppies between three and 14 weeks of age.

While an absence of exposure has lasting and substantial detrimental impact, interactions necessary for adequate socialization need not be robust in intensity or proximity. In other words, a little bit goes a long way when it comes to making positive, lasting impressions (Figure 6.3). See Box 6.1 for quick socialization tips. For example, Scott and Fuller (1965) revealed that as little as twice weekly, 20-minute encounters with a human provided adequate social exposure for most laboratory-raised puppies. In addition, daily contact with handlers during feeding was enough human contact to avoid significant fear in all breeds except basenjis (Scott and Fuller 1965). Numerous retrospective studies, namely surveys of adult dog owners, have linked undesirable adult dog behaviors (e.g. aggression, separation anxiety, hyperactivity, and increased fear responses) to negative or absent experiences during the socialization period (Appleby et al. 2002; Blackwell et al. 2013; Duxbury et al. 2003). In addition, puppies removed from their dam and littermates prior to six weeks of age had higher odds of displaying destructiveness, excessive barking, fearfulness on walks, reactivity to

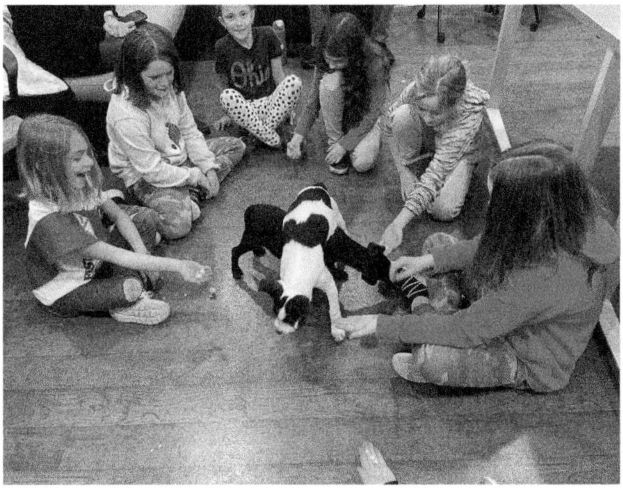

Figure 6.3 An eight-week-old puppy gains social experience with children through gentle interactions with a visiting Girl Scout troop. To ensure a positive experience, the girls allow the puppy to approach them and offer small bits of palatable food.
Source: Meghan E. Herron (Author).

Box 6.1 Socialization: Quick Tips on How and When

- Include the puppy in activities, events, locations, and social networks that the puppy will be involved with as an adult.
- Prioritize introductions with people and animals with whom your puppy will interact as an adult.
- When possible, avoid having the puppy be picked up by unfamiliar people. Rather, allow the puppy to approach and retreat from people and other animals at their own pace. Most puppies will approach on their own if given the time to do so.
- Many puppies will avoid novel inanimate objects. Allow puppies to approach and retreat at their own pace.
- Consider opportunities for the puppy to interact with other puppies and socially astute adult dogs, especially prior to 16 to 20 weeks of age.
- Puppy socialization classes may begin as early as seven to eight weeks of age, as long as age-appropriate vaccinations have been administered at least seven days prior to the first class.
- Maintain a focus on quality over quantity. Approximately one to three new stimuli per week is likely adequate.
- This may mean reducing the intensity and/or frequency of the experience so that it can be positive for the puppy.

noises, toy possessiveness, food possessiveness, and attention-seeking (Pierantoni et al. 2011).

Significant physical maturation occurs during the socialization phase. There are increases in mobility, conspecific play, and investigation beyond the whelping pen (Figure 6.4). Limited only by their developing physical abilities, puppies in their socialization period are likely to approach and investigate human beings and other animals (Scott and Fuller 1965). In a more recent study of twenty-five puppies raised in typical household environments, all of them, eight of whom were under 13 weeks of age, approached a non-interactive stranger regardless of whether the person was oriented toward or away from the puppy (Flint et al. 2018). In a study of six to seven-week-old Border Collie puppies (N = 134), almost all the puppies approached a crouched stranger who called them by name and spoke to them in a

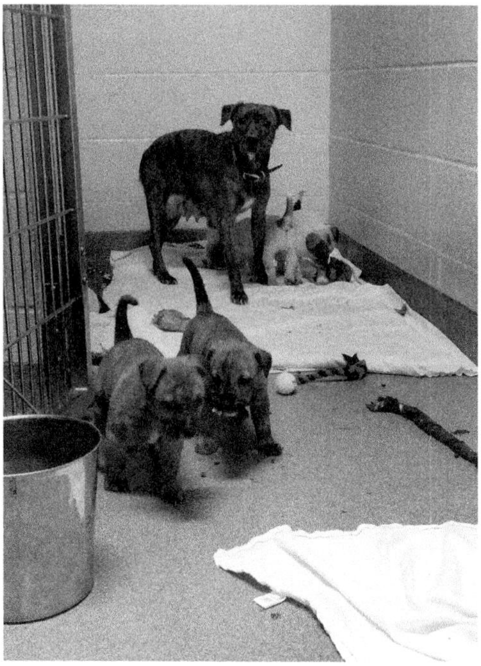

Figure 6.4 Puppies in the socialization period will leave the nest more and more as each week progresses, engaging in play with toys and each other as well as beginning to explore their environment. *Source:* With permission from Chelsea Craig.

friendly manner; however, there was a great deal of variation in how quickly and enthusiastically the puppies did so (Riemer et al. 2013). Most puppies (N = 91) approached within 10 seconds, while eighteen puppies approached within 20 seconds and fourteen within 45 seconds. Nine puppies did not approach the experimenter at all. Thus, typical puppies between six weeks and roughly three months of age should readily approach unfamiliar people.

Due to the domestic dog's capacity to form strong bonds with humans, puppies in this age range also display evidence of innate social cognition skills (Udell and Brubaker 2016). A study of three-hundred-seventy-five retrievers demonstrated that eight-week-old puppies were already adept at attending to human communication (Bray et al. 2020). These puppies responded accurately to a human pointing gesture 70% of the time and readily gazed toward human faces when spoken to. Interestingly, variation in sociocognitive aptitude can be observed from this early age and remains stable into adulthood (Bray et al. 2021; Helton and Helton 2010; Udell et al. 2010; D'Aniello and Scandurra 2016). While these effects are at least partly heritable, with genetic factors accounting for 43% of variation in dogs (Bray et al. 2020), most puppies will demonstrate attention to certain human gestures and verbal communication without any prior training.

Fear Periods

The work of Fox and Stelzner (1966a) has often been extrapolated to indicate a **fear period** between eight and nine weeks of age. However, a critical evaluation of the origins of this period yields tenuous support for such a narrow window of additional sensitivity. In the pioneering, yet ultimately preliminary work of Fox, Stelzner, and others (1966a), puppies were exposed to a control or shock condition upon approaching an unfamiliar experimenter at various timepoints between five and 13 weeks of age. Puppies exposed to the shock condition at five to six or 12–13 weeks of age initially reacted to the stimulus but recovered to approach the experimenter. However, half of those exposed to the shock condition between eight and nine weeks of age (n = 4) formed a lasting negative impression and refused to approach the experimenter ever again. Based on these findings, it has been carried forth in the literature that traumatic experience has the greatest effect around eight to nine weeks of age. However, as the original authors discussed, individual differences in personality and level of attachment toward humans are plausible explanations for the divergent responses of eight to nine-week-old puppies. While further studies would be ideal to best interpret this data, it is safe to say that some individual puppies may be more drastically impacted by trauma than others. In addition, trauma may also have a profound impact at ages outside this narrow window of time.

Juvenile Period

The **juvenile period** begins as the socialization period wanes and ends with the onset of **sexual maturity**. Although this phase is understudied, it is likely that this period of continued growth and development is equally sensitive to experiences and may have lasting impact on behavior. In one study, lack of exposure to urban environments (e.g. well-trafficked roads, pedestrians, and other dogs) between three and six months of age was associated with aggression toward unfamiliar people and avoidance of unfamiliar people and dogs, as well as apprehension related to sounds and other environmental stimuli, getting into the car, and going on walks (Appleby et al. 2002). Several studies have investigated working dog success and reported associations between experiences during the juvenile period and adult behavior based on owner and handler surveys and behavioral assessments (Foyer et al. 2014; Harvey et al. 2016; Serpell and Duffy 2016; Gazzano et al. 2008c). Therefore, the juvenile period should be considered an extension of the socialization phase and prioritized as such.

Sexual Maturity

Considered the onset of puberty, the age at which domestic dogs begin sexual maturity ranges from six to nine months of age, with variation based on size, breed, and individual differences. Miniature and small breeds tend to reach full sexual maturity earlier, around six to seven months, in comparison to 18 or even 24 months for some giant breed dogs. At the onset of sexual maturity, dogs and puppies are capable of reproduction. This period is also marked by the expression of sexually dimorphic physical and behavioral traits. The total array of sexually dimorphic behaviors in dogs is not universally agreed upon but includes urination posture and marking, mounting, roaming, and inter-male aggression (Hart and Eckstein 1997).

Several studies have demonstrated that sexually dimorphic behaviors respond to castration (McGuire 2019; McGreevy et al. 2018; Palestrini et al. 2021; Maarschalkerweerd et al. 1997; Neilson et al. 1997; Hopkins et al. 1976). McGuire (2019) reported a decrease in urine marking in shelter dogs post-castration while Palestrini et al. (2021) found that mounting and roaming decreased significantly in their observed population of 15 dogs. These studies agree with earlier work on the effect of castration on reducing urine marking, mounting, roaming, and aggression between male dogs (Hopkins et al. 1976; Maarschalkerweerd et al. 1997; Neilson et al. 1997).

Recent data regarding the impact of castration on aggression is conflicting. A survey of more than thirteen thousand respondents revealed that neither gonadectomy nor age at gonadectomy were associated with aggressive behavior toward familiar people or dogs (Farhoody et al. 2018). In this study, there was a low but significant increase in the odds of moderate or severe aggression toward strangers for all gonadectomized dogs compared with intact dogs. Further, Palestrini et al. (2021) reported a trend but no statistical significance in aggression toward familiar human household members after castration. Neilson et al. (1997) found aggression toward unfamiliar people had a less than 1% chance of improvement post-castration, while aggression toward housemate dogs and family members was diminished in about 25% of the population. Based on the current literature, castration should not be recommended as a primary or sole treatment for aggression.

Data regarding age of gonadectomy and its effect on behavior are challenging to interpret for many reasons. Most of the literature is retrospective in nature, no studies have randomly assigned dogs to different ages of gonadectomy, and all have significant confounding variables. The current breadth of literature is reviewed here with the caveat that numerous unanswered questions remain.

Many sheltering organizations perform prepubertal gonadectomy per the Association of Shelter Veterinarians' Guidelines for Spay-Neuter Programs (2016). Given that almost a quarter of dogs are adopted from shelters and humane societies, many patients will have been spayed or neutered prior to adoption. In a study of two-hundred-sixty-nine shelter dogs, Howe et al. (2001) reported that prepubertal gonadectomy, defined as prior to 24 weeks of age, did not result in an increased incidence of behavioral problems. In another study, behavioral benefits of early-aged gonadectomy included reduced frequency of separation anxiety, escape behaviors, and inappropriate elimination when frightened in both male and female dogs (Spain et al. 2004). However, Spain et al. (2004) also reported a correlation between decreasing age of gonadectomy and increased noise phobia in both males and females, and in male dogs, excessive vocalization was correlated with an earlier age of gonadectomy. Further, aggression toward family members was more frequent in male dogs castrated at less than 5.5 months of age (Spain et al. 2004).

Two studies looked at Canine Behavior Assessment and Research Questionnaire (C-BARQ) scores relative to age of gonadectomy (Starling et al. 2019; McGreevy et al. 2018) and reported that some expressions of anxiety and aggression decreased with increasing age of gonadectomy. However, earlier age of spay was correlated with reductions in howling and chewing, as well as improved retrieval and recall (Starling et al. 2019). In castrated male dogs, a reduction in howling and urine marking was reported (McGreevy et al. 2018).

There is conflicting information regarding the age of spay and urinary issues in female dogs. One study reported that female dogs spayed prior to three months of age may have an increased risk of urinary incontinence (Spain et al. 2004). However, Stöcklin-Gautschi et al. (2001) reported that half as many (9.7%) female dogs spayed before their first heat cycle had urinary incontinence as compared to those spayed after their first estrus. Howe et al. (2001) found no difference in urinary incontinence in female dogs spayed before or after 24 weeks of age.

Regardless of the age of gonadectomy, there appear to be no negative impacts on trainability, and retention in the home may be improved in spayed and neutered dogs (Serpell and Hsu 2005; Spain et al. 2004; Kustritz 2002; Howe et al. 2001). In summary, the age of gonadectomy may have limited behavioral relevance for most pet dogs.

Social Maturity

Social maturity is a time when dogs demonstrate their full repertoire of adult dog behavior. The timeframe of social maturity in dogs is not well defined in the literature, and little data exists about this developmental period. Anecdotally, social maturity may be reached somewhere in the range of 18–36 months of age. This timeframe may have some parallels to post-pubertal development described in other species. In humans, it has been demonstrated that the prefrontal cortex undergoes a prolonged course of maturation after puberty and into early adulthood (Nelson and Guyer 2011; Amlien et al. 2016). It is in this transition from adolescence to adulthood that humans may be diagnosed with mental health concerns (Solmi et al. 2022). Similarly, it is in young adulthood that dogs may be most likely to exhibit behavioral health concerns, which place them at risk for relinquishment (Protopopova and Gunter 2017; Salman et al. 1998). While further research on this period is warranted, clinical evidence suggests that dogs' responses to stimuli may change as they progress through social maturity, with a transition from avoidant manifestations of fear in puppyhood to more overt signs of fear aggression in adulthood. For example, a dog who, as a puppy, barked and retreated in response to a stranger may start to move forward in a more offensive manner by barking, lunging, and snapping (even biting) as they become more socially mature.

Neonatal: Pups experience rapid neurological development but are entirely dependent on the dam. Short, gentle handling bouts by humans during this period may improve resiliency in response to stressors, although the degree to which it may influence future behavior remains unknown.

Transitional: The transitional period is brief, lasting approximately one week. It is marked by the opening of the eyes and ear canals and expanding motor function. Social play behavior with littermates and interest in solid food begin although the puppy-dam relationship is still the primary source of nourishment and comfort.

Socialization: Between approximately three weeks to three months, the socialization period marks a time when small amounts of experience may be very meaningful and when total absence of social exposure has profound consequences. Families of puppies in this sensitive period may be directed toward the following recommendations, although they should be informed that experiences during the socialization period may not override the effects of genetics, epigenetics, nor particularly notable experiences for the puppy prior to three weeks and past three months of age.

If concerns arise, look to improve quality, *not* frequency.

Juvenile: The juvenile period begins around three months of age and ends at the onset of sexual maturity, which varies based on breed or size of the dog. Experiences during the juvenile period are likely to influence future behavior, along with the hormonal and cognitive changes that occur during this time. Consider the juvenile phase as an extension of the socialization period.

Sexual maturity: This is the age range when dogs can reproduce and may start to demonstrate sexually dimorphic behavior, such as urine marking, mounting, roaming, and conspecific aggression. However, many of our canine patients may have undergone prepubertal gonadectomy, making this phase much less remarkable.

Social maturity: This is a time when dogs demonstrate their full repertoire of adult dog behavior. For example, a puppy who seemed shy may demonstrate fear-motivated aggression as an adult. Dogs are at increased risk of relinquishment between one and two years of age. Therefore, clients should be invited to share concerns over their dog's behavior, counseled on ways to manage problem behaviors, or provided with contact information for reputable behavior specialists.

Veterinary Care

Appropriate and timely veterinary visits are essential for the physical health of the growing puppy. They also coincide with behavioral development milestones, which can inform expectations of and interactions with puppy patients and provide opportunities for education and early interventions if behavioral concerns arise.

First Puppy Visits

These initial veterinary visits often occur during the sensitive period of socialization and at an age when long-lasting fearful memories can be formed. Therefore, the utmost caution should be taken so as not to scare the puppy and to allow for the most pleasant visit possible. There is also evidence to indicate that allocating time and resources to the initial puppy visit has a lasting impact. Spending one hour offering behavioral advice regarding normal puppy development and basic training resulted in improved behavior for the dogs as adults (Gazzano et al. 2008a); specifically, clients receiving advice reported less aggression toward unfamiliar people and dogs, house soiling, mounting, excessive play behavior, mouthing, and begging for food.

The first veterinary visit allows the clinician and staff to evaluate the puppy's response to an unfamiliar environment with a variety of social and non-social stimuli. Puppies in this age range are likely to approach and investigate human beings and other animals (Flint et al. 2018; Riemer et al. 2013; Scott and Fuller 1965). It is important to note that in these studies, experimenters were stationary, for example, quietly seated on the floor or crouched while calling the puppy. Based on these studies, allowing the puppy to approach on its own may be most comfortable for the puppy and informative to the care team. It may be worthwhile to document the puppy's speed and demeanor of approach in the medical record.

A puppy's investigation of people should not, however, be interpreted as being comfortable with restraint. According to Riemer et al. (2013), all but two puppies struggled and most vocalized when gently cradled in a dorsally recumbent position by a person seated on the floor. These same puppies also varied in their responses to veterinary examination, with 38% being passive and tolerant, 28% mouthing or licking, 25% attempting to escape, and 9% exhibiting a combination of both escape behaviors and interaction with the handler. Social puppies who exhibited rapid approach, tail wagging, jumping up, pawing, and rolling over were more likely to be interactive versus showing a passive response during handling. Thus, indications of a puppy's comfort with handling include being wiggly, mouthy, and playful with staff. On the other hand, puppies who freeze may be easy to handle but are actually quite fearful. It is also important to consider that fearful puppies may be passive during restraint when they are young, but adult dogs may manifest their fear through active efforts to escape or aggression. See Chapter 11 for details on fight, flight, freeze, and fidget responses to stress/threats in dogs.

Whereas typical puppies are expected to approach unfamiliar people, most puppies exhibit avoidance of novel, non-social stimuli (Flint et al. 2018). The age at which avoidance is observed ranges from five to eight weeks of age and varies by breed (Morrow et al. 2015) but should subside by five to six months of age (Hansen et al. 2019). Extrapolating these data to the veterinary clinic setting, care team members should anticipate that the hospital environment and equipment may startle puppy patients, especially before four to five months of age. Introduce medical equipment to puppies slowly while providing palatable treats for counterconditioning and ample reassurance. If a puppy is alarmed by an item, exhibit patience and consider how essential it is to complete that task.

For some puppies, the location of examination and the presence of a familiar household member are meaningful. Several studies have reported the physiologic impact on canine blood pressure, heart rate, and temperature when dogs are examined away from the client (Mandese et al. 2021; Csoltova et al. 2017; Höglund et al. 2012). In addition, Mandese et al. (2021) reported higher fear, anxiety, and stress scores when dogs were examined in the treatment area. When placed on the examination table, most dogs exhibited signs of fear, especially trembling, crouched posture, and a tucked tail (Döring et al. 2009). In addition, more than 70% of dogs exhibited avoidance behaviors, manifesting as leaning away from the veterinarian, leaning into their familiar person, and/or attempting to jump off the table. Clients petting and talking to their dogs during examinations reduced the likelihood of the dog attempting to jump off the examination table (Csoltova et al. 2017). Based on these findings, it is recommended to perform initial puppy examinations and procedures with a family member present and consider alternatives to the examination table and treatment area. Please refer to Chapter 11 for additional handling tips to minimize fear, anxiety, and stress during puppy and adult veterinary visits.

Godbout and Frank (2011a) reported that puppies exhibiting anxiety at the initial veterinary visit exhibited similar signs one year later. Therefore, it is important to identify these outlier puppies early and use extra care in their handling.

Puppy Visit Checklist

- Allocate time during puppy visits to educate clients about behavior and reward-based training.
- Puppy-proof the exam room, removing access to trash cans or other items puppies might chew or consume.
- Set out toys and treats to encourage oral exploration of appropriate items.

- Select appropriately sized equipment (e.g. 25-gauge needles, pediatric stethoscope, etc.).
- When greeting, allow puppies to approach you rather than you approaching the puppy; document how quickly the puppy approaches.
- Consider performing your examination on the floor or on your lap.
- Encourage cooperation and condition a positive emotion with the experience by pairing handling and procedures with high-value, lickable treats.
- Give the puppy breaks during examination and in between procedures.
- Prioritize procedures and refrain from performing extraneous tasks (e.g. do not trim toenails, clean ears, etc. unless necessary).

Future Visits

Subsequent visits allow for behavioral reevaluation and comparison to previous visits. As the environment becomes less novel, the veterinary hospital acquires associations for the puppy, which may be positive, neutral, or negative. Fear conditioning serves as self-preservation, and dogs with prior negative experiences are more likely to exhibit fearful behavior at subsequent appointments (Döring et al. 2009). Whereas 10% of puppies under 16 weeks of age exhibit social avoidance, excessive locomotion, panting, and/or vocalization at their first veterinary visit (Godbout et al. 2007), 41–78.5% of adult dogs demonstrate evidence of fear in the veterinary clinic setting (Edwards et al. 2019a and 2019b; Mariti et al. 2017; Mariti et al. 2015; Döring et al. 2009; Stanford 1981). This indicates that many dogs have negative veterinary experiences during puppyhood and adolescence. Once dogs have developed a negative emotional association with the veterinary clinic, it can be difficult to reverse it. One study reported minimal improvement from weekly "happy visits" for adult dogs with existing veterinary-related anxiety (Stellato et al. 2019). Thus, the onus is on veterinary professionals to make puppy appointments as positive as possible. Prevention may have a more profound impact than trying to undo the negative impacts of frightening veterinary experiences.

Behavior Support for Clients

Puppy Classes

Studies have consistently identified that attendance in puppy class (Figure 6.5) improves trainability and response to cues (Gonzalez-Martinez et al. 2019; Kutsumi et al. 2013; Seksel et al. 1999). Puppy class attendance has also been associated with reductions in non-social fear, fear of noises, crate-related fear, and sensitivity to touch (Gonzalez-Martinez et al. 2019; Cutler et al. 2017). Aggression, compulsive behavior, destructive behavior, and excessive barking were reduced in dogs that attended puppy training before six months of age compared to dogs that never attended puppy classes (Dinwoodie et al. 2021).

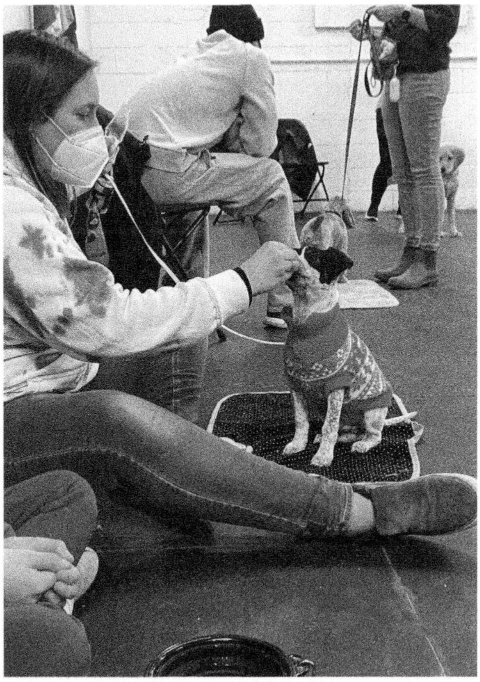

Figure 6.5 An appropriately designed puppy socialization class provides social exposure to people, other dogs, novel items, and body handling in a safe and controlled manner. *Source:* Meghan E. Herron (Author).

Several studies have reported how puppy class impacts inter-dog interactions. Puppies that attended puppy classes had exposure to a greater number of other dogs between 14 and 20 weeks of age as compared to puppies that did not attend classes (Cutler et al. 2017). Puppy class attendees were less likely to exhibit undesirable reactions to dogs from outside the household (Blackwell et al. 2008), more likely to exhibit friendly approaches toward unfamiliar dogs (Martin, unpublished thesis), and have a reduced likelihood of inter-dog aggression within the household (Gonzalez-Martinez et al. 2019). Similarly, studies have evaluated puppy class attendance as it relates to interactions with unfamiliar people. Puppies that attended puppy classes received exposure to a greater number of people between 10 and 20 weeks of age as compared to those with no class attendance (Cutler et al. 2017). Puppy class attendance has been associated with more positive responses to strangers (Kutsumi et al. 2013) and reduced aggression toward unfamiliar people (Casey et al. 2014). Clients who did not attend puppy classes had increased odds of reporting problem behaviors in their dogs at nine months of age (Lord et al. 2020). Retention within the home has been documented as a potential benefit of puppy class enrollment (Schulkey and DePorter 2017; Duxbury et al. 2003).

There is evidence to indicate that puppies may attend training and/or socialization classes prior to completion of their vaccine series. One study found that two-hundred-seventy-nine vaccinated puppies attending socialization classes were at no greater risk of Parvovirus infection than vaccinated non-attendees (Stepita et al. 2013). Per the 2008 AVSAB Position Statement on Puppy Socialization, puppies may start puppy socialization classes as early as seven to eight weeks of age if they have received age-appropriate vaccinations at least seven days prior to the first class. The American Animal Hospital Association (AAHA) Canine Vaccination Guidelines (2017) can serve as a framework for developing puppy-class vaccine protocols.

In summary, attendance at socialization classes offers many potential long-term behavioral benefits that may outweigh physical health risks, which can be mitigated with timely vaccinations.

Identifying Behavior Support

There is an extensive amount of information and misinformation to be found regarding puppy behavior and training (Browne, et al. 2017). Searching on their own, clients will find many options for behavior modification and training support, some of which are considered more humane than others (Kuhl et al. 2022). It is our job as veterinarians to steer clients toward humane training that is based on science and supported by the literature. We now know that positive reinforcement training is less stressful than aversive training and has been associated with improved human-animal interactions (Vieira de Castro et al. 2020; Ziv 2017; Deldalle and Gaunet 2014), while behavioral interventions associated with confrontational techniques have been associated with aggression (Herron et al. 2009). The effectiveness of reward-based training has also been demonstrated in several studies (Blackwell et al. 2012; Haverbeke et al. 2008; Hiby et al. 2004). With appropriate guidance from their veterinarian and puppy class instructors, clients are less likely to utilize positive punishment with their dogs (Lord et al. 2020; Cutler et al. 2017).

Trainers who utilize humane methodologies may identify themselves as force-free, reward-based, or LIMA (least intrusive, minimally aversive). They may also highlight their reliance on positive reinforcement techniques and indicate that they do not utilize positive punishment. There are several organizations with which dog trainers may be affiliated or through which dog trainers may become certified. See Chapter 12 for a breakdown of training certifications and professional organizations whose techniques are supported by the current scientific body of literature.

Managing Typical Puppy Behaviors

Oral Behaviors

Mouthing

Mouthing is normal for puppies regardless of size, origin, breed, and sex and may be first observed during conspecific interactions around three weeks of age (Godbout and Frank 2011b; Pal 2010). Mouthing also persists into young adulthood, with a taper after about one year of age (Waite et al. 2021). It is important to note that excessive mouthing is unlikely to be associated with future aggression (Godbout and Frank 2011b; Scott and Fuller 1965). Godbout and Frank (2011b) followed sixty-one puppies, thirty-eight of whom mouthed excessively, until three years of age. Retention of puppies in the household was not affected by the presence of mouthing behavior in puppyhood, and there was no significant difference between puppies who mouthed excessively and those that did not in the development of aggression at one or three years of age.

From a functional perspective, one small study reported that mouthing was maintained by attention (Waite and Kodak 2022). Thus, teaching a puppy that there are other ways (e.g. bringing a toy, sitting, and lying down) to obtain attention and providing that attention at a satiating frequency may be important tools. It is also worth mentioning that clients may inadvertently ignore their puppy when it is behaving calmly. Thus, there may be a benefit to the clients initiating attention when the puppy is spontaneously offering independent behavior (e.g. self-directed play, resting, etc.). Commonly recommended interventions include high-pitched vocalization when mouthing is too hard, ceasing interactions, and redirecting (e.g. to play with an appropriate toy or chew item). These are not well studied but can be effective means of interrupting mouthing in the moment. While evidence is lacking to indicate how play with other dogs impacts mouthing toward humans, the authors recommend ensuring the puppy has the opportunity for regular conspecific play to meet its social needs. Such interactions may serve to satisfy the puppy's desire for oral play and allow the puppy to learn elements of bite inhibition from other dogs.

Chewing

The transition from suckling to chewing motions correlates with the timing of deciduous dentition eruptions (Ikuno 1989), and the frequency of chewing may be greater in dogs under one year of age (Arhant et al. 2021). In a survey of over a thousand dog owners, 94% offered chewable items to their dogs, and less than 3% of dogs were reported to chew on household items daily (Arhant et al. 2021). In this same study, chewing was most likely to occur during social isolation and changes in routine, and the need for veterinary treatment related to ingesting foreign material was only reported by 3.6% of the clients studied. Recommended management strategies for chewing include limiting access to inappropriate items (e.g. puppy proofing the home) and providing an array of suitable chew items of varying sizes, textures, and edibility. Crating or confinement at times when the family cannot supervise the puppy's chewing behaviors may be warranted. Please see the online materials for Chapter 6 for information on crate/confinement training.

Resource Guarding

Sharing is not a strong tendency in dogs, and some amount of resource guarding is part of the normal behavioral repertoire of domestic canines (Miklosi 2014). However, resource guarding is considered a problem by most people (Pirrone et al. 2015) and can be demonstrated related to food, chewing items, toys, and procured items. A survey study of 4,857 dogs identified associations that can guide our puppy training strategies (Jacobs et al. 2018). Aggression related to resource guarding may be reduced by teaching puppies to relinquish items in exchange for a treat (e.g. trade cue) and by adding palatable food to the puppy's dry food during meals. It is important to highlight that this study found that removing the food dish during meals may increase resource guarding. Similarly, it is important that clients teach the puppy to trade non-food items (e.g. chew toys, paper products, and client belongings) for a treat instead of grabbing the item from the puppy's mouth.

Take Home Points

- Mouthing behaviors are not predictive of aggression in adulthood.
- Most puppies will outgrow their mouthing by age one. In the meantime, teach the puppy that there are other ways to get attention (e.g. sitting, bringing a toy) and offer adequate play time with other dogs.
- Chewing may be increased when adult teeth are erupting and when puppies are socially isolated. Offer puppies a variety of toys to meet their need for chewing. When not supervised, confine puppies to reduce their risk of chewing something inappropriate.
- Taking the food bowl away may increase the risk of resource guarding. Allow the puppy to eat undisturbed or drop a few high-value treats near the puppy when they are eating.
- Teach the puppy a trade cue by having them relinquish items for a treat. Refrain from grabbing objects from the puppy's mouth.

Excitable Behaviors

Jumping

Clients find excitable behaviors to be a source of great frustration. Shabelansky and Dowling-Guyer (2016) reported that jumping was noted most when owners arrived home and during play; however, mealtimes rarely triggered jumping. This may reflect the ritualized nature of interactions during mealtimes, which may be replicated in other interactions. From a functional perspective, jumping was maintained by verbal or tactile owner attention and/or access to tangible reinforcers, such as a ball, plush toy, or application of the leash (Pfaller-Sadovsky et al. 2019; Dorey et al. 2012). Differential reinforcement (e.g. offering the known reinforcer when the dog was not jumping) was one strategy utilized to reduce the frequency of jumping in this study. Extrapolation of this work implies that our clients may be well served to increase predictability of their interactions with their puppy by offering praise, petting, toys, and any outcome desired by the dog (e.g. being let outside, having a leash put on) when the dog is spontaneously not jumping and ensuring that attention, enrichment, and exercise are offered at a frequency that meets their puppy's needs.

Mounting

Sexual play, manifesting as mounting, clasping, and pelvic thrusting, is normal and begins to develop when puppies are five to six weeks of age (Pal 2010; Scott and Fuller 1965). The current literature regarding gonadectomy implies that mounting is reduced by castration but unaffected by spaying. Palestrini et al. (2021) reported that 60–70% of intact males mounted, whereas 20% exhibited mounting nine months after neutering. In this same study, mounting behavior was not affected by ovariohysterectomy in thirty-three female puppies or adult dogs. From a management of perspective, mounting of other dogs may be ignored if it does not result in aggression. In many dogs, mounting (be it of other dogs, humans, or inanimate objects) is a manifestation of stress, and as such, treatment strategies may need to be focused on anxiety reduction in contexts where mounting is observed. Options may include anxiolytic medication, provision of food enrichment to help the dog self-soothe, or avoidance of the stressful scenario altogether.

Barking

Barking has various functions in canine communication, including serving as an alert, expressing distress, and soliciting play (Yin 2002). Excessive barking, however, can be unnerving to the client and a reason for concern in the developing dog. Risk factors for nuisance barking include removal from the dam and litter before six weeks of age, herding breeds, age less than one year, and residing in a multi-dog household (Cross et al. 2009; Pierantoni et al. 2011). Excessive barking when alone may be related to underlying separation or confinement anxiety and should be treated accordingly. Excessive barking in the presence of family members may be attention-seeking in nature and/or driven by underlying hyper-attachment. Thus, management of excessive barking requires an understanding of the dog's motivation. Bark collars, such as those that deliver a shock, aversive sound, or spray in response to vocal cord vibration, are not recommended, as these devices do not address underlying motivation. For barking related to attention, the recommendations are similar to other excitement-related behaviors, including teaching the puppy alternative strategies for gaining attention (e.g. sitting quietly) and ensuring attention and enrichment are offered at a frequency that meets their puppy's needs.

Take Home Points

- Whenever possible, ignore excitable behaviors (e.g. jumping, and barking) and reinforce the puppy (e.g. with treats and attention) when they spontaneously offer calmer behavior (e.g. four paws on the floor or sitting quietly even for a few seconds).
- To encourage self-soothing behavior, offer the puppy a toy or food-enrichment item during times of transition, such as when the client leaves or arrives home; when the puppy is confined; and when clients are not able to focus their attention on the puppy.
- Dogs exhibiting excessive mounting of people and other dogs should be evaluated for underlying anxiety.
- Nuisance barking may be related to underlying anxiety or attention seeking. Bark collars should not be utilized, as management should focus on addressing the motivation for barking and ruling out underlying anxiety.

Elimination Behaviors

Housetraining is an imperative skill for puppies, as dogs that soil the home may be two to four times more likely to be relinquished to a shelter (Scarlett et al. 2002). The process of housetraining is based on the unlikelihood that dogs will soil their sleeping area. By three to four weeks of age, puppies crawl away from the nest to urinate and defecate (Scott and Fuller 1965), and by eight weeks of age, puppies may have developed a preferred elimination location for defecation (Ross 1950). At birth, puppies have normal digestive motility patterns (Milla 1988). The gastrocolic reflex predicts that a puppy will need to defecate shortly after eating. Colloquially, it is estimated that a puppy needs to urinate on a schedule based on age in months, such that, for example, a two-month-old puppy needs to eliminate every two hours and a three-month-old puppy needs relief every three hours, and so on.

In a survey of completeness of housetraining in seven-hundred-thirty-five dogs, 67% of small dogs (<9.0 kg) and 95% of large dogs (>18 kg) were considered fully housetrained (Learn et al. 2020). The most-commonly exhibited signals dogs offered to alert clients of their need to go outside were standing at the door and staring at someone within the household. According to Yeon et al. (1999), many house-soiling problems are caused by incomplete housetraining and should improve with behavior modification. Recommendations include more frequent elimination breaks, accompanying the dog to the preferred elimination area, positive reinforcement for eliminating appropriately (e.g. verbal praise and a treat), close supervision via tethering the dog to the owner, crate training, and ensuring that dogs are not punished for accidents after the fact.

For puppies, there is limited information regarding the average age of complete housetraining. In adult dogs, most were considered housetrained one month after adoption from a shelter, and adopters who received counseling regarding housetraining were more likely to identify their dog as housetrained (Herron et al. 2007). Thus, advice regarding housetraining should be offered by veterinary staff. Reasonable clinical housetraining guidelines include frequent elimination breaks, especially following meals, naps, and play; positive reinforcement for appropriate elimination; close supervision; confinement when not supervised directly; and avoidance of punishment. When challenges arise with housetraining, it may be helpful to have clients keep a log of elimination habits for several days to a week, during which time they take the puppy out approximately every 2 hours when they are home and note whether urination or defecation occurs at each break, as well as when and where accidents are found. Logging may identify temporal or spatial trends in the puppy's elimination habits that can guide adjustments to the housetraining plan. Puppies who do not respond to the aforementioned housetraining strategies warrant medical follow-up and/or evaluation for underlying anxiety. See the online materials for Chapter 6 for a sample client handout on housetraining best practices.

Take Home Points

- Take puppies out to eliminate after meals, naps, and playtime.
- Puppies need to eliminate frequently, so they should be taken out about every two to four hours until they are four to six months of age. Offer a potty pad or litter box as an alternative when you are unable to take the puppy out frequently.
- To avoid accidents, puppies should be under close supervision or in a safe confinement space.
- Puppies who are repeatedly having accidents despite reasonable housetraining strategies should be evaluated for underlying behavioral or physical concerns.

Separation-Related Behaviors

Distress during social isolation is normal for puppies. By six to seven weeks of age, laboratory-raised puppies demonstrated intractable vocalization when socially isolated in an unfamiliar location (Scott and Fuller 1965). This is an adaptive behavior that serves to alert the dam and ensure the puppy's safety (Cohen and Fox 1976). More recent studies have reported elevations in cortisol in response to social separation at five weeks of age (Nagasawa et al. 2014). In puppies less than three months, social isolation manifests as vocalizing, yawning, scratching, lip licking, and orienting to the environment, with only a small portion of puppies exhibiting significant distress (Cannas et al. 2010; Frank et al. 2007). In both studies, there appeared to be no significant difference in behavior between crated and uncrated puppies, suggesting that crating may not provide substantial comfort.

It is important to be mindful that puppies are entering new households during periods of time when their behavioral and endocrinologic responses to social isolation are substantial. General recommendations may include creating a safe space for the puppy with comfortable bedding that could replicate the sensation of curling up with conspecifics, food or toy enrichment items, and a separate area for elimination (e.g. potty pads). Ensuring the puppy's area maintains a consistent temperature may reduce thermal stress in puppies younger than four weeks and provide physical comfort to older puppies.

Provision of auditory stimuli may be beneficial. Classical music and audio books may reduce stress in kenneled dogs (Brayley and Montrose 2016; Kogan et al. 2012; Wells et al. 2002). One study assessed the response to heartbeat sounds in adult dogs (Fukuzawa and Kajino 2018). Heartbeat sounds have not been evaluated in puppies but have been reported to be beneficial in human infants (Kawakami et al. 1996; Kurihara et al. 1996); therefore, it may be reasonable to offer puppies a stuffed animal with heartbeat sounds (e.g. Snuggle Puppy® [Smart Pet; Love, MI, US]).

Creating opportunities for puppies to feel safe when alone is something we can discuss with clients at early puppy visits. Encourage clients to create a safe space as described above. Then, introduce short periods of confinement when the owner is home to observe the puppy's response prior to leaving the puppy home alone for the first time. The puppy may be set up for success by practicing confinement when the puppy is tired, not hungry, and has very recently been taken out to eliminate. Offer a food-puzzle toy or chew to encourage self-soothing (Figure 6.6).

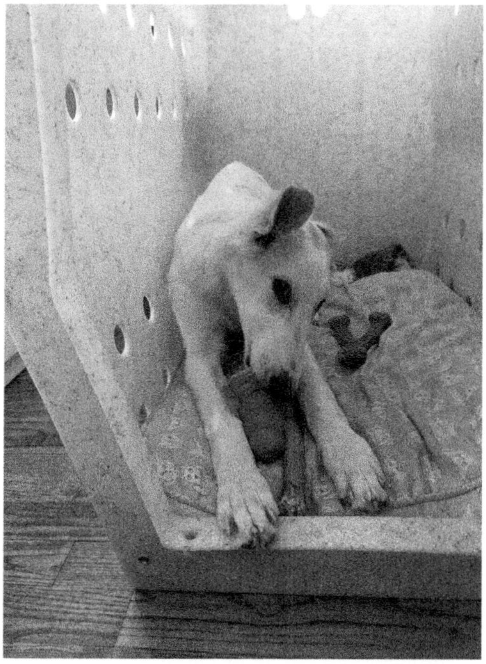

Figure 6.6 Food-stuffed puzzle toys and chew outlets can provide long-lasting entertainment and help create a positive emotional response to confinement training. *Source:* Photo credit: Heather Luedecke.

Puppies who exhibit persistent distress when confined and/or when socially isolated warrant further support. Even with the best preparation, separation anxiety may still develop (Herron et al. 2014). Refer to Chapter 16 for details on setting puppies up for successful separation time, as well as the diagnosis and treatment of separation-related disorders.

Take Home Points

- Some amount of separation distress is normal when puppies are initially removed from their dam and litter mates.
- Set puppies up for success by creating a safe confinement space (e.g. crate or pen) with comfortable bedding that could replicate the sensation of curling up with conspecifics, food or toy enrichment items, and a separate area for elimination (e.g. potty pads).
- Practice short periods of confinement when the someone is home and can observe prior to leaving the puppy home alone.
- Repeated and protracted episodes of vocalizing, destruction, and escape efforts are not

Red Flag Puppies – Some puppy behavior concerns need to rise to the level of immediate attention. The examples below outline behaviors that are beyond typical and may indicate underlying medical or behavioral pathologies.

- Puppies removed from their dams and/or littermates prior to six weeks of age and bottle-fed puppies should be identified and monitored closely. It may be ill advised to bottle-feed puppies when a dam is deemed unadoptable from a behavioral standpoint. Good maternal care offers puppies their best opportunity for normal development.
- Puppies who do not approach new people: Most puppies between the ages of five weeks and three months readily approach a stationary and friendly unfamiliar person.
- Puppies who pant, pace, attempt to flee, or snap during veterinary visits: These puppies should be identified for targeted intervention. Social puppies are likely to be playful and may be mouthy during a physical examination, but they should not appeared stressed.
- Juveniles who avoid novel, non-social stimuli: Persistent fear of non-social stimuli, especially beyond four to five months of age, is not typical.
- Puppies avoiding conspecific play: Whether reported at home or noted during puppy class, these puppies should be identified and monitored closely for dog-dog problems later in life.
- Puppies who exhibit protracted vocalization and/or physically active manifestations of anxiety (e.g. efforts to escape confinement

or pacing) when alone: This behavior is not typical for puppies over three months of age. These puppies should be identified and behavior support implemented.
- Puppies who repeatedly urinate and/or defecate in an appropriately sized crate when confined for an appropriate length of time relative to the puppy's age: These puppies should be evaluated for underlying anxiety, physical illness, and congenital abnormalities.

typical. These puppies should be further evaluated for the potential for underlying separation or confinement anxiety.

Conclusion

Canine behavior is shaped and influenced by many factors, including genetics, epigenetics, and experiences during early life through adulthood. Developmental periods during early life are marked by significant motor, cognitive, and social changes, which influence the way the puppy perceives and responds to the world. Early life experiences may have lasting effects on behavior into adulthood; therefore, it is important that breeders, clients, animal shelterers, and veterinary professionals provide quality experiences, taking care not to overwhelm or scare puppies. A well-versed veterinary team can be uniquely poised to serve as sources of expertise that may improve long-term behavioral outcomes. Further, the veterinarian and staff can identify any red flags during routine puppy visits and provide guidance and early intervention to treat the problem, preserve the human-animal bond, and retain the puppy in the home and in the practice.

References

American Veterinary Society of Animal Behavior (2008). Position statement on puppy socialization. https://avsab.org/resources/position-statements/ (accessed May 1, 2022).

Amlien, I.K., Fjell, A.M., Tamnes, C.K. et al. (2016). Organizing principles of human cortical development--thickness and area from 4 to 30 years: insights from comparative primate neuroanatomy. *Cereb. Cortex* 26: 257–267.

Appleby, D.L., Bradshaw, J.W.S., and Casey, R.A. (2002). Relationship between aggressive and avoidance behaviour by dogs and their experience in the first six months of life. *Vet. Rec.* 150: 434–438.

Arhant, C., Winkelmann, R., and Troxler, J. (2021). Chewing behaviour in dogs – a survey-based exploratory study. *Appl. Anim. Behav. Sci.* 241: 105372.

Association of Shelter Veterinarians' Veterinary Task Force to Advance Spay-Neuter, Griffin, B., Bushby, P.A. et al. (2016). The association of shelter veterinarians' 2016 veterinary medical care guidelines for spay-neuter programs. *J. Am. Vet. Med. Assoc.* 249: 165–188.

Bacon, W.E. and Stanley, W.C. (1970a). Avoidance learning in neonatal dogs. *J. of Comparative and Physiol. Psychol.* 71 (3): 448.

Bacon, W.E. and Stanley, W.C. (1970b). Reversal learning in neonatal dogs. *J. Comparative and Physiol. Psychol. 70* (3p1): 344.

Battaglia, C.L. (2009). Periods of early development and the effects of stimulation and social experiences in the canine. *J. Vet. Behav.* 4: 203–210.

Blackwell, E.J., Bradshaw, J.W.S., and Casey, R.A. (2013). Fear responses to noises in domestic dogs: prevalence, risk factors and co-occurrence with other fear related behaviour. *Appl. Anim. Behav. Sci.* 145: 15–25.

Blackwell, E.J., Bolster, C., Richards, G. et al. (2012). The use of electronic collars for training domestic dogs: estimated prevalence, reasons and risk factors for use, and owner perceived success as compared to other training methods. *BMC Vet. Res.* 8: 93.

Blackwell, E.J., Twells, C., Seawright, A., and Casey, R.A. (2008). The relationship between training methods and the occurrence of behavior problems, as reported by owners, in a population of domestic dogs. *J. Vet. Behav.* 3: 207–217.

Bray, E., Sammel, M., Cheney, D. et al. (2017). Effects of maternal investment, temperament, and cognition on guide dog success. *Proc. Natl. Acad. Sci.* 114 (34): 9128–9133.

Bray, E.E., Gnanadesikan, G.E., Horschler, D.J. et al. (2021). Early-emerging and highly heritable sensitivity to human communication in dogs. *Curr. Biol.* 31 (e5): 3132–3136.

Bray, E.E., Gruen, M.E., Gnanadesikan, G.E. et al. (2020). Cognitive characteristics of 8- to 10-week-old assistance dog puppies. *Anim. Behav.* 166: 193–206.

Brayley, C. and Montrose, V.T. (2016). The effects of audiobooks on the behaviour of dogs at a rehoming kennels. *Appl. Anim. Behav. Sci.* 174: 111–115.

Browne, C.M., Starkey, N.J., Mary Foster, T., and McEwan, J.S. (2017). Examination of the accuracy and applicability of information in popular books on dog training. *Soc. Anima. Soc. Sci. Stud. Hum. Exp. Other Anim.* 25 (5): 411–435.

Canine Vaccination Guidelines (2017). American Animal Hospital Association. https://www.aaha.org/aaha-guidelines/vaccination-canine-configuration/vaccination-canine/ (accessed 04 January 2022).

Cannas, S., Frank, D., Minero, M. et al. (2010). Puppy behavior when left home alone: changes during the first few months after adoption. *J. Vet. Behav.* 5: 94–100.

Casey, R.A., Loftus, B., Bolster, C. et al. (2014). Human directed aggression in domestic dogs (*Canis familiaris*): occurrence in different contexts and risk factors. *Appl. Anim. Behav. Sci.* 152: 52–63.

Cohen, J.A. and Fox, M.W. (1976). Vocalizations in wild canids and possible effects of domestication. *Behav. Processes* 1: 77–92.

Cross, N.J., Rosenthal, K., and Phillips, C.J.C. (2009). Risk factors for nuisance barking in dogs. *Aus. Vet. J. 87* (10): 402–408. https://doi.org/10.1111/j.1751-0813.2009.00484.x.

Csoltova, E., Martineau, M., Boissy, A., and Gilbert, C. (2017). Behavioral and physiological reactions in dogs to a veterinary examination: owner-dog interactions improve canine well-being. *Physiol. Behav.* 177: 270–281.

Cutler, J.H., Coe, J.B., and Niel, L. (2017). Puppy socialization practices of a sample of dog owners from across Canada and the United States. *J. Am. Vet. Med. Assoc.* 251: 1415–1423.

D'Aniello, B. and Scandurra, A. (2016). Ontogenetic effects on gazing behaviour: a case study of kennel dogs (Labrador Retrievers) in the impossible task paradigm. *Anim. Cogn.* 19: 565–570.

Deldalle, S. and Gaunet, F. (2014). Effects of 2 training methods on stress-related behaviors of the dog (*Canis familiaris*) and on the dog–owner relationship. *J. Vet. Behav.* 9: 58–65.

Dietz, L., Arnold, A.-M.K., Goerlich-Jansson, V.C., and Vinke, C.M. (2018). The importance of early life experiences for the development of behavioural disorders in domestic dogs. *Behaviour* 155: 83–114.

Dinwoodie, I.R., Zottola, V., and Dodman, N.H. (2021). An investigation into the impact of pre-adolescent training on canine behavior. *Animals (Basel)* 11 (5): 1298.

Dorey, N.R., Tobias, J.S., Udell, M.A.R., and Wynne, C.D.L. (2012). Decreasing dog problem behavior with functional analysis: linking diagnoses to treatment. *J. Vet. Behav.* 7: 276–282.

Döring, D., Roscher, A., Scheipl, F. et al. (2009). Fear-related behaviour of dogs in veterinary practice. *Vet. J.* 182: 38–43.

Duxbury, M.M., Jackson, J.A., Line, S.W., and Anderson, R.K. (2003). Evaluation of association between retention in the home and attendance at puppy socialization classes. *J. Am. Vet. Med. Assoc.* 223 (1): 61–66.

Edwards, P.T., Hazel, S.J., Browne, M. et al. (2019a). Investigating risk factors that predict a dog's fear during veterinary consultations. *PLoS One* 14: e0215416.

Edwards, P.T., Smith, B.P., McArthur, M.L., and Hazel, S.J. (2019b). Fearful fido: investigating dog experience in the veterinary context in an effort to reduce distress. *Appl. Anim. Behav. Sci.* 213: 14–25.

Elliot, O. and Scott, J.P. (1961). The development of emotional distress reactions to separation, in puppies. *J. Genet. Psychol.* 99: 3–22.

Farhoody, P., Mallawaarachchi, I., Tarwater, P.M. et al. (2018). Aggression toward familiar people, strangers, and conspecifics in gonadectomized and intact dogs. *Front. Vet. Sci.* 5: 18.

Flint, H.E., Coe, J.B., Serpell, J.A. et al. (2018). Identification of fear behaviors shown by puppies in response to nonsocial stimuli. *J. Vet. Behav.* 28: 17–24.

Fox, M.W. (1971). Overview and critique of stages and periods in canine development. *Dev. Psychobiol.* 4: 37–54.

Fox, M.W. and Stelzner, D. (1966a). Approach/withdrawal variables in the development of social behaviour in the dog. *Anim. Behav.* 14: 362–366.

Fox, M.W. and Stelzner, D. (1966b). Behavioural effects of differential early experience in the dog. *Anim. Behav.* 14: 273–281.

Foyer, P., Bjällerhag, N., Wilsson, W., and Jensen, P. (2014). Behaviour and experiences of dogs during the first year of life predict the outcome in a later temperament test. *Appl. Anim. Behav. Sci.* 155: 93–100.

Foyer, P., Wilsson, E., and Jensen, P. (2016). Levels of maternal care in dogs affect adult offspring temperament. *Sci. Rep.* 6: 19253.

Frank, D., Minero, M., Cannas, S., and Palestrini, C. (2007). Puppy behaviours when left home alone: A pilot study. *Appl. Anim. Behav. Sci.* 104: 61–70.

Freedman, D.G., King, J.A., and Elliot, O. (1961). Critical period in the social development of dogs. *Science* 133: 1016–1017.

Fukuzawa, M. and Kajino, S. (2018). Auditory stimuli as environmental enrichment tool for family dogs. *Int. J. Biol.* 10: 19.

Gazzano, A., Mariti, C., Alvares, S. et al. (2008a). The prevention of undesirable behaviors in dogs: effectiveness of veterinary behaviorists' advice given to puppy owners. *J. Vet. Behav.* 3: 125–133.

Gazzano, A., Mariti, C., Notari, L. et al. (2008b). Effects of early gentling and early environment on emotional development of puppies. *Appl. Anim. Behav. Sci.* 110: 294–304.

Gazzano, A., Mariti, C., Sighieri, C., Ducci, M., Ciceroni, C., & McBride, E. A. (2008c). Survey of undesirable behaviors displayed by potential guide dogs with puppy walkers. *Journal of Veterinary Behavior: Clinical Applications and Research: Official Journal of: Australian Veterinary Behaviour Interest Group, International Working Dog Breeding Association*, *3*(3), 104–113. https://doi.org/10.1016/j.jveb.2008.04.002

Godbout, M. and Frank, D. (2011a). Persistence of puppy behaviors and signs of anxiety during adulthood. *J. Vet. Behav.* 6: 92.

Godbout, M. and Frank, D. (2011b). Excessive mouthing in puppies as a predictor of aggressiveness in adult dogs. *J. Vet. Behav.* 1: 93.

Godbout, M., Palestrini, C., Beauchamp, G., and Frank, D. (2007). Puppy behavior at the veterinary clinic: a pilot study. *J. Vet. Behav.* 2: 126–135.

González-Martínez, Á., Martínez, M.F., Rosado, B. et al. (2019). Association between puppy classes and adulthood behavior of the dog. *J. Vet. Behav.* 32: 36–41.

Guardini, G., Bowen, J., Mariti, C. et al. (2017). Influence of maternal care on behavioural development of domestic dogs (*Canis*

Familiaris) living in a home environment. *Animals (Basel)* 7 (12): 93.

Hansen, W.C., van der Bijl, W., and Temrin, H. (2019). Dogs, but not wolves, lose their sensitivity toward novelty with age. *Front. Psychol.* 10: 2001.

Hart, B.L. and Eckstein, R.A. (1997). The role of gonadal hormones in the occurrence of objectionable behaviours in dogs and cats. *Appl. Anim. Behav. Sci.* 52: 331–344.

Harvey, N.D., Craigon, P.J., Blythe, S.A. et al. (2016). Social rearing environment influences dog behavioral development. *J. Vet. Behav.* 16: 13–21.

Haverbeke, A., Laporte, B., Depiereux, E. et al. (2008). Training methods of military dog handlers and their effects on the team's performances. *Appl. Anim. Behav. Sci.* 113: 110–122.

Helton, W.S. and Helton, N.D. (2010). Physical size matters in the domestic dog's (*Canis lupus familiaris*) ability to use human pointing cues. *Behav. Processes* 85: 77–79.

Herron, M.E., Lord, L.K., and Husseini, S.E. (2014). Effects of preadoption counseling on the prevention of separation anxiety in newly adopted shelter dogs. *J. Vet. Behav.: Clin. Appl. Res.*: Official J. Aus. Vet. Behav. Int. Group, Intern. Work. Dog Breed. Assoc. *9* (1): 13–21. https://doi.org/10.1016/j.jveb.2013.09.003.

Herron, M.E., Shofer, F.S., and Reisner, I.R. (2009). Survey of the use and outcome of confrontational and non-confrontational training methods in client-owned dogs showing undesired behaviors. *Appl. Anim. Behav. Sci.* 117: 47–54.

Herron, M.E., Lord, L.K., Hill, L.N., and Reisner, I.R. (2007). Effects of preadoption counseling for owners on house-training success among dogs acquired from shelters. *J. Am. Vet. Med. Assoc. 231* (4): 558–562.

Hiby, E., Rooney, N., and Bradshaw, J. (2004). Dog training methods: their use, effectiveness and interaction with behaviour and welfare. *Animal Welfare 13* (1): 63–69.

Höglund, K., Hanås, S., Carnabuci, C. et al. (2012). Blood pressure, heart rate, and urinary catecholamines in healthy dogs subjected to different clinical settings. *J. Vet. Intern. Med.* 26: 1300–1308.

Hopkins, S.G., Schubert, T.A., and Hart, B.L. (1976). Castration of adult male dogs: effects on roaming, aggression, urine marking, and mounting. *J. Am. Vet. Med. Assoc.* 168: 1108–1110.

Howe, L.M., Slater, M.R., Boothe, H.W. et al. (2001). Long-term outcome of gonadectomy performed at an early age or traditional age in dogs. *J. Am. Vet. Med. Assoc.* 218: 217–221.

Ikuno, S. (1989). Development of chewing center at transition period from sucking to chewing. *Shoni. Shikagaku. Zasshi.* 27: 595–606.

Jacobs, J.A., Coe, J.B., Pearl, D.L. et al. (2018). Factors associated with canine resource guarding behaviour in the presence of people: a cross-sectional survey of dog owners. *Prev. Vet. Med.* 161: 143–153.

Kawakami, K., Takai-Kawakami, K., Kurihara, H. et al. (1996). The effect of sounds on newborn infants under stress. *Infant Behav. Dev.* 19: 375–379.

Kogan, L.R., Schoenfeld-Tacher, R., and Simon, A.A. (2012). Behavioral effects of auditory stimulation on kenneled dogs. *J. Vet. Behav.* 7: 268–275.

Kuhl, C.A., Lea, R.G., Quarmby, C., and Dean, R. (2022). Scoping review to assess online information available to new dog owners. *Vet. Rec.* 190 (10): e1487.

Kurihara, H., Chiba, H., Shimizu, Y. et al. (1996). Behavioral and adrenocortical responses to stress in neonates and the stabilizing effects of maternal heartbeat on them. *Early Hum. Dev.* 46: 117–127.

Kustritz, M.V.R. (2002). Early spay-neuter: clinical considerations. *Clin. Tech. Small Anim. Pract.* 17: 124–128.

Kutsumi, A., Nagasawa, M., Ohta, M., and Ohtani, N. (2013). Importance of puppy training for future behavior of the dog. *J. Vet. Med. Sci.* 75: 141–149.

Learn, A., Radosta, L., and Pike, A. (2020). Preliminary assessment of differences in completeness of house-training between dogs based on size. *J. Vet. Behav.* 35: 19–26.

Lord, M.S., Casey, R.A., Kinsman, R.H. et al. (2020). Owner perception of problem behaviours in dogs aged 6 and 9-months. *Appl. Anim. Behav. Sci.* 232: 105147.

Lyons, D., Parker, K., and Schatzberg, A. (2010). Animal models of early life stress: implications for understanding resilience. *Develop. Psychobiolo.* 52: 616–624.

Maarschalkerweerd, R.J., Endenburg, N., Kirpensteijn, J., and Knol, B.W. (1997). Influence of orchiectomy on canine behaviour. *Vet. Rec.* 140: 617–619.

Mandese, W.W., Griffin, F.C., Reynolds, P.S. et al. (2021). Stress in client-owned dogs related to clinical exam location: a randomised crossover trial. *J. Small Anim. Pract.* 62: 82–88.

Mariti, C., Pierantoni, L., Sighieri, C., and Gazzano, A. (2017). Guardians' perceptions of dogs' welfare and behaviors related to visiting the veterinary clinic. *J. Appl. Anim. Welf. Sci.* 20: 24–33.

Mariti, C., Raspanti, E., Zilocchi, M. et al. (2015). The assessment of dog welfare in the waiting room of a veterinary clinic. *Anim. Welf.* 24: 299–305.

McGreevy, P.D., Wilson, B., Starling, M.J., and Serpell, J.A. (2018). Behavioural risks in male dogs with minimal lifetime exposure to gonadal hormones may complicate population-control benefits of desexing. *PLoS One* 13: e0196284.

McGuire, B. (2019). Effects of gonadectomy on scent-marking behavior of shelter dogs. *J. Vet. Behav.* 30: 16–24.

McMillan, F.D. (2017). Behavioral and psychological outcomes for dogs sold as puppies through pet stores and/or born in commercial breeding establishments: Current knowledge and putative causes. *J. Vet. Behav.* 19: 14–26.

Miklosi, A. (2014). *Dog behaviour, evolution, and cognition*. Oxford University Press.

Milla, P.J. (1988). Gastrointestinal motility disorders in children. *Pediatr. Clin. North Am.* 35: 311–330.

Morrow, M., Ottobre, J., Ottobre, A. et al. (2015). Breed-dependent differences in the onset of fear-related avoidance behavior in puppies. *J. Vet. Behav.* 10: 286–294.

Nagasawa, M., Shibata, Y., Yonezawa, A. et al. (2014). The behavioral and endocrinological development of stress response in dogs. *Dev. Psychobiol.* 56: 726–733.

Neilson, J.C., Eckstein, R.A., and Hart, B.L. (1997). Effects of castration on problem behaviors in male dogs with reference to age and duration of behavior. *J. Am. Vet. Med. Assoc.* 211: 180–182.

Nelson, E.E. and Guyer, A.E. (2011). The development of the ventral prefrontal cortex and social flexibility. *Dev. Cogn. Neurosci.* 1: 233–245.

Pal, S.K. (2010). Play behaviour during early ontogeny in free-ranging dogs (*Canis familiaris*). *Appl. Anim. Behav. Sci.* 126: 140–153.

Palestrini, C., Mazzola, S.M., Caione, B. et al. (2021). Influence of gonadectomy on canine behavior. *Animals (Basel)* 11 (2): 553.

Parker, K.J. and Maestripieri, D. (2011). Identifying key features of early stressful experiences that produce stress vulnerability and resilience in primates. *Neurosci. Biobehav. Rev.* 35 (1466–1483): 60.

Pfaller-Sadovsky, N., Arnott, G., and Hurtado-Parrado, C. (2019). Using principles from applied behaviour analysis to address an undesired behaviour: functional analysis and treatment of jumping up in companion dogs. *Animals (Basel)* (12): 9, 1091.

Pierantoni, L., Albertini, M., and Pirrone, F. (2011). Prevalence of owner-reported behaviours in dogs separated from the litter at two different ages. *Vet. Rec. 169* (18): 468. https://doi.org/10.1136/vr.d4967.

Pirrone, F., Pierantoni, L., Mazzola, S.M. et al. (2015). Owner and animal factors predict the incidence of, and owner reaction toward, problematic behaviors in companion dogs. *J. Vet. Behav.* 10: 295–301.

Pirrone, F., Pierantoni, L., Pastorino, G.Q., and Albertini, M. (2016). Owner-reported aggressive behavior towards familiar people may be a more prominent occurrence in pet shop-traded dogs. *J. Vet. Behav.* 11: 13–17.

Protopopova, A. and Gunter, L.M. (2017). Adoption and relinquishment interventions at the animal shelter: a review. *Anim. Welf.* 26: 35–48.

Riemer, S., Müller, C., Virányi, Z. et al. (2013). Choice of conflict resolution strategy is linked to sociability in dog puppies. *Appl. Anim. Behav. Sci. 149* (1-4): 36–44.

Ross, S. (1950). Some observations on the lair dwelling behavior of dogs. *Behaviour* 2: 144–162.

Salman, M.D., New, J.G. Jr., Scarlett, J.M. et al. (1998). Human and animal factors related to relinquishment of dogs and cats in 12 selected animal shelters in the United States. *J. Appl. Anim. Welf. Sci.* 1: 207–226.

Scarlett, J.M., Salman, M.D., New, J.G., and Kass, P.H. (2002). The role of veterinary practitioners in reducing dog and cat relinquishments and euthanasias. *J. Am. Vet. Med. Assoc.* 220: 306–311.

Schulkey, R. and Deporter, T., (2017). Evaluation of the association between attendance at veterinary hospital-based puppy socialisation classes and long-term retention in the home. In: *Proceedings of the 11th International Veterinary Behaviour Meeting*. p. 100. CABI.

Scott, J.P., Bronson, F., and Trattner, A. (1968). Differential human handling and the development of agonistic behavior in basenji and shetland sheep dogs. *Dev. Psychobiol.* 1: 133–140.

Scott, J.P., Stewart, J.M., and DeGhett, V.J. (1974). Critical periods in the organization of systems. *Develop. Psychobiol.* 7: 489–513.

Scott, J.P. and Fuller, J.L. (1965). *Genetics and the Social Behavior of the Dog: The Classic Study*. The University of Chicago Press.

Seksel, K., Mazurski, E.J., and Taylor, A. (1999). Puppy socialisation programs: short and long term behavioural effects. *Appl. Anim. Behav. Sci.* 62: 335–349.

Serpell, J. and Duffy, D. (2016). Aspects of juvenile and adolescent environment predict aggression and fear in 12-month old guide dogs. *Frontiers in Veterinary Science* 3: 49.

Serpell, J.A. and Hsu, Y.A. (2005). Effects of breed, sex, and neuter status on trainability in dogs. *Anthrozoos A Multidiscip. J. Inter. People Anim.* 18: 196–207.

Serpell, J., Duffy, D., and Jagoe, J.A. (2017). Becoming a dog: early experience and the development of behavior. In: *The Domestic Dog: Its Evolution, Behavior and Interactions with People*, 2e. Cambridge University Press.

Shabelansky, A. and Dowling-Guyer, S. (2016). Characteristics of excitable dog behavior based on owners' report from a self-selected study. *Animals* 6: 22.

Solmi, M., Radua, J., Olivola, M. et al. (2022). Age at onset of mental disorders worldwide: large-scale meta-analysis of 192 epidemiological studies. *Mol. Psychiatry* 27: 281–295.

Spain, C.V., Scarlett, J.M., and Houpt, K.A. (2004). Long-term risks and benefits of early-age gonadectomy in dogs. *J. Am. Vet. Med. Assoc.* 224: 380–387.

Stanford, T.L. (1981). Behavior of dogs entering a veterinary clinic. *Appl. Anim. Ethol.* 7: 271–279.

Stanley, W.C., Bacon, W.E., and Fehr, C. (1970). Discriminated instrumental learning in neonatal dogs. *J. Comparative and Physiol. Psychol. 70* (3p1): 335.

Starling, M., Fawcett, A., Wilson, B. et al. (2019). Behavioural risks in female dogs with minimal lifetime exposure to gonadal hormones. *PLoS One* 14: e0223709.

Stellato, A., Jajou, S., Dewey, C.E. et al. (2019). Effect of a standardized four-week desensitization and counter-conditioning training program on pre-existing veterinary fear in companion dogs. *Animals (Basel)* 9 (10): 767.

Stepita, M.E., Bain, M.J., and Kass, P.H. (2013). Frequency of CPV infection in vaccinated puppies that attended puppy socialization classes. *J. Am. Anim. Hosp. Assoc.* 49: 95–100.

Stöcklin-Gautschi, N.M., Hässig, M., Reichler, I.M. et al. (2001). The relationship of urinary incontinence to early spaying in bitches. *J. Reprod. Fertil. Suppl.* 57: 233–236.

Udell, M.A.R., Dorey, N.R., and Wynne, C.D.L. (2010). The performance of stray dogs (*Canis familiaris*) living in a shelter on human-guided object-choice tasks. *Anim. Behav.* 79: 717–725.

Udell, M.A.R. and Brubaker, L. (2016). Are dogs social generalists? Canine social cognition, attachment, and the dog-human bond. *Curr. Dir. Psychol. Sci.* 25: 327–333.

Vieira de Castro, A.C., Fuchs, D., Morello, G.M. et al. (2020). Does training method matter? Evidence for the negative impact of aversive-based methods on companion dog welfare. *PLoS One* 15: e0225023.

Waite, M. and Kodak, T. (2022). Owner-implemented functional analyses and reinforcement-based treatments for mouthing in dogs. *Behav. Anal. Pract.* 15: 269–283.

Waite, M.R., Harman, M.J., and Kodak, T. (2021). Frequency and animal demographics of mouthing behavior in companion dogs in the United States. *Learn. Motiv.* 74: 101726.

Weinstock, M. (2008). The long-term behavioural consequences of prenatal stress. *Neurosci. Biobehav. Rev.* 32: 1073–1086.

Wells, D.L., Graham, L., and Hepper, P.G. (2002). The influence of auditory stimulation on the behaviour of dogs housed in a rescue shelter. *Anim. Welf.* 11: 385–393.

Yeon, S.C., Erb, H.N., and Houpt, K.A. (1999). A retrospective study of canine house soiling: diagnosis and treatment. *J. Am. Anim. Hosp. Assoc.* 35: 101–106.

Yin, S. (2002). A new perspective on barking in dogs (*Canis familaris*). *J. Comp. Psychol.* *116* (2): 189–193. https://doi.org/10.1037/0735-7036.116.2.189.

Ziv, G. (2017). The effects of using aversive training methods in dogs—a review. *J. Vet. Behav.* 19: 50–60.

7

The Development of Behavior and the Shaping of the Human–Animal Bond

Cats

Kersti Seksel

Adjunct Professor in Veterinary Behaviour, University of Queensland, Australia

Introduction

Lithe and smooth, they move around their world with elegant grace. They purr contentedly, sit on laps, rub around legs, and generally appear to enjoy the company of the people with whom they share the home. This can make them very attractive to many people as companions. So how does a feline embryo develop into such a fabulous pet?

Feline behavior is crafted by a number of factors, including genetics, what the cat learns from past experiences, particularly those that occur during early development, as well as the environment in which the cat finds itself at any given time. **Epigenetics** (modification of gene expression without changing the DNA sequence) also plays a key role. With just the right combination of nature and nurture, cats develop into loving creatures and provide companionship that is unique from that of other domesticated species.

To enjoy a feline friendship to its fullest, one must appreciate that cats retain a number of ancestral behaviors that can be challenging to manage in the indoor environment. Even when the stars align both genetically and environmentally, cats may still behave in ways that their human families do not appreciate. Normal but nuisance behaviors, such as counter surfing/lounging, early morning wake-up calls, late night mad moments, running up and down the hallway, scratching furniture, pouncing on people, or climbing up curtains, are not an uncommon phenomenon in kittens and young cats.

Although these behaviors may be neurotypical (normal) for the cat, they can be misunderstood, leaving people to misinterpret and inappropriately manage them. This mishandling of feline behavior leads to a deterioration of the human–animal bond and, sadly, may result in cats losing their home. It is our role as veterinarians to understand natural feline behavior and development so that the bond between our clients and their cats can flourish.

It starts with good parenting.

The cat's journey through development and growth to becoming a well-mannered cat begins with the breeder. Breeders should know which queen to breed with which tom and base their selection on the best evidence that science can provide. Understanding how to look after and handle the queen and the tom, both physically and psychologically, before mating, is essential. For queens, what happens before, during, and after pregnancy is important. As an **altricial** species, kittens are born blind and practically deaf, and with limited ability to move and regulate body temperature, they are

Introduction to Animal Behavior and Veterinary Behavioral Medicine, First Edition. Edited by Meghan E. Herron.

Companion website: www.wiley.com/go/introductiontoanimalbehavior

totally dependent on their mother for survival. Thus, the role of the queen cannot be underestimated. Breeders should also know how to help build resilience in the kittens, as well as to raise them appropriately before they go to their new homes, providing good litter box hygiene, ample social experiences, and keeping them with their queen and littermates until at least 12 weeks of age, if possible.

Animal shelters also bear responsibility for building resiliency in the kittens for whom they care. This is particularly relevant regarding orphaned kittens. Just as with other species, good maternal behavior is essential for healthy kitten development, putting orphans or early-weaned kittens at a physical and behavioral disadvantage (Ahola et al. 2017). In the case of bottle-fed kittens, if there are no infectious disease concerns, cross-fostering with another litter and queen may be of great benefit. Quality time spent with a healthy, kitten-friendly adult cat is the next best surrogate when cross-fostering is not an option. As the shelter environment is typically not one that can provide the complex social experiences necessary for adequate **socialization**, kittens should ideally be adopted into their new homes between eight and nine weeks of age, or the litter can be placed in a foster home that can provide socialization.

Once the kitten goes to a new home, the new family needs to be educated about how best to look after both the physical and mental health of the kitten. Both are important if cats are to make good companions. Unfortunately, the focus of veterinarians has previously been on physical wellness (vaccinations, deworming, and nutrition). While the physical aspects of feline health are an essential component of client education, behavioral health education may be what saves more feline lives. Studies have shown that cats are surrendered, abandoned, or euthanized due to unwanted behavior more than they are due to infectious diseases. Helping clients develop realistic expectations of what a kitten can and should do at all stages of its development helps prevent behavioral mismanagement and, ultimately, keeps cats happier and in their homes longer.

Appropriate maternal care goes a long way toward successful kitten development, but quality time spent with littermates can also help shape good social behavior. This leads to the debate regarding whether it is better to obtain two kittens or just one at a time. The benefits of two kittens, particularly litter mates, are many. They will keep each other company while their human family is out. They may also share similarly strong play/prey instincts and can, as such, amuse each other at dawn when their human family wants to sleep. Young, related cats are more likely to live amicably long-term, compared to older, unrelated cats. However, if the two kittens do not get along, problems can arise later. This conflict is most likely to occur when cats reach sexual and/or social maturity as this is when the litter may dispel and naturally leave their natal group. If one of the kittens grows to be a large male and the other a small female, a mismatch of strength and resource-holding potential may arise, leading to **misdirected play** or social status-related aggression issues. Making sure that there is always an environment of plenty will be important so that there is minimal need for conflict.

Developmental Periods

Understanding the developmental periods of the cat is the first step in understanding why cats do what they do. This knowledge is important to help kittens grow into great cats that make great companions for not only the people they live with but also the other animals they may meet during their lifetime. The development of a kitten from a totally dependent neonate, with a limited ability to perceive and respond to stimuli, to an independent cat with a fully developed physiology that can care for itself, hunt, and interact with members of its own species as well as members of other species, happens relatively rapidly. Yet the process

Table 7.1 Developmental period in cats by age.

Developmental period	Age
Prenatal	conception–birth
Neonatal	0–9 days
Transitional	9–14 days
Socialization	2–7 (9) weeks
Juvenile	7 weeks–5 months
Sexual maturity	5–9 months
Social maturity	3–4 years
Senior	10–15 years
Geriatric	15+ years

is very complex, and there are many factors that may disrupt the process. There are several periods of development that have been documented in cats (Table 7.1). Events that occur within each period may have a significant influence on the behavior of the cat. This means that these periods are not rigidly fixed and vary with the individual cat.

Prenatal Period

Although it has only relatively recently been discussed, the **prenatal period** is significant in the kitten's development. The stages involved in prenatal development signify an enormous amount of change. The first steps in the fertilization of an ovum involve several processes, each of which results in a new stage in the development of the kitten. From there, it develops into an embryo, which will implant in the lining of the uterus. This occurs roughly two weeks after fertilization. As cats are multiparous, this process is repeated by multiple zygote-morulas, possibly even from mating with different males.

The uterine environment experienced by the kitten during pregnancy has also been shown to have extensive effects on its behavior and development. Research has shown that queens who were malnourished during their pregnancy spent less time mothering their kittens (Simonson 1979). In addition, kittens from queens who were fed a low-protein diet during late gestation and through lactation were found to be more emotional and to move and vocalize more frequently than kittens from queens who were fed what was considered a balanced and complete diet (Gallo et al. 1980). These kittens also lost their balance more often, had poor social attachment, and fewer social interactions with the queen.

Other research has shown that at four months of age, male kittens of malnourished queens exhibited more aggressive play behaviors and that both the male and female kittens had motor deficits (Simonson 1979). This is postulated to have been due to a lack of protein in the queen's diet, especially in the latter stages of pregnancy. In another study, when queens were restricted to half of their nutritional requirements, the kittens had growth deficits in some brain regions, including the cerebrum, cerebellum, and brain stem (Smith and Jensen 1977). As these areas initiate and coordinate movement and actions, this deficiency leads to many issues in development. Delays were observed in the following areas of development, including suckling, eye opening, crawling, general posture, walking, running, playing, and climbing, all part of important kitten behavior. All that said, much research on the impact of diet on epigenetics is ongoing. The microbiome is also an area that is increasingly being investigated with more studies being conducted to further elucidate the impact on the developing cat.

Neonatal Period

The **neonatal period** starts at birth and lasts until approximately nine days of age. The queen initiates nursing and elimination during this period and into the next. At this point, kittens are totally dependent on the mother for their survival (Figure 7.1). Eating and sleeping are their most significant activities. On average, kittens in the first week of life spend about

(a) (b)

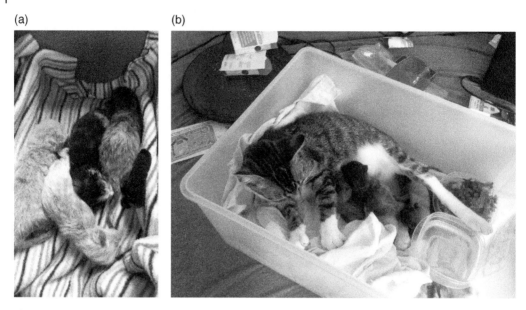

Figure 7.1 Neonatal kittens (a) are born blind and deaf with limited locomotor abilities. They use their sense of smell and touch to find nourishment (b). *Source:* With permission from Ashley Friend (a), With permission from Sara Flax (b).

four hours per day suckling. As kittens are born with their eyes closed and poor hearing, they rely on their sense of smell, touch, and ability to detect warmth to navigate their world. Hearing starts to develop around day 5 after birth. Although the eyes are shut, many visual reflexes (e.g. blink reflex) may be present even before birth. As the neonatal kitten cannot regulate its own body temperature, the ability to detect a thermal gradient is important for survival. Teat localization is done using their sense of smell, which is present at birth. However, although kittens do not vocalize much, they will purr when suckling and cry in response to physical discomfort (Kolb and Nonneman 1975).

As kittens are born neurologically immature, movement is limited at birth, and the legs are not strong enough to support their body weight until about the second week of life. However, kittens are able to right themselves if they are pushed onto their back, as this righting ability develops 10 days before birth. Perineal stimulation is necessary for elimination. This means that bottle-raised kittens must be stimulated in order to urinate and defecate – typically through the use of a warm, moistened washcloth.

Transitional Period

During the **transitional period,** rapid physical and behavioral changes occur, and the kitten develops a degree of independence from the queen. The kitten can crawl and walk awkwardly, and the eyes open around 7–10 days of age. The ears are now fully open, and the kitten starts to orient to sound. The teeth erupt, the kitten starts to ingest solids, and the sense of smell is fully developed by three weeks of age (Bateson 2014).

Kittens who were separated from their mother and hand-raised from two weeks of age appear to be more fearful and aggressive toward people and other cats. They are also more sensitive to novel stimuli, their ability to learn is poor, and they tend to have poor social and parenting skills later (Ahola et al. 2017). These effects may be attenuated, at least in part, if kittens are hand-reared in a home with other neurotypical cats so that they can learn by observing other felines.

Socialization Period

Socialization is strongly tied to the neurologic and physical development of the kitten. However, the socialization process is not just confined to kittenhood but continues throughout the life of the cat. A cat's socialization as a kitten can play a role in how they socialize with new individuals as an adult cat.

The **socialization period** is thought to last from approximately two to about seven weeks of age, although many clinicians believe it could be as late as nine weeks of age. Therefore, this is one important distinction from dogs as the period of socialization appears to both begin and end earlier in cats. However, as social play peaks between 9 and 14 weeks of age, it has been suggested that this may not always be the case, and the timing of this period is thought to also vary according to the individual, the breed, and experiential factors. During this period, the kitten becomes more independent, and this is usually the time that a kitten might go to its new home.

By the time the kitten is four weeks of age (Figure 7.2), hearing is fully developed. Depth perception is present, although visual acuity continues to improve until about 16 weeks of age. The air righting ability is equivalent to that of an adult cat by the time the kitten is six weeks of age. By seven weeks of age (Figure 7.3), kittens can maintain body temperature as well as the adult cat can.

During this period play develops, and several types have been recognized (social, object, and locomotory play). Social play starts around 4 weeks of age and peaks at around 9–14 weeks of age. After 14 weeks of age, more active play starts, and the kittens learn to play fight, and social fighting may occur.

Object and locomotory play starts at 6 weeks of age and peaks at around 16 weeks of age. By the time the kitten is six to seven weeks of age, adult-like locomotion is present. At seven to eight weeks of age, object play with eye–paw coordination is developing (Figure 7.4). Single kittens play more with objects and with their mothers compared with kittens in litter. Object play appears to be more prominent in male kittens and females with male littermates (Barrett and Bateson 1978).

Young kittens start to eat solids and will eat what the queen eats, thus establishing taste preferences (Figure 7.5). The time of weaning

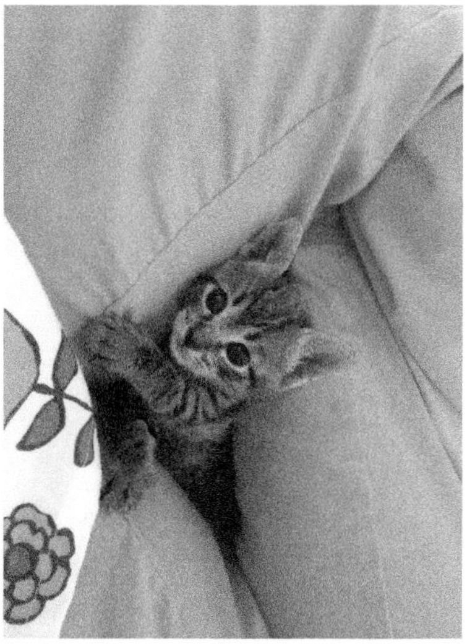

Figure 7.2 A four-week-old kitten can see and hear, allowing socialization with people and animals as well as habituation to objects and with handling. *Source:* Photo credit: Sara Flax.

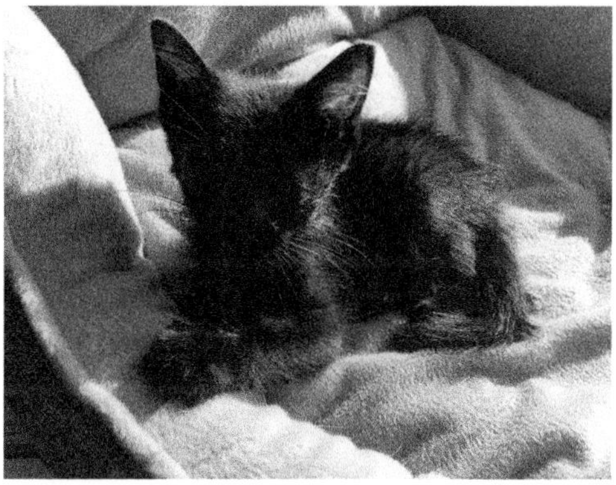

Figure 7.3 A seven-week-old kitten can maintain body temperature without huddling close to her dam and littermates. *Source:* Meghan E. Herron.

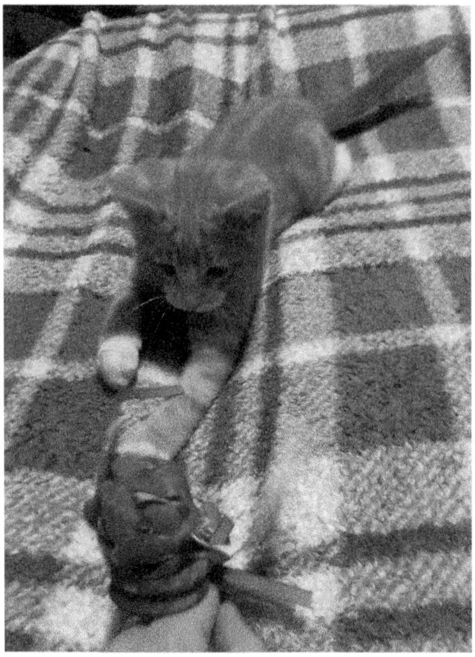

Figure 7.4 An eight-week-old kitten is developing eye–paw coordination through object play.
Source: With permission from Ashley Friend.

has been shown to affect the behavior of kittens with early-weaned kittens (from four weeks of age) showing predatory behavior earlier than usual, while late-weaned kittens (from nine weeks of age) developed predatory behavior later and were less likely to kill prey (Tan and Counsilman 1985).

From around the time the kittens turn three weeks of age, the queen starts to teach them the rudiments of predation. By the time the kittens are around five weeks of age, early, independent predatory behavior is seen. While early observational experience with predation enhances predatory skills and affects prey species preferences, cats will still be driven to hunt even if they never witness another cat hunting, capturing, or consuming their prey.

At four weeks of age, kittens can recognize the chirps of their mother when recordings of their mother's chirps, meows, and the same sounds made by other cats are played.

By five to six weeks of age, the kitten has full voluntary control of elimination, digging, and covering feces and urine on loose soil. The **gape** (flehmen) response begins to appear around five weeks of age and is similar to that of an adult (Figure 7.6) by seven weeks of age.

Fearful reactions to threatening stimuli may begin to be displayed by six weeks of age. Individual differences in behavior begin during the second month of life, due to genetic influences and different early environments.

Increased handling (mild stress) appears to speed development (Lyons et al. 2010). Between three and nine weeks of age, human contact and handling are very important so that the kitten develops socially acceptable behaviors. Thus, regular, gentle handling and

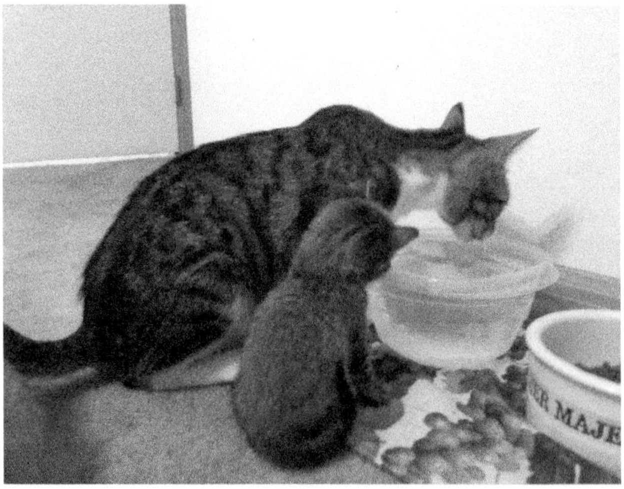

Figure 7.5 A four-week-old kitten observes his mother eat and drink, establishing early taste preferences.
Source: With permission from Sara Flax.

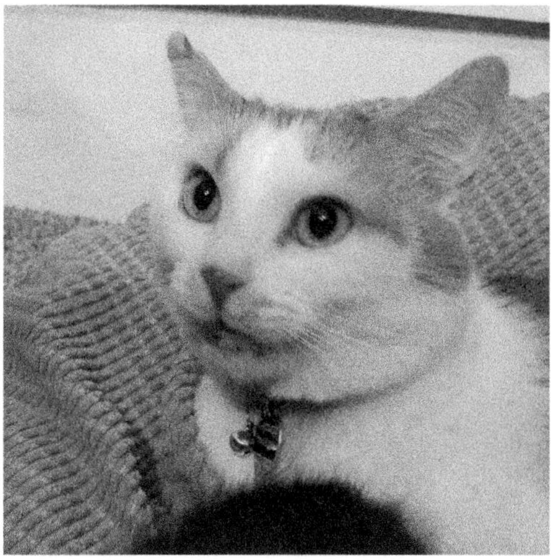

Figure 7.6 An adult cat gapes when smelling a new cat. This allows her to move pheromones into her vomeronasal organ via the ducts just behind her canine teeth. This behavior starts in kittens as young as five weeks of age. *Source:* With permission from Dr. Sara Bennett.

very mild routine restraint (such as picking up and holding) of the kitten should be practiced before the kitten reaches three months of age, and preferably it should start as early as possible, even from birth.

It is also important that the kitten is exposed to various novel stimuli in a nonthreatening manner during this sensitive period of development. The most receptive time for socializing kittens with humans and other species is between two and seven weeks of age, and the more handling by people is done, the less likely it is that fear of humans will develop (Collard 1967; Wilson et al. 1965). It appears that if kittens are to become social pets, then it is important to have human contact prior to seven weeks of age.

This is therefore also the best time to start socialization classes. Most behaviorists now believe that kitten socialization classes (when properly taught) are beneficial, and kitten socialization classes are suggested in the American Association of Feline Practitioners (AAFP) feline behavior guidelines, see Box 7.1 and Figure 7.7.

Box 7.1 Kitten socialization classes:

These classes are offered to kittens aged 8–12 weeks, allowing for 4–6 kittens (maximum) to interact and gain mutually beneficial social experiences. In class, kittens are also exposed to veterinary handling, various textures, and obstacles, as well as the various people attending class. In addition to valuable social experiences, kittens benefit from their caregivers' ability to ask questions, bring up concerns, and learn weekly lessons regarding cat health and behavior. Such classes are typically offered in a veterinary or other similar clinical space that can be fully sanitized before and after class, and all kittens should be health screened and appropriately vaccinated for their age by a licensed veterinarian at least seven days prior to the start of class.

Juvenile Period

The juvenile period is considered to last until sexual maturity. Although the basic behavioral patterns do not change during this time, there are gradual improvements in motor skills and coordination and the kittens become increasingly independent.

The juvenile period is associated with the kittens becoming ready to disperse. They also become fully independent from their mother for their food needs. Play and exploration of inanimate objects and locomotory play begin to escalate at approximately 7–8 weeks of age and peaks at approximately 18 weeks of age.

Social play is most prevalent from about 4–14 weeks of age. Social play begins to take on aspects of predation in the third month. Object play may be social or solitary, and may consist of pawing, stalking, leaping, and biting of objects and securing them with the paws. This type of play simulates a variety of aspects of the predatory sequence.

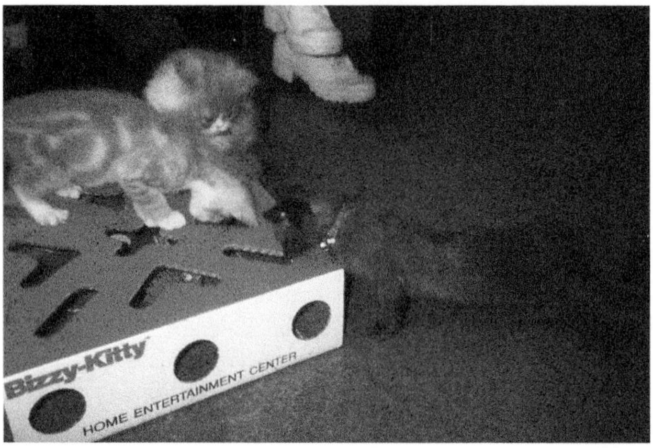

Figure 7.7 Kittens gain positive experiences with handling, new people, and other pets in kitten socialization classes. *Source:* With permission from Kersti Seksel.

The juvenile period is considered finished with the onset of puberty when sexual reproduction is possible. Female kittens may show their first signs of estrus between 3.5 and 12 months of age, although first estrus typically occurs at five to nine months. Earlier signs of estrus can be influenced by environmental factors, such as being born in the early spring, exposure to mature tomcats, presence of other female cats in estrus, or periods of increasing light. However, this also depends on the cat's body weight and may also vary depending on whether they are born in the northern or southern hemisphere. The juvenile period for male kittens is finished when they start to produce viable sperm at around 8–12 months of age. However, they are not considered to be psychologically mature at this age as social maturity does not occur until at least three years of age.

Cats are seasonally polyestrous so during the breeding season several periods of sexual receptivity occur. Queens are induced ovulators, that is, they do not ovulate unless mated and one queen may mate with several males during this time.

Sexual Maturity and Social Maturity

The adult period is characterized by the onset of sexual maturity and continues until the end of life. **Sexual maturity** is variable between breeds, with oriental breeds being sexually receptive as early as four months of age, while in other breeds it usually occurs between five and nine months of age.

Although cats can reproduce at sexual maturity, sexual maturity is not equivalent to **social maturity**. Social maturity refers to the development of adult social behavior and interactions with other cats and is believed to occur between 36 and 48 months of age. Social maturity includes defense of territory. It takes longer for cats than dogs to reach social maturity as it is thought that they must develop physically and mentally sufficiently to cope in an adult society.

Seniors

Cats are considered seniors when they are over 10 years of age and geriatric once over 15 years of age. While the aging process affects different cats in different ways, there are common changes that are indicative of advancing age. Among these is a loss of muscle mass and change in body carriage. Cats may begin to lose muscle tone over their backs, with muscle atrophy and loss also apparent around painful joints like hips affected by degenerative joint disease. They may slow down their activity, but most cats should remain active in their golden years. Both mental and cognitive abilities have been shown to decline with age (Gunn-Moore et al. 2007; Sordo and Gunn-Moore 2021). However, how much decline occurs depends on the individual cat.

Personality

The way that an individual tends to display characteristic behavior patterns, thoughts, and feelings is described as *personality*.

The ability of a cat to socialize with humans appears to be due to its inherited personality. Some research has shown that there are genetically "friendly" (bold) and genetically "unfriendly" (timid) characteristics. This part of the personality is paternally influenced, meaning the personality type of the father will have a stronger influence on his offspring's behavior than the personality type of the mother (Reisner et al. 1994). This predisposition means that some cats may never be very confident around humans, regardless of the amount of socialization they receive. However, regular handling from birth, until seven to nine weeks of age, can increase the likelihood of a well-socialized cat. Even 15 minutes a day is thought to be beneficial, and this effect is more profound for the timid kittens (Karsh and Turner 1988).

Variability in feline personality has important implications as to how well a cat will satisfy its human caretaker's expectations for a relationship with the cat. Bold, noisy cats are not valued by everyone, and some owners find it hard to cope with a timid cat that is not friendly to people.

Setting Up for Success

Armed with all this information, how can we set up for success so that the new kitten in the home becomes the companion that their new family wants? If pets are to be good companions for their human family, then we need to meet their needs, both physical and behavioral.

Basic *Physical* Needs: Food, Water, Latrine, Shelter

Food – Cats need food. The food should meet the nutritional requirements of the cat and be balanced and complete. Cats are obligate carnivores or *hyper-carnivorous*. This means that they rely on nutrients found only in animal products. As hunters, cats consume prey that contains high amounts of protein, moderate amounts of fat, and a minimal amount of carbohydrates, and this should be reflected in their diet.

When cats eat, they generally eat alone. As hunters, they only catch small prey, so it is not enough to share with others. Their willingness to eat together is often mistaken to mean that the cats like each other, but, in fact, they eat together because they have to, not because they want to. When they are hungry, they may eat together but if given the choice they will eat in turns.

Water – Cats need water, but most prefer not to drink next to where they eat. They need a water station well away from their food bowl. As hunters, they would not want to contaminate their water source with where they may disembowel their prey. Many people report that their cat drinks from the dogs' water bowl, the sink, or the saucer below the pot plants. This is just a reflection of the cat's evolutionary development and need for survival. One study involving household cats suggests cats prefer water of a cooler temperature (Tatliağiz and Akyazi 2023). Some cats also prefer running water and a water source that allows their whiskers not to touch the sides (Figure 7.8).

Latrine – Cats need a place to toilet. Litter trays/boxes should be large enough so that when the cat circles to dig a hole, the cat's tail should not touch the sides. Although many cats will tolerate a smaller tray, a human preference, when things go wrong – think *bigger* tray. Cats, like people, also like clean latrines. So cleaning, not just scooping out the solids, at least daily when the kitten arrives, is a good idea. After all, people prefer toilets that are flushed after use, and it makes good sense for hygiene reasons and parasite control for cats to prefer the same.

Although some cats will tolerate sharing a litter tray with a familiar cat, some will not, so multiple trays may be necessary. Some cats

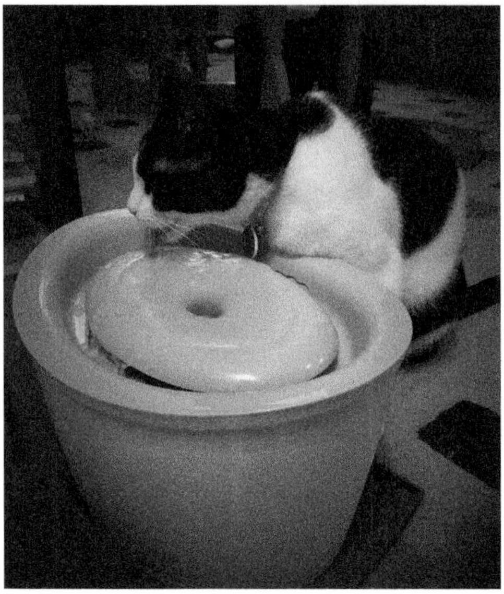

Figure 7.8 A cat drinks from a running water fountain. She can drink without letting her whiskers touch the sides of a bowl. *Source:* With permission from Dr. Andrea Y. Tu.

prefer to defecate in one tray and urinate in another, so again several trays may be necessary. The trays should not be placed next to each other but in different locations in the home.

People tend to have preferences for type of toilet paper, so it should not come as any surprise that cats also have preferences for litter type and depth. This may relate back to their evolutionary ancestors and parasite control.

The litter tray also needs to be easily accessible for the cat. It should be located in a low-traffic area. Litter trays should not be located up or down a set of stairs or hidden in the basement, which makes it harder to access. The sides of the litter tray should be easy for the kitten to climb over, so getting access to the latrine is not a challenge.

Some cats prefer open trays, so they can see what dangers may be around, while other cats prefer covered trays. Regardless, the litter tray should be large, clean, easily accessible for the cat, and should contain a litter type the cat prefers. See Chapter 13 for greater detail on litter box management and troubleshooting problems.

Shelter – Cats need places to rest and sleep. They may be the same place, but generally, they are different. Just like humans may rest on the couch after a long day at work, but sleep overnight in their bed, cats tend to have consistent preferences for resting and sleeping, and those places are often not the same.

Basic Behavioral Needs: Hunting, Chewing, Scratching, Viewing

Hunting – Cats are natural-born predators, but not all cats hunt. Most cats have an instinct to focus, stalk, and chase small, quickly moving objects/animals. When appropriate opportunities to rehearse this sequence are not provided, cats, especially kittens, will literally pounce on the next best thing, wreaking havoc on other pets and, sometimes, people in the home. It is, hence, essential that families provide hunting outlets through safe and appropriate hunting and play.

Toys that allow the cat to use its natural instincts to hunt and pounce allow cats to exercise both their minds and bodies. Instead of feeding meals just from a food bowl, some of the cat's food can be used to stimulate both the body and the brain (Figure 7.9). Searching for food around the house, hidden up high, or from food-dispensing puzzle toys provides this exercise for the cat. Games and toys should be challenging but not a source of frustration for the cat. They should also be safe for the cat to use, with no sharp edges or parts that could be ingested while the cat investigates. See Box 7.2 for insight on the use of laser pointers with cats.

Toys for cats need not be expensive or complex. Cats like to get into cardboard boxes, paper bags, and happily play with scrunched-up paper (Figure 7.10). Cats love to run and pounce but play should not involve the use of human hands, fingers, feet, or toes. Cats are carnivores, so dangling "meat" in front of them as a play object should be avoided. The use of

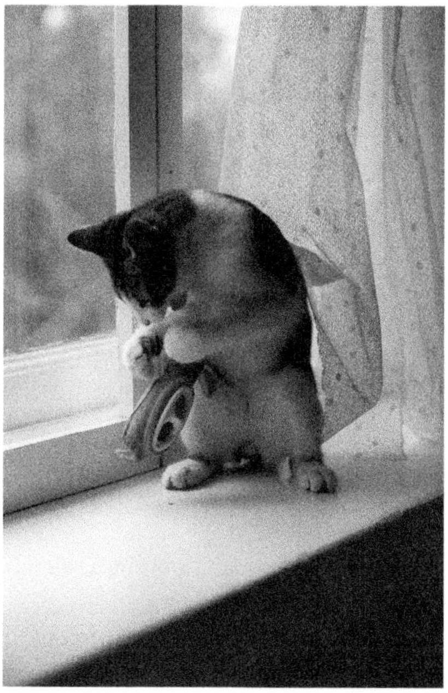

Figure 7.9 An interactive feeding toy (Indoor Hunting Feeder [Doc & Phoebe's Cat Co.; Camden, NJ, US]), allows this cat to hunt for a portion of her daily food in a way that allows her to express her natural feeding instincts. *Source:* With permission from Sarah Millet.

toys that move on poles or dangle from doors are much safer option.

Cats are crepuscular, which means that they are most likely to be active at dusk and dawn. This is the best time for the humans in their family to play with them. Cats play in short active bursts so this does not have to be for prolonged periods, but it should be aerobically active.

Some cats, particularly wild-crossed breeds, such as Bengals, have high exercise needs that correlate to when and how long they might hunt in the wild. The house is their playground, and when that household cannot provide ample space for exercise, a little creativity can go a long way. Treats or toys tossed down a long hallway (yes, many cats WILL play fetch!), extended-length wands that prompt a cat to run from one side of the room to the other, and exercise wheels can provide extended physical exercise as needed (Figure 7.11).

Box 7.2 Box

Laser pointers can provide endless fun for our feline friends, but some cats take the game a bit too far. A recent study showed a correlation (not necessarily causation) between laser pointer games and compulsive light-chasing behavior in cats (Kogan and Grigg 2021). Further research is needed to explore the depth of this correlation, but caution should be exercised when engaging in laser pointer play. Some clinicians speculate that the endless chasing of an object that cannot be physically captured overstimulates the "seeking" pathways in the brain without a clear or defined end or "capture." Without a final shutoff, the cat may begin seeking lights to chase elsewhere, focusing compulsively on reflections and other light sources. To provide more finality at the end of a game of laser pointer chase, the light should lead the cat to a treat or beloved small toy before shutting off the light. This allows the cat to "capture" a physical object and complete the predatory sequence.

Chewing – The propensity to chew and/or consume plants or other household items varies greatly between individual cats. As obligate carnivores, there is no physiological need for cats to consume plant material, yet almost all cats do so at some point in their lives. Whether this is in response to gastrointestinal upset or an attempt at antiparasitism remains unclear. Regardless, families taking in cats should be aware that their cats may be attracted to household plants and remove those that may be toxic or fatal. The American Society for the Prevention of Cruelty to Animals® (ASPCA®) offers an A–Z list of plants and their potential for toxicity – see Toxic and Non-Toxic Plants (aspca.org).

While many household plants are indeed safe, most families do not wish to see their beloved plants destroyed. Keeping ornamental

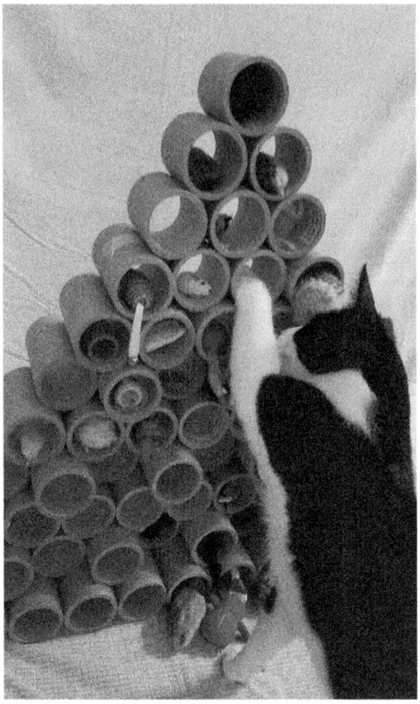

Figure 7.10 This homemade tower is comprised of cardboard tubing. Toys and treats hidden inside the tubes can provide hours of investigative fun for a cat. *Source:* With permission from Deborah Crosier.

plants out of reach and offering safe, appealing alternatives should help keep destructive chewing below the nuisance level. Examples include cat grass, catnip plants, and wheat grass. Some cats can be quite destructive – chewing plants to their roots or even pulling them up by their roots. It may be of benefit financially to grow such plants at home so they can be replenished frequently (Figure 7.12).

Scratching – Cats need places to scratch. Scratching serves two main purposes – nail maintenance and communication. When cats hook their nails onto a rough surface, they pull and then shed the outer layer of the nails. This is essential in keeping nails sharp and preventing overgrowth/nails from growing into the foot pads. Scratching also allows for both visual and pheromonal communication. Cats apply pressure with their foot pads as they scratch, allowing for ample pheromone deposition in the scratched area. The tattered mess left on posts (or furniture) gives a visual signal to other cats, prompting them to investigate the deposited pheromones. Pheromones are nonvolatile chemicals (see Chapter 4) and, as such, linger for days on surfaces. This allows for long-lasting interspecies communication. Scratching posts may be vertical or horizontal, depending on the cat's individual preferences (Figure 7.13). But key characteristics are substrate, stability, height (length), and location.

- **Substrate** – The most appealing material covering the post or mat is one that allows the nails to hook, rip, and tear, leaving a

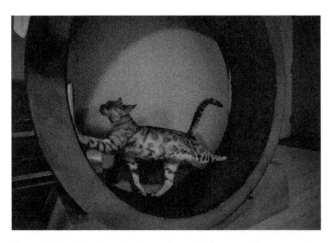

Figure 7.11 Exercise wheels, such as this homemade carpeted one, allow high-energy cats an outlet for their physical exercise needs. *Source:* With permission from Sheri Johnson.

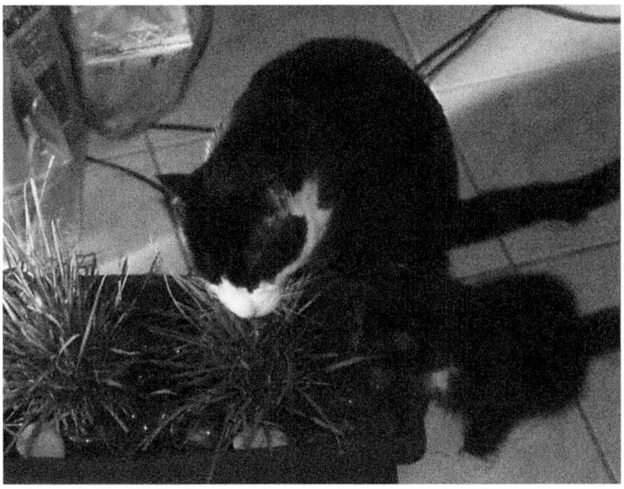

Figure 7.12 Cat-safe plants, such as these homegrown cat grasses, allow cats to engage in normal chewing behavior without risk of toxicity. *Source:* With permission from Kersti Seksel.

tattered display or mess. Examples of appealing substrates include sisal, shag carpet, and corrugated cardboard. Posts should not be replaced when they look tatty as that is when it has most meaning for the cat. It would be like someone deleting all of your emails and so you have no record of what was sent or received!

- **Stability** – Posts need to be stable, not tipping or wobbling when the cat uses it. For vertical posts, this means a sturdy, wide base, and for horizontal posts, it means a secure attachment to the floor or base surface. They need to withstand the torque placed on them when the cats put pressure on them to release the outer nail layers.
- **Height or length** – Vertical posts need to be high enough and horizontal posts long enough to allow for full extension of the front limbs when scratching. The height of a couch back or the length of a stair width are good places to start.

Location – The post should be in a place where the cat spends time and in a spot that is readily visible. This is likely why corners of couches or recliners in the dead center of a living room are popular scratching targets. Often cats will scratch after napping or resting, making placement near resting areas appealing.

Viewing – Cats feel safest up high in secure areas on the periphery of rooms (Ellis et al. 2013). This allows for a safe vantage point of their environment, away from the hustle and bustle of the household and other pets in the home. Only the most confident of cats will be found lounging on the floor in the middle of a room. Elevated resting platforms placed near windows also allow an entertaining outside view, expanding their mental stimulation options beyond the indoors (Figure 7.14). Some timid cats also prefer resting places out of view and may hide under beds or covered furniture (hidey-holes). Offering places for concealment in elevated areas may further increase their comfort and allow them to come out from hiding more often.

Keep in mind that if appealing elevated areas are not provided, cats will make do with what they have. This typically means counter-lounging, perching on top of refrigerators, backs of furniture, and other household items. This may not be an issue for families who do not mind little cat paws in their eating places. Countertops are prime resting real estate for most cats as they are elevated, close to food and family, and are often near windows or have access to sunny lounging spots. Resting platforms/perches need to be just as appealing, if not more appealing than the counters

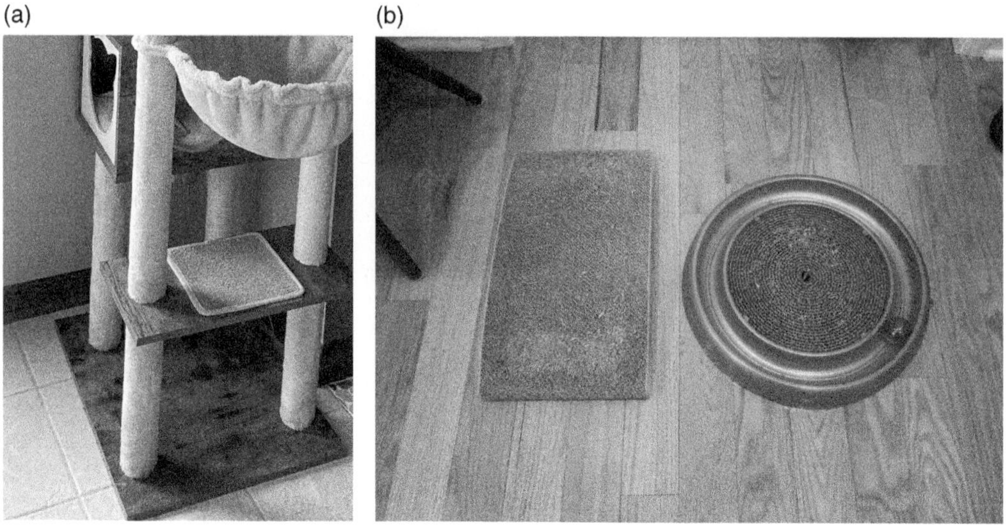

Figure 7.13 Scratching posts should be stable and large enough to allow for maximum stretch when scratching. Both vertical (a) and horizontal (b) options should be offered until preferences are established/known. *Source:* (a) Meghan E. Herron, (b) With permission from Carlo Siracusa.

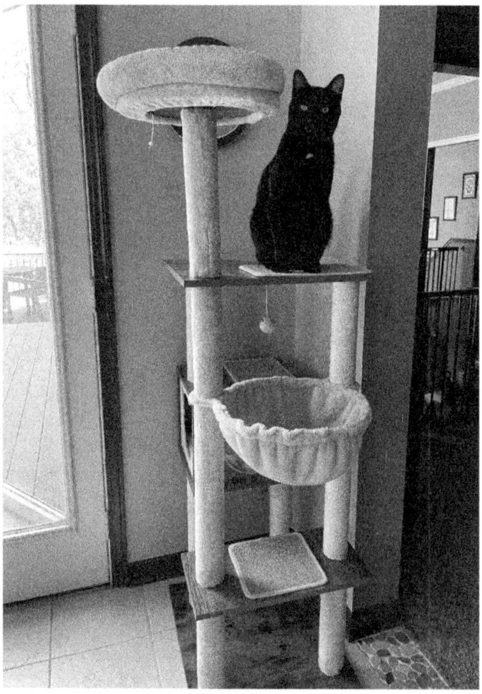

Figure 7.14 High resting platforms allow cats a safe vantage point. Placing them on the periphery of a room near windows will increase their appeal. *Source:* Meghan E. Herron.

and located near or in the kitchen area (Figure 7.15) if we expect them to be utilized. In winter, having a cat heating pad in high-up resting places can prove useful to encourage the cat to use these areas.

Indoor Versus Outdoors

One might read the above recommendations for meeting the cat's needs and find that the great outdoors likely meets these needs readily and easily. Our clients must consider whether to keep their new kitten strictly indoors or to allow access to the outdoors. Opinions vary as to what is best, but there is no doubt that an indoor-only cat is safer. In fact, cats allowed outdoor access have been shown to have a shorter lifespan than cats who are strictly kept indoors (Ragan 2003). This is likely due to the inherent risks of outdoor life, including being hit by a car, fights with an unfamiliar or roaming cats, exposure to infectious diseases and ectoparasites, and falling victim to local predators (foxes, coyotes, hawks, alligators, and crocodiles.). Provided the cat's needs, behavioral and environmental, are met, cats

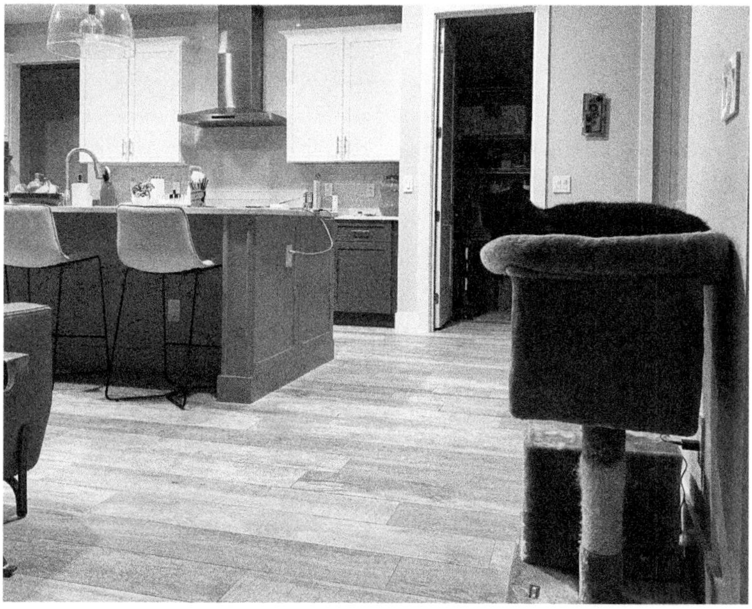

Figure 7.15 Countertops are prime lounging spots for many cats. To encourage these cats to lounge elsewhere, resting areas should be in proximity to where the family spends time and of the same height as the countertop (or higher). Daily treats to reward perching in this area will help reinforce the behavior. *Source:* With permission from Lisa Radosta.

can live very happily indoors only. If the cat is allowed indoor and outdoor access when young, it can be more difficult to keep the cat strictly indoors later. If needed, teaching a cat to walk on a harness can be a good way to allow indoor cats access to the outdoors safely.

Setting Up for Success – Living with Multiples

Feline social systems differ vastly from those of canines and humans, often setting feline families up for unrealistic or unmet expectations. People may feel their older cat needs a "friend" and consider getting a new overly exuberant and playful kitten as a companion. Cats have not evolved (generally) to have prolonged social contact with others and bringing in a young, active cat may be the last thing a senior cat wants. Cats are, indeed, social animals, and many thrive in the multi-cat environment, but most are not as socially obligated as dogs and people tend to be.

Cats tend to time-share real estate, but they do not often share resources. They need to have access to their own food, water, resting, and sleeping areas, and they prefer their own toileting area. All resources should be located in what they consider to be their core territory (core area). Regardless of the number of cats in the household, each cat needs their behavioral needs met in a way that can be accomplished without always having to share that resource with another cat. Think of these cats as "me me me, mine mine mine and now now now". If the human family understands this about cats, then the potential for problems is minimized. Therefore, resources should be plentiful.

The key words for new feline introductions are slow and gradual. How cats will get along for life is directly correlated with how well their introduction went at the start of cohabitation (Levine et al. 2005). Typically, the newcomer is kept in a separate space from the resident cat(s) where all basic physical and behavioral needs are met. They are introduced to the rest of the social group gradually, starting with scent exchange, then controlled visual access to each other, and then supervised physical time together. One should not proceed with the next step unless the previous step has been calm and without tension, fear, or stress. See Chapter 14 for more information on managing inter-cat aggression issues and setting up multiples for success.

Veterinary Experiences

To keep kittens healthy, they need regular veterinary attention, including annual to biannual wellness visits and additional exams throughout the year for any problems that arise. Ideally, kittens should learn that veterinary visits are not stressful and can even be fun. As described in Box 7.1, socialization classes within the veterinary clinic are a good way to help the kitten gain social experience as well as to help the kitten's family learn all about felines, and why they do what they do.

Kittens also need to learn that being placed in their carrier leads to a positive experience and not always a trip to a place that might be stressful such as the vet or a cattery for boarding. Leaving the cat carrier out in the home for the kitten to explore and become familiar with is a good way to start. Feeding tasty treats in the carrier and leaving favored toys inside it can entice a kitten not only to enter the carrier but also to linger, perhaps even rest or sleep there. Leaving it out in an area where the family spends time is a good way for the humans to remember to toss treats into the carrier daily, and for the kitten to grow up seeing the carrier as part of daily life – not something that just comes out once a year for veterinary visits. If possible, cats should never be forced into the carrier, as the cat is already stressed when it goes into the carrier, which will make travel to the vet as well as the vet visit itself more difficult. See Appendix B and Chapter 11 for more information on carrier comfort and safe transport.

Clients can also work on teaching kittens that nail trims need not be stressful. Using rewards and slowly habituating kittens to have first one paw handled, and then another will lead to more compliance with nail trims later. Once the kitten accepts the paws being touched, the client can work on retracting the claws, using rewards such as tiny, tasty treats, and very quiet praise.

Popular culture suggests that cats are "self-cleaning" and do not need to be washed or brushed. However, some cats will need to be bathed at some stage during their life, either because they develop a skin disease or soil themselves somehow. Hairless or fine-haired cats, such as the Sphinx and Rex, will require regular bathing to cut down on yeast accumulation and dark-colored oil accumulation. Creating a positive experience with bathing, and using treats and toys early on, will save the client from a lifetime of struggle. If bathing a cat, it is best not to just submerge them in water, but to use a handheld shower attachment and use warm water. If the shower is held close to the cat's body, and moved slowly along the cat's back, it should feel like a gentle warm massage to the cat.

Long-haired cats often need brushing and grooming so that they do not develop mats. The hair on their paws needs regular trimming to prevent litter clumping/accumulation and subsequent litter box issues. Teach clients to always brush in the same direction as the fur grows, not against it, and to brush slowly, but firmly, as if giving the cat a massage. Grooming sessions should be kept brief as there is no need to groom the whole cat at once if the cat is not enjoying the experience. Tasty treats throughout help establish this experience as positive and cats will be more compliant as adults. If the kitten is taught to accept these husbandry procedures when it is young, it can make life much easier for the cat as well as the cat's human family later in life.

"Red Flag" Kitties – When Nuisance is not Normal

If all the needs of the cat have been adequately and appropriately met and the kitten still behaves in an unacceptable manner, it may be time to seek professional help. If the kitten does not use its litter tray, bites or scratches excessively, hides all the time, or destroys and ingests nonfood items, then it is the veterinarian's job to triage the problem and to rule out any medical causes for the behavior, especially pain. If a medical contribution for the behavior is not detected, or if once resolved the behavior persists, referral to a behavior professional may be warranted. This is especially true if the general practitioner does not feel behavioral treatment is within their area of comfort or expertise. See Chapter 12 for details on behavioral triage. Anxiety disorders can be recognized at a young age, so in the interests of the cat's and the family's welfare management, treatment, and referral options should be discussed as soon as possible.

Conclusion

Behavior is a product of learning, genetics, and environmental factors. As discussed in Chapter 2, the behavior of domesticated cats is stunningly similar to that of their wild counterparts. This means that many of their natural or "normal" behaviors can be quite a nuisance to their human families if they are not given appropriate outlets for the behaviors they are driven to perform, or when their basic physical and behavioral needs are not met. While it is important to recognize that there are developmental differences between breeds, individual personality also affects the way a cat behaves. Finally, a good understanding of developmental periods helps us to cement the bond between companion cats and their human family, hopefully decreasing relinquishment and euthanasia. This knowledge helps veterinarians give sound advice, preserve cat welfare, and secure the future of cats as human companions.

References

Ahola, M.K., Vapalahti, K., and Lohi, H. (2017). Early weaning increases aggression and stereotypic behaviour in cats. *Nat. Sci. Rep.* 7: 10412.

Barrett, P. and Bateson, P. (1978). The development of play in cats. *Behaviour* 66: 106.

Bateson, P. (2014). Behavioural development in the cat. In: *The Domestic Cat: The Biology of its Behaviour*, 3e (ed. D. Turner and P. Bateson), 13. Cambridge: Cambridge University Press.

Collard, R.R. (1967). Fear of strangers and play behavior in kittens with varied social experience. *Child. Dev.* 38: 877–891.

Ellis, S.L., Rodan, I., Carney, H.C. et al. (2013). AAFP and ISFM feline environmental needs guidelines. *J. Feline Med. Surg.* 15 (3): 219–230.

Gallo, P.V., Werboff, J., and Knox, K. (1980). Protein restriction during gestation and lactation: development of attachment behavior in cats. *Behav. Neural Biol.* 29: 216.

Gunn-Moore, D. Moffat, K, Christie, LA. Cognitive dysfunction and the neurobiology of ageing in cats *J. Small Anim.* 2007 48, 546–553 DOI: https://doi.org/10.1111/j.1748-5827.2007.00386.x

Ragan, P. and Humane Society of the United States (HSUS) (2003). *A Safe Cat is a Happy Cat.* Washington, DC: Ragan, P., Humane Society of the United States, (HSUS).

Karsh, E.B. and Turner, D.C. (1988). The human-cat relationship. In: *The Domestic Cat: The Biology of its Behaviour*, 1e (ed. D.C. Turner and P.P.G. Bateson), 157–177. Cambridge: Cambridge University Press.

Kogan, L.R. and Grigg, E.K. (2021). Laser light pointers for use in companion cat play: association with guardian-reported abnormal repetitive behaviors. *Animals* 11 (8): 2178.

Kolb, B. and Nonneman, A.J. (1975). The development of social responsiveness in kittens. *Anim. Behav.* 23: 368.

Levine, E., Perry, P., Scarlett, J., and Houpt, K.A. (2005). Intercat aggression in households following the introduction of a new cat. *Appl. Anim. Behav. Sci. 90* (3-4): 325–336.

Lyons, D.M., Parker, K.J., and Schatzberg, A.F. (2010). Animal models of early life stress: implications for understanding resilience. *Dev. Psychobiol.* 52: 616–624.

Reisner, I.R., Houpt, K.A., Erb, H.N., and Quimby, F.W. (1994). Friendliness to humans and defensive aggression in cats: the influence of handling and paternity. *Physiol. Behav.* 1119–1124.

Simonson, M. (1979). Effects of maternal malnourishment, development and behavior in successive generations in the rat and cat. In: *Malnutrition, Environment and Behavior*, 133–160. Ithaca, NY: Cornell University Press.

Smith, B. and Jensen, G. (1977). Brain development in the feline. *Nutr. Rep. Int.* 16: 487.

Sordo, L. and Gunn-Moore, D.A. (2021). Cognitive dysfunction in cats: update on neuropathological and behavioural changes plus clinical management. *Vet. Rec.* 188: e3. https://doi.org/10.1002/vetr.3.

Tan, P.L. and Counsilman, J.J. (1985). The influence of weaning on prey-catching behaviour in kittens. *Z Tierpsychol.* 70: 148.

Tatliağiz, Z. and Akyazi, I. (2023). Investigation of the effect of water temperature on water consumption of cats. *J. Istanbul Vet. Sci. 7* (1): 50–54.

Wilson, M., Warren, J.M., and Abbott, L. (1965). Infantile stimulation, activity, and learning by cats. *Child. Dev.* 36: 843–853.

8

The Development of Behavior and the Shaping of the Human–Animal Bond

Horses

Katherine A. Houpt[1] *and Sharon Madere*[2]

[1] *Cornell University, College of Veterinary Medicine, Ithaca, NY, USA*
[2] *International Association of Animal Behavior Consultants (IAABC), Cranberry Township, PA, USA*

Introduction

Foals are a delight to watch as they meet the world, their mother, humans, and eventually, other horses. It is during this time that caretakers can shape the future of the foals by introducing common husbandry procedures such as grooming, hoof care, and leading. The importance of suckling promptly after birth, and knowledge of other normal behaviors such as coprophagia, are essential concepts regarding foal raising. This chapter will review these concepts, walk you through important developmental periods in horses, and provide tips that have proven helpful in reducing the stress of training.

The Neonatal Period

Foals are usually born in the early morning hours, probably as a predator defense strategy. It is important for the clinician to recognize that the mare will act normally until the hour before foaling – at this point, she will stop eating. The mare licks the newborn foal during the first hour after its delivery (Figure 8.1). The function of licking is to dry the foal, which is wet with uterine fluids, and to stimulate respiration and muscular activity. Some clinicians hypothesize that licking may help in foal recognition, but olfactory recognition also plays a strong role.

The foal is **precocious,** meaning it can stand, walk, and follow its mother within hours of birth. Foals are also born with full vision and hearing capabilities. The foal will initially struggle to stand but usually succeeds within the first hour (Figure 8.2a–c).

Once the foal is standing, it will immediately try to find the udder (Figure 8.3a–c). This is easier for pony foals than for the longer-legged horse foals. The latter have to flex their forelegs in order to be level with the ends of the teats. The visual cue the foal is using to locate nourishment is the underline of her belly, so the foal will often approach the axial rather than the inguinal junction of the mare's body and limbs.

Whereas a pony foal will usually suckle within 30 minutes, a thoroughbred takes up to 60 minutes (Rossdale 1967). Finding the udder and suckling is essential for the foal, not only for calories but also for antibodies because the equine placenta allows no antibodies to reach the foal. Without colostrum, the foal will have no immunity. The other time-sensitive factor is the period when antibodies can be carried across the intestinal wall and into the bloodstream. The intestine of the foal gradually loses

Introduction to Animal Behavior and Veterinary Behavioral Medicine, First Edition. Edited by Meghan E. Herron.

Companion website: www.wiley.com/go/introductiontoanimalbehavior

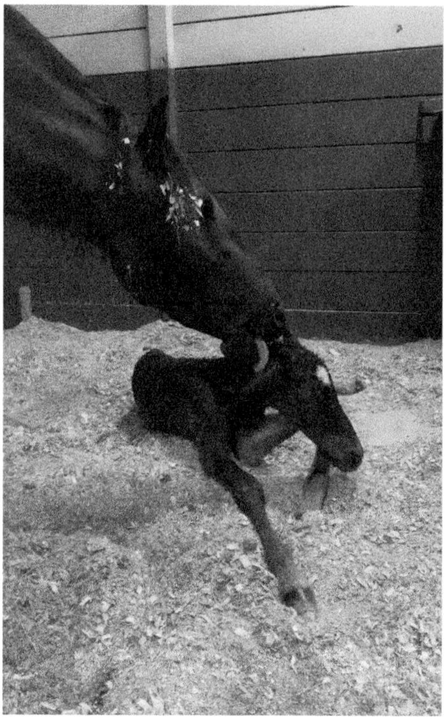

Figure 8.1 A mare licks a newborn foal to clean off uterine fluids and to stimulate respiration and muscular activity.

its ability to absorb antibodies over the first 24 hours after birth when gut closure is complete. Once the foal has found the udder, it with suckle every 15 minutes around the clock for the first few days and is still suckling once an hour at 6 months of age. The foal spends the rest of its time lying down, playing, and grazing.

The foal will lie down soon after birth but seems to find that a difficult task, often flexing its limbs, then standing up again and falling down. The foal will sleep in lateral recumbency for 15% percent of its daily time budget, decreasing to 2% at 40 weeks. Resting in sternal recumbency occupies another 15% and does not decrease as rapidly as lateral recumbency (Boy and Duncan 1979) (Figure 8.4). When awake, the foal will follow the mare.

Coprophagia

Coprophagia is a normal foal behavior and clients need to be aware that it is not a sign of abnormality. The dam's feces are preferentially consumed over their own, or the feces of others (Figure 8.5). The purpose of this behavior is

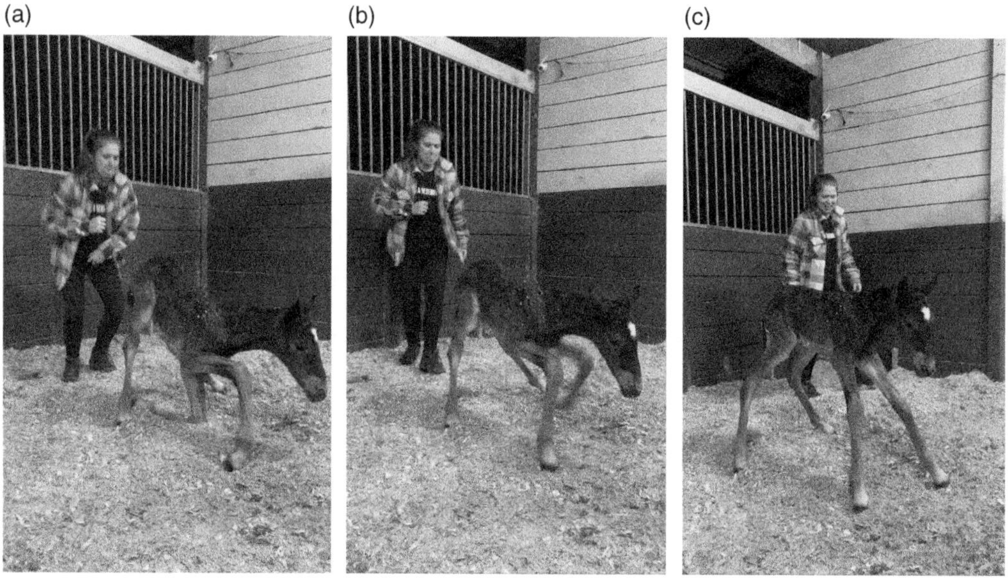

Figure 8.2 (a–c) A foal standing for the first time. First one forelimb flexes (a), then both forelimbs flex (b), and then all limbs are extended (c).

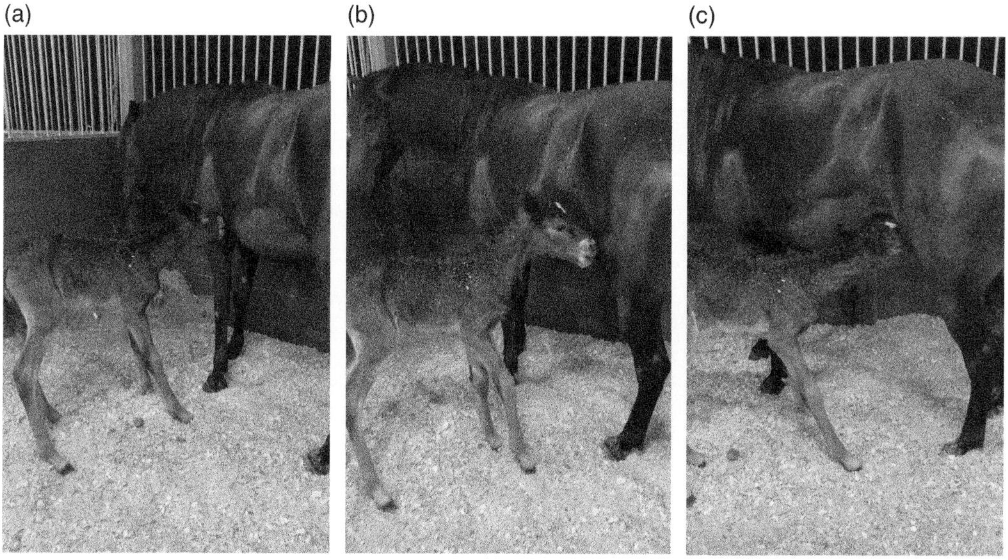

Figure 8.3 (a–c) A foal finds the utter. First, the foal approaches the mare's axilla (a), then the inguinal fold (b), and then finds the utter and suckles (c).

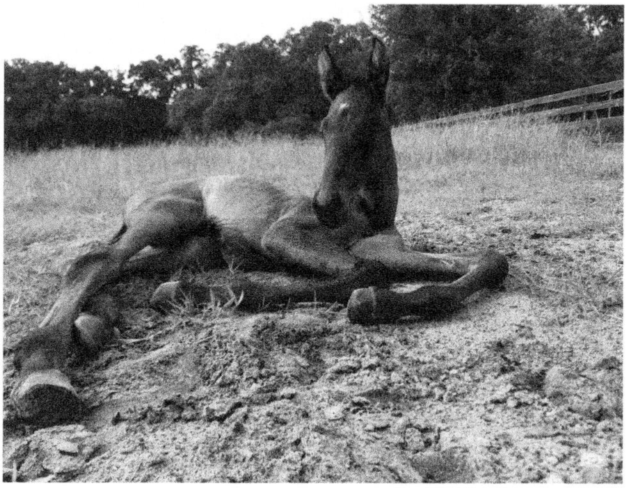

Figure 8.4 A foal rests in lateral recumbency.

unclear. Some clinicians suggest that foals consume the mare's feces to add her intestinal microbiome to their own (Crowell-Davis and Caudle 1989).

The precise age of the socialization period has not been identified in horses. To determine a socialization period, mares and foals would have to be isolated from all human contact from birth for several weeks and the behavior of those foals toward humans would have to be compared with that of foals exposed to humans from birth. Because foals are so precocial, the development period is probably condensed into hours after birth rather than weeks as in carnivores. We do know that the attachment to the dam is greatest at about four weeks and declines after that. Meanwhile, the mare's attachment to the foal declines from birth onwards. How long does it take for the mare to bond with the foal, and how long after delivery is she willing to accept a foal? These questions have been answered in ruminants. Goats, for example, will accept a kid up to an hour after delivery and need only five minutes to form the bond. To determine this in horses, we would need to take foals away from mares at birth, and then present the foals to the mother at different time periods – 30 minutes after delivery, one hour after delivery, and so on.

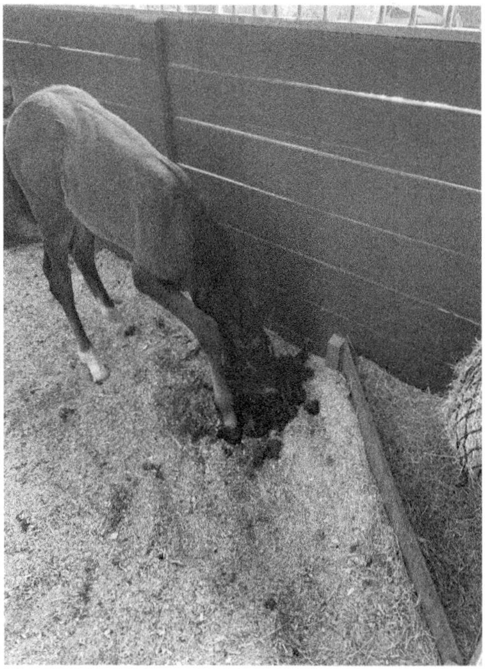

Figure 8.5 The consumption of feces by the foal is a normal behavior.

Mare–Foal Communication

Most mare–foal communication is vocal. The mare and foal nicker to one another. The mare is calling the foal to her, and the foal is requesting milk. Nickering persists in adult horses when they wish to be fed. When out of visual contact, mares and foals will neigh, and the mare neighs more to her own than any other foal, whereas the foal does not discriminate (Wolski et al. 1980). When a foal is frightened by another horse, or even by its mother, it will open and close its mouth while retracting its lips (Figure 8.6). While the term for this expression is **snapping**, it is not an aggressive gesture. More likely it is an appeasement gesture signaling that the foal is immature. In fact, if a horse exhibits snapping behavior to another horse, it suggests they are not fully mature, or that they have learned to fear the horse to which they are directing the snapping.

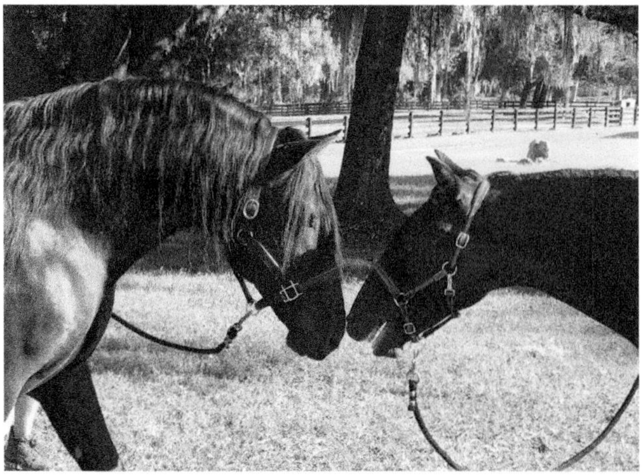

Figure 8.6 A foal engages in snapping behavior by opening and closing the mouth with lips retracted as an appeasing gesture to an older horse.

Early Training

Imprint Training

"Imprint" training was a technique popularized by the late Robert Miller, DVM. It involves handling the foal all over, slapping the hooves, and handling the tail, ears, hooves, and mouth as soon after birth as possible. The hypothesis was that this **flooding** of early handling would render the foal easier to handle for the rest of its life. Since then, this hypothesis has not been substantiated and researchers now recognize that such early interference with the foal–mare bonding may have undesirable consequences. Studies have shown *no benefit* to early imprint training. In fact, there was little difference in resistance to handling between imprint-trained foals and their controls (Williams et al. 2002; Simpson 2002). Handling a young horse at any age over the first year will improve its tractability, rendering the animal easier to handle, indicating that there is nothing unique about neonatal handling. The danger of handling a foal right after birth is that the mare may not form a bond with the foal, leading to lack of passive transfer of immunity and potential foal rejection. Another safer technique is handling the *dam* (brushing and hand feeding) daily for the first weeks of the foal's life. One study found that this positive handling of the mare in the presence of the foal resulted in a more tractable foal (Henry et al. 2005). Furthermore, Søndergaard and Jago (2010) found that although early handling (10 minutes, 3 times a day, for the first 2 days after birth) did not affect the foals' responses to freeze branding, the dams of handled foals were less active in keeping their foals close, and the handled foals themselves had a smaller flight distance from humans. In summary, positive handling of the mare in the presence of the foal may have longer-lasting effects than handling of the foal itself.

Halter Training

A crucial part of early handling is halter training. This has a lot more benefits than "imprint" training and uses positive reinforcement to teach foals to accept handling. It is important to use very small steps/approximations to help the foal understand and feel confident with the process of having a halter put on its head. In the beginning, the halter is held simply for the foal to investigate. As the foal touches the halter with its nose, the trainer "marks" the behavior with a conditioned reinforcer (see Chapter 5 for a review) and then offers the desired reward – scratching (Figure 8.7a). This is repeated several times. Then the halter is lifted to the foal's head, again the trainer marks, scratches, and removes the halter (Figure 8.7b). Gradually, the halter is put over the nose, and then the neck strap is lifted behind the ears. With each repetition, the halter is briefly placed and then immediately removed so as not to overwhelm the foal. Finally, the halter is buckled in place (Figure 8.7c).

Using Positive Reinforcement

Positive Reinforcement, as discussed in Chapter 5, is the addition of any desirable stimulus that increases the likelihood of a specific behavior. In order to use positive reinforcement training, we must first identify something that the foal greatly desires. In the early weeks and months, scratching is ideal. We can offer scratches in various places to determine which place the foal likes best. Favorite locations often include the line of the shoulder, the neck crest, chest, and rump. Preferences may change from week to week. To test, offer the scratch; if the foal enjoys it, it will stand, and you will usually see a stretch of the neck and/or scrunching of the upper lips. Take a couple of steps back away from the foal. If they come towards you, you know they liked it! Positive reinforcement is most effectively used with a "marker" signal (**conditioned reinforcer**), similar to clicker training with dogs. Many horse trainers will use a "tongue pop" sound, or a specific word said in a quick and consistent way, such as "good!" or "yes!" The marker sound is made, followed

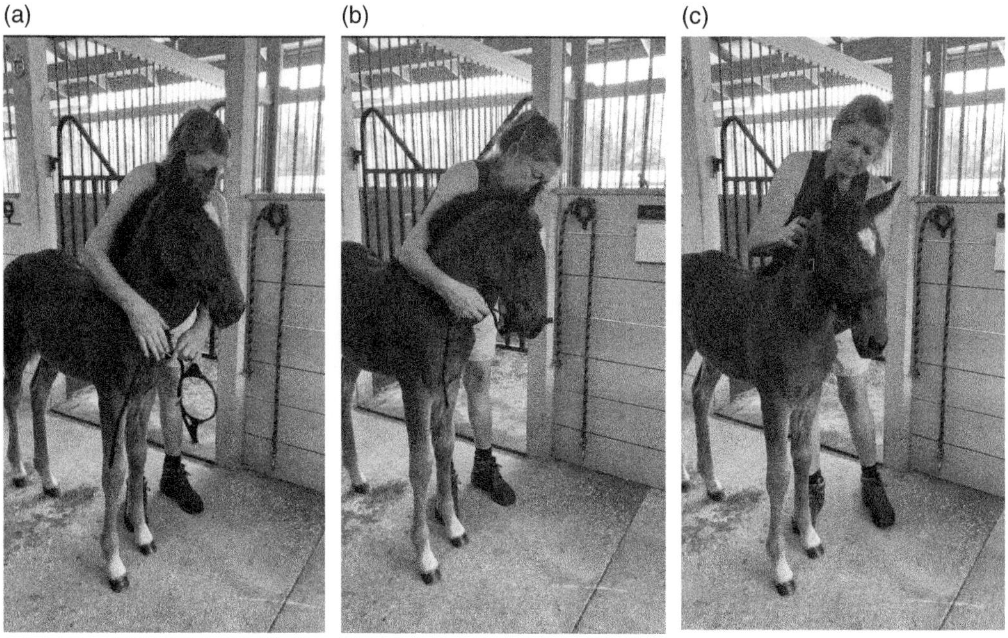

Figure 8.7 (a–c) Halter training with a foal. First, the handler offers and rewards for the tolerance of gentle restraint (a), then the handler places the halter just over the muzzle of the foal (b), then the halter is fastened, (c) and the foal is rewarded with scratches.

immediately by the scratching. Figure 8.8 indicates how much a young filly enjoys scratching long before she would enjoy solid food.

Feeding Behavior

Grazing begins as exploratory behavior. The foal will put anything into its mouth and soon learn that grass is tastier than its mother's tail or the fence rail (Figure 8.9).

When foals and mares are kept on pasture, grazing increases from 8% of the daily time budget at one week of age to 60% of the daytime budget at six months of age (Crowell-Davis et al. 1985). The foal grazes when the mare grazes, which probably ensures that they know which plants are safe to eat.

Play

The first form of foal play centers on the dam. The foal will pull at her mane and tail and gallop around her. The foal will gradually be willing to move farther and farther from the mare, to explore or simply to gallop. By three weeks, the foals gradually begin to play with one another, and solitary play declines by two months. That is the time when sex differences between colts and fillies first arise. Fillies like to mutually groom. Colts like to play-fight by rearing up, striking, and mounting (Crowell-Davis et al. 1987). In addition to mounting, colts also exhibit **flehmen** – aspirating nonvolatile material into their vomeronasal organ. This behavior peaks at three to four weeks, about the time the mare would be expected to come into foal heat (Crowell-Davis and Houpt, 1985).

Social Preference Development

Feral mares may have preferred associates – usually their dam's preferred associate or her foal – but fillies usually leave their natal bands and will have little choice in which mares are added to her band by the lead stallion. Colts

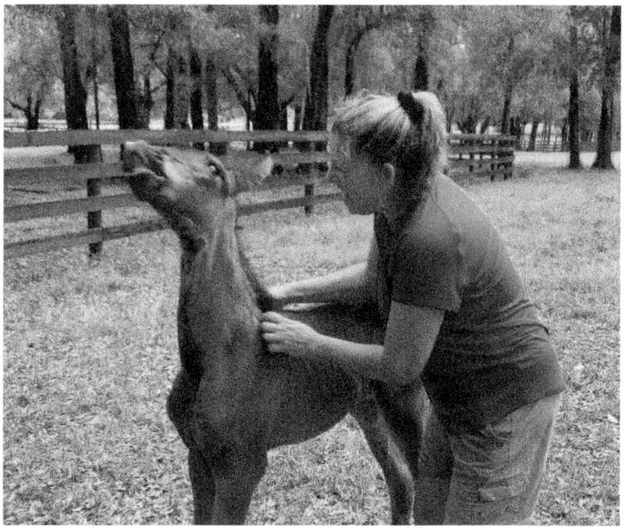

Figure 8.8 A young filly enjoys scratching as a reward for desirable behavior. At this age scratching is a more powerful reinforcer than solid food.

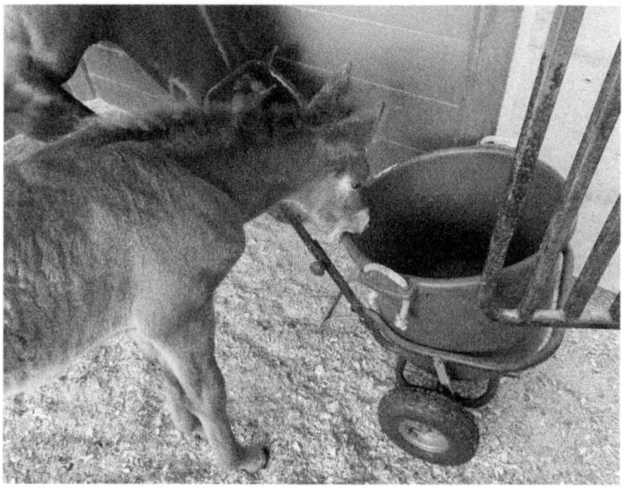

Figure 8.9 Exploratory mouthing behaviors are a normal way for a foal to explore the environment.

will have been driven from their natal bands by their sire and will join a bachelor group where they may form associations with other colts, but eventually, they will leave to form their own bands where, although they may prefer the company of one of their mares to another, the breeding season will affect that. Domestic horses have no choice as to their preferred associates. We place stage horses together and can only hope that friendly rather than agonistic attachments will form. When horses do develop friendly relationships, they may seek comfort in preferred associates and many behavioral issues related to isolation may improve if preferred associate relationships can form.

Sick Foals

Although the maximum number of hours or days that a foal can be separated from its dam before she fails to recognize it is not fully clear, we do know that sick foals may be rejected if the mare cannot see the foal during those early hours. When a foal is ill and/or receiving medical treatment, the mare and foal should share a stall. If needed, the mare can be restrained in such a way that she does not interfere with the foal's medical treatments.

In some cases, the mare is so protective of her foal that treatments are dangerous for the humans involved. This scenario is best approached through classical conditioning – the client can groom the mare and/or give her treats out of sight while the foal is being treated.

Foal Rejection

Foal rejection is a problem of primiparous mares. A few mares may reject foal after foal, but most are not repeat offenders and will accept their second foal. A foal may be rejected because the mare is afraid of it, because she does not want her udder touched, or because she is offensively aggressive to it. There seems to be a breed and strain predisposition in the Egyptian strain of Arabians (Juarbe-Díaz et al. 1998). At least some mares that reject are overly sensitive to touches in the inguinal fold region and desensitization to handling that area before foaling would forestall rejection. Although alprazolam has been used in one case report to successfully treat foal rejection (Wong et al. 2015), it is usually necessary to restrain the mare for at least a week or two so she cannot bite or kick the foal, allowing the foal to suckle every 15 minutes. Treatment with acepromazine may help tranquilize her and stimulate prolactin release. See Chapter 17 for more details on foal rejection or foal-directed aggression.

The Orphan Foal

The best treatment for an orphan foal is to provide a nursing mare replacement. There may be mares whose newborn foals have recently died, in which case the orphan can be introduced gradually, usually with a barrier between the foal and the surrogate until she accepts it. There are commercial farms that provide lactating mares for this purpose. Another method is to induce lactation in a mare using sulpiride, a phenothiazine tranquilizer that stimulates prolactin release (Daels 2002). Prolactin will not only stimulate milk production but also general maternal behavior. Milk production is only half the battle though. Oxytocin is necessary for a female to form a bond with a newborn and allow nursing. The natural stimulus for oxytocin release is vaginal stimulation by the foal during the birthing process. In order to simulate this, deep pressure vaginal message is performed for 5–10 minutes. At that point, the orphan foal can be introduced, and the mare will sniff it and, typically after a squeal or two, accept it. A large breeding farm should have sulpiride-treated mares ready during foaling season, in case a surrogate mother is needed.

If a foster mother is not available, caregivers should try to find an equine companion (even geldings can be profoundly helpful) who will provide comfort and also teach the foal what is acceptable behavior. In addition to an adult, the orphan should be exposed to other foals so that they can run and play, practicing adult life skills. The foal should not be encouraged to play with humans because as foals grow, they can become dangerous as they rear and strike during play.

Weaning

Natural weaning of foals takes place shortly before the birth of the next foal, which is typically at 11 months. If the dam does not have another foal, she may let the (now yearling) foal suckle indefinitely. Artificial weaning is often performed at four to six months of age. This is stressful and may lead to oral stereotypies, such as cribbing. Small groups of breeders are beginning to reconsider this tradition and delaying weaning until 9–11 months of age. There are many ways to wean foals. Simply remove the mare and leave the foal alone in a stall, or paddock, or wean two or more foals together in a stall. In another method, the mare and foal are put in adjacent stalls so that they can see and hear one another, but not nurse. Some suggest weaning a group of foals with an adult gelding. Perhaps the least stressful is gradual and interval weaning. "Gradual" refers to soft separations of mare and foal for very brief periods of time, for instance in adjacent stalls, beginning at about four months of age. As the months go by, the goal is to gradually increase time apart, up to two hours, while both mare and foal stay calm. Another, and probably the least stressful method, is "interval" weaning, in which the horses are on pasture and the mother of the oldest foal is removed. The following week, the mother of the second oldest foal is removed. The foals remain in a familiar location and have one another for companionship and play. This results in the smallest percentage of foals developing oral stereotypies (Nicol et al. 2005).

One way to do gradual weaning is to briefly separate the mare and foal into adjacent stalls with open grills, just long enough for each to eat their daily grain ration. Then the foal is immediately returned to the mare before either becomes anxious or stressed. Alfalfa hay can also be provided in each stall to facilitate lower stress levels (Figure 8.10a,b). Gradually, the time apart is increased, until by nine months of age, the mare and foal are content to be separated for two hours or more. Distance can also be increased by using stalls across the aisle from each other, or even further apart in the barn. In addition, brief periods of separation in adjacent or nearby pastures can be introduced (Figure 8.11). It is important that both the mares and foals have highly desirable grass or alfalfa to help distract and calm. The first pasture separation usually lasts just a few minutes. Mares and foals should be closely observed and reunited prior to the onset of increased stress. The key is to make these short separations easy and non-anxiety-inducing.

The time after weaning seems to be an important one for social interactions with other horses. In the authors' experiences, horses, particularly colts who were isolated from other horses during the period from weaning to two or three years of age, seem to have problems relating to other horses. In a natural situation, the colts would join a bachelor band where they would spend most of their non-foraging time play-fighting.

The male who is most dominant would be the first to acquire mares and, by that time, he is five years old. By the time he is 10, he would have lost his mares, indicating how short a stallion's reproductive career is (Berger 1986).

(a) (b)

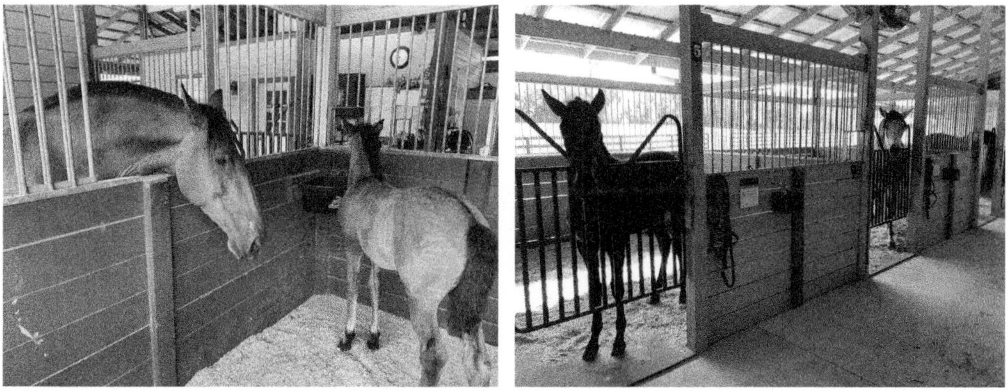

Figure 8.10 (a–b) Gradual weaning can be accomplished by feeding the mare and foal in separate stalls, but keeping visual contact with one another. They can be separated by adjacent stalls (a) or separated with an empty stall in between (b).

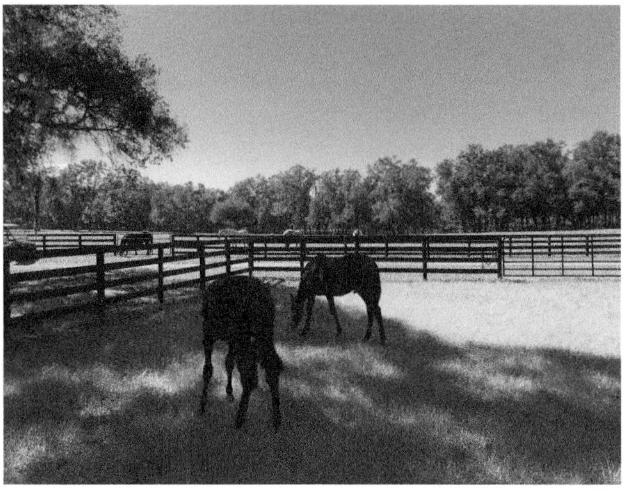

Figure 8.11 Another option for gradual weaning is to keep the mare and foal in separate pastures but maintain visual contact with each other.

Predicting Adult Behavior

It would be valuable to be able to predict adult behavior, and some steps have been made in that direction. Fearfulness in foals can be measured by quantifying their reaction to novel objects. Alerting (focusing on object with head and neck raised) behavior is consistent from foal hood to at least three years old (Christensen et al. 2020).

Additional Problem Prevention Tips

- Leave mares undisturbed for the first day once the foal is suckling, but do spend time brushing and feeding the mare over the next few days to accustom the foal to humans.
- Teach foals to wear a halter and to lead. This is easily accomplished by allowing the foal to follow the mare while holding the lead line.
- Practice handling foals' hooves, using **classical conditioning** with scratching, to create a positive association with what will become a necessary routine later in life.
- Teach foals to walk into a trailer at an early age, start with them following the mare, and then have them being led on their own as they age.
- Create a positive association with veterinary handling by associating the presence of the veterinarian, as well as touch by the veterinarian, with something the foal enjoys, such as scratching and, later, alfalfa hay or carrots.

References

Berger, J. (1986). *Wild Horses of the Great Basin: Social Competition and Population Size*. Chicago, IL: University of Chicago Press.

Boy, V. and Duncan, P. (1979). Time-budgets of Camargue horses I. Developmental changes in the time-budgets of foals. *Behaviour* 71: 187–201. https://doi.org/10.1163/156853979X00160.

Christensen, J.W., Beblein, C., and Malmkvist, J. (2020). Development and consistency of fearfulness in horses from foal to adult. *Appl. Anim. Behav. Sci.* 232: 105106. https://doi.org/10.1016/j.applanim.2020.105106.

Crowell-Davis, S. and Houpt, K.A. (1985). The ontogeny of flehmen in horses. *Anim. Behav.* 33: 739–745. https://doi.org/10.1016/S0003-3472(85)80005-1.

Crowell-Davis, S.L. and Caudle, A.B. (1989). Coprophagy by foals: recognition of maternal feces. *Appl. Anim. Behav. Sci. Neth.* 24 (3): 267–272.

Crowell-Davis, S.L., Houpt, K.A., and Carnevale, J. (1985). Feeding and drinking behavior of mares and foals with free access to pasture and water. *J. Anim. Sci.* 60: 883–889. https://doi.org/10.2527/jas1985.604883x.

Crowell-Davis, S.L., Houpt, K.A., and Kane, L. (1987). Play development in Welsh pony (*Equus caballus*) foals. *Appl. Anim. Behav. Sci.* 18: 119–131. https://doi.org/10.1016/0168-1591(87)90186-9.

Daels, P. (2002). Induction of lactation in non-foaling mares and growth of foals raised by mares with induced lactation. *Theriogenology*, Proceedings of the 8th International Equine Reproduction Symposium on equine Reproduction. 58: 859–861. https://doi.org/10.1016/S0093-691X(02)00859-2.

Henry, S., Hemery, D., Richard, M., and Hausberger, M. (2005). Human–mare relationships and behaviour of foals toward humans. *Appl. Anim. Behav. Sci.* 93: 341–362. https://doi.org/10.1016/j.applanim.2005.01.008.

Juarbe-Díaz, S.V., Houpt, K.A., and Kusunose, R. (1998). Prevalence and characteristics of foal rejection in Arabian mares. *Equine Vet. J.* 30: 424–428. https://doi.org/10.1111/j.2042-3306.1998.tb04513.x.

Nicol, C.J., Badnell-Waters, A.J., Bice, R. et al. (2005). The effects of diet and weaning method on the behaviour of young horses. *Appl. Anim. Behav. Sci.* 95: 205–221. https://doi.org/10.1016/j.applanim.2005.05.004.

Rossdale, P. (1967). Clinical studies on the newborn thoroughbred foal. I. Perinatal behaviour. *Br. Vet. J.* https://doi.org/10.1016/S0007-1935(17)39702-6.

Simpson, B.S. (2002). Neonatal foal handling. *Appl. Anim. Behav. Sci.* 2–4: 303–317.

Søndergaard, E. and Jago, J. (2010). The effect of early handling of foals on their reaction to handling, humans and novelty, and the foal–mare relationship. *Appl. Anim. Behav. Sci.* 123: 93–100.

Williams, J.L., Friend, T.H., Toscano, M.J. et al. (2002). The effects of early training sessions on the reactions of foals at 1, 2, and 3 months of age. *Appl. Anim. Behav. Sci.* 2: 105–114.

Wolski, T.R., Houpt, K.A., and Aronson, R. (1980). The role of the senses in mare-foal recognition. *Appl. Anim. Ethol.* 6: 121–138.

Wong, D.M., Alcott, C.J., Davis, J.L. et al. (2015). Use of alprazolam to facilitate mare-foal bonding in an aggressive postparturient mare. *J. Vet. Intern. Med.* 29: 414–416. https://doi.org/10.1111/jvim.12510.

9

Bovine Communication, Handling, and Restraint

Kathryn L. Proudfoot

University of Prince Edward Island, Sir James Dunn Animal Welfare Centre, Atlantic Veterinary College, Charlottetown, PEI, Canada

Introduction

Humans and cattle interact regularly in both the beef and dairy industries. As a veterinarian, you will likely encounter situations where you may need to handle or restrain cattle in ways they may not always find comfortable. This chapter describes best practices for handling and restraining cattle, drawing on examples from both beef and dairy animals. The Chapter will begin with a summary of how cattle perceive their world, communicate their emotions, and can be affected by human behaviors. This foundational information is critical to understanding why certain handling and restraint techniques are preferable to others. Then, a summary of handling and restraint practices that aim to mitigate stress and negative emotions in cattle will be discussed. The Chapter will end with examples of real-world challenges with cattle restraint and handling.

If you remember anything from this Chapter, it should be that when cattle are calm, they are easier to move (Grandin 2019). It is possible for you, as a human handler, to maintain a positive relationship with the animals that you work with, allowing for smooth handling and restraint without the use of unnecessary force. If you use correct techniques, cattle can be moved without shouting, hitting, or prodding. Using positive rather than negative behaviors toward cattle can improve each interaction you have with them and can lead to a positive human-animal relationship (Rault et al. 2020).

How Cattle Perceive Their World

Cattle experience the world very differently than humans do. It is important to recognize this difference when attempting to move or restrain them. In this section, we will focus on vision, hearing, and tactile sensations in cattle, as these are most critical to understand when working with cattle.

Vision

Due to the placement of their eyes, cattle have wide-angle vision that allows them to see around themselves without having to turn their heads (Figure 9.1) (Adamczyk et al. 2015; Prince 1977). Thus, cattle have a wide field of monocular vision (about 330°) and a rather narrow field of binocular vision (25–50°), resulting in poor depth perception. Thus, it is difficult for cattle to tell how deep something is, and this can make them startle when there are shadows or high contrast objects in their visual field (Grandin 2019).

Introduction to Animal Behavior and Veterinary Behavioral Medicine, First Edition. Edited by Meghan E. Herron.

Companion website: www.wiley.com/go/introductiontoanimalbehavior

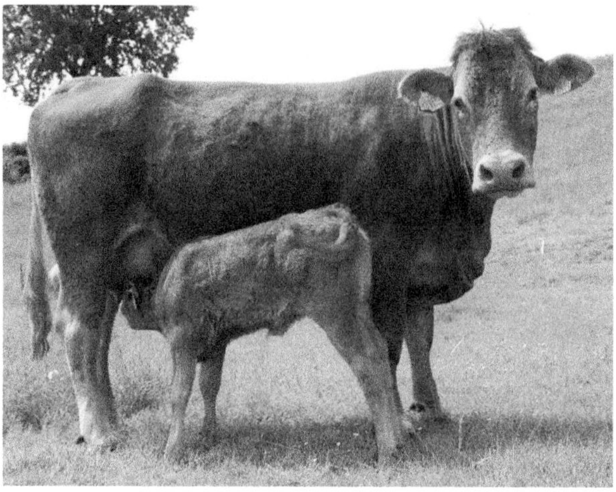

Figure 9.1 A vigilant beef cow with her calf. Notice how the cow's eyes are far apart, giving her a wide visual field. The dam is pointing her hear and ears toward the camera person, suggesting that she is vigilant and aware of their presence. Handling new mothers can be challenging, as they may express aggression toward a handler to protect their newborns. *Source:* Jai79/Pixabay.

Despite having expansive peripheral vision, cattle have a "blind spot" directly behind them (Figure 9.2) (Grandin 2019). As prey animals, cattle pay more attention to moving objects than static objects, however, sudden movements can startle them. Handlers should avoid abruptly entering an animal's blind spot, as this can also startle them. Standing in the animal's visual field, waiting for an animal to turn their head toward you, or gently resting your hand on their back can reduce the chance that you will startle them.

Hearing

Cattle have very sensitive hearing due to their large pinnae. They also have a larger hearing range compared with humans and are thus more sensitive to high-pitched sounds (Adamczyk et al. 2015; Heffner and Heffner 1983). Despite having large ears that can be moved to point in front and almost completely behind them, cattle are poor at localizing sounds (Heffner and Heffner 1992).

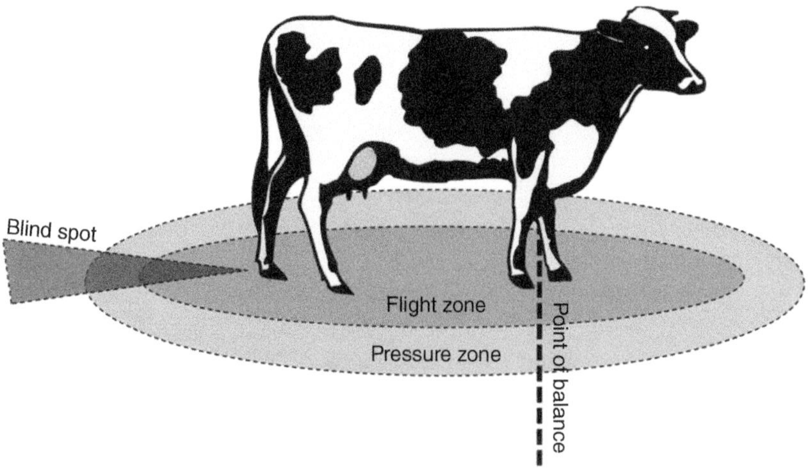

Figure 9.2 The blind spot, pressure zone, flight zone, and point of balance on a dairy cow. The placement of each of these features is different for each animal.

This poor localization may make cattle more fearful of unexpected sounds as they cannot clearly determine where the sound is coming from. It may seem easy to resort to making loud noises to get cattle to move, but this can be stressful for them (Pajor et al. 2003), likely because the sound is amplified. It is also important to avoid using high-pitched, loud sounds and instead use low-pitched, normal speaking voices around cattle to avoid causing stress (Hemsworth and Coleman 2010).

Tactile Sensation

Like all mammals, cattle likely experience a wide range of painful stimuli (Remnant et al. 2017; Weary et al. 2006). Here, pain will be defined by the International Association for the Study of Pain as "an unpleasant sensory and emotional experience associated with, or resembling that associated with, actual or potential tissue damage." Despite an abundance of research on painful procedures in cattle (e.g. castration, branding, and disbudding/dehorning), there is surprisingly little research on assessing pain during routine handling and restraint. Using tools such as an electric prod is very likely to cause pain in cattle (Pajor et al. 2003) and result in behavioral signs of stress (Simon et al. 2016), so it should be avoided unless the safety of the animal or the handler is in jeopardy. Cattle may also experience pain during restraint if the pressure is too localized to one area of the body (Grandin 2019). In contrast, gentle tactile stimuli, such as stroking, can help some animals remain calm during handling and veterinary examinations (Lürzel et al. 2015; Schmied et al. 2010).

How Cattle Communicate Their Emotions

This section will review what we know about emotions (affect) and communication in cattle. As a handler, you should be prepared to recognize signs of both negative and positive affective states in animals and adjust your behavior depending on the situation. For example, recognizing when an animal is experiencing fear or pain allows you to take caution and adjust your behavior when attempting to move or restrain them. Understanding what causes negative affect in cattle can also help caretakers mitigate stress associated with handling and general management.

Signals of Affect in Cattle

Animals cannot tell us how they feel with words, but they can show us how they feel with their facial features, posturing, and behavior. A full description of how we interpret affect in animals is outside of the scope of this chapter but can be found in several review papers (Ede et al. 2019; Paul et al. 2005). Briefly, affect can be described in terms of both valence (positive versus negative) and level of intensity or arousal. For example, a beef steer that has just come across a predator will experience fear, a negative, high arousal state. A dairy cow that has just eaten a large meal and has gone to lie down likely experiences a feeling of calmness, a positive, low arousal state.

Signals of High Arousal and Stress in Cattle

When an animal experiences a threat or perceived threat in their world, they may initiate a "stress response." Here we will define "stress" as "real or perceived environmental demands ('stressors') that can be appraised as threatening or benign, depending on the availability of adaptive coping resources to an individual" (McEwen and Gianaros 2010). The hallmarks of a stress response include activation of the autonomic nervous system and of two main biological pathways: the sympathoadrenal medullary pathway (SAM) pathway and the hypothalamic-pituitary-adrenal (HPA) pathway (axis). These pathways result in marked changes in the animal's physiology, including (but not limited to) the release of hormones such as epinephrine, norepinephrine, and glucocorticoids (e.g. cortisol), increased heart rate, increased respiration rate, and pupil dilation (Sapolsky et al. 2000). This response is adaptive, as it prepares the animal to escape from the threat (e.g. by fleeing, fighting, or staying completely still). However, chronic stress can result in negative downstream effects in cattle and other animals (Proudfoot and Habing 2015).

Although stress is often associated with negative affect, the physiological changes associated with a stress response cannot often be distinguished between positive and negative affective states (Boissy et al. 2007). Thus, animals experiencing high arousal positive and negative states, such as excitement and fear, may show similar physiological indicators of arousal.

Signals of Negative Affect in Cattle

Cattle experience a range of negative emotions, but not all are easy to detect. As prey animals, cattle may hide some negative feelings, such as pain (Weary et al. 2006). However, pain in ungulates can be recognized through some pain-specific behaviors that differ by the source of pain (Adcock and Tucker 2017). For example, a lame dairy cow will limp as she is walking (Flower and Weary 2009), and a beef calf that has just been castrated will flick his tail and spend less time exhibiting normal behavior like feeding (Meléndez et al. 2017). Painful stimuli can also be startling to cattle. For example, beef cattle that are prodded with an electric shock are at high risk of vocalizing, stumbling, and falling during restraint in a chute (Simon et al. 2016). Animals experiencing pain may be more difficult to handle due to restricted mobility and a reduced motivation to behave normally.

Fear is another affective state that handlers should recognize, as human behavior is one source of fear in cattle (Rushen et al. 1999c). Fear is defined as the emotional response of an animal to the perception of danger (Boissy 2015) and is one of the most studied negative states in cattle. Although it is not possible to directly measure fear in cattle, we can use behavioral and physiological indicators that are likely associated with fear. It should be noted that there are many limitations to our interpretation of all these measurements, as we can only make assumptions about what the animals are experiencing. That said, two behavioral tests (approach and aversion) are often used to assess if an animal may be fearful of humans. In an approach test, a handler will stand in the home pen or test pen with the animal, and researchers will measure the latency for the animal to approach the handler, the time spent near the handler, the latency to interact with the handler, and the number of interactions with the handler (Breuer et al. 2000). It is assumed that an animal that is more fearful of humans will take a longer time to approach and interact with the handler, as well as spend less time near the handler compared with an animal that is less fearful of humans.

Aversion tests have been used to determine if cattle will avoid certain handling techniques, such as hitting and yelling, that may contribute to their fear of human handlers. "Aversion" is defined as animals generally try to escape from, or avoid, situations that result in the experience of negative emotions (Pajor et al. 2000, 2003). Researchers have used Y-mazes and aversion learning tests to determine if cattle avoid certain handling practices, potentially due to fear. In a Y-maze, the animal is introduced to different handling techniques or nothing at the end of each arm of the "Y" and is then asked to choose which arm to walk down (Pajor et al. 2003). If an animal chooses the arm with nothing over the arm with a handling technique (e.g. yelling or hitting), then we may assume that the handling technique is averse to the animal and may result in fear. In an "aversion learning" test, cattle learn to associate their environment (e.g. a "race" or pathway; Pajor et al. 2000) with certain handling practices, and then are brought back to that environment later for testing. If an animal associates a pathway with a negative handling experience, they may show signs of aversion, including their reluctance or force needed to get them to walk down the path.

Behaviors and physiological indicators of stress have also been used to assess fear in cattle, as a fearful animal is likely experiencing a stress response. For example, **flight distance** is sometimes measured to indicate fear, using the distance between an animal and a handler when the animal will step away (Hemsworth et al. 2000). Behaviors that indicate increased vigilance (e.g. raising their heads or moving their ears forward) and physiological responses (e.g. increased heart rate, urination and defecation, vocalizations, etc.) have been measured to assess fear in dairy cows and calves (Battini et al. 2019; Rushen et al. 1999b; Welp et al. 2004). Showing eye whites can also indicate negative, high arousal states, though this response is not specific to fear as it may also indicate other negative emotions like frustration and high arousal positive emotions like excitement (Battini et al. 2019; Lambert [Proctor] and Carder 2017). Behavior at milking is also often measured to indicate a cow's response to handling; for example, researchers have measured kicks, steps, and flinches of dairy cows in the milking parlor as indicators of fear toward humans (Breuer et al. 2000). Cattle experiencing intense fear toward humans may also show aggressive behaviors, such as lowered heads, flaring nostrils, and pawing at the ground (Sheldon et al. 2009).

Handlers should also recognize when cattle are experiencing low arousal negative states, such as malaise associated with sickness. Like all mammals, cattle show adaptive changes in behavior when they become ill (Hart 1988); these "sickness behaviors" are meant to help the body respond and recover from illness. For example, dairy cows with mastitis (an infection of the udder) spend less time grooming and spend more time idle compared with healthy animals (Fogsgaard et al. 2012). Beef cows with bovine respiratory disease (BRD) will eat and groom less compared to healthy animals (Toaff-Rosenstein et al. 2016).

Cattle likely also experience other negative affective states, such as frustration, anxiety, or boredom, during routine handling and restraint. However, there has been little research assessing these other states in cattle.

Signals of Positive Affect in Cattle

Recognizing signs of positive affect can also aid in a cattle handling, though less research has been done on this topic. That said, there are still some indicators that can help handlers determine if cattle are in a positive state. For example, play behavior can indicate a high arousal positive state (Boissy et al. 2007), especially in young animals like calves. Play behavior, such as running, jumping, and kicking can also indicate absence of negative affect such as pain in dairy calves (Mintline et al. 2013). Rumination in adult cattle is also thought to be associated with positive affect, as it declines during period of stress and sickness (King et al. 2017; Schirmann et al. 2011). Cattle in a low arousal, positive state will also have less eye white visible and relaxed ear postures (e.g. ears loosely hung downwards) (Proctor and Carder 2014). They may also be engaging in normal behaviors, such as lying down, grazing or feeding, socializing, and grooming. That said, an inactive animal may not always be in a positive state of mind, as it has also been associated with low arousal negative states such as boredom (Hintze et al. 2020).

Green, Yellow, and Red Zones

Table 9.1 shows the three "zones" that cattle may enter when being handled. Each zone is associated with an affective state, including both arousal and valence. Handlers should be wary that this table is meant to generalize behavior across individuals; however, there is substantial variation in how individual animals respond to handlers (Petherick et al. 2009).

An animal in the "Green" zone is in a low arousal, positive affective state. These animals are the safest and easiest to handle. Cattle in

Table 9.1 Three "zones" indicating different affective states, including valence and arousal, in cattle.

Zone	Affective state (arousal, valence)	Examples of behavioral signs (these will differ between animals)
Green	Low arousal, positive	Lying in sternal or lateral recumbency Grazing, feeding Socializing, grooming Ruminating Relaxed ear postures
Yellow	Medium to high arousal, positive or negative	Vigilance (head and ears pointed to handler), Fidgeting Females showing signs of estrus (high activity, mounting) Eye whites Fleeing from handler, attempting to escape Defecation/urination Playing, running, bucking Vocalizations
Red	High arousal, negative	Pawing at ground Flaring nostrils Following handler Head lowered toward handler Eye whites

the "Yellow" zone can either be in a medium arousal positive or negative affective state. These animals are more difficult to handle because they are likely experiencing high arousal and a physiological stress response. Animals in the yellow zone can be handled; however, it is ideal to try to bring the level of arousal down as much as possible before handling. It is thought that it can take 20–30 minutes for cattle to calm down and their heart rates to come back to normal after becoming frightened (Grandin 2019). Cattle in the "Red" zone are in a high arousal negative affective state and are at the greatest risk of showing aggression toward a handler. Aggression toward humans is rare in cattle but is most common in new mothers protecting their offspring (Turner and Lawrence 2007), bulls (uncastrated males) (Sheldon et al. 2009), and cattle with little previous human interaction (e.g. calves raised on range) (Boivin et al. 1994).

Missing from Table 9.1 are animals in a low arousal, negative state. These animals do not fit cleanly into one of the three "zones," although they are likely more difficult to handle than those in the "green" zone. An animal in a low arousal, negative state is experiencing emotions or moods like malaise or depression and is likely to show sickness behaviors. These animals may be experiencing pain or discomfort and should be handled with special care and patience.

Impact of Human Handlers on Cattle Affective States

Your goal as a cattle handler should be to keep the cattle in the "Green" zone. As a veterinarian, you may need to cause some pain or discomfort (e.g. providing a vaccination or a blood draw) as part of routine examinations, so it is especially important for you to ensure that the cattle under your care do not associate you with the high arousal, negative emotion they may be experiencing.

Impacts of Negative Handling on Cattle

Tests of cattle aversion have been used to determine what human behaviors cattle consider negative. For example, using the Y-maze described earlier, dairy cows were provided with the choice to approach handlers using different handling techniques; researchers then measured which techniques the cows avoided (Pajor et al. 2003). Cows were most likely to avoid handlers associated with hitting, shouting, and the use of an electric prod. This result is not surprising, as hitting and the electric prod both likely cause cows to be startled and experience pain, while shouting likely causes cows to startle and experience fear due to their sensitive hearing. Similarly, using the "aversive learning" test, dairy cows learned to associate walking down a pathway with either aversive or gentle handling (Pajor et al. 2000). When cows were brought back to that pathway, the cows that had been previously handled aversively took longer to walk through the path compared to those that were previously handled gently. Cows were able to associate negative handling with the pathway, and thus began to experience fear in the pathway even with the lack of negative human behavior.

These negative behaviors can have broad impacts on cattle learning, memory, behavior, physiology, and productivity. A main concern with negative handler behavior is that the animal will begin to associate the handler with a negative affective state. Indeed, research has shown that dairy cows and calves can recognize individual handlers and remember who treats them poorly (de Passillé et al. 1996; Rushen et al. 1999b). For example, in one study, cows were either handled by a handler that treated them gently or aversively (Rushen et al. 1999b). Researchers then asked the handlers to stand near the cows in the milking parlor and recorded the behavioral and physiological responses of the cows; when the aversive handler was in the parlor, cows had 70% more residual milk (e.g. they did not let as much milk down) than when the gentler handler was in the parlor.

Negative handling can have clear impacts on animal productivity, including carcass quality in beef cattle and milk production in dairy cattle. For example, beef cattle that were prodded with an electric prod within 15 minutes of slaughter were found to have tougher meat compared with those that were not prodded (Warner et al. 2007), and pre-slaughter stress due to poor handling was associated with "dark cutting beef," considered poorer quality meat (Ferguson and Warner 2008). In a study using dairy cattle, researchers found that cow behaviors indicative of fear of humans were correlated with milk yield and composition (Breuer et al. 2000). In a similar study, researchers recorded the behaviors of handlers on 66 dairy farms and found that cows on farms where handlers showed the most negative interactions showed indicators of fear toward humans (using an approach test) and lower milk yield compared to those on farms with more positive interactions (Hemsworth et al. 2000).

Impacts of Positive Human Behavior

Positive handler behavior can have the opposite effect on cow behavior and productivity of negative behaviors. For example, researchers have found that gentle stroking of dairy heifers reduced fear of humans, measured using avoidance tests (Lürzel et al. 2015). Stress responses of dairy cows during routine veterinary examinations can be reduced by previous positive handling as well as by a person providing positive, gentle interactions during the procedure (Waiblinger et al. 2004). Dairy cows that experienced positive behavior from milkers stepped and kicked less during milking and had higher milk yield compared to those that experienced negative behaviors from handlers (Hanna et al. 2009). In beef cattle, gentle touching from a handler in early life reduced flight distance and cortisol at slaughter and resulted in better quality meat (Probst et al. 2012).

Table 9.2 Positive cattle handling techniques to stay in the "Green" zone.

Positive "low-stress" cattle handling techniques
• Wait for an animal to calm down before moving them.
• Check pathways, milking parlors, and chutes for visual distractions (e.g. objects, high contrast shadows, or poor lighting).
• Use slow, confident movement and principles of flight zones, pressure zones, and the point of balance to get an animal to move in the desired direction.
• Move cattle in a pair or group when possible to reduce stress due to isolation and to encourage social facilitation.
• Focus on making the animal's first experience with you or a new place as positive as possible.
• Avoid using electric prods or other tools that cause pain unless the safety of the handler or animal is in jeopardy.
• Do not "force" the animal to move – instead "guide" them.
• Use positive reinforcement (e.g. grain or hay) to help make the experience positive for the animal.

Source: Adapted from Grandin (2019).

Cattle Handling and Restraint

To avoid some of the side effects of negative handling, it is critical to use "low-stress" techniques when moving and restraining cattle (Table 9.2). As a handler and veterinarian, your knowledge of cattle sensation, perception, and affective states can help you recognize when an animal is in the "Yellow" or "Red" zone, enabling you to use techniques that bring the animal back down to the "green" zone.

Natural Cattle and Herd Behavior that Influence Handling

As herd animals, cattle feel safe and protected when they are in the company of other cattle. They will also naturally follow each other due to social facilitation and following behavior – when one cow starts walking in a certain direction, other cows are likely to follow (Grandin 2019). Attempts to isolate one animal from their herd will lead to a physiological stress response (Rushen et al. 1999a), likely due to a high arousal negative states like fear or panic (Grandin and Shivley 2015). Thus, one way to make handling easier is to move a pair or group of animals together, as they will naturally follow each other (Figure 9.3).

Cattle are also creatures of habit and like to have consistency in their environments. Thus, any kind of novelty will initially be stressful for cows and may make them difficult to handle. If possible, habituating the animal to the novel environment can help reduce their fear. Indeed, dairy heifers that were trained to enter a milking parlor before calving had less stepping and kicking during milking, showed less eye whites, and had more relaxed ear postures during the milking after calving compared to those that did not have training (Kutzer et al. 2015).

Cattle may also become startled if there are novel objects in their visual field as you are moving them. For example, Temple Grandin recommends that handlers remove objects such as dangling ropes, clothing hung on a fence, swinging objects like chains, or objects that create high contrasts or shadows (Grandin 2019). If an animal does become startled at an object or other visual distraction, Grandin recommends letting the animal investigate the object to determine that it is safe before attempting to move the animal forward. It is also helpful

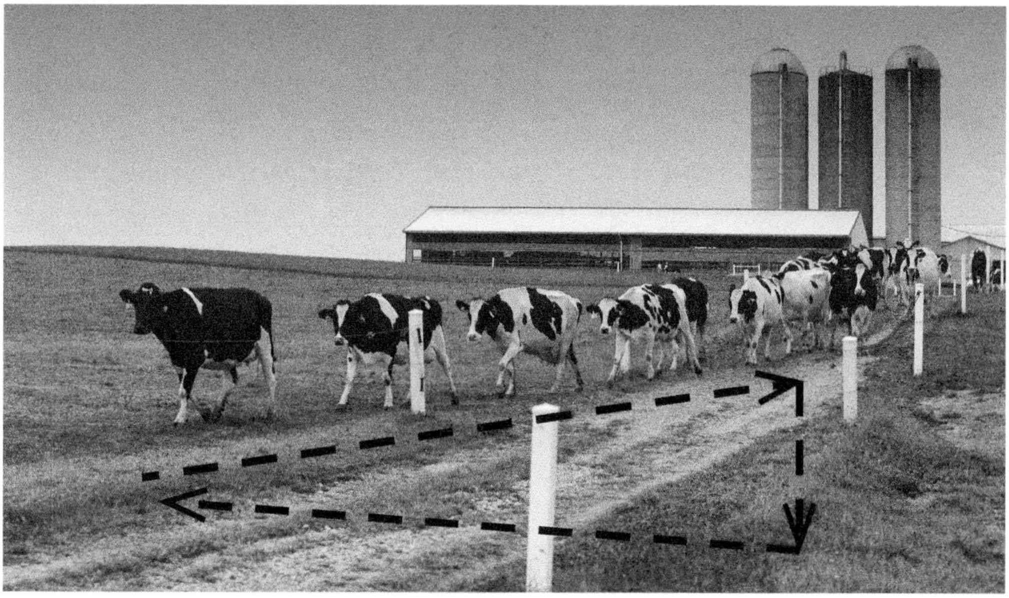

Figure 9.3 Dairy cows following each other out of the barn to pasture. Cattle are herd animals and are easier to handle when they can follow other cows. The arrows show the path that a human handler could take to move the animals forward using principles of flight/pressure zones and the point of balance. *Background image source:* David Mark/Pixabay.

to avoid having novel humans stand in front of cattle, as this can also cause them to be startled.

Principles of Cattle Movement

Before moving cattle, it is important to know three main principles: **flight zones**, **pressure zones,** and the **point of balance** (refer back to Figure 9.2). The "flight zone" is the animal's personal space; if you enter that zone, then the animal will flee or run away from you. The "pressure zone" is outside of the flight zone; as a handler, you can slowly move into this zone to guide the cow to move away from you. It is important to not move too quickly toward cattle, as you may enter their flight zones, causing them to become more difficult to handle. Instead, take slow steps in and out of the pressure zone to get the cow to slowly move away from you. Another way to think of this is putting yourself at the "edge of the flight zone" when moving cattle (Grandin 2019).

The size of flight and pressure zones will depend on the animal's individual personality (also called temperament), their breed, their stage of estrus, their experience with humans, and several other factors. For example, dairy heifers that were handled aversively by humans had larger flight zones compared to those that were handled more gently (Breuer et al. 2003). Cattle with less experience with humans, such as beef cattle on range, will likely have larger flight zones compared to animals that have had frequent (positive) interactions with humans (Grandin 2019).

The point of balance, located near the shoulder of cattle, can be used to direct cows once you have them moving (Kilgour 2019). If a handler is standing behind the point of balance, the animal gets the signal to move forward. If the handler is standing in front of the point of balance, the animal gets the signal to move backwards. Thus, if a handler wants to move an animal forward, they should step into the pressure zone/edge of the flight zone behind the point of balance. If you find that the animal keeps backing away from you instead of moving forward, you are likely standing in front of their point of balance.

The point of balance can also be used to move a group of cattle forward (Figure 9.3). A handler attempting to move beef cattle into a chute, dairy cattle into a milking parlor, or animals moving single file indoors or outdoors can quickly but calmly walk past the point of balance in the opposite direction (e.g. start in front of the animal and walk along their side) this can encourage the whole group to move forward (Grandin 2019). When the handler reaches the last animal, they can move out of the flight and pressure zones and then walk back to where they started.

Restraint and Facility Design

Restraining cattle is often necessary for veterinary procedures. However, restraint can be stressful and leave a negative impression of you and the procedure in the animal's memory. Indeed, restraint is often used in research as a model to study stress and fear in cattle and may be difficult for cattle to get used to. For example, beef heifers that were restrained in a squeeze chute in five-minute periods every week for three weeks showed increasing levels of serum cortisol across time, suggesting that the calves were becoming sensitized rather than habituated to restraint (Chen et al. 2016). It should be noted that the animals in this study were not previously acclimated to humans and likely had negative, painful experiences in the past with restraint (e.g. for branding and vaccinations). Thus, it is critical to avoid negative experiences with restraint, especially when cattle are young.

Dairy cattle are often restrained using headlocks. A benefit of this method of restraint is that the head locks are usually positioned behind their feed, giving the cows a frequent and positive association with putting their heads through the device. That said, dairy cattle can still become fearful when they are restrained in a headlock, and this can be novel to young cattle. Moreover, restraining dairy cows in headlocks for prolonged periods of time should be avoided, as this may increase their chance of becoming lame.

Factors associated with the design of the handling facility can impact how animals respond to both handling and restraint. For example, non-slip flooring is encouraged throughout all handling facilities where animals are moved or restrained. Adding solid sides to chutes and pathways can also help reduce visual distractions such as shadows (Grandin 2019). Using curved instead of straight alleyways may also help reduce stress in beef cattle, especially after they exit a squeeze chute (Simon et al. 2016).

The Power of Positive Reinforcement

Our job as handlers should not be to *force* cattle to behave according to our own will, regardless of how it affects them. Instead, we should focus on *guiding* them to choose to move in the way we desire, using the principles explained in this chapter. Moreover, we should try to make all handling experiences as positive as possible for the cattle under our care.

Positive reinforcement can be used to help cattle associate positive affective states with handlers, handling, and even painful procedures. For example, researchers trained dairy heifers to voluntarily put their heads into a headlock to receive a sham injection using grain as a reward (Lomb et al. 2021). The heifers that were trained had fewer negative reactions to an actual injection compared with control animals. Similarly, grain is frequently used to attract dairy cows to automatic milking systems (e.g. robots that milk cows without humans) to help the animals associate the system with positive affective states (von Kuhlberg et al. 2021). Although intensive training may not be practical for dairy and beef operations, the use of positive reinforcers like hay and grain should always be available when animals are restrained or moved into novel, potentially stressful environments.

Cattle Handling in the Real World

As useful as the tips provided in this chapter may be, the real world is seldom so simple. Unfortunately, negative handling of cattle can become a "culture" on some farms, requiring a significant amount of effort to change people's behavior. As a veterinarian, one of your responsibilities is to model good behavior. If you avoid using negative behavior toward cattle and instead use techniques like flight/pressure zones, social facilitation, and positive reinforcement, this can have an impact on your clients. You should also be aware of the regulations or "best practices" for cattle handling that may exist for the animals you are working with, such as through the National Dairy F.A.R.M. Program (www.nationaldairyfarm.com) and Beef Quality Assurance (www.bqa.org). As the veterinarian, you may also be asked to train stockpeople on how to handle and restrain animals.

The Effect of Handler Skills, Attitude, and Personality on Their Behavior

Three factors that influence whether someone uses positive handling techniques with cattle are their skills, attitude, and personality. Training handlers to have good skills is an important step in ensuring that animals under their care are treated appropriately. However, a handler's behavior toward animals is strongly influenced by their attitudes toward animals. For example, researchers provided handlers on 31 dairy farms with an attitude survey, and found that those with higher scores (e.g. more positive beliefs about animals) showed more positive behavior directed toward the cattle (Breuer et al. 2000). Handler attitudes may also have downstream effects on the productivity of cows; researchers found that dairy cows on farms with handlers that held positive beliefs about cows had higher milk production compared to cows on farms with handlers that held more negative beliefs (Fukasawa et al. 2017).

A handler's personality may also influence their treatment of animals under their care. For example, researchers identified two handling styles related to personality in dairy farm workers: (1) positive (calm/patient, positive interactions) and (2) negative (dominating/aggressive, insecure/nervous) and measured the impact of these styles on dairy calf behavior (Ellingsen et al. 2014). The handlers with positive handling styles had calves that were more friendly, content, and sociable, whereas those handlers with negative handling styles were considered more nervous, frustrated, and fearful.

Animal Handling Training On-farm

Training handlers to improve both their skills and attitudes can benefit the welfare of the cattle under their care. For example, training stockpeople on beef farms can improve both their behavior and beliefs toward animals (Ceballos et al. 2018). A training program for dairy stockpeople that targeted cognitive-behavioral intervention resulted in stockpeople expressing more positive beliefs about handling cows and showing fewer negative tactile interactions with cows compared to those that did not receive training (Hemsworth et al. 2002). In addition, the cows on farms where handlers received training had shorter flight distances and higher milk yields compared to those on farms without training.

Despite research showing benefits of animal handling training, researchers in Minnesota found that only 30% of dairy farmers surveyed in the state had some form of animal handling training (Sorge et al. 2014). Of those with training, 42.6% of farmers reported that they learned animal handling skills from a family member. Dairy producers reported that they understand good handling skills are important, but time limitations, language and cultural barriers, as well as a lack of perceived resources were considered challenges to training handlers.

Conclusion

Whether you plan on becoming a bovine practitioner or not, it is important for all veterinarians to know how to safely work around cattle. Understanding how cattle interpret the world and signal their emotions can help you change your behavior and better adapt to their needs. Decades of research have shown that using the right handling techniques can help veterinarians and other animal handlers avoid causing negative affective states in beef and dairy cattle. Forcing cattle to move where we want them to using whatever means, including techniques that cause pain and distress, is unnecessary and an animal welfare concern. Instead, we should refocus on creating more positive interactions and relationships between humans and the cattle under their care.

References

Adamczyk, K., Górecka-Bruzda, A., Nowicki, J.P., and Gumułka, M. (2015). Perception of environment in farm animals – a review. *Ann. Anim. Sci. 15* (3): 565–589. https://doi.org/10.1515/aoas-2015-0031.

Adcock, S.J.J. and Tucker, C.B. (2017). Painful procedures: when and what should we be measuring in cattle? In: *Advances in Cattle Welfare* (ed. C. Tucker), 157–198. Elsevier https://doi.org/10.1016/B978-0-08-100938-3.00008-5.

Battini, M., Agostini, A., and Mattiello, S. (2019). Understanding cows' emotions on farm: are eye white and ear posture reliable indicators? *Animals* 9 (8): 477. https://doi.org/10.3390/ANI9080477.

Boissy, A. (2015). Fear and fearfulness in animals. *Q. Rev. Biol. 70* (2): 165–191. https://doi.org/10.1086/418981.

Boissy, A., Manteuffel, G., Jensen, M.B. et al. (2007). Assessment of positive emotions in animals to improve their welfare. *Physiol. Behav. 92* (3): 375–397. https://doi.org/10.1016/J.PHYSBEH.2007.02.003.

Boivin, X., le Neindre, P., Garel, J.P., and Chupin, J.M. (1994). Influence of breed and rearing management on cattle reactions during human handling. *Appl. Anim. Behav. Sci. 39* (2): 115–122. https://doi.org/10.1016/0168-1591(94)90131-7.

Breuer, K., Hemsworth, P.H., Barnett, J.L. et al. (2000). Behavioural response to humans and the productivity of commercial dairy cows. *Appl. Anim. Behav. Sci. 66* (4): 273–288. https://doi.org/10.1016/S0168-1591(99)00097-0.

Breuer, K., Hemsworth, P.H., and Coleman, G.J. (2003). The effect of positive or negative handling on the behavioural and physiological responses of nonlactating heifers. *Appl. Anim. Behav. Sci. 84* (1): 3–22. https://doi.org/10.1016/S0168-1591(03)00146-1.

Ceballos, M.C. et al. (2018). Impact of good practices of handling training on beef cattle welfare and stockpeople attitudes and behaviors. *Livest. Sci. 216*: 24–31. https://doi.org/10.1016/J.LIVSCI.2018.06.019.

Chen, Y., Stookey, J., Arsenault, R. et al. (2016). Investigation of the physiological, behavioral, and biochemical responses of cattle to restraint stress. *J. Anim. Sci. 94* (8): 3240–3254. https://doi.org/10.2527/JAS.2016-0549.

de Passillé, A.M., Rushen, J., Ladewig, J., and Petherick, C. (1996). Dairy calves' discrimination of people based on previous handling. *J. Anim. Sci. 74* (5): 969–974. https://doi.org/10.2527/1996.745969X.

Ede, T., Lecorps, B., von Keyserlingk, M.A.G., and Weary, D.M. (2019). Symposium review: scientific assessment of affective states in dairy cattle. *J. Dairy Sci. 102* (11): 10677–10694. https://doi.org/10.3168/JDS.2019-16325.

Ellingsen, K., Coleman, G.J., Lund, V., and Mejdell, C.M. (2014). Using qualitative behaviour assessment to explore the link between stockperson behaviour and dairy calf behaviour. *Appl. Anim. Behav. Sci. 153*: 10–17. https://doi.org/10.1016/J.APPLANIM.2014.01.011.

Ferguson, D.M. and Warner, R.D. (2008). Have we underestimated the impact of pre-slaughter stress on meat quality in ruminants? *Meat Sci. 80* (1): 12–19. https://doi.org/10.1016/J.MEATSCI.2008.05.004.

Flower, F.C. and Weary, D.M. (2009). Gait assessment in dairy cattle. *Animal 3* (1): 87–95. https://doi.org/10.1017/S1751731108003194.

Fogsgaard, K.K., Røntved, C.M., Sørensen, P., and Herskin, M.S. (2012). Sickness behavior in dairy cows during *Escherichia coli* mastitis. *J. Dairy Sci. 95* (2): 630–638. https://doi.org/10.3168/JDS.2011-4350.

Fukasawa, M., Kawahata, M., Higashiyama, Y., and Komatsu, T. (2017). Relationship between the stockperson's attitudes and dairy productivity in Japan. *Anim. Sci. J. 88* (2): 394–400. https://doi.org/10.1111/ASJ.12652.

Grandin, T. (2019). *Livestock Handling and Transport*. CABI https://www.cabi.org/bookshop/book/9781786399151/.

Grandin, T. and Shivley, C. (2015). How farm animals react and perceive stressful situations such as handling, restraint, and transport. *Animals 5* (4): 1233–1251. https://doi.org/10.3390/ANI5040409.

Hanna, D., Sneddon, I.A., and Beattie, V.E. (2009). The relationship between the stockperson's personality and attitudes and the productivity of dairy cows. *Animal 3* (5): 737–743. https://doi.org/10.1017/S1751731109003991.

Hart, B.L. (1988). Biological basis of the behavior of sick animals. *Neurosci. Biobehav. Rev. 12* (2): 123–137. https://doi.org/10.1016/S0149-7634(88)80004-6.

Heffner, R.S. and Heffner, H.E. (1983). Hearing in large mammals: horses (*Equus caballus*) and cattle (*Bos taurus*). *Behav. Neurosci. 97* (2): 299–309. https://doi.org/10.1037/0735-7044.97.2.299.

Heffner, R.S. and Heffner, H.E. (1992). Hearing in large mammals: sound-localization acuity in cattle (*Bos taurus*) and goats (*Capra hircus*). *J. Comp. Psychol. (Washington, D.C.: 1983) 106* (2): 107–113. https://doi.org/10.1037/0735-7036.106.2.107.

Hemsworth, P. and Coleman, G.J. (2010). *Human-Livestock Interactions: The Stockperson and the Productivity and Welfare of Intensively Farmed Animals*, 1–194. Cambridge, MA: CABI https://doi.org/10.1079/9781845936730.0000.

Hemsworth, P.H., Coleman, G.J., Barnett, J.L., and Borg, S. (2000). Relationships between human-animal interactions and productivity of commercial dairy cows. *J. Anim. Sci. 78* (11): 2821–2831. https://doi.org/10.2527/2000.78112821X.

Hemsworth, P.H., Coleman, G.J., Barnett, J.L. et al. (2002). The effects of cognitive behavioral intervention on the attitude and behavior of stockpersons and the behavior and productivity of commercial dairy cows. *J. Anim. Sci. 80* (1): 68–78. https://doi.org/10.2527/2002.80168X.

Hintze, S., Maulbetsch, F., Asher, L., and Winckler, C. (2020). Doing nothing and what it looks like: inactivity in fattening cattle. *PeerJ 8*: e9395. https://doi.org/10.7717/PEERJ.9395.

Kilgour, R. (2019). *Livestock Behaviour: A Practical Guide*. Boca Raton, FL: CRC Press.

King, M.T.M., Dancy, K.M., LeBlanc, S.J. et al. (2017). Deviations in behavior and productivity data before diagnosis of health disorders in cows milked with an automated system. *J. Dairy Sci. 100* (10): 8358–8371. https://doi.org/10.3168/JDS.2017-12723.

Kutzer, T., Steilen, M., Gygax, L., and Wechsler, B. (2015). Habituation of dairy heifers to milking routine—effects on human avoidance distance, behavior, and cardiac activity during milking. *J. Dairy Sci. 98* (8): 5241–5251. https://doi.org/10.3168/JDS.2014-8773.

Lambert (Proctor), H. S., & Carder, G. (2017). Looking into the eyes of a cow: can eye whites be used as a measure of emotional state?

Appl. Anim. Behav. Sci., *186*, 1–6. https://doi.org/10.1016/J.APPLANIM.2016.11.005

Lomb, J., Mauger, A., von Keyserlingk, M.A.G., and Weary, D.M. (2021). Effects of positive reinforcement training for heifers on responses to a subcutaneous injection. *J. Dairy Sci. 104* (5): 6146–6158.

Lürzel, S., Münsch, C., Windschnurer, I. et al. (2015). The influence of gentle interactions on avoidance distance towards humans, weight gain and physiological parameters in group-housed dairy calves. *Appl. Anim. Behav. Sci. 172*: 9–16. https://doi.org/10.1016/J.APPLANIM.2015.09.004.

McEwen, B.S. and Gianaros, P.J. (2010). Central role of the brain in stress and adaptation: links to socioeconomic status, health, and disease. *Ann. N. Y. Acad. Sci. 1186*: 190–222. https://doi.org/10.1111/j.1749-6632.2009.05331.x.

Meléndez, D.M., Marti, S., Pajor, E.A. et al. (2017). Effect of band and knife castration of beef calves on welfare indicators of pain at three relevant industry ages: I. Acute pain. *J. Anim. Sci. 95* (10): 4352–4366. https://doi.org/10.2527/JAS2017.1762.

Mintline, E.M., Stewart, M., Rogers, A.R. et al. (2013). Play behavior as an indicator of animal welfare: disbudding in dairy calves. *Appl. Anim. Behav. Sci. 144* (1–2): 22–30. https://doi.org/10.1016/J.APPLANIM.2012.12.008.

Pajor, E.A., Rushen, J., and de Passillé, A.M.B. (2000). Aversion learning techniques to evaluate dairy cattle handling practices. *Appl. Anim. Behav. Sci. 69* (2): 89–102.

Pajor, E.A., Rushen, J., and de Passillé, A.M.B. (2003). Dairy cattle's choice of handling treatments in a Y-maze. *Appl. Anim. Behav. Sci. 80* (2): 93–107. https://doi.org/10.1016/S0168-1591(02)00119-3.

Paul, E.S., Harding, E.J., and Mendl, M. (2005). Measuring emotional processes in animals: the utility of a cognitive approach. *Neurosci. Biobehav. Rev. 29* (3): 469–491. https://doi.org/10.1016/J.NEUBIOREV.2005.01.002.

Petherick, J.C., Doogan, V.J., Holroyd, R.G. et al. (2009). Quality of handling and holding yard environment, and beef cattle temperament: 1. Relationships with flight speed and fear of humans. *Appl. Anim. Behav. Sci. 120* (1–2): 18–27. https://doi.org/10.1016/J.APPLANIM.2009.05.008.

Prince, J. (1977). The eye and vision. In: *Dukes Physiology of Domestic Animals* (ed. M. Swensen), 696–712. Cornell University Press.

Probst, J.K., Spengler Neff, A., Leiber, F. et al. (2012). Gentle touching in early life reduces avoidance distance and slaughter stress in beef cattle. *Appl. Anim. Behav. Sci. 139* (1–2): 42–49. https://doi.org/10.1016/J.APPLANIM.2012.03.002.

Proctor, H.S. and Carder, G. (2014). Can ear postures reliably measure the positive emotional state of cows? *Appl. Anim. Behav. Sci. 161* (1): 20–27. https://doi.org/10.1016/J.APPLANIM.2014.09.015.

Proudfoot, K. and Habing, G. (2015). Social stress as a cause of diseases in farm animals: current knowledge and future directions. *Vet. J. 206*: 15–21. https://doi.org/10.1016/j.tvjl.2015.05.024.

Rault, J.-L., Waiblinger, S., Boivin, X., and Hemsworth, P. (2020). The power of a positive human–animal relationship for animal welfare. *Front. Vet. Sci. 7*: 590867. https://doi.org/10.3389/FVETS.2020.590867.

Remnant, J.G., Tremlett, A., Huxley, J.N., and Hudson, C.D. (2017). Clinician attitudes to pain and use of analgesia in cattle: where are we 10 years on? *Vet. Rec. 181* (15): 400. https://doi.org/10.1136/VR.104428.

Rushen, J., Boissy, A., Terlouw, E.M.C., and de Passillé, A.M.B. (1999a). Opioid peptides and behavioral and physiological responses of dairy cows to social isolation in unfamiliar surroundings. *J. Anim. Sci. 77* (11): 2918–2924. https://doi.org/10.2527/1999.77112918X.

Rushen, J., de Passillé, A.M.B., and Munksgaard, L. (1999b). Fear of people by cows and effects on milk yield, behavior, and heart rate at milking. *J. Dairy Sci. 82*: 720–727. https://doi.org/10.3168/jds.S0022-0302(99)75289-6.

Rushen, J., Taylor, A.A., and de Passillé, A.M. (1999c). Domestic animals' fear of humans and its effect on their welfare. *Appl. Anim. Behav. Sci. 65* (3): 285–303. https://doi.org/10.1016/S0168-1591(99)00089-1.

Sapolsky, R.M., Michael Romero, L., and Munck, A.U. (2000). How do glucocorticoids influence stress responses? Integrating permissive, suppressive, stimulatory, and preparative actions. *Endocr. Rev. 21* (1): 55–89. https://doi.org/10.1210/er.21.1.55.

Schirmann, K., Chapinal, N., Weary, D.M.M. et al. (2011). Short-term effects of regrouping on behavior of prepartum dairy cows. *J. Dairy Sci. 94* (5): 2312–2319. https://doi.org/10.3168/jds.2010-3639.

Schmied, C., Boivin, X., Scala, S., and Waiblinger, S. (2010). Effect of previous stroking on reactions to a veterinary procedure: behaviour and heart rate of dairy cows. *Interact. Stud. 11* (3): 467–481. https://doi.org/10.1075/IS.11.3.08SCH.

Sheldon, K.J., PhD, G.D., EdD, W.E.F., and PhD, J.L.A. (2009). Bull-related incidents: their prevalence and nature. *J. Agromedicine* 14 (3): 357–369. https://doi.org/10.1080/10599240903042024.

Simon, G.E., Hoar, B.R., and Tucker, C.B. (2016). Assessing cow–calf welfare. Part 2: risk factors for beef cow health and behavior and stockperson handling. *J. Anim. Sci. 94* (8): 3488–3500. https://doi.org/10.2527/JAS.2016-0309.

Sorge, U.S., Cherry, C., and Bender, J.B. (2014). Perception of the importance of human-animal interactions on cattle flow and worker safety on Minnesota dairy farms. *J. Dairy Sci. 97* (7): 4632–4638. https://doi.org/10.3168/JDS.2014-7971.

Toaff-Rosenstein, R.L., Gershwin, L.J., and Tucker, C.B. (2016). Fever, feeding, and grooming behavior around peak clinical signs in bovine respiratory disease. *J. Anim. Sci. 94* (9): 3918–3932. https://doi.org/10.2527/JAS.2016-0346.

Turner, S.P. and Lawrence, A.B. (2007). Relationship between maternal defensive aggression, fear of handling and other maternal care traits in beef cows. *Livest. Sci. 106* (2–3): 182–188. https://doi.org/10.1016/J.LIVSCI.2006.08.002.

von Kuhlberg, M.K., Wensch-Dorendorf, M., Gottschalk, J. et al. (2021). The effects of a training program using a phantom to accustom heifers to the automatic milking system. *J. Dairy Sci. 104* (1): 928–936. https://doi.org/10.3168/JDS.2020-18715.

Waiblinger, S., Menke, C., Korff, J., and Bucher, A. (2004). Previous handling and gentle interactions affect behaviour and heart rate of dairy cows during a veterinary procedure. *Appl. Anim. Behav. Sci. 85* (1–2): 31–42. https://doi.org/10.1016/J.APPLANIM.2003.07.002.

Warner, R.D., Ferguson, D.M., Cottrell, J.J. et al. (2007). Acute stress induced by the preslaughter use of electric prodders causes tougher beef meat. *Aust. J. Exp. Agric. 47* (7): 782–788. https://doi.org/10.1071/EA05155.

Weary, D.M., Niel, L., Flower, F.C., and Fraser, D. (2006). Identifying and preventing pain in animals. *Appl. Anim. Behav. Sci. 100* (1–2): 64–76. https://doi.org/10.1016/J.APPLANIM.2006.04.013.

Welp, T., Rushen, J., Kramer, D.L. et al. (2004). Vigilance as a measure of fear in dairy cattle. *Appl. Anim. Behav. Sci. 87* (1–2): 1–13. https://doi.org/10.1016/J.APPLANIM.2003.12.013.

10

Equine Communication, Handling, and Restraint

Jeannine Berger[1] *and Kathryn Holcomb*[2]

[1] *Sacramento Veterinary Behavior Services, Vacaville, CA, USA*
[2] *University of California, Davis, School of Veterinary Medicine, Davis, CA, USA*

Introduction

Equine veterinarians evaluate and treat horses whose responses to veterinary procedures range from calm to highly agitated. Fortunately, most interactions go well. However, even normally compliant horses may behave differently when they are in pain, are fearful, or when a procedure is uncomfortable or invasive. As large prey animals, horses may react to frightening situations with their natural flight response, potentially injuring themselves and the people around them. Understanding how to communicate, handle, and restrain a horse safely and effectively in ways that either prevent the horse's emotional state from elevating to a difficult level, or de-escalate a challenging situation, is critical to promoting a positive experience for all.

The keys to dealing with potentially difficult situations when handling horses are understanding how situations escalate and recognizing the signs of escalation with associated emotional states; recognizing equine body language that is predictive or indicative of those states; and using knowledge, tools, and skills to humanely prevent or de-escalate high emotions. This chapter presents a practical tool to assess signs of calm or escalation; describes skills, equipment, and procedures to safely handle and restrain horses with examples of their application; and discusses psychotropic medications that may be useful for handling and restraint of horses.

Body Language and Emotional States

A wild horse's survival depends upon rapid recognition and removal of the threat, whether by fleeing (creating distance) or fighting (aggression). Domestic living and positive socialization with proper training familiarize horses with many otherwise frightening things, but the fight-or-flight instinct will always be present. Any transition can evoke this response, including a change of speed, direction, gait, and adding or removing a stimulus. In these situations, a behavioral and emotional progression from calm to fight-or-flight mode may take place. When the handling of a horse goes wrong, the situation can escalate rapidly and result in injuries to the human as well as the horse. With almost 100 years of combined experience working with horses in various settings, the authors know first-hand how quickly even a seemingly calm situation

Introduction to Animal Behavior and Veterinary Behavioral Medicine, First Edition. Edited by Meghan E. Herron.

Companion website: www.wiley.com/go/introductiontoanimalbehavior

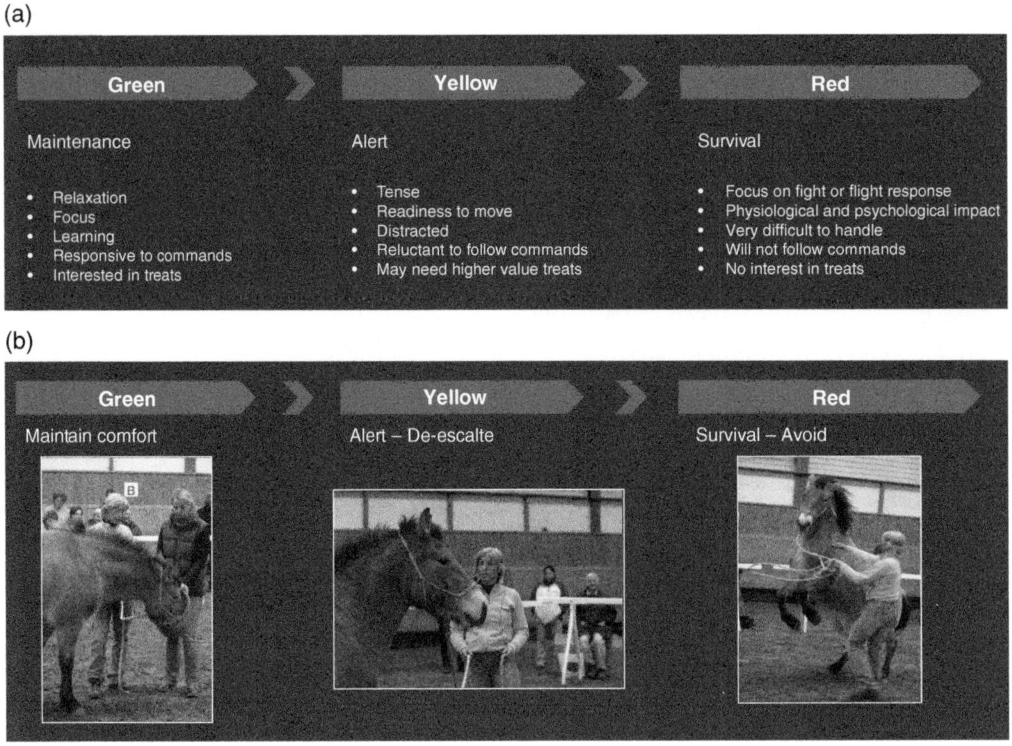

Figure 10.1 The emotional states (a) correlate with the zones of escalation (b) and are divided into three categories: "green" indicates the horse is in a state of comfort and handling may continue; "yellow" indicates the horse is sensing danger and immediate steps to de-escalate the emotional state are needed; "red" indicates that the horse is in survival mode and handling should be avoided. Further provocation could be very dangerous for the handler and the horse.

can turn. This progression can be described by specific zones (emotional states, Figure 10.1a), where each zone is characterized by recognizable body language. The Zones of Escalation tool (Figure 10.1b) offers handlers an important, practical tool to help them evaluate the state of the horse and make decisions about handling that animal in a safe way that promotes its welfare.

The Green Zone

The green zone is the calm zone. In this zone, the horse is emotionally quiet and feels safe. A good mental picture of the green zone is of relaxed horses grazing in a pasture or resting in their paddock. Their heads and necks are held in a middle position, below their withers (Figure 10.2a), or are down for grazing (Figure 10.2b). Ears are relaxed, and tails may be swishing calmly and rhythmically at insects. They may be walking, rolling, allogrooming, dozing, or sleeping. These are some natural maintenance behaviors horses perform when there is no threat (McDonnell 2003).

A horse in this zone being led or held by a person also keeps the head and neck in a middle position, and has relaxed ears, eyes, and tail. The neck and tail of the horse being led would swing gently in rhythm with the steps. The horse focuses on the handler, willingly follows cues, and is seemingly easy to handle. They change gaits easily from standing still to walking to trotting in hand when cued and will accept treats gently if offered. The heart and respiration rates are in the normal range (Box 10.1).

This is the preferred zone for veterinarians when handling horses. In this zone, the horse is in an emotional state that allows handling and procedures such as vaccinations or

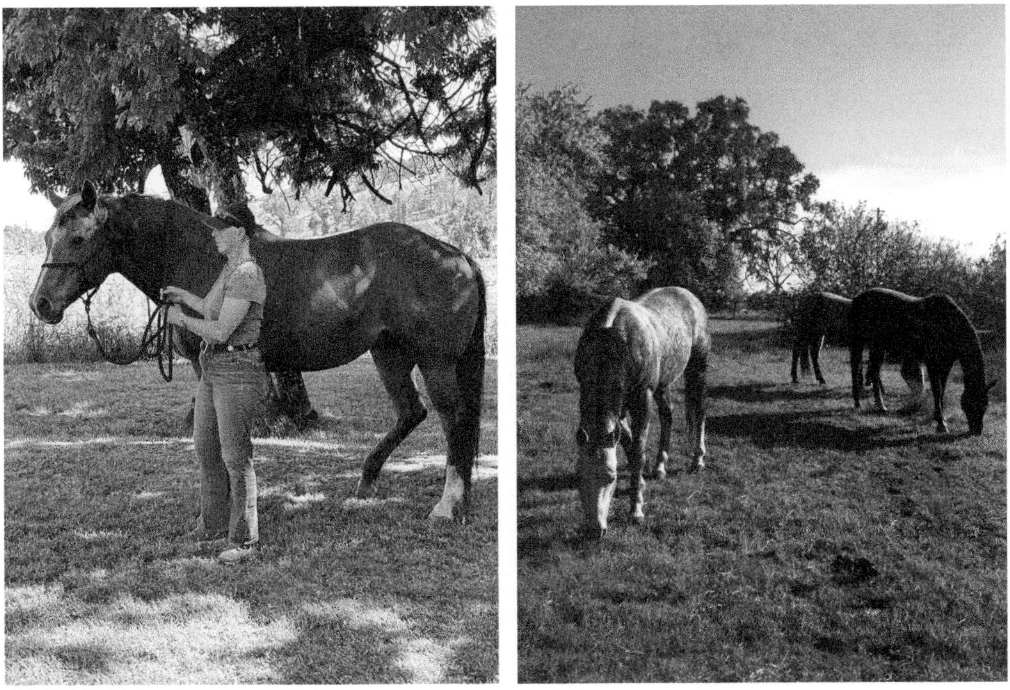

Figure 10.2 The green zone: A horse in the green zone on halter (a) has relaxed ears and has the head held in a middle position, below the withers. Horses in the green zone on pasture (b) are relaxed and grazing. *Source:* Jeannine Berger.

Box 10.1 Normal resting ranges for equine vital signs
Heart rate: 28–40 beats/minute Respiration rate: 10–14 breaths/minute Rectal temperature: 99–101 °F (37.2–38.2 °C)

lameness evaluations to be performed safely. A common veterinary need is to walk, trot, turn, and halt horses in hand during a lameness exam. Whereas the client may be asked to lead the horse for such an exam, it is critical that the veterinarian assess what emotional state the horse is in before proceeding.

The Yellow Zone

In the yellow zone, the first stage of escalation, the horse has become more alert and evaluates whether any change in the environment should be perceived as a positive opportunity, a threat, or something that can be ignored. Escalation to the yellow zone moves the horse to a more aroused mental state that is not necessarily bad yet calls for an equally more attentive presence from the handler. If not in a fear state, the horse may even be more responsive to verbal or visual cues from the handler. The horse may become frightened by an unfamiliar person or location, from the tension of people present, from the equipment needed for a procedure, from the procedure itself, or for other reasons. In this alert state, the horse makes a decision: remain and calm down (return to the green zone)? Stay alert and curious, and explore the opportunity (remain in the yellow zone)? Or prepare to escape or fight off a potential threatening stimulus (escalate to the red zone)?

The visual image of a horse in the yellow zone would include a head held high, ears

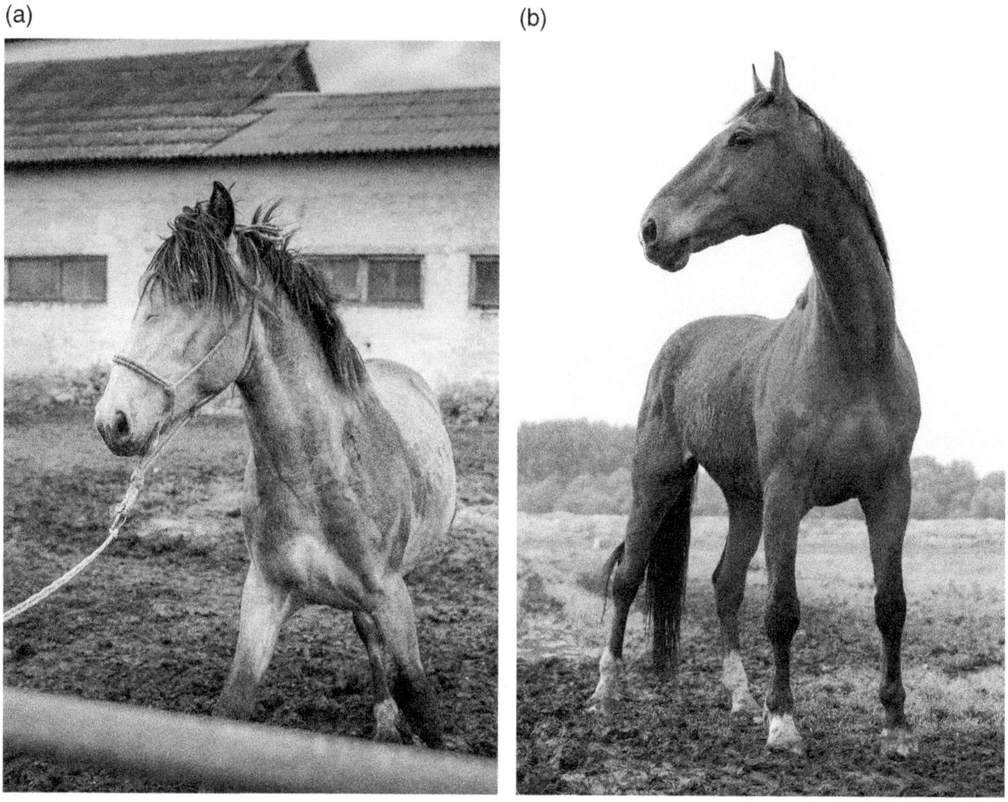

Figure 10.3 Horses in the yellow zone are sensing a threat and preparing to flee (or fight, if necessary). The head is held high to maximize peripheral visual input as they scan for danger. Muscles are tense, and they may balk or be hesitant to move forward toward what they find threatening (b). *Source:* ahavelaar/AdobeStock (a) and shymar27/AdobeStock (b).

pointed toward the object, eyes scanning the environment, and nostrils wide (Figure 10.3a,b). The muscles are increasingly tense; the tail may be moving from side to side or up and down faster, or it may be raised or tucked against the body. The heart and respiration rates increase above resting ranges. The horse may defecate multiple times. Horses in this state may choose multiple strategies to cope with the emerging tension – some appear frozen in place while others show opposite behaviors, stepping around and fidgeting quickly but not (yet) trying to leave the situation. Stressed horses may snort or blow, a very loud and quick exhalation of breath; this is their sound of alarm (McDonnell 2003).

If this stage is reached when handling a horse, the potential for injury to the horse and people increases. The handler should be alert and ready for any movement of a fear or flight response. If the horse has reached this level, the goal of the handler should shift from a focus on the exam to a focus on de-escalating the horse's emotional state, returning to the green zone as quickly as possible. However, in this heightened state, the horse's focus may no longer be on the handler but on whatever caused the alarm. Maintaining focus on the handler and/or responding to cues or requests they responded to easily in the green zone may be difficult now. Redirecting the horse's focus to something positive can help to recover the horse's attention. This may encompass offering higher value treats, giving a cue for simple, easily performed behaviors (such as stepping back), or repositioning the situation by giving the horse a short break or taking a walk. In some cases, it is helpful to move to a different location or even return the horse to the stall to rest and calm down before starting over. Observing whether or not a horse is willing to take treats during handling is useful in gauging relaxation, focus, and the current emotional zone. A fear-eliciting stimulus should never be used to get the horse's attention, as that might lead to a freeze response (at best) or an escalated flight response. The key is to use the change in emotional state as valuable information, rather than ignore it and try to continue and force the procedure. Reposition, rethink, and restart!

The Red Zone

If horses in the yellow zone perceive the threat as real and action is required for survival, they enter the red zone. The fight or flight response is fully activated, and the horse's emotional state is one intent on survival, where the horse becomes difficult and even dangerous to handle. This is a physiological and psychological response in which handlers rarely have much immediate influence. The horse has decided either to attempt escape (flight) or confront (fight) the perceived danger. The horse is emotionally and mentally incapable of following cues and has no interest in treats.

The body language of a horse in the red zone includes a head held high, ears pinned forward or directed toward a threat, snorts, and other alarm vocalizations. This horse is prepared for fight (Figure 10.4a) or flight (Figure 10.4b). These horses become increasingly difficult to handle because they are focused on survival and are not likely to follow any cues or to be interested in taking treats. The behavior of

(a) (b) (c)

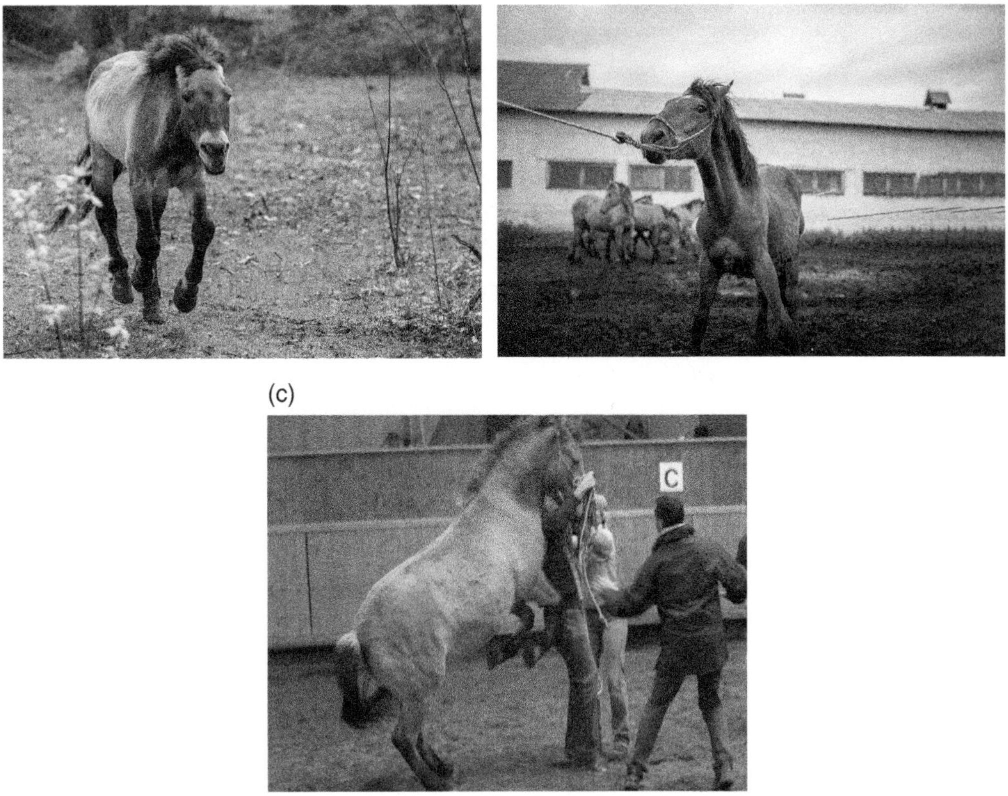

Figure 10.4 Horses in the red zone: These horses are starting to use aggression (a) or flee (b) a situation they perceive to be a threat. Horses who cannot escape may rear (c) and strike, which can be dangerous to handle. *Source:* Jodi/AdobeStock (a), shymar27/AdobeStock (b), Jeannine Berger (c).

horses in the red zone can include violent movements. They may suddenly bolt and leave the situation in any manner possible. The dangers in this situation are many. The horse may knock the handler down or pull them off their feet, break equipment, or even crash through barriers. If tied, the horse could pull back, potentially injuring their neck, falling, and/or suffering other injuries. The horse that is unable to flee what is perceived to be a life-threatening situation may then choose to fight by biting, kicking, rearing, and/or striking (Figure 10.4c).

In this stage, redirecting or encouraging the horse to focus on anything other than the threating stimulus typically fails. The best strategy is to move the horse to a safe place, and sometimes the handlers just need to remove themselves. Safety for both the handler and the horse should have priority. As with the yellow zone, never use a fear- or pain-eliciting stimulus on a horse in the red zone, as that is likely to further escalate. If you can identify the trigger for the red zone response, avoid it. For example, if the trigger is an external stimulus, such as a loud noise, the handling or the exam could be performed in a different, quieter location or with another calm horse close by. If the handling itself triggered such a strong emotional response, then medications should be considered before attempting such handling again. If time allows, a desensitization and counterconditioning plan should be put in place to alleviate the stress of future exposure.

Tools, Handling Skills, and Procedures

Tools

When we handle a horse for any type of intervention, perhaps to pick up a hoof or take a temperature, we want to apply some form of restraint to control the horse's movement and keep the handler safe. A variety of equipment is available to help us safely handle and restrain horses. Whatever equipment the hander chooses, it should be humane and should improve rather than harm the human-animal bond. Hence, any tools should help to keep horses in the green zone or return them to the green zone as quickly as possible.

Halters and ropes are the most basic pieces of equipment for working with horses. Halters are available in many sizes and can be made from a variety of materials. Most commonly, they are made of leather, nylon web, nylon, or cotton rope (Box 10.2), and sometimes combinations of one or more of these (Figure 10.5a–c). The halter should be clean, fit well, and be made of good quality material. All pieces should be in good repair with any hardware free of dirt or rust. Lead ropes of various lengths and materials are commonly attached to the chin part of the halter. The attachment between the halter and the rope can be either a loop or a metal clasp. The rope should be clean, made from good quality material, and in good condition. The length should be at least 10 feet long for safety but can be longer in the case a horse needs lunging in addition to leading.

Gloves, whether of leather or another material, can be helpful tools to protect the hands. Gloves are controversial in some equestrian circles, reasoning that they could allow a more forceful approach than necessary. Of course, medical gloves are important for maintaining a clean environment and preventing transmission of disease and should always be changed between client horses.

Treats – highly digestible small food items varying from low to high value, should be readily available when handling horses for medical procedures, regardless of whether the procedures are truly painful or not. Treats are commercially available in many sizes and flavors and even include low-starch varieties for horses with metabolic conditions. Sugar cubes, pieces of carrots, and apples are traditional favorites. For handling, treats should be small. Carrots or apples can easily be cut into small 1 × 1 cm or dime-sized pieces. Using the small

(a)

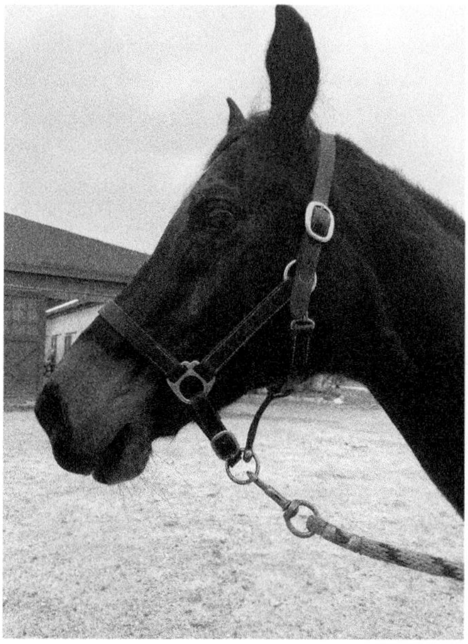

(b)

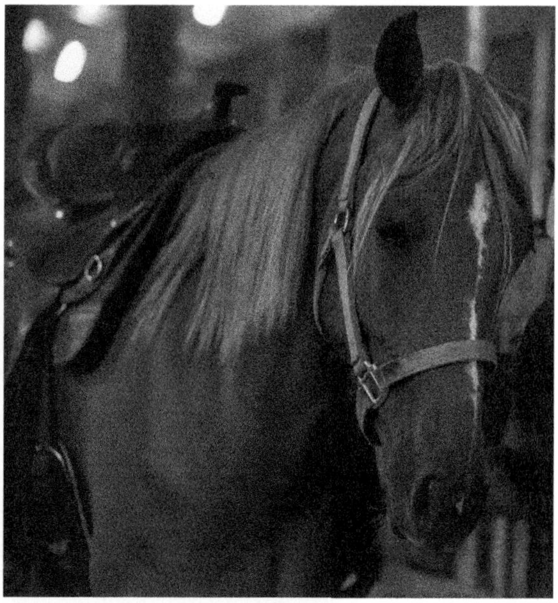

(c)

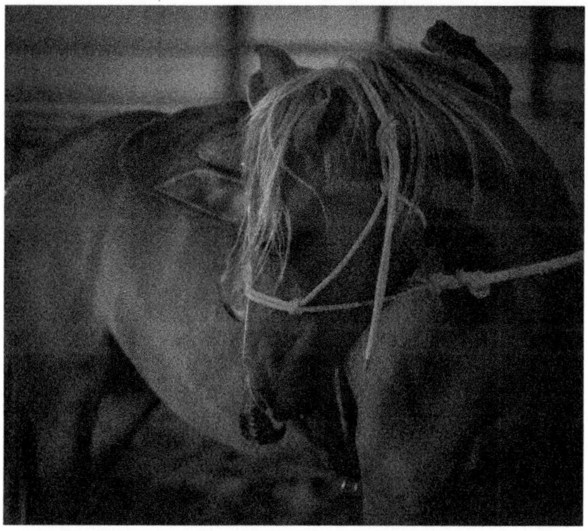

Figure 10.5 Halters are available in many sizes and from many materials, including leather (a), nylon web (b), and cotton rope (c). *Source:* Jeannine Berger (a), With permission from Jill Sackman (b and c).

size helps keep the animal interested, engaged, and leaves a positive association, promoting learning by causing a dopamine surge. Full-size carrots, apples, larger or harder treats can be helpful during a longer-lasting procedure, such as an intramuscular injection. It will give the horse something positive to engage with and distract from the actual needle poke that could be painful. However, for some horses, it is better to reward them after the fact for remaining calm by applying true positive reinforcement (see Chapter 5) rather than using the treat as a distraction.

Treat holders – Treats can be carried in jackets or pant pockets, but treat bags similar to those used in the dog training world are

Box 10.2 Rope Halters

Good rope halters, made from high quality sailing-type rope, are a popular alternative to leather and web halters. They are more adjustable, making them easier to fit to horses of various sizes. Because they do not contain any metal pieces, any pressure applied travels smoothly along a single type of material from the handler to the horse.

A rope halter is lighter than a leather or nylon halter, thereby placing less passive pressure on the horse's head. The result is that less pressure needs to be applied by the handler (active pressure) to signal the horse to move. Rope halters can be "sharper" if too much pressure is applied, so they must be used with caution and the principles of negative reinforcement in mind.

Regardless of halter type, based on the understanding of negative reinforcement as a technique to teach behaviors, only the minimum amount of pressure should be applied to it, with immediate release of that pressure the moment the horse responds in the desired way.

In some cases, handlers attach a chain to the lead rope. The chain is threaded through the halter and clipped to the opposite side, so that the chain lays over the bridge of the nose or is inserted in the mouth, applying pressure to the gums of the upper lip of the horse. Called "stud chains" (Figure 10.6), they are sometimes used in stallions or horses with handling challenges. The chain will amplify any pressure applied to the lead rope, applying pain to a sensitive part of the horse's mouth. By eliciting pain, the horse may seem more manageable, at least for the moment, in order to avoid the inflicted pain. The authors of this chapter acknowledge that the use of chains for handling is common in many equestrian venues, but it is challenging not to inflict pain or induce fear with their use. Handlers should recognize that the compliance they achieve with this tool is one of fear and not one of relaxation.

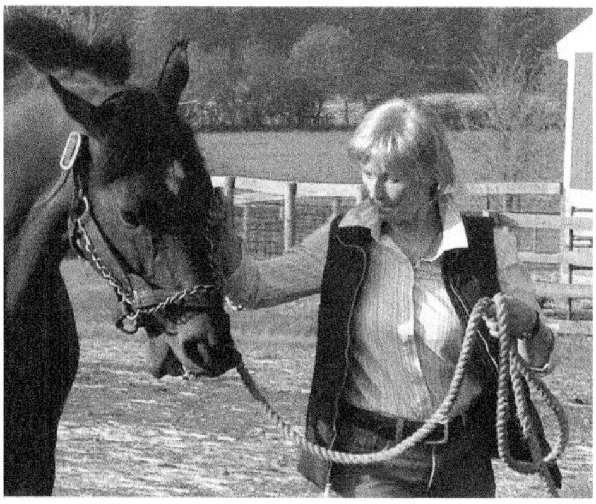

Figure 10.6 A metal "stud" chain can be threaded through the halter and clipped to the other side. While this is a commonly used control device, its effectiveness is based on pain and physical discomfort in the horse's mouth, causing inhibition of behavior. This is not to be mistaken for relaxation. *Source:* Jeannine Berger.

recommended. A useful type of treat bag has a clip that can easily be opened or closed and includes a belt so it can be worn around the waist. If there is a concern with wearing the treats on the body of the handler, treats can be placed in a bucket, and a helper can provide the food when appropriate (Figure 10.7).

Whips, sticks, and flags are extensions that are used at times to help move an animal when lunging or sending (see later). While these tools can be useful, they also are used too often as punishment tools. If not used appropriately, they can easily be ignored, at best or worse, inflict pain, and lead to fear and the deterioration of the human-animal bond. An alternate use of a flag or stick would be to use them as targets for the horse to touch with their nose. This encourages forward movement and teaches horses to engage in a calm behavior with their mouths (a nice alternative to biting if that is an issue). Target sticks of various materials have become more and more

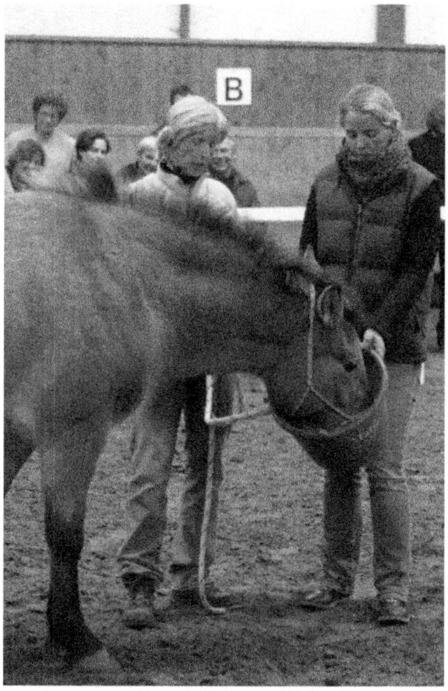

Figure 10.7 A hand-held bucket serves as a treat holder to provide positive reinforcement for desirable behavior, as well as to countercondition a positive emotional response to medical procedures. *Source:* Jeannine Berger.

mainstream in horse training as they can help in many different ways. For example, a target trained horse can be led into a trailer by following the target stick and be rewarded for walking forward, rather than being whipped for not entering the trailer.

This list of handling tools is not complete, as there are many more the practitioner may use when assessing and treating horses. For example, for a horse that spooks at the sight of needles, one may block vision by cupping a hand over the eye or even placing a covered fly mask, driving blinkers, or a medical eye protection mask. In cases of a horse with a bite history, a handler may place a grazing muzzle for protection, similarly to a dog basket muzzle. Prior to the availability of medical restraint, veterinarians and horsemen alike used hobbles to restrain horses. However, those tools can be dangerous and have mostly lost their application, thankfully.

Handling Skills

Veterinarians and students must learn and practice how to handle a horse effectively and safely. In many cases, it may be best to let the client handle, lead, or even lunge the horse, but in some cases, the client is not available or able to do so safely. Knowing how to best approach, handle, lead, or lunge a horse is a necessary skill for any equine veterinarian. This section presents practical, hands-on methods for those less familiar with handling horses.

Approaching the Client Horse

The manner in which the veterinarian approaches the horse can establish a positive atmosphere for the appointment, setting it up for success. Keep in mind that veterinarians are not usually people the horse sees on a daily basis. Consider that the activities and procedures we do with horses contradict their nature and their ethology (McGreevy et al. 2018). The horse may welcome the veterinarian or instead view them as a stranger and potential threat, especially if previous veterinary care was invasive or aversive. The veterinarian should take a few moments to quietly "greet" the horse, speaking to it quietly and calmly.

As the veterinarian greets the horse, they should determine what zone that horse is in. Ideally, no procedures take place unless the horse is in the green zone. To make that judgment, the horse can be asked for some simple cues and the handler can gauge responsiveness: step back, step left or right, lower his head, etc. Another easy technique is placing a hand on the large muscles, such as the neck or shoulder. The feel of a relaxed horse is quite different from a horse that is tense. Observation of heart and respiration rates can also be used.

If the horse is not in the green zone but instead in yellow or even red, take some time to assess why. Are they reacting to a new person? Is the location unfamiliar or loud? Is the horse in pain? Were they just unloaded from the trailer and they are not used to being hauled? Is fear of veterinarians the real issue? The client can be helpful by sharing any history and the horse's usual demeanor.

Approach and Retreat

If the horse is loose in a stall or paddock and reluctant to allow anyone near, an approach-and-retreat process can be used to encourage the horse to approach the handler willingly. See online materials for a video example.

Equipment: Halter and lead rope, treats, bucket, or treat bag.

Safety: The veterinarian or other handler should always be positioned between the horse and the exit door or gate.

1) Begin by standing quietly to observe the horse's body language and assess the current zone. This allows the horse to assess the handler, too.
2) Take a step toward the horse. If the horse makes any positive change in behavior, stop or even step back. This is a form of negative reinforcement where the handler's retreat is the reward. For example, if the horse is facing away, any movement in the direction of the handler should be rewarded, even turning the head toward the handler at first. If the horse is moving, a moment of standing still should be rewarded.
3) Repeat as needed until the horse either approaches the handler or the handler can approach the horse and the halter can be placed.
4) If the horse is close enough, giving a treat at the same time (positive reinforcement) can increase the probability of the desired behavior to recur. If the horse is too far away or is not ready to take a treat from the hand, then the treat can be gently tossed toward the horse into a bucket or even on the ground.
5) Proceed at a rate that never raises the level of tension in the horse.
6) The horse learns that they have some control over the situation by how they react, and they begin to associate good things with the veterinarian (classical conditioning) while also being reinforced for the desired behavior.

Note: The handler must be careful when using reinforcement not to accidentally reward unwanted behavior.

Approach and Haltering

Hopefully when the veterinarian arrives, the horse is already caught, haltered, and will be presented by the client in a controlled fashion. However, it is not uncommon that the client is not available or cannot catch the horse, and the veterinarian is tasked with this job. A successful equine veterinarian must be able to safely approach, catch, and halter a horse in a stall or paddock.

When approaching a horse, you must first get the horse's attention. This can be done by calling their name, making a clucking noise, or even shaking a treat or grain bucket. The goal is for the horse to face you. Never directly approach a horse that has its hind end turned toward you. Remember, horses are prey species, and in a large area, a quick approach from behind may cause the horse to bolt. If there is no space, such as in a stall, the potential to get kicked or run over if the horse turns quickly is too high. Once the horse faces the handler, the handler should stop or even take a step backwards, thereby negatively reinforcing the horse's attempt to look at or approach the handler. If the horse is friendly or curious, they may even approach the handler. At that point, it is helpful to have a treat ready for the horse.

Always approach from the front. The best position is at a 45° angle toward the point of the left shoulder of the horse. Gently reach out toward the neck and scratch the horse, if they allow, at the neck or the withers. When approaching a horse, always avoid stepping toward the horse behind the withers. That can not only spook a horse but can also drive the horse forward and away from you. Avoid stepping beyond the point of the shoulders until you have taken time to ensure the horse is relaxed and in the green zone. The horse could kick out at any time and if you are behind the point of the shoulder, you may get hurt. Being prepared to halter the horse means to have the unbuckled or untied halter and the rope neatly in the left hand when approaching the horse. Stand between the head and the shoulder of the horse on the left side, which is the side on which the halter is fastened once on the horse (Figure 10.8). However, generally, horses should be taught to be approached comfortably from both sides.

Ideally, as a next step, the horse willingly lowers the head to a height where the handler can easily reach it with the right arm over the horse's neck. Holding the rope and halter in the left hand, the handler then reaches with the right arm over the horse's neck while the left hand passes the longer strap (poll strap) of the halter under the neck to be grasped by the right hand (Figure 10.9a). At this point, the buckle or loop side of the halter is in the handler's left hand and the long strap (poll strap) in the right (Figure 10.9b). The handler then lifts the halter to allow the nose to slip gently into the nose loop (Figure 10.9c). The handler then brings the poll strap over the poll with the right hand, with both hands meeting at the left side of the horse's face to buckle or tie the halter on the left side of the horse's head (Figure 10.9d). By using this method, the handler never needs to let go of the halter or change hands. The circle formed by the left hand, halter, and right arm over the neck holding the long strap also offers a bit of control should the horse attempt to move away.

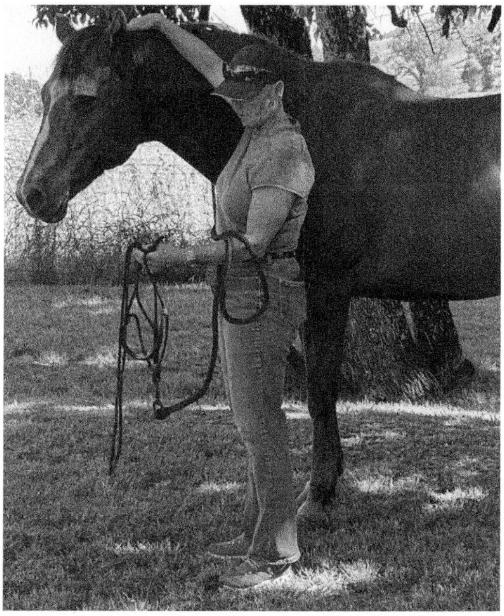

Figure 10.8 As the handler approaches a horse to place a halter, they stand between the head and the shoulder, facing the same direction, with the halter unbuckled or untied with the rope neatly in the left hand. *Source:* Jeannine Berger.

In a less desirable method, when haltering tall horses or horses that will not easily lower their heads, the handler uses the right hand to flip the longer strap (poll strap) over the horse's neck from below. This can cause the long strap of the halter to hit the horse in the face or eye and cause injury or an aversion that may lead to the horse lifting the head even higher up the next time (yellow zone). If this method is being used because the horse raises his head too high for the handler, he can be taught to lower his head.

Once the halter is safely in place, the handler will attach the clip of the lead rope to the ring or loop beneath the horse's jaw, if not already attached. The handler then folds the rest of the rope and either holds it in their left hand or places it over their left arm. This positions the lead rope, ready to control the horse.

WARNING: *Never* wrap or loop the lead rope around your hand or arm, as the horse could pull away, causing injury to the handler by tightening around the hand or arm. In a similar caution, do not let the end of the lead rope lay on the ground where a horse or handler could step on it or become tangled in it.

Leading

Once the horse is caught and the halter is securely in place, we usually want to lead the horse either a few steps forward or backwards.

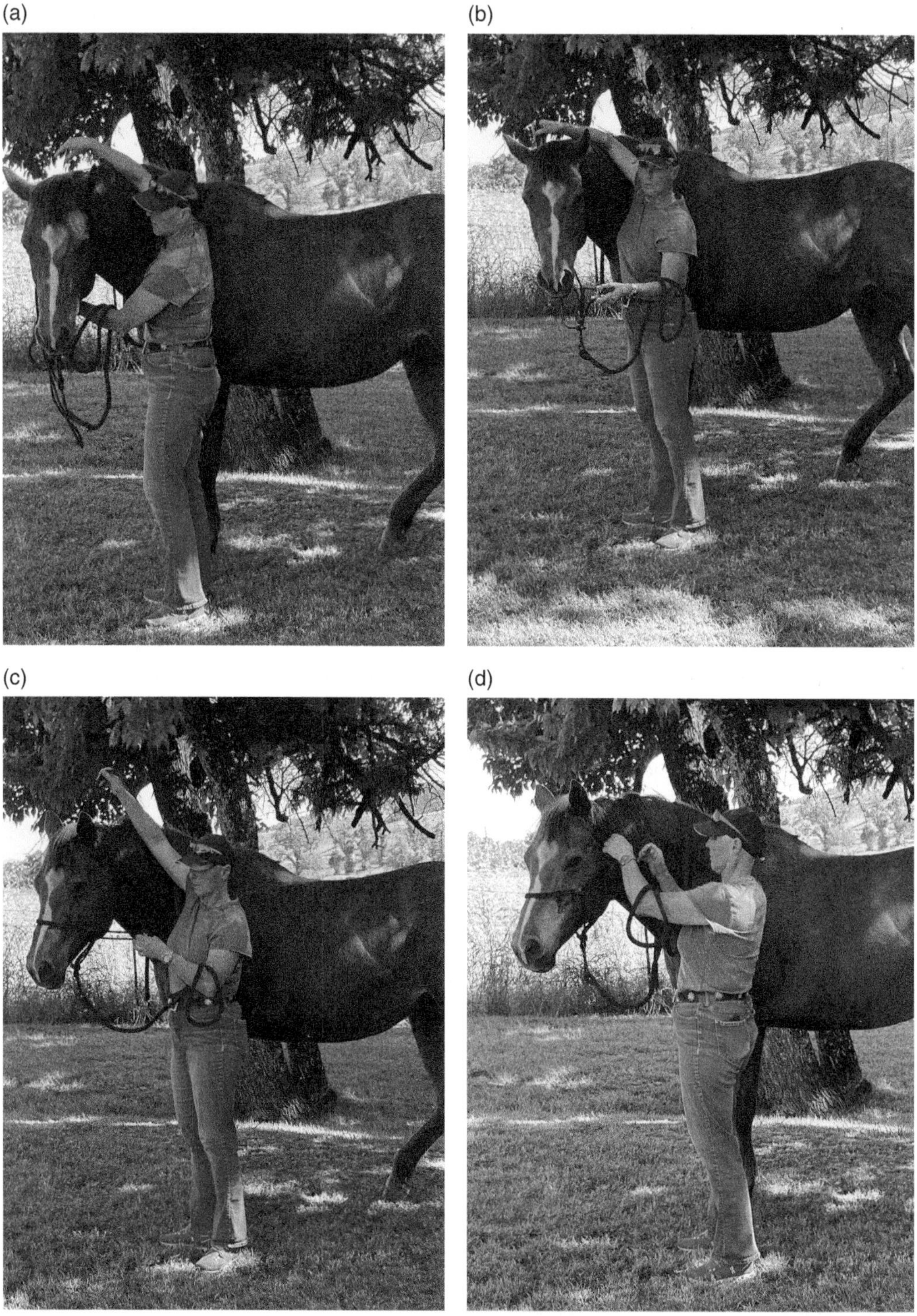

Figure 10.9 Holding the rope and halter in the left hand, the handler reaches with the right arm over the horse's neck while the left hand passes the poll strap of the halter under the neck of the horse to be grasped by the right hand (a). At this point, the buckle or loop side of the halter is in the handler's left hand and the poll strap is in the right (b). The handler then lifts the halter to allow the nose to slip gently into the nose loop (c). The handler then brings the poll strap over the poll with the right hand, with both hands meeting at the left side of the horse's face to buckle or tie the halter on the left side of the horse's head (d).

When leading a horse, the handler should be on the left side of the horse, holding the lead rope a few inches below the rope/halter intersection, usually with the right hand. The left hand should then hold the rope 20–30 inches further down, with the tail end folded as described above. Maintaining slack in the rope is very important. Tension or contact should be applied to the rope/halter only when the horse is asked to perform a behavior such as stepping forward, sideways, or backward. A horse can feel the tension of the handler through the rope and halter, and if the handler grips tightly, the horse's prey animal instinct may engage, causing the horse to feel trapped and sense danger. The horse may then react by escalating into the yellow zone, such as by raising the head, pulling, or running forward or backward.

To begin walking, the handler and horse should both be facing in the intended direction. The handler applies a little pressure to the rope with the right hand and may use a verbal cue ("walk on" and tongue clicks are common). As the handler steps forward, the horse should also take its first step forward. The handler should release tension immediately when the horse steps forward with the handler, and verbal praise can be given. The release of that pressure is the negative reinforcement, and the verbal praise is the positive reinforcement. If the horse does not take a step, the handler needs to either wait a little longer until the horse responds to the pressure or increase the intensity slightly, such as with a little more pressure on the lead, or apply a little pressure toward the hind end of the horse. The pressure that is applied to drive a horse forward needs to be directed toward the hip of the horse. This can be done with the end of the rope using the left hand if the rope is long enough or with a helper that stands behind the drive line, or in some cases, it can be helpful to use a stick, flag, or whip as an extension of the arm for support (not to punish or scare the horse). There is an imaginary vertical line that divides the horse at the level of approximately the withers; pressure applied in front of this line may slow a horse down; pressure applied behind that point generally drives a horse forward. This line is sometimes referred to as the **driving line** (Figure 10.10).

If the horse takes more steps than the handler intends to and gets ahead of the handler, the handler needs to slow the horse down or even stop it to regain control. In some cases, it helps to ask the horse to take a step backwards and then start over. When walking next to a horse, the handler should make sure to match

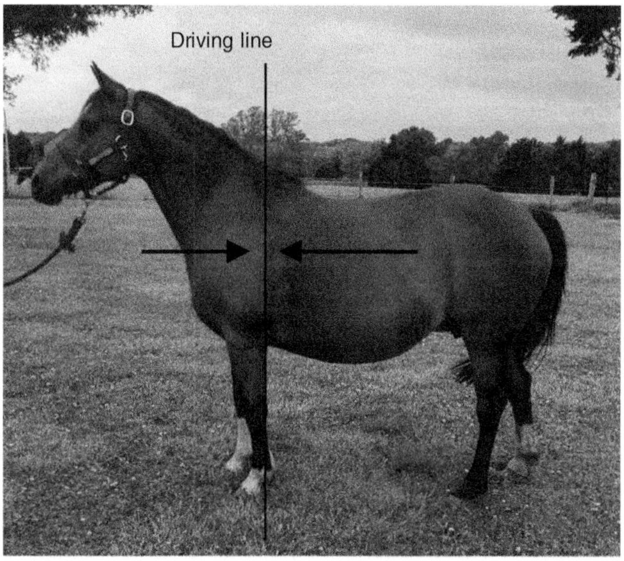

Figure 10.10 The driving line on a horse is just at the point of the withers (shoulder). Pressure applied caudal to the line will cause the horse to move forward, whereas pressure applied cranial to the line will cause the horse to move backwards. *Source:* With permission from Jill Sackman.

their step to the stride of the horse. A bigger horse may have a bigger stride or walk naturally faster.

Often, equine exams are best started at the head once the horse is safely haltered and in a relaxed state. It is always advised to have an assistant handle the head of the horse, standing on the same side as you are examining. The assistant stays with the horse's head for the duration of your exam. When you are ready to move caudal to the point of the shoulders, gently scratch the horse, speak in a calm voice, and keep physical contact as you move to inspect different parts of the body. The concept of keeping in constant physical contact is known as a **touch gradient** and helps to prevent startle. Repeatedly putting hands on and off of a horse, as well as slapping or patting the horse, can elicit startle and agitation. The same is true for auscultation. Rather than taking your stethoscope on and off of the body, keep it in contact with the skin and slowly slide it into the different places you wish to auscultate. Keep your body close to the horse, especially around the pelvic limbs, and avoid standing directly behind the horse's rear end. When you need to move to the other side of the horse, either walk around the front or, if you choose to walk behind, let the handler know that you are switching sides and keep a hand on the rump and slide from one side of the body to the other, keeping close. If a horse kicks you while you are right up against them, you may just get pushed out of the way, whereas at an arm's length away, you may get seriously injured. Remember, the assistant holding the lead rope should remain on the same side of the horse as the clinician so they can keep awareness of any potentially uncomfortable interactions and are ready to steer the hind end immediately away from the clinician if needed. In this case, the handler directs the head toward the clinician so that the rump swings away from them. When examining the legs of the horse, never hover down or kneel; always stay on your feet, bending at the hips and keeping your head up. Let your hands glide along the body down the extremity all the way to the hooves for safety.

For lameness exams, horses are often examined in hand at a trot. Sudden changes in behavior or body language have been shown to be possible indicators of orthopedic pain. Hence, you should examine horses at all gaits in a straight line as well as in a circle to the left and the right, in hand and under saddle, to fully evaluate lameness. The handler should begin by leading the horse at the walk in a straight line and on the lunge and see how easily the horse leads, turns, and stops before adding speed or transitioning to the trot. If the horse asked to trot starts going too fast, slow down to a walk or stand still and try again. Stay calm during this process.

Turning: To make a turn when leading a horse from the left side, the handler should turn the horse to the right, away from themselves, to avoid being stepped on or run over. The horse needs to slow down so the handler can be on the outside of that turn. This is safer than turning left, which brings the horse around the handler on the outside, where the horse can easily run over them.

Halting: To slow down, the handler should slow their own walk and put slight downward or backward pressure on the lead rope, possibly using a verbal cue ("whoa" or "ho," drawn out rather than a sharp single tone), and then come to a halt. The horse should also come to a halt when the handler's feet stop. If the horse keeps walking, slightly more pressure should be added to the lead rope until the horse stops, and then immediately the pressure must be released. Once control over stop, go, and turn is confirmed, the handler's walking speed can increase to the point where the horse begins to trot.

Sending: A handler can safely lead a horse in the desired direction or to a location in most cases, such as into a stall or into a large trailer for transport. However, in some situations, leading a horse may not be safe, and sending the horse is the better choice. For example, the handler should not lead the horse into narrow spaces, such as a trailer, if there is not enough room for the handler to be next to the horse and safely exit. Entering stocks with the horse is also dangerous; the handler should always remain on the outside of the bars of the stock, even if there is an opening in the front. If space prevents leading the horse into stocks from the outside, the handler can send the horse instead.

In this method, the handler does not walk with the horse but sends the horse forward from a location or a stationary position into or toward a spot, such as into a stall, a trailer, or stocks. This maneuver is a little more advanced and requires a horse that is very responsive to pressure on the halter and easily steps forward when asked to do so. The handler must understand and be attentive to the movement of the horse and direction of travel to prevent getting into an unsafe position where the horse runs past the handler, or the handler loses control of the horse and could get kicked or stepped on.

The handler begins by facing the horse, perpendicular to the direction of travel, with the horse looking toward the direction of travel. The handler holds the rope in the left hand, lifts the hand, and uses the rope to apply a little pressure directed to the halter while lifting the right hand to send or drive the horse forward. Using this method to send a horse into a trailer, the handler would gently lay the free end of the lead rope over the horse's back as it enters so the horse does not step on it. Once the horse steps forward, the handler needs to feed more rope from the left hand or step along with the horse so as not to suddenly apply pressure to the halter when the horse moves forward (see online materials for video examples).

Lunging in a Circle

Lunging is a method of exercising the horse in a circle, both directions, with or without a rider. It initially looks like sending, where the handler may walk in a straight line with the horse. However, while lunging, the horse continues the movement in a circle around the handler, who stays at the center of the circle, rotating as the horse goes around in either clockwise or counterclockwise direction. The basic equipment needed is the halter, a lunge line (commonly 30 feet long, flat nylon or cotton webbing), and often a lunge whip. A lunge whip is a whip handle with a longer string attachment to be able to apply pressure behind the drive line to aid forward movement if needed. Veterinarians can use lunging to view the horse's movement for lameness, or to evaluate the cardiovascular system of the horse during or after exercise. The horse can perform all gaits – walk, trot, and canter – on the lunge line when trained properly. Alternatively, a round pen can also be useful to free lunge (no lunge line) a horse that has not yet learned to move nicely on the lunge line or to evaluate a horse without the attachments.

Picking up Hooves

Most horses are taught to lift their feet to inspect the bottom of the hooves, to remove dirt, and to trim or put shoes on. Various types of cues are used and, therefore it may take several tries until the horse recognizes the request from an unfamiliar handler. For some, just running the hand down the leg signals the horse to pick up that foot. For others, the cue may be pulling fetlock hairs or gently squeezing the fetlock, the back of the lower cannon bone, the chestnut on the inner front leg, or the hock. A few horses respond to verbal cues, such as "hoof" or "up." Being pushed by the handler's body weight toward the center of the horse's body, to shift the weight onto the other legs, is another cue used in young or untrained horses.

To begin, an assistant should hold the horse. The veterinarian or handler should stand beside the horse's shoulder, facing the rear. As a safety measure, the handler can maintain contact between their own shoulder and the horse's body and may also use this contact to help shift the horse's weight to the opposite leg. They will then put the hand closest to the horse on its shoulder for front hooves

(Figure 10.11a), or on the hip for hind hooves. Then run the hand down the medial aspect of the leg slowly to reach the hoof (Figures 10.11b and 10.12a). Once the hoof is lifted, the handler should cup the hoof with one hand, leaving the other hand free for whatever task is at hand, such as cleaning, checking for stones, or viewing injuries (Figures 10.11c and 10.12b). Once the handler is finished inspecting the hoof, the hoof should be gently placed back on the ground and not just dropped. If the hoof is just dropped, the horse could be caught by surprise and hit the tip of the hoof capsule, potentially inflicting pain and possibly leading to aversion to having their feet picked up.

Measuring Body Temperature

When it is necessary to take a horse's temperature, the tip of a digital thermometer is placed into the horse's rectum. Safety is always important in activity around horses and is doubly important when working near the hind end. Prepare the thermometer by lubricating it with petroleum jelly or soapy water. Turn on the digital thermometer before you insert it. Depending if the handler is left- or right-handed the recommended process is: Standing on the left side of the horse (can be done from the right side by just reversing the directional instructions) and facing to the rear, the handler puts the left hand on the horse's back and slowly slides it down over the croup toward the top of the tail (Figure 10.13a). This touch gradient approach lets the horse know the handler is approaching a potentially sensitive area. Going slowly allows the horses to either stay in the green zone or, if the horse gets uncomfortable, let the handler either slow down, stop, or step away in order to de-escalate and not get hurt. As with lifting a hoof, maintaining contact between the handler and horse's body increases the safety factor. Do not grab the tail from the top, because the harder the handler grabs the tail, the harder the horse will clamp the tail down. The correct way is to gently scratch the top of the tail and the area next to the anus, slip the hand slowly and gently under the tail, and lift the tail with the back of your hand (Figure 10.13b). By doing so, most horses will lift the tail, and the handler can then gently slip the thermometer into place (Figure 10.13c). The handler should either continue holding the end of the thermometer to prevent it from being pushed out or, preferably, there should be a string and a clip attached to the thermometer that can easily be attached to the tail hairs until the temperature is ready to be read. An electronic thermometer will sound a tone when it reaches the horse's body temperature. Once done, gently slide the thermometer out and scratch the tail or the side of the croup of the horse as a reward.

Injections

Most horses, at some point in their lives, will need an injection. Medication can either be injected into a vein or into the muscle. This can be uncomfortable or even mildly painful. Hence, it is critical to learn the right techniques for injection. This will not be covered here and must be learned elsewhere. We will, however, teach the correct approach to injections with the hope of maintaining a horse in the green zone.

Intravenous (IV) injections to the jugular vein: The handler will stand on the side of the horse they are most comfortable with between the shoulder and the middle of the neck. The handler can apply a little pressure to the jugular vein at the base of the neck, and if the horse stands still, the handler should stop the pressure for a moment (negative reinforcement). The handler may even choose to give a small treat to reward the horse. Either way, a treat should always be given after an injection to create a positive memory of this procedure. It will pay off in the long run. After the location for the injection has been chosen, the area over the vein can be tapped or pinched lightly (desensitization) to again see the horse's response to a mildly aversive process and

(a)

(b)

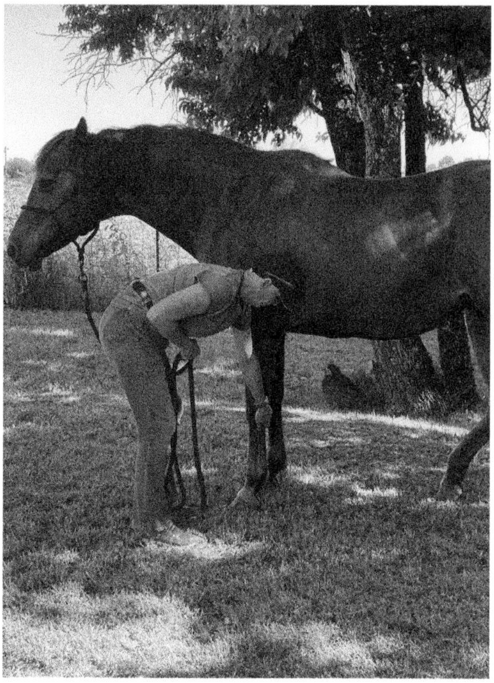

(c)

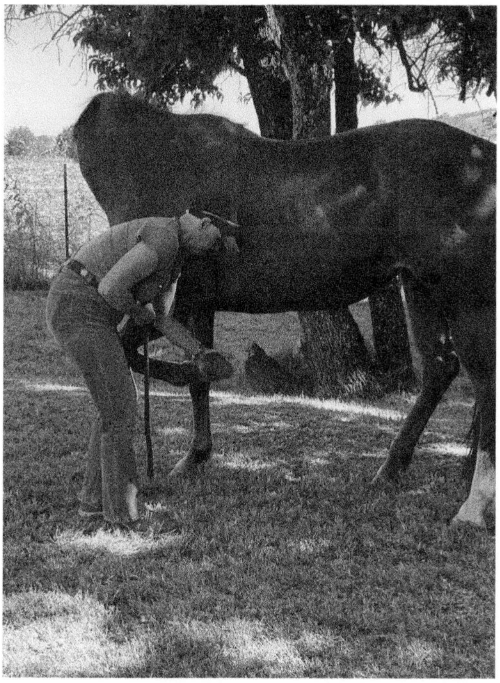

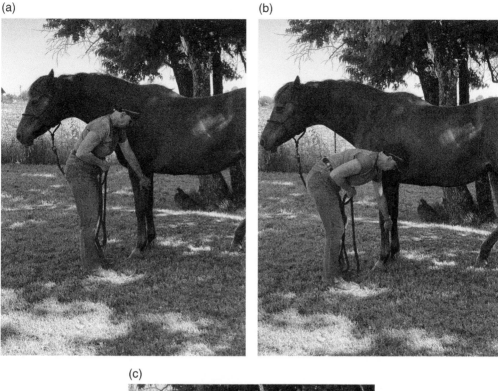

Figure 10.11 The handler inspects a front hoof by standing directly to the side of the front leg, placing a hand on the shoulder, while facing the rear end of the horse (a). Next, the handler will slowly slide their hand down the medial aspect of the limb, putting a small amount of pressure on the "chestnut" or medial carpus, which should signal the horse to lift the hoof (b). Finally, the handler cups the hoof with one hand in order to inspect/trim the hoof with the other hand (c). *Source:* Jeannine Berger.

(a) (b)

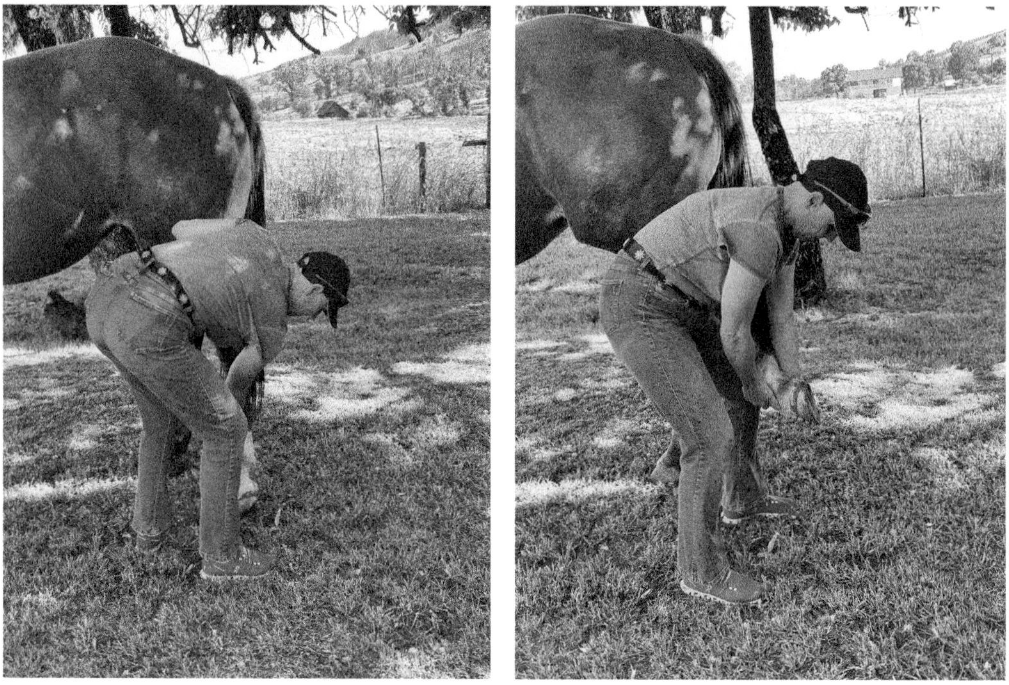

Figure 10.12 The handler will slowly slide their hand down the limb, which should signal the horse to lift the hoof (a). Then the handler cups the hoof and leans it on the leg closest to the horse (b). *Source:* Jeannine Berger.

prevent startle from a sudden needle poke. Again, if the horse stands still and allows this without changing its emotional zone, the process can be stopped briefly and rewarded. Once the handler has confirmed that the horse is likely to stand still, the needle should be moved into the vein with a quick but smooth movement.

Avoid multiple needle sticks. It is easier to reposition the needle once under the skin than it is to stick a horse multiple times. If the horse jerks or tries to move away, stay with the horse, keeping the needle in place. One of the main mistakes the authors have observed when teaching inexperienced handlers is that they poke, the horse jerks or moves the head, and the handler stops – negatively reinforcing the horse for moving away. Beginners would do well to practice their technique first on a horse that is easy to inject.

Intramuscular (IM) injections: These are very similar to the process described above. The area of injection is larger, but the approach is very similar. When injecting into the neck muscle, stand as described above and tap or pinch the skin a few times (desensitization) before injecting the needle deep into the muscle. When completed, gently retract the needle and reward the horse with a treat.

Procedures Aversion

De-escalation: When a horse is not comfortable with handling during any of the procedures discussed above or has formed a negative association, the process must be slower, with more intermediary steps from start to finish, and with the introduction of high value rewards.

We will use a process of desensitization and counterconditioning (see Chapter 5 for

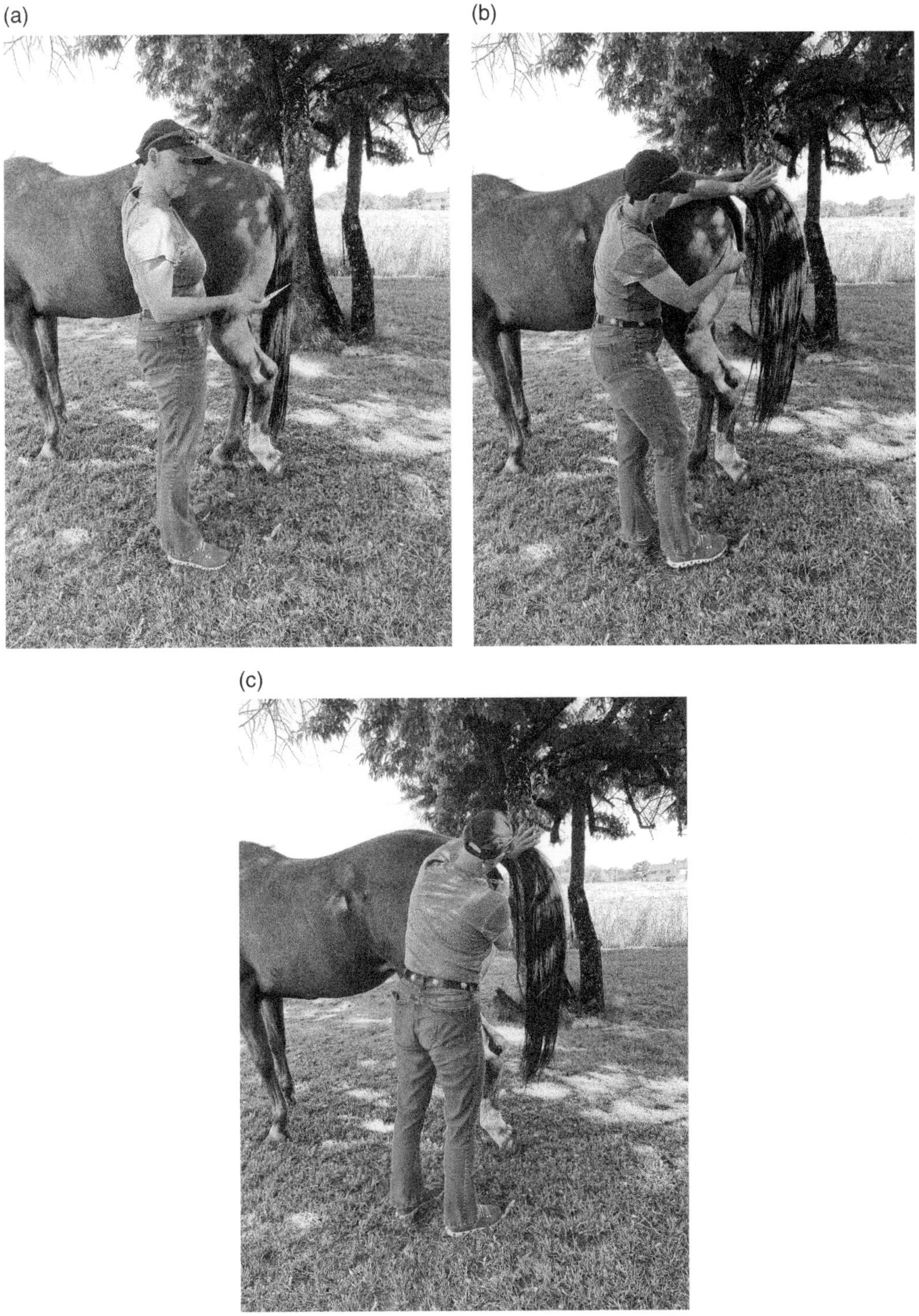

Figure 10.13 Taking the temperature of a horse: the handler stands against the side of the rear leg, keeping in contact while gently scratching the base of the tail (a). Next, the handler gently slides the hand closest to the horse down the proximal aspect of the tail to lift it (b). Finally, the handler inserts the thermometer with the opposite hand to get a temperature reading (c). *Source:* Jeannine Berger.

definitions) in the example of working with a needle-shy horse:

Step 1. Teach the horse to stand still using positive reinforcement and treats.
Step 2. Teach the horse to stand still when a person with a needle and a syringe approaches. If the horse remains still, give it a treat and step back.
Step 3. Follow the same process to teach the horse to stand still when handler stands beside its neck holding the needle and syringe.
Step 4. Teach the horse to remain still when the handler touches the horse's neck.
Step 5. Have a jackpot ready for when the horse is all the way desensitized to the step where we can insert the needle through the skin. This can be a bucket with grain, a whole apple or carrot to bite, or a larger hard treat.

It is important to stop every time the horse stands still while we are going stepwise through the process until we can insert the needle. Repeat steps 1–4 in between injections to keep the positive emotional response fresh.

Medications to Aide in Handling

Increasing compliance in handling with help of **psychotropic medication** is not a new concept in the horse industry. Medications given in various forms can make horses easier to handle or even to ride. A variety of medications can be used for that purpose. In this section, we want to explore why and how to use such medications to possibly keep the handler safe, to improve the welfare of horses, especially when we are performing brief and possibly mildly aversive procedures, or to deal with a horse with severe fears or anxiety about certain procedures. We will discuss some key diagnostic principles and examine realistic expectations for treatment with psychotropic medications in horses.

A word of caution: a sedated horse is less reactive to stimuli and may be less responsive to cues. Riding a sedated horse can be dangerous. Because this chapter focuses on veterinary handling, we will not address medicating horses for riding.

The term psychopharmacology stems from three Greek words: *psyche* meaning soul or mind; *pharmacon* meaning drug; and *logos* meaning study. The use of psychotropic medications in horses remains somewhat controversial due to the lack of understanding of and need for more research in equine psychopharmacology. Nonetheless, some drugs have been prescribed by veterinarians and explored by riders, owners, and trainers to calm horses. Most of these medications are prohibited for competition and racing in order to promote the welfare of sport horses and in fairness to other competitors. Many can and will be detected with sophisticated testing practices that are continuously being developed.

Psychotropic medications produce changes in behavior and/or motivation. They may prove useful in some behavioral cases for short-term restraint and in conjunction with a behavior modification plan. Rarely does the use of a short-term medication alone provide the necessary long-term change in emotional or motivational state. Drug selection requires an accurate assessment of the situation and the individual horse, as well as comprehensive understanding of the available and effective drugs that are safe to use to facilitate the behavioral treatment plan.

Restraining a horse for a procedure is, in most cases, a brief and temporary event, and many horses do not require medical intervention, especially if proper (calm) handling techniques and positive learning theory are applied. However, in some cases, horses are either fearful of handling or have already had negative experiences. Their fear and anxiety may be elevated to a level where they enter a yellow or even red emotional state very quickly. If such stressful events cannot be avoided or delayed and safely managed with behavior modification, using medications to alleviate fear and distress may be warranted. A fast onset, short-acting medication can be helpful if used before the event to make the event less stressful and safer for the horse and the handler. This will allow for best practices and the most effective care while avoiding aggravation of the situation in the future. Ignoring horses' fear, anxiety, and stress may decrease their welfare significantly and may lead to development of medical and behavioral problems and reduced tractability.

Assessing welfare on an individual basis and addressing the animal's emotional needs are of utmost importance in guiding treatment decisions. Body language and interactions during and away from such a stressful event need to be observed in order to decide if, when, and what kind of medications should be used. Watch for indicators such as changes in the body language, reduced ease of handling, and refusal to follow cues.

Some medications are labeled for horses, whereas others are human-grade and, when prescribed for horses, are considered "off label" use. The effects and side-effects of human-grade medications on horses are still poorly understood. Hence, the prescriber of such medications must understand the functions relative to the neurotransmitters associated with their use as well as the neurophysiology, including the mechanisms within the cell (electrical) and at the nerve ending (chemical) that can be affected. With this knowledge, side effects can be better understood or anticipated.

Examples of Drugs used in Horses and Their Effect on Neurotransmission

There are several drugs that affect glutamate and gamma-aminobutyric-acid (GABA). These amino acids can be classified as excitatory or inhibitory based on the responses evoked and are generally fast-acting. GABA is synthesized from glutamate and is the major inhibitory neurotransmitter. These chemicals have important functions in the central nervous system. The drugs are generally in the class of the benzodiazepines and can be used in a newborn foal for restraint or the treatment of acute convulsions caused by neonatal maladjustment syndrome. In adult horses, diazepam is commonly used as part of a preoperative sedative protocol, to treat seizures or idiopathic epilepsy and is prescribed in some breeding stallions due to its beneficial effect on reducing sexual inhibition.

There are also medications which work on the various monoamines (dopamine, norepinephrine, serotonin, epinephrine, melatonin, and/or histamine). In the mammalian brain, serotonergic neurons are located in the limbic system, hence its involvement in anxiety-related disorders. These medications are generally in the class of the selective serotonin reuptake inhibitors (SSRIs) or tricyclic antidepressants (TCAs) and, while sometimes used in horses, have a slower onset, usually taking effect over several weeks. They could prove useful with a long-term behavior modification approach, where a behavioral treatment plan is designed to alleviate certain fears, anxiety, or phobias. However, these medications would most likely not be useful when immediate relief is needed during handling or restraint.

Beta-blocking drugs such as propranolol seem to be useful in treating human fears, especially those associated with situational anxieties. However, to date, they have not been proven useful to treat situational anxiety in horses. More unwanted side effects are reported than positive effects (Cenani et al. 2017).

Phenothiazine derivatives, such as acepromazine, have historically been used to achieve tranquilization in horses. This medication works by reducing the initiation of motor activity in the brain's basal ganglia, slowing down movement. It produces very reliable sedation without ataxia, with predictable dose-dependent effects. For separating a mare from a foal that needs surgery, acepromazine is excellent, and the mare can continue eating – a benefit not available with other drugs. It is also useful for trailering anxious horses (S. Spier, personal communication). However, due to the sedative effect and possible lack of learning in that state, this drug is not very effective for behavioral therapy. WARNING: Acepromazine may cause priapism in horses that can last for hours. Acepromazine should always be used with caution, especially in stallions, as it can cause permanent paralysis of the penis retractor muscle. The phenothiazine derivative, fluphenazine, has also been used in horses, but its popularity has decreased due to causing significant unwanted side effects and being a prohibited drug before and during competition.

Gabapentin has been used for neuropathic pain (Davis et al. 2007), and its anti-anxiety properties have recently been discovered. Many published studies report the positive effect on dogs and cats (see Chapter 21). Few studies exist, though, on the use of gabapentin to treat anxiety disorders in horses. Researchers looking at pharmacodynamic effects of gabapentin in horses found that the oral bioavailability of gabapentin (2.5–10 mg/kg PO q12h) was relatively low, did not produce noticeable effects in the sedation score, and did not affect cardiovascular parameters significantly (Terry et al. 2010). Gabapentin has been used alone or in combination with other anti-anxiety medications, and benefits have been demonstrated for use with behavior modification therapy. It has a molecular structure similar to that of the neurotransmitter GABA but does not act like a GABA mimetic. Until very recently, there was no evidence for the ability of gabapentin to influence the functioning of either GABA receptors or GABA re-uptake mechanisms. It acts by mediating voltage-dependent calcium ion influx by inhibiting certain calcium channels in the cell (Dirikolu et al. 2008). NOTE: Gabapentin has been placed on the controlled substance list in some states.

Trazodone is a triazolopyridine derivative that inhibits the reuptake of serotonin (5-HT) and blocks the histamine and alpha-1-adrenergic receptors. The full spectrum of trazodone's mechanism of action is not fully understood and would be considered off-label use in horses. Trazodone is in the category of SARI (5-HT antagonist and reuptake inhibitors) drugs with other members being phenylpiperazine, etoperidone, lorpiprazole, and mepiprazole. Recently, the pharmacokinetics of oral trazodone has been evaluated in horses (Knych et al. 2017). Trazodone has been shown to be rapidly absorbed after oral administration, with a fairly short half-life of approximately seven hours. Studies show, the effect of oral trazodone in modifying behavioral responses was dose-dependent, emphasizing the need to adjust the dose based on the horse's response (Davis et al. 2018). Interestingly, this same study showed that some horses developed a tolerance and subsequent lack of drug effect following 14 or 21 days of use (Davis et al. 2018). Adverse effects attributed to trazodone are dose-dependent and include oversedation, muscle fasciculations, ataxia, sweating, and transient arrhythmias lasting up to 12 hours (Davis et al. 2018, Moss et al. 2021).

Detomidine hydrochloride is an alpha-2 agonist that produces calming, sedation, muscle relaxation, ataxia, and analgesia and can be administered transmucosally, intravenously, or intramuscularly (Dai et al. 2020). The FDA-approved oromucosal gel Dormosedan® is a sedative that can be safely administered by horse owners with a dosing syringe, and its absorption is achieved through the mucous membranes. Clients should wear gloves to prevent self-absorption. Oral (sublingual) administration of detomidine (0.06 mg/kg body weight) has been shown to produce profound sedation 45 minutes after administration (Gardner et al. 2010). Sublingual doses of detomidine gel (0.03 mg/kg body weight)have been shown to reduce fear and anxiety associated with loud noises in horses.

Medications can be very helpful to make horses safer, change their behavior, and/or aid in behavior modification. Veterinarians should consider if there is a medication that can help ease the stress of the horse and make any situation as safe as possible. That said, medicating horses should not be used to make up the gap in your handling skills. Those of us in this field must learn and hone our ability to read and respond to the emotional states of horses, utilize handling tools early, often, and appropriately, and know when to stop and make a plan, rather than pushing forward just to meet client demands. Mastering these skills and knowing how medication can augment the tools you have to offer will help you perform your job safely and humanely.

References

Cenani, A., Brosnan, R.J., Madigan, S. et al. (2017). Pharmacokinetics and pharmacodynamics of intravenous romifidine and propranolol administered alone or in combination for equine sedation. *Vet. Anaesth. Analg.* *44* (1): 86–97.

Dai, F., Rausk, J., Aspegren, J. et al. (2020). Use of detomidine oromucosal gel for alleviation of acute anxiety and fear in horses: a pilot study. *Front. Vet. Sci.* *7*: 573309.

Davis, J.L., Posner, L.P., and Elce, Y. (2007). Gabapentin for the treatment of neuropathic pain in a pregnant horse. *J. Am. Vet. Med. Assoc.* *231* (5): 755–758.

Davis, J.L., Schirmer, J., and Medlin, E. (2018). Pharmacokinetics, pharmacodynamics and clinical use of trazodone and its active metabolite *m*-chlorophenylpiperazine in the horse. *J. Vet. Pharmacol. Ther.* *41* (3): 393–401.

Dirikolu, L., Dafalla, A., Ely, K.J. et al. (2008). Pharmacokinetics of gabapentin in horses. *J. Vet. Pharmacol. Ther.* *31* (2): 175–177.

Gardner, R.B., White, G.W., Ramsey, D.S. et al. (2010). Efficacy of sublingual administration of detomidine gel for sedation of horses undergoing veterinary and husbandry procedures under field conditions. *J. Am. Vet. Med. Assoc.* *237* (12): 1459–1464.

Knych, H.K. et al. (2017). Pharmacokinetics and selected pharmacodynamics of trazodone following intravenous and oral administration to horses undergoing fitness training. *Am. J. Vet. Res.* **78** (10): 1182–1192.

McDonnell, S. (2003). *The Equid Ethogram: A Practical Field Guide to Horse Behavior*. Lexington, KY: Eclipse.

McGreevy, P., Christensen, J.W., von Borstel, U.K., and McLean, A. (2018). *Equitation Science*. West Sussex, England: Wiley.

Moss, A.L., Hritz, R.L., Hector, R.C., and Wotman, K.L. (2021). Investigation of the effects of orally administered trazodone on intraocular pressure, pupil diameter, physical examination variables, and sedation level in healthy equids. *Am. J. Vet. Res.* **82** (2): 138–143.

Terry, R. et al. (2010). Pharmacokinetic profile and behavioral effects of gabapentin in the horse. *J. Vet. Pharmacol. Ther.* **33** (5): 485–494.

11

Canine and Feline Communication, Restraint, and Handling

Meghan E. Herron[1], Allison Shull[2], Traci Shreyer[3], and Susan Barrett[4]

[1] *Gigi's, Canal Winchester, OH, USA*
[2] *ASPCA Cruelty and Recovery Center, Columbus, OH, USA*
[3] *Purdue University, The Croney Research Group, West Lafayette, IN, USA*
[4] *Small Animal Clinical Private Practice, VCA Morris Animal Hospital, Lancaster, OH, USA*

Foreword by Candace Croney, PhD

The quality of handling animals receive can profoundly influence both their sense of safety when interacting with people and their perceptions of the environments in which such interactions occur. The emotional states animals consequently experience influence their physiological and behavioral responses, and ultimately, their welfare. The importance, therefore, of ensuring that animals are handled gently, consistently, and efficiently cannot be understated. Consistently delivering Low Stress Handling® (https://cattledogpublishing.com/lsh/), however, can be challenging. This can be particularly troublesome in clinical settings, where animals may be ill, injured, or distressed due to transport, separation from familiar people and conspecifics, and handling in unfamiliar environments by personnel whose time constraints may create pressure to work too rapidly for the animal's comfort. Unsurprisingly, many animals respond to these sorts of stressors with fear expressed through behaviors that can frustrate even the most experienced handlers. When handlers lose patience and behave in ways that elicit even greater fear responses in animals, they may trigger a feedback cycle, elegantly outlined by Grahame Coleman and Paul Hemsworth (2010) that potentially worsens the quality of each subsequent handling interaction. Thus, clinicians (and students) may come to dread seeing the "difficult dog," the "evil cat" or the "stubborn donkey" and these characterizations in and of themselves may set the stage for interactions and handling that are aversive to both parties.

How might things be different if handlers instead more accurately viewed these same animals as confused, afraid, or painful, and were prepared with a well-conceived plan to reduce or avoid these negative affective states? Having observed and directly experienced the effects of suboptimal handling, including with livestock and my own "fractious" cat, it became clear to me that teaching of Low Stress Handling® techniques might be enhanced by providing students opportunities to better connect animals' emotional states with their behavioral responses to handling, while simultaneously illustrating how managing the environment and our own emotional responses might facilitate more desirable outcomes. In other words, students (and all those who handle animals) might benefit from practicing empathetic handling, as well as pre-handling environmental troubleshooting and self-assessment to help reduce

Introduction to Animal Behavior and Veterinary Behavioral Medicine, First Edition. Edited by Meghan E. Herron.

Companion website: www.wiley.com/go/introductiontoanimalbehavior

arousal and distress in animals as well as themselves. Even better, students could develop proactive thought processes and strategies to create positive handling experiences and welfare outcomes. This approach laid the groundwork for the inaugural teaching of Low Stress Handling® of companion and livestock animals to first-year veterinary students at The Ohio State University's College of Veterinary Medicine. Each interaction during handling laboratories began with an environmental and handler evaluation, and a collaboratively developed handling plan that was patient-centric and, in anticipation of potential problems, was designed to be revised as needed. These and other foundational scientific concepts form the basis for the following chapter on Low Stress Handling®.

Introduction

Low Stress Handling®, created by Dr. Sophia Yin, may be a new concept for many practitioners, yet the basic principles follow the oath taken by every veterinarian upon graduation as part of the "prevention and relief of animal suffering" (American Veterinary Medical Association 2022). The commitment to ensuring the emotional wellbeing of the patient should equal that shown to the physical wellbeing of the animals under a veterinarian's care. Furthermore, as dog and cat bites are a substantial cause of injury in a veterinary practice setting (Drobatz and Smith 2003; August 1988; Volk et al. 2014; Jeyaretnam et al., 2000), handling animals in a safe and effective manner is essential in reducing the costs associated with personnel injury. Many of us groan when we see a "difficult" dog or cat on our schedule; "this is going to be a stressful appointment." If this is how you feel, imagine how the animal, as well as the client and your staff, are feeling. Client polls suggest the perceived fear and distress an animal feels because of a veterinary visit is a top reason why people avoid bringing their pet to see the veterinarian (Kry and Casey 2007, Volk et al. 2014). Would not it be great if we all could feel differently – better? This chapter will help you change such problematic visits into the positive encounters they can be, as well as prevent them from developing in the first place. Benefits of Low Stress Handling® include the enhancement of patient welfare, increase in job satisfaction, the bonding of clients to the practice, enhancement of staff, patient, and client safety, and reduction of time and resources spent on subsequent visits (Yin 2009). You will also have more valid physical data on your patient (e.g. temperature, heart rate, blood pressure, and respiratory rate), and a more complete physical exam.

Keep in mind that Low Stress Handling® may be a new concept for your clients. Previous veterinary care for their pets may have included a "get it done" mentality in which each dog was held down for nail trims and each cat was scruffed and stretched with one-size-fits-all techniques. Frequently, this restraint was done "in the back," preventing the client from seeing how the visit actually transpired. We have all heard a technician, covered in fur and scratches; announce in a chipper tone, "She did great!" as the disheveled cat is presented back to the client. For years, we have been keeping this secret from the clients and bearing the burden that so many pets are fearful and/or fear-aggressive in the clinic setting. It is time to enlist our clients to help their pets cope with veterinary care, and help the veterinary team enjoy better work satisfaction and safety. Although not every situation or procedure is appropriate to conduct in a tiny examination room with the client present, sharing honest feedback with them is essential in gaining buy-in and making the next visit better.

During her tenure at The Ohio State University Veterinary Medical Center, applied animal behaviorist and animal welfare expert, Dr. Candace Croney, designed an assessment and plan system for clinicians, students, and staff based on Dr. Sophia Yin's ten principles of handling, to utilize before ever placing hands on a patient (Yin 2009). The four main parts include:

1) Assess the environment
2) Assess the patient's comfort level and indicators of intent
3) Assess yourself
4) Make a handling plan

Based on the information you gather in the first three assessments, you can create a successful handling plan and proceed in a safe and effective manner. Remember that no single visit will go exactly as planned; your goal as a practitioner should be to make the visit in front of you go as well as it can, document the visit, and modify the plan to help the patient's next visit go even better. This is the *practice* of veterinary medicine, not the *perfection* of it! By moving the needle incrementally toward lower stress, your entire practice should gradually become easier for your patients, clients, and team.

Step 1: Assess the Environment

The goal here is to set up an exam site that is comfortable for the patient (Yin 2009). When performing this assessment, one must consider how the patient perceives and interprets everything around them. What an animal sees, smells, feels, tastes, and hears can have dramatic effects on its well-being and emotional state (Morgan and Tromborg 2007). Furthermore, multiple noxious stimuli can lower the threshold for fear and aggression, making it essential to minimize the pet's exposure to them at each step. Animals with previous frightening or painful veterinary visits may be classically conditioned to associate any or all the surrounding stimuli with a negative emotional response (fear) (Mazur 2016; Yin 2009). Part of the setup of the environment requires that you identify and remove patients' known triggers for fear and aggression. The authors use behavioral wellness screening surveys (see Chapter 12) to facilitate this, especially for new patients.

Maximize Visual Comfort

Bright and/or constant light can be stressful for animals (Morgan and Tromborg 2007; Veranič and Jezernik 2001; Pollard and Littlejohn 1994). The presence of the tapetum lucidum allows certain species to perceive light in higher abundance than humans, making what people consider soft lighting seem brighter and aversive (Gunter 1995; Miller and Murphy 1995). Consider 60-watt bulbs in exam rooms and treatment areas to provide softer lighting. Mimic natural light cycles for hospitalized patients, and avoid fluorescent lights as they flicker at a rate that can be detected by animals but not humans. Keep quick and sudden movements to a minimum, as animals may startle or suddenly feel threatened. If animals are not tolerating subtle movement, it may help to restrict their visual intake using towels or other visual blocking aids, such as a ThunderCap (Thunderworks, Duram). You can use towels to cover a cat's head during all parts of the exam and procedures that do not involve the head (Yin 2009). Provide additional comfort by covering cats' carriers in the clinic with a towel until you are ready to work with them (Yin 2009). If housing cats in a cage, provide a hiding option, such as a box or a partially covered cage front, so that they can remove themselves from visual stimuli and have the perception of being concealed (Carlstead et al. 1993; Yin 2009; Kry and Casey 2007). The sight of dogs or other cats in the hospital is highly likely to be stressful (Yin 2009).

Admit fearful or fear-aggressive dogs and cats through a side or back entrance to reduce visual contact with other animals and strangers (Yin 2009). This is helpful from a welfare standpoint, both for the patient you are admitting and for the patients waiting in the lobby or treatment areas. If your clinic has several corners and blind spots (as most do), it may help to enlist the help of a "scout" who can walk ahead and ensure a clear path as you walk a reactive patient to the desired, quiet location. Keep the patient walking or held directly at your side, keeping yourself between the patient and the center of the hallway where triggering people or animals may suddenly appear (Figure 11.1a,b). If your patient is walked or held out ahead of you, the trigger may reach them before it reaches you, and you will have little ability to control the situation or intervene (Figure 11.1c,d) (Yin 2009).

Finally, consider ditching the white coat. The bright, light-reflective material can be

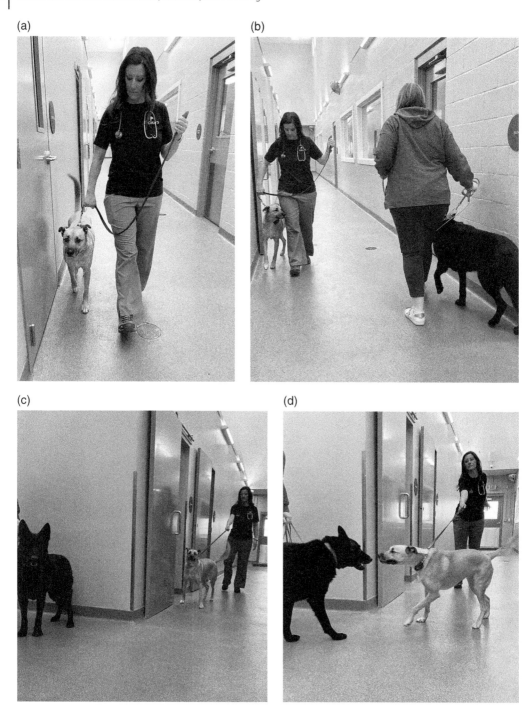

Figure 11.1 When walking any patient, but especially a reactive dog, you will have better control over preventing an altercation when passing people or other patients if you keep them at your side and away from the center of the hallway. Keeping your body between your patient and anyone passing allows you to keep a buffer and distance between your patient and potential triggers (a) (b). Allowing the patient to walk out ahead or in the center of the hallway allows too much potential for exposure/interaction with triggers, and by the time it happens, it may be too late to intervene (c) (d). *Source:* With permission from Aditi Czarnomski.

jarring to some patients. Furthermore, animals may make visual associations with stimuli in the veterinary clinic, including the attire of the veterinary clinicians and staff, with a frightening experience (aka the "white coat effect") (Belew et al. 1999). These animals may respond better without exposure to this fear-eliciting stimulus (Crowell-Davis 2007).

Maximize Auditory Comfort

Speak softly and sparingly around animals to help them stay calm. As animals begin to exhibit symptoms correlated with elevated stress when ambient sounds approach 85dB (Anthony et al. 1959) – keeping noise levels at or below 60dB is preferable. Along these same lines, avoid reprimands or using harsh or punitive tones of voice, regardless of the animal's behavior, as this is likely to increase stress and may exacerbate aggression (Herron et al. 2009). Take care when opening and closing metal hospital cages and kennels to minimize the loud, often resonating clang of metal hitting metal.

Studies demonstrate that music has various effects on the emotional states of animals. For example, classical music and reggae have been shown to increase behaviors associated with relaxation in animals (Kogan et al. 2012; Bowman et al. 2017), while "hard rock" and "heavy metal" music have been shown to cause behaviors associated with stress (Kogan et al. 2012). Your clinic can play classical music playlists or commercial recordings that might be calming, such as Through a Dog's Ear (Sounds True, Inc., Louisville, CO, USA), on overhead sound systems during the day. Staff members who prefer hard rock should use personal sound devices and wear headphones so as not to expose the animals to this style of auditory stimulation. To further mask sudden noises that may be startling and potentially stressful, such as barking dogs and people talking or moving in the adjacent hallway or room, sources of noise cancellation, such as white noise, can be utilized in addition to music (Yin 2009).

Maximize Olfactory Comfort

Olfactory processing in the brain has a direct and widespread influence on the parts of the forebrain that affect odor discrimination, emotion, and memory, making the degree of negative emotional association potentially more powerful than for other sensory stimuli (Bear et al. 2015). Allow time for the chemical smell of cleaning agents to dissipate after disinfecting an exam room between patients. This is also important for cage cleaning, as placing an animal in a cage that has not fully dried after cleaning will expose them to harsh chemical scents. When selecting disinfectant agents, consider those that do not contain bleach or ammonia, such as accelerated hydrogen peroxide products (Rescue® [Virox Technologies, Inc., Oakville, ON, USA]). Try to use alcohol sparingly, if at all, during procedures, as the strong scent is potentially aversive to animals. If an animal has had a previous frightening experience associated with the smell of alcohol, it may have a conditioned negative emotional response when exposed to this smell at subsequent visits (Mazur 2016; Yin 2009).

Wipe down exposed surfaces, such as the floors, walls, and cabinets, after stressed animals, as they have likely deposited scents and pheromones associated with fear and alarm which may indicate the environment is dangerous (Bekoff 1979; Stoddart 1980). For this reason, avoid leaving stressed animals in common areas, such as the lobby or waiting area, for prolonged periods (Yin 2009). Be sure not to share towels between animals, as the scents and pheromones associated with fear and alarm will transfer between patients. Minimize exposing cats to canine odors by having designated cat-only exam and waiting rooms (Figure 11.2a,b) and/or wiping down and airing out rooms between canine and feline patient, as the smell of a potential predator may induce a stress response (Takahashi et al. 2005; Yin 2009). Be aware that these scents can transfer to and linger on clothing and other handling tools, such as "cat gloves" and

(a)

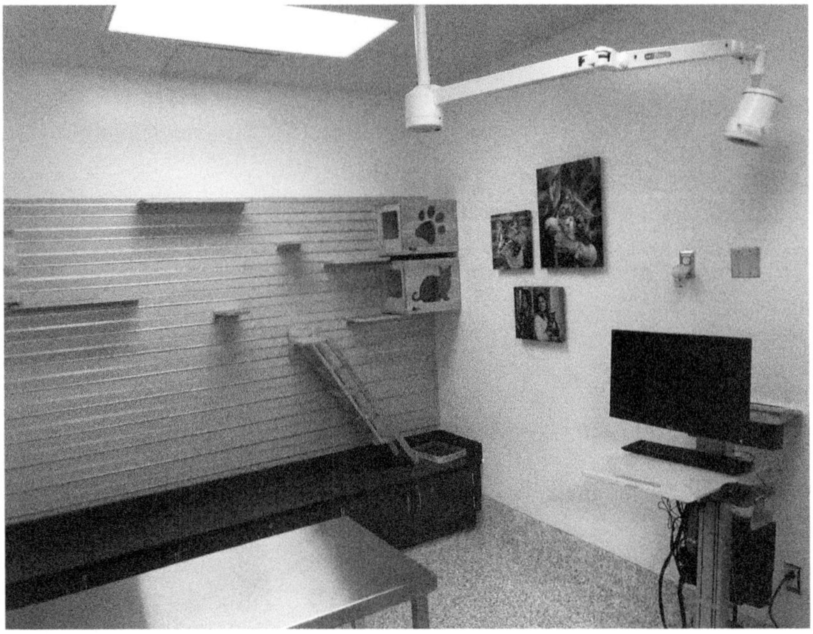

(b)

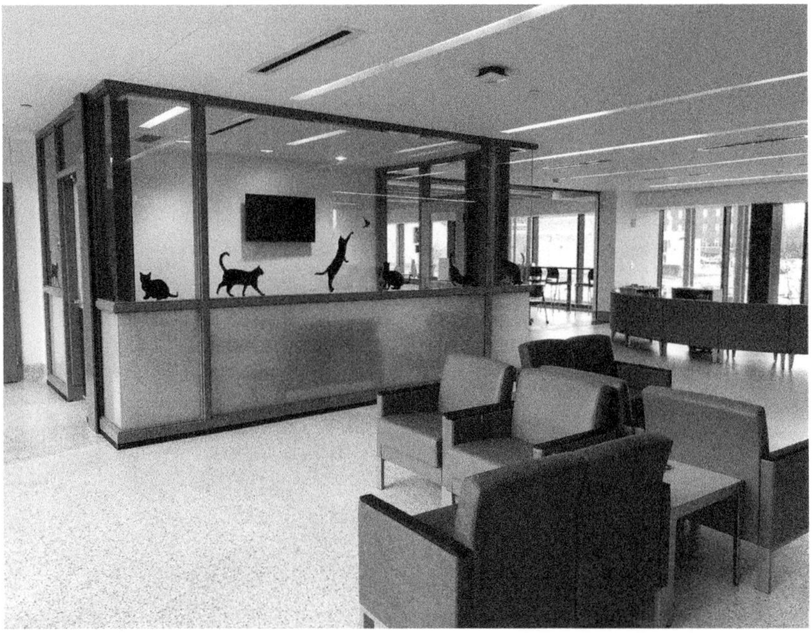

Figure 11.2 Designating exam rooms (a) and waiting areas (b) for cats prevents the stress-elevating scents of dogs and allows you to cater the room set up and design in a more feline-friendly manner. *Source:* The Ohio State University Veterinary Medical Center lobby and exam room, Meghan E. Herron.

muzzles. Hospitalized cats should be housed separately from dogs and their scent, as recent biomedical studies have demonstrated that exposure to predators or predator cues (such as scents) can induce "sustained psychological stress" that is directly comparable to chronic stress from PTSD in humans (Clinchy et al. 2013).

Utilize calming pheromones (discussed in Chapter 4) [FELIWAY; ThunderEase with ADAPTIL (Ceva Animal Health, Lenexa, KS, USA)] in exam rooms (Figure 11.3) and treatment wards, on towels, tables, bandanas, and your own clothing, to provide a signal of safety for the animal and to reduce stress (Yin 2009). Synthetic pheromone products have been shown to reduce signs associated with fear and anxiety in the veterinary setting (Mills et al. 2006; Siracusa et al. 2010). Animals are sensitive to the pheromones of animals within their same species only and, as such, will not respond to pheromone products based on other species. This makes it possible to utilize both canine and feline pheromone products in the same vicinity. Please note that pheromone spray should be applied a few minutes prior to the animal interacting with the fabric; the initial spray is overwhelming for the noses of humans and animals alike!

Utilize calming scents, such as lavender and chamomile, when handling and housing animals, as they have been shown to increase behaviors associated with relaxation (Wells 2006). Essential oils can be dabbed on bedding, and handlers can use mildly scented lotions on their hands prior to handling.

Maximize Tactile Comfort

Avoid placing animals on cold, slippery surfaces. Cover metal exam tables and scales with towels, no-slip mats, or soft foam covering, such as the Ezee-Visit Pet Vet Mat (Ezee-Visit Pet Vet Mat, Limington, ME, USA; Figure 11.4), to provide a warmer, more comfortable tactile experience (Yin 2009). Use a padded mat if you must place animals into recumbency on the floor. In cages and kennels, you can place soft bedding to promote rest, to provide warmth, and to prevent cats from resting in their litter box (Crouse et al. 1995). Cats appear to prefer polyester fleece bedding, over towels and other mat types, which are easily washable between patients (Hawthorne et al. 1995).

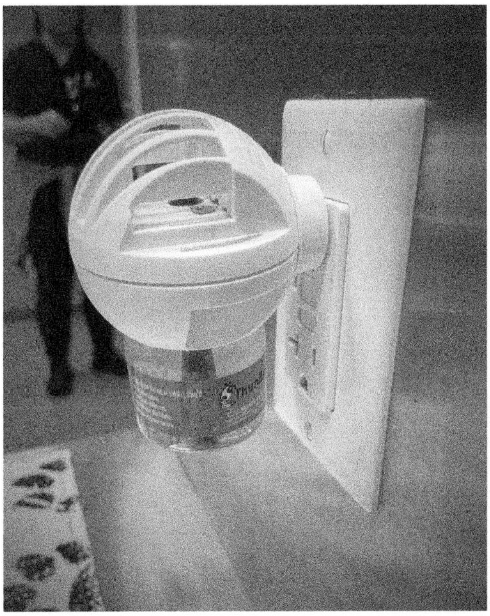

Figure 11.3 A ThunderEase, powered by ADAPTIL (Ceva Animal Health, Lenexa, KS, USA), diffuser containing appeasing pheromones sits in an exam room outlet in order to provide comfort throughout the exam experience. *Source:* Meghan E. Herron.

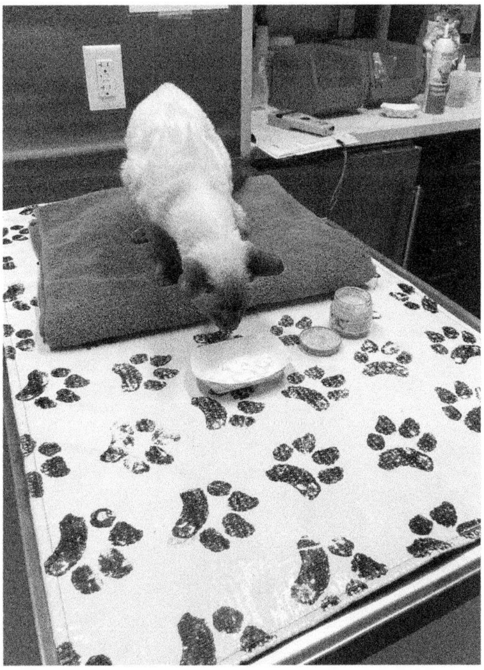

Figure 11.4 The Ezee-Visit Pet Vet Mat® provides a non-slip surface that can be readily disinfected and is available in exam table and scale sizes. *Source:* Meghan E. Herron.

When handling animals, avoid overstimulating touch. While some pets enjoy petting, others may find it frightening or uncomfortable. For pets that solicit or appear comfortable with petting, pet with a light touch and in the direction of hair growth. Limit petting of cats to the head and neck, as long strokes down the back and abdomen may increase arousal and aggression. Whenever possible, utilize the Fear Free's **Touch gradient** (TG), a concept first described by Dr. Sophia Yin (Yin 2009). TG aims to minimize the abrupt starting and stopping of touch with animals. This is best accomplished by keeping a gentle hand on the patient in a non-sensitive or socially invasive area for the duration of the exam and all procedures. When you are ready to examine more sensitive areas on the patient, gently slide your hands toward the area of interest so that the patient is eased into the interaction and is not suddenly started with an invasive or painful touch (Figure 11.5) (Yin 2009). When possible, food should be used for counterconditioning when examining these areas (Yin 2009). You can apply this same concept to thoracic auscultation – start with gentle placement of your stethoscope on the dorsum of the chest. Then slowly slide your stethoscope into the regions you wish to auscultate and slowly apply the needed pressure for maximum auditory access. See the online materials for video examples of TG.

Lidocaine-based topical analgesics help reduce pain associated with injections, fine needle aspirates, ear cleanings, etc. This is especially true in cats, where a contact time of 20 minutes reduces struggling during jugular catheterization – at least in sedated cats (Wagner et al. 2006). Dogs appear to require a longer skin contact time (60 minutes) to achieve similar analgesia (van Oostrom and Knowles 2018). Application of topical analgesics may be most helpful and practical if you apply them to your surgical patients at intake, rather than waiting until the time of induction.

Maximize Gustatory Comfort

Palatable food is a powerful means of mitigating stress and changing the underlying emotional state of the animal from one of fear to a state of pleasure. Offering food may help keep our patients from feeling stressed or fearful and from displaying undesirable, defensive behaviors. Utilize food for counterconditioning (see Chapter 5) when possible and safe, keeping in mind that the more palatable the food is from the animal's perspective, the greater the effect on conditioning a positive emotional response (Yin 2009). Disguise bitter-tasting medications with a coating of tasty food or an empty gelatin capsule prior to administration,

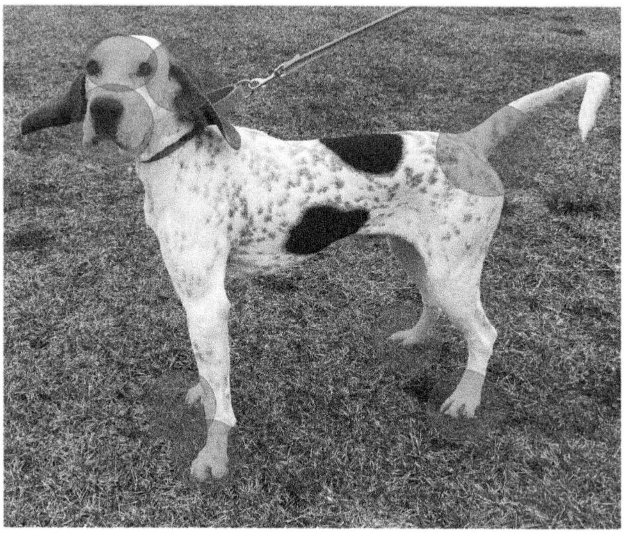

Figure 11.5 Areas of a dog's body that are more sensitive to handling and may be perceived as more socially invasive when touched include the ears, eyes, oronasal area, feet, and rectum (think "handling hot zones"). Exams are best performed using a touch gradient where the clinician starts in a more comfortable area of the body and gradually moves toward these more sensitive areas. *Source:* With permission from Alyssa Wright.

especially for cats. Long-term medications can be compounded into flavored liquids or treats that can more easily be disguised in tasty food. If direct pill administration is absolutely necessary, utilize a pill administrator or "pill gun" so that contact with the tongue is minimized.

Maximize Thermal Comfort

Cats' ability to thermoregulate is directly affected by their housing environment. This is an especially important factor for hospitalized cats, as in this small and limited environment they may be unable to express temperature regulating activities (Stella and Croney 2016). The thermoneutral zone for domestic cats is 86–98°F (NRC 2006). Yet most hospitals are maintained closer to 68–75°F (author experience). Work with your staff to find housing options that you can reasonably maintain at this warm, ideal temperature and provide opportunities for cats to behaviorally thermoregulate, such as provision of warm bedding, resting areas, and boxes, that will enable them to cope with the environment more readily (Stella and Croney 2016) (Figure 11.6).

Maximize the Comfort of Familiarity

Many animals are less anxious and tolerate veterinary handling better with a familiar person present (Stellato et al. 2020), likely because animals feel safer in proximity to familiar members of their social group. This is a concept known as **social buffering**. There are several practice management advantages to having the client watch the appointment that go beyond the comfort level of the animal: enhanced trust in the practitioner/team, value added since the client can see and hear your expertise, and more efficient care plans since you can discuss findings in real-time. On one hand, you may feel reluctant or embarrassed to have a client witness the patient coping poorly with the veterinary visit; however, the authors have found it advantageous in several ways. First, when the client witnesses the use of appropriate handling, you can avoid the accusation that your handling created the fear. Second, many clients have handling ideas ("maybe if you tried singing to him. . .") of varying effectiveness. In the best case, the handling ideas may help the animal; more often, trying them in real-time avoids the extra time spent explaining what did not work in the treatment room, only to try what the client suggests to no avail. Finally, there is simply no substitute for the client seeing their pet's distress to help create buy-in for pre-visit medications, muzzles, restraint, or injectable sedation. More than once, the authors have been told by a client that they would not have believed their pet was so fearful or

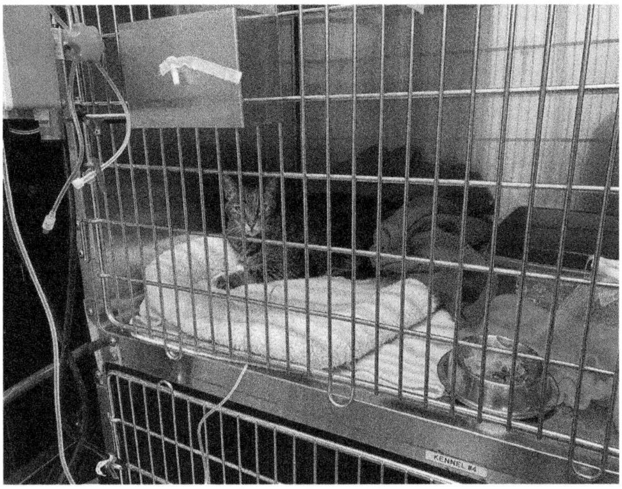

Figure 11.6 The provision of cat bedding that traps warmth in hospital housing areas will help cats maintain a thermoneutral body temperature. *Source:* Jeannine Berger.

fear-aggressive without seeing it themselves. And remember that not every pet is fearful – having the client watch their pet glide seamlessly through a venipuncture without noticing, due to your skilled low-stress approaches, is the finest client retention tool around.

Despite the many advantages of having the client present for the visit, their presence should be mindfully manipulated. A fearful, agitated, or punishing family member may escalate the animal's fear and aggression – a result of **social referencing** (Merola et al. 2012, 2015). Also, some clients become queasy at the sight of needles or blood and may need to leave the room during certain interactions. It is also worth noting that some animals show less aggression away from their familiar caretakers. Keep in mind pets that show less aggression when separated from their people are not necessarily less fearful or less stressed. Often without social group facilitation, stressed animals cope by retreating or freezing, even though they are still feeling threatened. While an animal that freezes may be easy to handle at this particular visit, if the animal learns that freezing does not end the negative interaction, it may be less apt to freeze at subsequent visits, or even handling bouts within the same visit, and may become increasingly difficult to handle. Avoid taking advantage of animals in this emotional state and mitigate stress as you would for animals with more active coping mechanisms, as their well-being is just as threatened.

In addition to client presence, the location of your examination and/or procedures also makes a difference. Griffin, Mandese, and colleagues in two separate studies (2021) found that stress signals were higher for dogs and cats examined in an open treatment area without their owners compared to those who were examined in an isolated exam room with their owner present. This study showed clinically significant, consistent, and directionally symmetrical increases when dogs and cats were examined in the common treatment area (Griffin et al. 2021; Mandese et al. 2021). When physical exam locations are highly stimulating/stressful, pets may experience increased stress and anxiety, with detrimental effects on clinical assessments and behavioral welfare.

For hospitalized patients or patients whose household members are not available or able to be present during the exam or procedures, try to pair patients with as familiar a handler as possible. Many clients can identify clinicians, technicians, and assistants with whom their pet is familiar. Maximize that person's contact time with that specific patient whenever possible. Clearly, you will not always have the same staff present. The good news is Grigg et al. (2022) found that having a new handler spend a brief period allowing the patient to establish short-term familiarity in addition to utilizing Low Stress Handling® techniques reduced patient stress.

Step 2: Assess the Patient's Comfort Level and Indicators of Intent

Understanding how to read and interpret patient body language may be the single most important skill necessary in recognizing and reducing fear and anxiety as well as keeping handlers, patients, and clients safe (Yin 2009). Animals communicate with each other, as well as humans, through changes in body posture, eye contact, movement, and vocalization. This is vastly different from inter-human communication, and understanding the difference requires experience and skill. Human caretakers must recognize the intent of the animal and react appropriately. This means a continuous observation of patient information and adjusting to that data as aspects, such as procedure location, level of patient pain, patient position, invasiveness, or restraint, can and will change. Since multiple parties within the practice will engage with the patient throughout the visit, it becomes critical to train everyone within the practice (from the receptionist to the veterinarian) to effectively read even the slightest changes in body language. The earlier you recognize fear and anxiety, the sooner you can implement mitigation strategies, making them more likely to work and to work with the least amount of effort. Such training requires effort, but in the authors' experience, this practice-wide foundation pays dividends over time and helps with client retention. Outlined in Figure 11.7a,b are the Fear Free™, LLC Fear, Anxiety and Stress Scales. These scales are one example used to illustrate body language indicators of intent coded as green, yellow, and red and a score of 0–5, with "0" being an indication of no FAS and "5" being an indication of high or extreme levels of FAS. Familiarity with these scales helps staff record and communicate regarding patient FAS in a consistent and objective manner. Keeping body language posters for clients to read will help them better understand what their pet is trying to communicate and gain fluency in how your staff communicates regarding their pet's emotional state. These scales can also be used when considering pre-visit pharmaceuticals, chemical restraint, and pain management (see Chapters 21 and 22 for more details). Keep in mind that these scales are behavioral indicators of an animal's current emotional state in response to the surrounding stimuli, are subject to change at a moment's notice, and are not a static reflection of the animal's underlying personality or temperament.

Step 3: Assess Yourself

Your body language and how you adjust it in response to cues from your patient can have dramatic effects on an animal's stress and comfort levels (Yin 2009). What humans perceive as a friendly, benign interaction may actually be threatening from the animal's perspective. As primates, humans utilize forward and ventral approaches, direct eye contact, and outstretched hands to convey friendliness and affection. Dogs and cats, on the other hand, rarely use forward, ventral contact in their communication and tend to take on more of a lateral, indirect approach, avoiding direct eye contact, and, therefore, may feel threatened by direct, frontal approaches (Yin 2009). This is especially evident when greeting a conspecific outside of the familiar social group or when a pet is sensitive and/or fearful. For example, a dog who greets another unfamiliar dog with a direct stare, putting its face in the other dog's face, or putting its head on top of the other dog's head or neck will be perceived as threatening, causing the other dog to either retreat, freeze, or show defensive aggression. What this means is that there is a miscommunication between human displays of affection and animal perceptions of threat. Animals become frightened, and humans get hurt.

During the first few moments of the veterinary visit, briefly greet the patient using the non-threatening body language described below, then engage with the client to clarify the reason for the visit, or have a bit of small talk, before touching/handling the patient (Yin 2009). This allows the patient to acclimate to your presence as a "normal" human before you become a "veterinarian." This is also a good time to toss treats to assess the patient's emotional state (lack of eating is an indication of stress) and to start the process of **counterconditioning** (more below).

Non-threatening human body language and behavior toward dogs (Yin 2009):

- Turn your body to the side, rather than toward the dog directly.
- Avoid prolonged direct eye contact, averting your gaze when possible.
- If safe, squat by bending at the knees, rather than at the waist, keeping your torso upright, and keeping yourself turned to the side (Figure 11.8a).
- Avoid squatting down with animals whose body language indicates they may come forward in an aggressive manner, as this puts you at risk of being bitten in the face or knocked over.
- Avoid bending over or leaning forward toward the dog – as you lean in the image you project becomes larger and more threatening.
- Hold your hand at your side, patting your leg gently and holding your palm open. If the dog approaches allow the dog to sniff and investigate. If the dog shows "green" body language and comes closer, you can gently pet under the chin and neck area and slowly move into the desired examination position (Figure 11.8b).

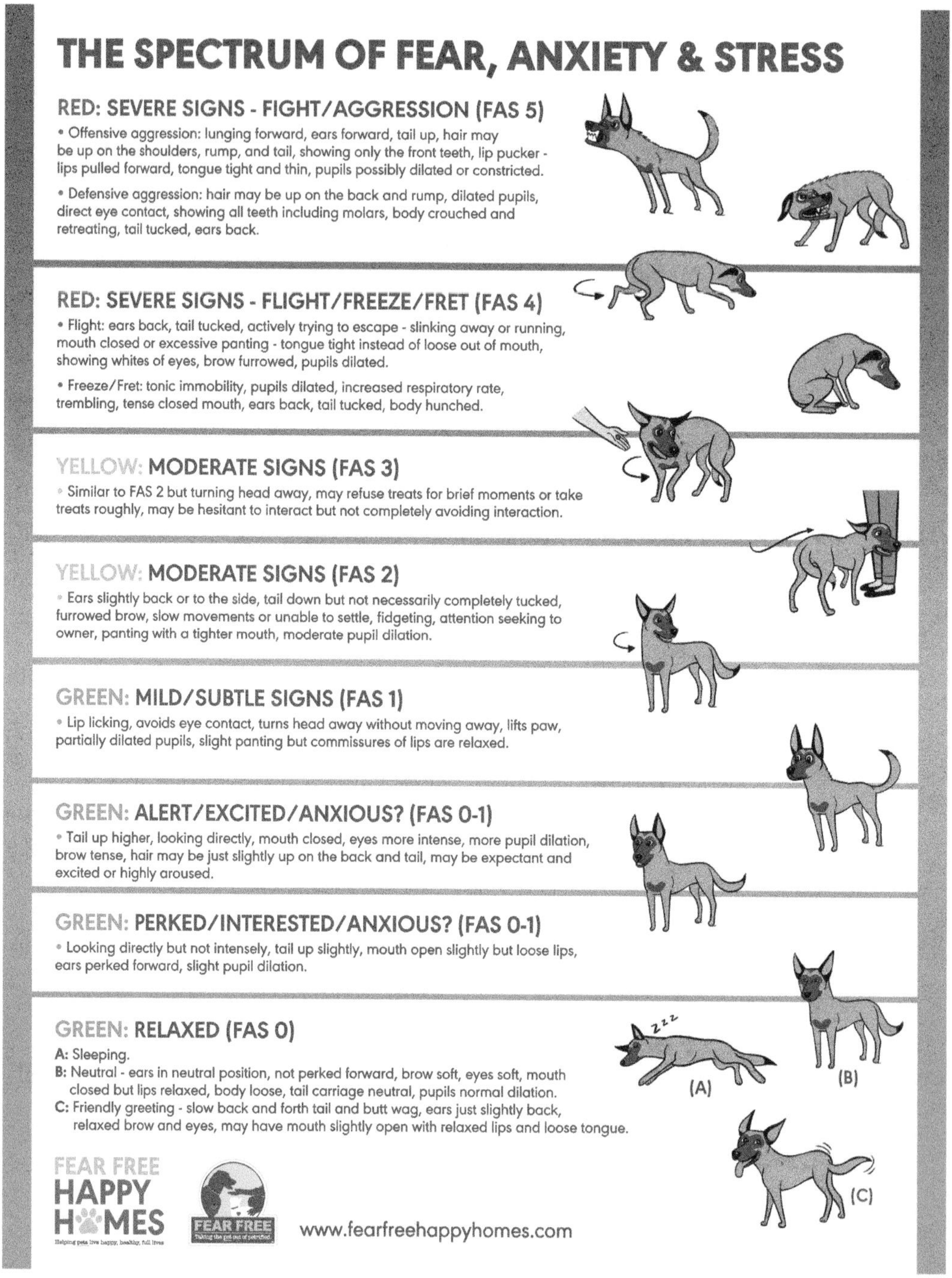
THE SPECTRUM OF FEAR, ANXIETY & STRESS
RED: SEVERE SIGNS - FIGHT/AGGRESSION (FAS 5)
• Offensive aggression: lunging forward, ears forward, tail up, hair may be up on the shoulders, rump, and tail, showing only the front teeth, lip pucker - lips pulled forward, tongue tight and thin, pupils possibly dilated or constricted.
• Defensive aggression: hair may be up on the back and rump, dilated pupils, direct eye contact, showing all teeth including molars, body crouched and retreating, tail tucked, ears back.
RED: SEVERE SIGNS - FLIGHT/FREEZE/FRET (FAS 4)
• Flight: ears back, tail tucked, actively trying to escape - slinking away or running, mouth closed or excessive panting - tongue tight instead of loose out of mouth, showing whites of eyes, brow furrowed, pupils dilated.
• Freeze/Fret: tonic immobility, pupils dilated, increased respiratory rate, trembling, tense closed mouth, ears back, tail tucked, body hunched.
YELLOW: MODERATE SIGNS (FAS 3)
• Similar to FAS 2 but turning head away, may refuse treats for brief moments or take treats roughly, may be hesitant to interact but not completely avoiding interaction.
YELLOW: MODERATE SIGNS (FAS 2)
• Ears slightly back or to the side, tail down but not necessarily completely tucked, furrowed brow, slow movements or unable to settle, fidgeting, attention seeking to owner, panting with a tighter mouth, moderate pupil dilation.
GREEN: MILD/SUBTLE SIGNS (FAS 1)
• Lip licking, avoids eye contact, turns head away without moving away, lifts paw, partially dilated pupils, slight panting but commissures of lips are relaxed.
GREEN: ALERT/EXCITED/ANXIOUS? (FAS 0-1)
• Tail up higher, looking directly, mouth closed, eyes more intense, more pupil dilation, brow tense, hair may be just slightly up on the back and tail, may be expectant and excited or highly aroused.
GREEN: PERKED/INTERESTED/ANXIOUS? (FAS 0-1)
• Looking directly but not intensely, tail up slightly, mouth open slightly but loose lips, ears perked forward, slight pupil dilation.
GREEN: RELAXED (FAS 0)
A: Sleeping.
B: Neutral - ears in neutral position, not perked forward, brow soft, eyes soft, mouth closed but lips relaxed, body loose, tail carriage neutral, pupils normal dilation.
C: Friendly greeting - slow back and forth tail and butt wag, ears just slightly back, relaxed brow and eyes, may have mouth slightly open with relaxed lips and loose tongue.
zzz
(A)
(B)
(C)
FEAR FREE
HAPPY
HOMES
FEAR FREE
www.fearfreehappyhomes.com

Figure 11.7 Fear Free™, LLC Canine (a) and Feline (b) body language and indicators of escalating fear, anxiety, and stress. Note the color coding that utilizes "green" and an indication of low FAS signs and moves into "yellow" and then "red" as FAS levels increase. *Source:* Reproduced with permission, courtesy of Fear Free™, LLC.

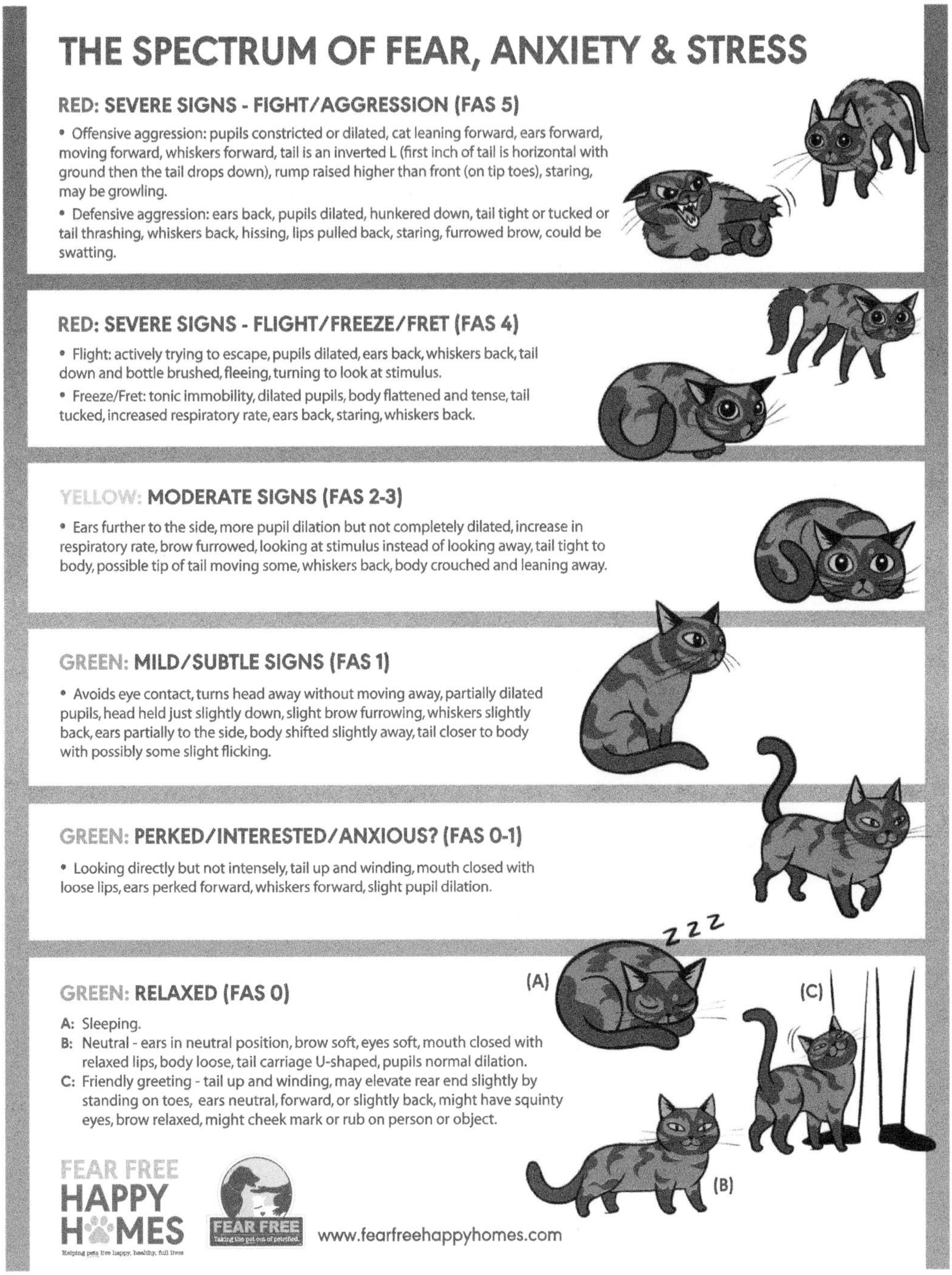
THE SPECTRUM OF FEAR, ANXIETY & STRESS
RED: SEVERE SIGNS - FIGHT/AGGRESSION (FAS 5)
• Offensive aggression: pupils constricted or dilated, cat leaning forward, ears forward, moving forward, whiskers forward, tail is an inverted L (first inch of tail is horizontal with ground then the tail drops down), rump raised higher than front (on tip toes), staring, may be growling.
• Defensive aggression: ears back, pupils dilated, hunkered down, tail tight or tucked or tail thrashing, whiskers back, hissing, lips pulled back, staring, furrowed brow, could be swatting.
RED: SEVERE SIGNS - FLIGHT/FREEZE/FRET (FAS 4)
• Flight: actively trying to escape, pupils dilated, ears back, whiskers back, tail down and bottle brushed, fleeing, turning to look at stimulus.
• Freeze/Fret: tonic immobility, dilated pupils, body flattened and tense, tail tucked, increased respiratory rate, ears back, staring, whiskers back.
YELLOW: MODERATE SIGNS (FAS 2-3)
• Ears further to the side, more pupil dilation but not completely dilated, increase in respiratory rate, brow furrowed, looking at stimulus instead of looking away, tail tight to body, possible tip of tail moving some, whiskers back, body crouched and leaning away.
GREEN: MILD/SUBTLE SIGNS (FAS 1)
• Avoids eye contact, turns head away without moving away, partially dilated pupils, head held just slightly down, slight brow furrowing, whiskers slightly back, ears partially to the side, body shifted slightly away, tail closer to body with possibly some slight flicking.
GREEN: PERKED/INTERESTED/ANXIOUS? (FAS 0-1)
• Looking directly but not intensely, tail up and winding, mouth closed with loose lips, ears perked forward, whiskers forward, slight pupil dilation.
ZZZ
GREEN: RELAXED (FAS 0)
(A)
(C)
A: Sleeping.
B: Neutral - ears in neutral position, brow soft, eyes soft, mouth closed with relaxed lips, body loose, tail carriage U-shaped, pupils normal dilation.
C: Friendly greeting - tail up and winding, may elevate rear end slightly by standing on toes, ears neutral, forward, or slightly back, might have squinty eyes, brow relaxed, might cheek mark or rub on person or object.
(B)
FEAR FREE
HAPPY
HOMES
Helping pets live happy, healthy, full lives
FEAR FREE
Taking the pet out of petrified.
www.fearfreehappyhomes.com

Figure 11.7 (Continued)

(a)

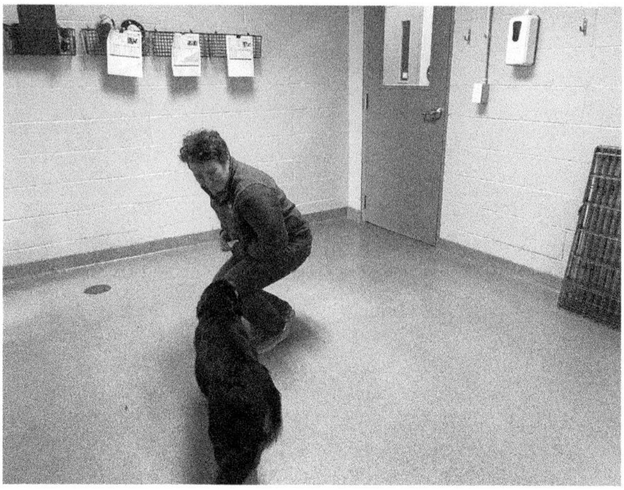

(b)

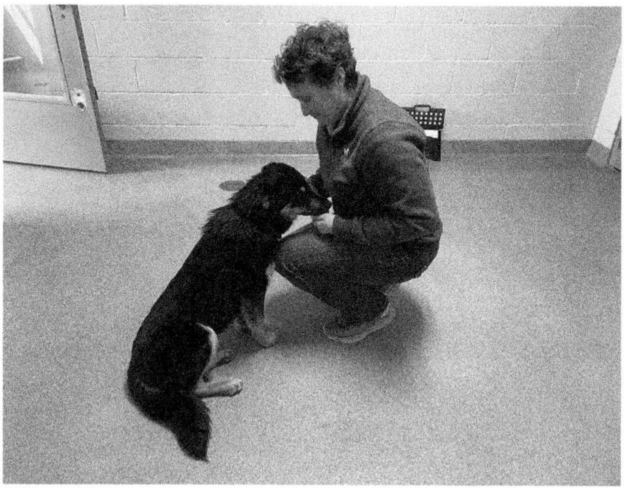

Figure 11.8 Utilizing a lateral, rather than forward approach to encourage a dog to approach you (a). Once the dog approaches, you can gently scratch under the chin to assess for comfort with touch before starting your exam (b). *Source:* Meghan E. Herron.

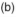

If the animal does not approach, despite your non-threatening approach, the animal may not be safe to handle, and further approach may lead to an aggressive response.

- If you need to move closer to the dog, do so from the side, rather than directly approaching the front of the dog, facing the same direction as the dog. Although many of us have been taught to examine a patient "nose-to-tail," the authors strongly suggest starting your exam at the shoulder of the animal and moving back to the head last, facing the same direction as the animal. This not only allows the patient to get accustomed to examination of a less socially invasive area of their body (refer back to Figure 11.5 for handling "hot zones") but also allows the veterinarian and handler to get a "feel" for how the patient is coping before handling the face and mouth.
- Avoid reaching out, petting on top of the dog's head, or suddenly grabbing for the collar. Make your movements more subtle and soft. Be aware that handling the feet, ears, tail, and rectum is socially invasive

from the animal's perspective and may be just as aversive as a physically painful procedure.

- Warning, if the dog does not approach you they are likely stressed, and the handler should anticipate that approaching the patient will increase the dog's stress level.
- Keep interactions as short as is practical, and attempt to perform examinations and procedures in one smooth process (e.g. examination, weight check, venipuncture, and vaccinations all at once rather than divided into three or four separate handling events).

Non-threatening body language and behavior toward cats (Yin 2009):

- Avoid direct eye contact or staring.
- Utilize toys or food to encourage the cat to approach you first (Figure 11.9). If the cat approaches and sniffs your hand, you can gently scratch under the chin and pet the side of the head if the cat shows "green" body language and appears to enjoy this type of touch.
- Pet along the sides of the head, neck, and body if the cat appears to enjoy it. Avoid petting caudal to the waist.
- Avoid looming over, reaching for, or putting your face into the face of a fearful cat.
- Stand to the side of the cat or from behind, rather than directly in front of the head, unless you are able to allow the cat to hide its head.
- Minimize hand gestures and move slowly and deliberately.
- Speak softly and sparingly.
- For cats in particular, keep interactions as short as is practical, and attempt to perform examinations and procedures in one smooth process (e.g. examination, weight check, venipuncture, and vaccinations all at once rather than divided into three or four separate handling events). Sometimes, taking breaks can make a world of difference.
- Avoid pulling cats toward you and never pull an animal by the scruff, tail or limbs during any part of your exam.
- Allow cats to hide in the bottom of the carrier and begin your exam here.

Assess your Language and Attitude toward the Patient

A great way to foster a Low Stress Handling® culture is to use language that is appropriate, accurate, and conducive to humane handling. Historically, many animals were labeled in a way that set up inherent conflict between the animal and the veterinary staff – we have all seen "Will Bite" or "Fractious" noted in the medical record or heard that a dog "hates men." The authors have witnessed an enormous change in veterinary student empathy toward patients just by encouraging more empathetic

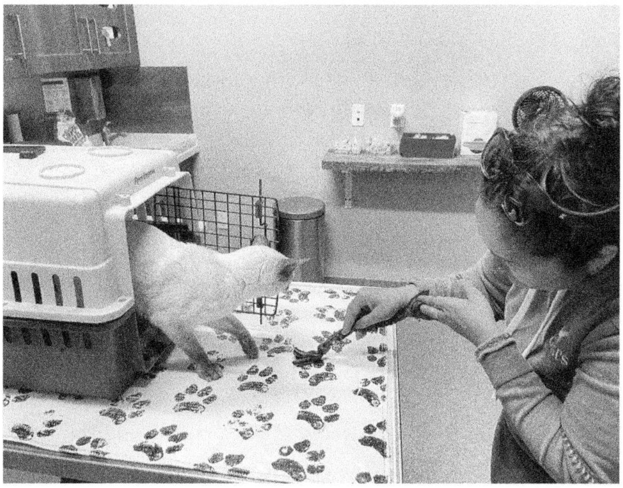

Figure 11.9 Example of utilizing a non-threatening approach with a toy at the start of a feline examination by enticing the cat to exit the carrier for a toy. *Source:* Meghan E. Herron.

verbiage. There is a subtle empathetic shift when you change the tone of just a few words. For example, substituting "blood draws are hard for him" for the historical "he hates blood draws" creates empathy and a desire to make things easier for the patient, rather than rolling up sleeves and preparing for a fight. Handlers who previously prided themselves on "wrangling mean cats" may find more comfort in hearing that their skills include reading and responding to fearful cats – note the inherent shift from going into battle (adversarial) to providing care for a struggling patient (compassionate). In fact, studies in livestock facilities show that the attitude of the handler directly relates to the way the animals are handled, as well as the stress levels of the animals (Hemsworth 2003). See Table 11.1 and Box 11.1 for commonly used words that affect patient handling and how rough handling negatively affects everyone involved.

When clients are coached to appropriately label the underlying reason, often fear, for their pet's behavior in the clinic setting, they are more apt to approve of Low Stress Handling® methods. If you believe your dog is being ornery when he will not allow a nail trim, pinning him down seems acceptable. On the other hand, if you recognize that your dog is panicking for the nail trim, it makes perfect sense to proceed slowly and cautiously, and perhaps even consider an anti-anxiety medication before the nail trim. Lastly, fear is a normal involuntary response to a perceived threat. While the veterinary profession's historic culture often discourages frank and honest discussion in this arena and discontinuation of dangerous handling, it is critical that handlers recognize when they are frustrated or fearful and that the hospital culture supports asking for help and assessing if or how to proceed.

Table 11.1 Commonly used terms that affect patient handling.

Inaccurate patient descriptors that result in poor handling	Accurate patient descriptors that promote more humane handling
Dumb	Confused
Stupid	Anxious, confused, or overwhelmed
Stubborn	Conflicted, confused, or in pain
Spiteful	Inadequately socialized
Evil	Fearful, panicked, highly distressed
Dominant	Uncertain, experiencing social distress
Mean	Distressed, fearful, protective of self

Source: Adapted by C. Croney from Hemsworth 2003.

Box 11.1

Fearful animals, frustrated handlers, and rough handling become a vicious cycle (Coleman et al. 1998; Yin 2009; Hemsworth and Coleman, 2010). Punishment makes fear-based behaviors worse, escalating the very behaviors you wish to eliminate. It also blunts the signalment of behavioral indicators of intent making handling more dangerous and is both contraindicated and unethical.

Unacceptable rough handling includes:

- Hitting and animal
- Kicking and animal
- Scruffing a dog
- Shoving or throwing an animal
- Verbally or physically threatening/intimidating and animal
- Moving or lifting an animal by the ears, tail, or limbs
- Forcing an animal to accept painful procedures without chemical restraint/analgesia

Step 4: Make a Handling Plan

Once you have completed your assessment of the patient's comfort, your approach, and the comfort of the environment, a careful handling plan can be designed and implemented (Yin 2009). Each handling plan should be unique to the individual patient and working environment, as well as everything you need to accomplish. The plan may then require adjustments depending on the patient's response. The efficacy of your handling plan can be objectively measured by both physiological and behavioral indicators. For success assessments must be made regularly (Table 11.2). Often, the initial planning and implementation are more time-consuming, but the payoff is that the patient will be more at ease, the clients will leave with a sense of satisfaction and trust, and subsequent visits should be much more efficient. After implementing a successful handling plan, we encourage you to keep a record of what worked well and how things can be improved in each patient's chart. That way, there is no reason to reinvent the wheel with each visit. This record also promotes communication within the practice. For example, if a patient has a FAS score of 1 when walking around the exam room, but quickly escalates to a 4 when placed on an exam table, documenting that this dog may do best examined on the floor will be helpful in keeping FAS low at future visits.

Most handling plans start with a critical consideration of what procedures need to be performed during the visit. If all procedures are not essential, it may be best to plan multiple visits of shorter duration with fewer procedures. Once the itinerary is established, then you can institute your plan for counterconditioning, the level of restraint, and the needed handling tools.

Guidelines for Organizing a Patient Handling Plan

Critically consider what must be done

- Critically consider what *needs* to be performed and what you *want* to perform (but is not critical) – must the procedure be done today, or at all? If the patient does not cope well today and the procedure is not critical, might it be appropriate to return with pre-visit pharmaceuticals on board? See Box 11.2 for more details.

Table 11.2 The efficacy of Low Stress Handling® can be objectively measured by both physiological and behavioral indicators.

Physiological measure you should see if your plan is going well:			
↓	Body temperature Heart rate Respiratory rate Blood pressure Pupil diameter	↓	Sweaty paws Excessive shedding Flushing
Behavioral measures you should see if your plan is going well:			
↓	Attempts to flee Fear related aggression Trembling Freezing/fearful body postures Displacement behaviors	↑	Affiliative behaviors Interest in food Improvement with each handling bout Relaxed body postures

Box 11.2

The *Needs* versus *Wants* Algorithm for Handling Patients. When making decisions regarding how to proceed with procedures in a patient demonstrating FAS, it helps to determine if the procedure is a want or a need and then use the patient's body language and behavior to dictate your next steps. Algorithm provided courtesy of Colleen Koch, DVM, DACVB.

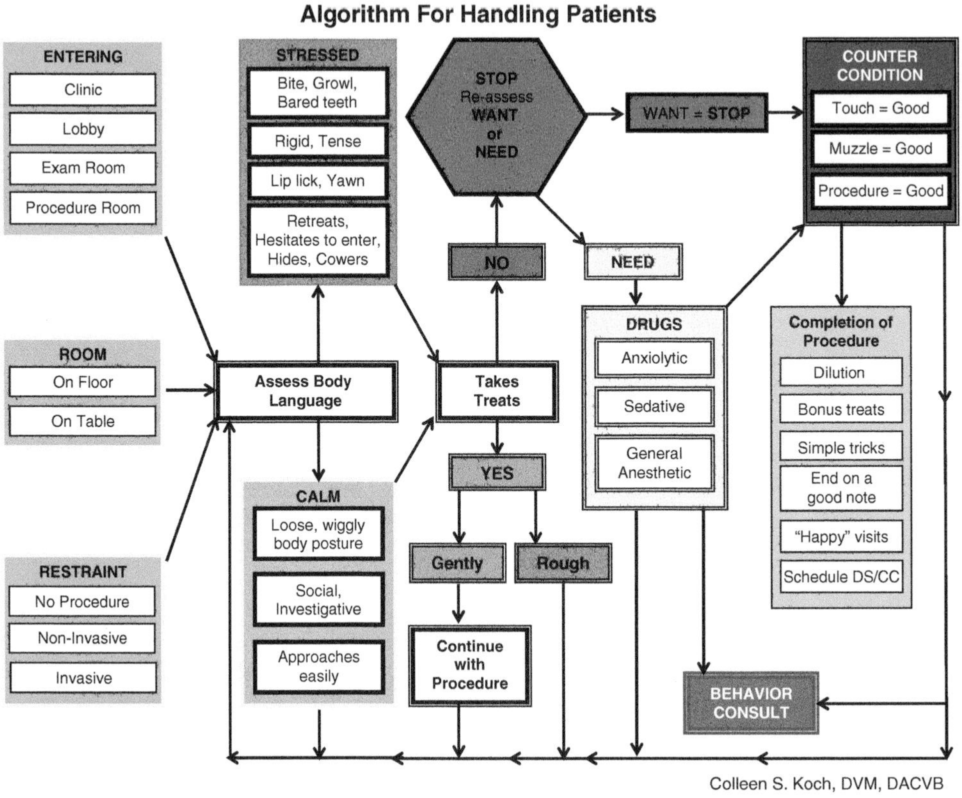

- Re-examine your clinic's typical "order of events." Does the technician or assistant *need* to remove the cat from the carrier, weigh them, and get a rectal temperature before your physical examination? Or would you prefer an examination and blood work first for the fearful geriatric cat?
- Determine if and what the patient can eat so that you can make a plan for counterconditioning that is appropriate and safe.
- Select the appropriate level of restraint (see below) for the individual patient and the procedure.
- Select any handling tools that will increase safety and decrease your patient's fear and arousal.
- Place the required procedures in order of *most important* to *least important* in the event the patient is unable to tolerate some of the procedures.

- Place those procedures in order of *least offensive* to *most offensive* so that early, difficult procedures do not inhibit your ability to complete later ones.
- Consider the level of pain, invasiveness, number of procedures, and how the patient is coping with minimal handling and consider chemical restraint (see Chapter 22) when it is unlikely the patient will be able to tolerate all the procedures.
- If there is a possibility that chemical restraint will be necessary, have it ready and waiting so that you can administer it before the animal becomes too aroused.
- Might pre-visit pharmaceuticals (PVPs) help facilitate the next visit? See Chapters 21 and 22 for detailed doses and mechanisms of action for common PVPs to help the patient cope with their visit.

It can be challenging to address many needs of a fearful patient in a limited appointment. Often, our clients will try to do "one stop shopping" with yearly visits, and with each procedure, a fearful patient's ability to cope may deteriorate despite our best efforts to minimize stress. Many times, something like a nail trim is the most stressful for the patient, yet it is also the most important to the client. Engaging the client in setting priorities is crucial. "Mr. Roe, we have a long list of things to address with Scrappy: yearly exam, express his anal glands, pull yearly bloodwork and heartworm test, assess several new skin masses, get him up to date on vaccines and trim his nails. Scrappy historically has been nervous with his veterinary visits and that's a lot to get done – we may exceed his ability to cope with all these things. Help me prioritize our list so I make sure we get the things that are most important to you completed today. We can schedule follow on appointments if needed, or alternatively we can sedate him today to make sure we can address everything without pushing him beyond what he can handle."

Utilizing Counterconditioning

Unfamiliar smells, sounds, and sights, as well as potentially threatening animals and people, assault our patients the moment they enter our care. On top of that, we perform unpleasant, sometimes painful procedures, often by force. As a result, many animals have been inadvertently conditioned to *fear* the veterinary setting. This *fear* often leads to dangerous and undesirable behavior toward humans in this setting.

Remember fear is not voluntary...

To combat the development of this fear or to alter an already established fear of the veterinary clinic settling, animal handlers can rely on counterconditioning. As discussed in Chapter 5, counterconditioning is a form of classical conditioning whereby an animal's negative emotional response (fear) to a given stimulus (veterinary setting) is changed to a positive one (pleasure) (Mazur 2016). To create this positive emotional response, we pair veterinary experiences with something that naturally elicits a positive emotional response in the animal – food. Palatable food is the easiest and most powerful means of establishing this association. This natural emotional wiring is what motivates animals to eat and survive. Counterconditioning is most effective in the clinic setting when the food is offered while the animal is still in a relaxed (FAS 0-1) state, just before and during the procedure, particularly for aversive procedures. Patients showing signs of stress (FAS 2-3) may need to be fed for the duration of the time they are handled to prevent escalation of fear and arousal. You can accomplish this by smearing sticky food onto a paper plate, Frisbee, the table, or the wall and allowing the patient to lick it. Monitor for signs of resource guarding (stiffening, growling, whale eye) if utilizing something not held directly in the handler's hand. Keep in mind the palatability of the food needs to be high to maximize the animal's interest in eating and increase the power of the positive emotional response. While petting and praise may be enjoyable to some animals, they do not serve as primary or automatic reinforcement of a positive emotional state in the way that palatable food does. Examples of procedures where you should use food for counterconditioning include injections, toenail trims, otoscopic exams, rectal temperature or palpation, restraint by a stranger, placement on an exam table or scale, microchip placement, and fine needle aspirates. Box 11.3 lists examples of palatable foods that can be used for counterconditioning in dogs and cats. See the online materials for video examples of counterconditioning during potentially aversive procedures in dogs and cats.

But am I just reinforcing "bad" behavior if I feed a patient who is aggressive toward me?

The answer is no, and here is why: Fear is an involuntary emotion, and aggression is merely a symptom of that underlying emotional state. Feeding an animal who is fearful (if you can lower their stress enough for them to be willing to eat) works to change (countercondition) the underlying emotion of fear to one that is more pleasant for the animal, such as pleasure, comfort, and/or joy. When animals are in a more positive emotional state, the motivation to utilize aggression for self-protection is alleviated, and the behavior, therefore, ceases. A good phrase to remember is *Pleasant emotions lead to pleasant behaviors*. This is not a voluntary process, but something that happens naturally and with time and repetition. This is different than feeding dogs when they offer a "sit" or if they capture a treat off the exam table after jumping up and grabbing it. In these cases, the dog is experiencing **operant conditioning** (see Chapter 5), where voluntary behaviors are reinforced. When dealing with fear and fear-based aggression, you must recognize the difference between these learning processes.

Box 11.3 Examples of palatable foods that can be used for counterconditioning in dogs and cats and the ideal times to use it:

Cats

Chicken or turkey baby food (without onions)
Canned tuna or chicken
Squeeze cheese
Canned cat food
Pill pockets® (Greenies, Franklin, TN, USA)
Pill Assist® for Cats (Royal Canin, St. Charles, MO, USA)
Temptations crunchy treats
Cat nip (ask owner if cat is calmed or aroused by it first)
Whipped cream
Churu®

Dogs

Chicken or turkey baby food
Whipped cream
Peanut butter (be mindful of human allergies)
Squeeze cheese
Kong Paste® (The Kong Company, Golden, CO, USA)
Braunschweiger (liverwurst)
Canned dog food
Pill Pockets® (Greenies, Franklin, TN, USA)
Pill Assist® – for dogs (Royal Canin, St. Charles, MO, USA)

Ideal Times to Use Food

- *First meeting* – continue to toss a few treats during history taking for anxious and fearful dogs and cats
- First *touch*
- *Socially invasive contact* – e.g. head, ears, mouth, feet, and rectum (Figure 11.5)
- *Painful activities or procedures* – injections, blood draw
- Any time you *change* location, handlers, or activity
- Feed *fearful and/or aggressive animals* continuously throughout handling

Should I reserve palatable food for my more difficult patients?

The answer is no, and here is why: The colloquial phrase *An ounce of prevention is worth a pound of a cure* could not be more accurate when describing this scenario. Utilizing food to set up a positive emotional association with the veterinary experience AT THE FIRST VISIT sets up the patient for long-term positive experiences and pleasant behaviors. We now know that early frightening experiences at the veterinary clinic are correlated with fear-based aggression later in a dog's life (Stellato et al. 2021), making it essential that we prevent fear memory consolidation from the start of a dog's veterinary experience.

Safe and Effective Restraint

Once you have organized the itinerary of procedures, you can coordinate a restraint plan for each procedure. Less invasive or socially threatening procedures (from the patient's perspective) tend to require less restraint, whereas more invasive and aversive procedures may require heavier restraint to provide a sense of security for the pet and safety for staff. There is often a tendency to over-restrain animals. Much of their stress then revolves around the restraint, rather than the procedure itself, begging the question of whether we are *creating* handling issues with classic restraint methods and in fact decreasing staff safety. The American Veterinary Medical Association' policy on the physical restraint of animals recommends the use of "the least restraint required to allow the specific procedure(s) to be performed properly." Scruffing and stretching cats is stressful and should be avoided; the combination of a "ring hold" around the head and a towel wrapping the rear limbs accomplishes the same goal with greater control and less patient stress (Figure 11.10) (Yin 2009). For procedures that require the cat to be still in lateral recumbency, the skillful use of towels provides a better experience for the patient and a safer experience for the handler. Lateral recumbency for dogs should be reserved only for procedures which require this positioning, such as orthopedic and neurologic exams. Most procedures can be performed with the dog in a standing or sitting position. Although the classic "bear hug" position has been used for large dogs in the past, requiring the restrainer to carefully navigate, putting their face very close to the patient's while wrapping an arm around the neck, the authors have achieved much greater control, safety, and patient compliance with a collar hold and the patient standing against a wall with the handler's leg against the dog's shoulder (see Figure 11.11) (Yin 2009). This keeps the handler at arm's length from the patient's face while exploiting a type of control (collar grab) to which many dogs are already accustomed.

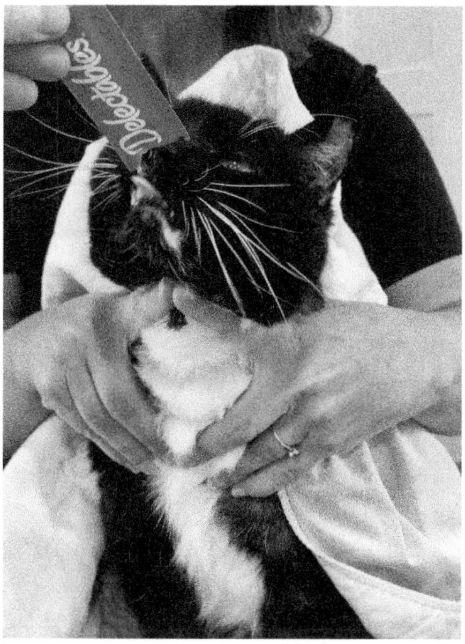

Figure 11.10 The "ring hold" provides head control by keeping the index fingers safely under the mandible. The towel provides comfort, controls the hind limbs, and offers greater protection when hands are slid underneath. The handlers' palms control the shoulders and side to side movement, while the middle fingers across the chest prevent forward movement. Sliding the brachium between the ring and little finger when in the sternal position limits the cat's ability to lift the front legs, rise and swat. See Yin (2009) for more on this hold and additional feline Low Stress Handling® options. Note: food used for counterconditioning. *Source:* Photo provided courtesy of Susan Barrett and Traci Shreyer.

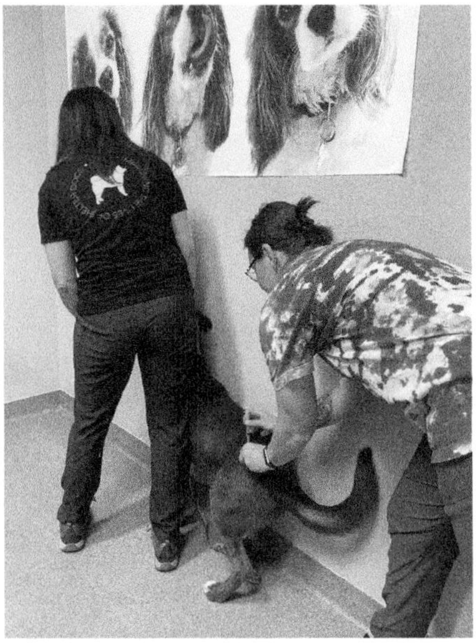

Figure 11.11 An assistant provides minimal restraint with a Low Stress Handling® collar hold on a dog prior to vaccination. For added security, she uses her legs and the wall to prevent movement and flailing while also feeding for counterconditioning. *Source:* Meghan E. Herron.

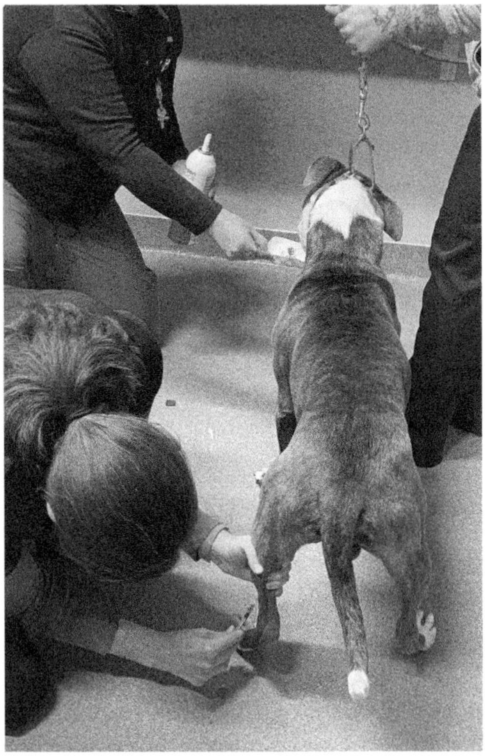

Figure 11.12 An example of venipuncture from a lateral saphenous vein using Low Stress Handling® concepts with a dog in a standing position. The handlers use collar restraint and start feeding prior to the needle insertion. They continue to feed until the blood draw is complete. *Source:* Meghan E. Herron.

Guidelines for Restraint

Use the least restraint that is necessary to safely perform the procedure, while maintaining a position that allows escalation of restraint or safe discontinuation of the procedure if not tolerated (Yin 2009). If you can utilize counterconditioning with food, often less restraint is needed. For example, dogs tolerate venipuncture from a lateral saphenous vein in a standing position well, especially when food is offered prior to inserting the needle (Figure 11.12). This negates the need to manipulate a dog into a position of lateral recumbency. Similarly, many cats will tolerate gently being turned into lateral recumbency for a medial saphenous venipuncture without being scruffed. When needed, you may add a towel which wraps and covers the head and neck and keep a hand gently on the neck so that greater restraint can be provided if necessary (Figure 11.13) (Yin 2009). When greater restraint is needed, support the animal well by providing firm, balanced restraint with global support around the patient (Figure 11.14) (Yin 2009). Prevent flailing by always keeping control of head and rear end (Yin 2009). When lateral recumbency is needed, move the patient slowly and steadily with full body support (Yin 2009). NOTE: If your patient is showing FAS 4–5 with minimal handling or your patient has a history of high FAS with a specific procedure, you may need to utilize chemical restraint early in the process as even the best of handling techniques may not adequately control or resolve FAS.

The Rule of 2 and 3

If a dog struggles in response to restraint for longer than three seconds (two seconds for cats), stop, reposition, and try again. Wait until the pet has relaxed and, preferably, starts eating, before beginning the procedure (Yin 2009). If after two to three attempts the patient does not relax and/or starts to get agitated or aggressive, stop altogether and consider whether the procedure is essential (Yin 2009). If it is essential, make a plan for chemical restraint. If it is non-essential, send the animal home and create a plan for a more successful visit the following day, including oral pre-visit pharmaceuticals and possibly an immediate injection of chemical restraint. Part of creating a successful subsequent visit may require having the pet visit the hospital at a low-traffic time, merely to enter the clinic, be offered food for counterconditioning, and then leave. This type of visit is often termed a "happy visit." These visits can be repeated and, as the animal tolerates it, more contact and handling can be applied in a systematic manner until the pet is comfortable enough to handle the restraint (Yin 2009). This systematic desensitization is best accomplished if you can keep the patient under the threshold of becoming fearful or stressed at each step. Proceeding too quickly or allowing the patient to go over threshold and become fearful can lead to sensitization, creating an even worse association.

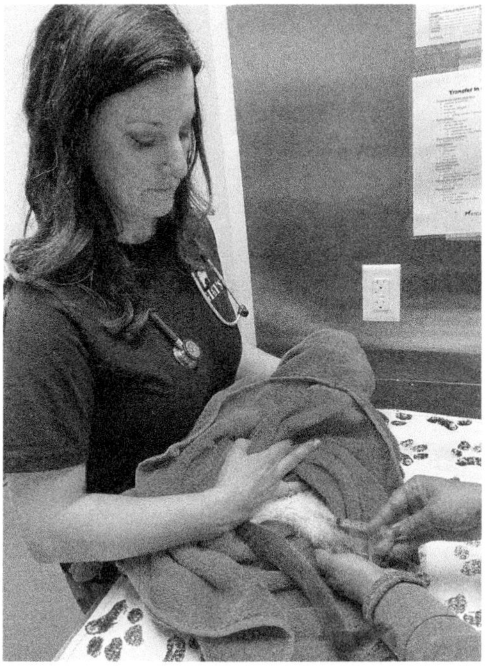

Figure 11.13 A towel wrap allows a cat to feel secure and concealed during medial saphenous venipuncture. *Source:* With permission from Aditi Czarnomski.

It is worth noting that the early introduction of handling tools, such a muzzle, can help maintain staff safety and comfort while simultaneously decreasing the need for heavy restraint. Although it should never be assumed that a muzzled patient cannot bite or scratch, a properly applied muzzle may make light restraint the only restraint required for some procedures and

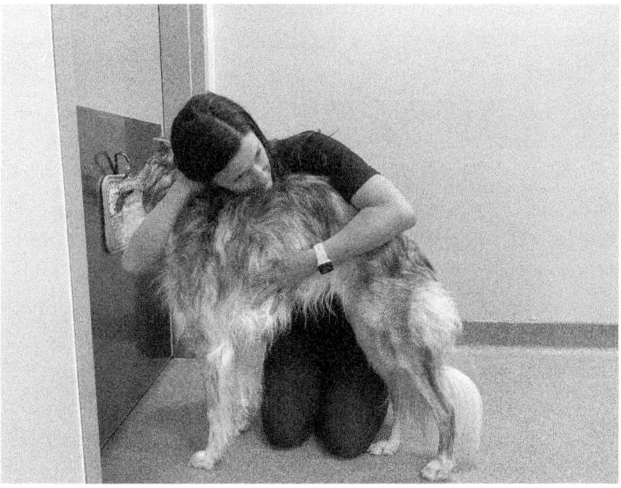

Figure 11.14 When greater restraint is needed, provide firm, balanced restraint that prevents flailing, putting pressure on the top, bottom, front, and sides of the dog's body. Ideally, the dog has an opportunity to eat for counterconditioning as shown here with a suction held lick plate. *Source:* Meghan E. Herron.

increase patient cooperation. A muzzle may also enable a client to safely stay close to the patient during certain procedures and allow you/them to safely feed throughout the procedure. Avoid performing painful or frightening procedures after muzzling, as this may permanently prohibit you from ever using this handling tool again. In this case, the muzzle will predict pain/fear and potentially be dangerous to place.

Pre-Visit Pharmaceuticals (PVPs)

Several short-acting medications are used to help patients cope with FAS during veterinary visits (see Chapters 21 and 22 for details). In practical terms, you will often identify that a patient is not coping well with a visit, and even though you may not be able to fully ameliorate their fear today, you may prescribe PVPs for a future visit – whether that is soon because today's goals could not be accomplished, or prior to next year's wellness visit. In the past, tranquilizers, such as acepromazine, that had no anxiolytic effect were routinely used for challenging patients. Changing the language around contemporary, anxiolytic medications may help alter client comfort with administering PVPs (Box 11.4). The authors find it helpful to explicitly tackle this misconception: "Mrs. Jones, I want to be clear that I'm not recommending sedation for Muffin because she's bad – in fact, I'm not recommending *sedation* at all. I see her struggling with all the weird things we need to do, and we can't explain to her that we're trying to help her. I'm suggesting a safe medication that takes away some of her anxiety before she comes to see us. It's cheap and side-effect free for most kitties. Next time may not be perfect either, but I'm hoping we'll see her show a little less fear when we give her vaccines, and hopefully not get more and more scared over time."

Box 11.4

Navigating client communication surrounding PVPs. Many clients have preconceived notions about psychotropic medications, and many would not take a medication themselves, let alone give it to their pets. Easing client concerns through mindful communication and gaining client buy-in will help you:

> *"Sometimes giving medications can be worrisome. There can be side effects, and I have chosen a drug to minimize those concerns. I can assure you I would only prescribe medication if I thought Nellie really needed it. We want to help her with her anxiety here at the clinic. We can do a trial dose and see what you think. You can let me know if you think it's helping or not, and we'll plan further from there."*

Chemical Restraint

Chemical restraint allows for safe and effective handling without causing the patient emotional distress. Avoid waiting for the animal to become aggressive or highly agitated before considering the use of chemical restraint (Yin 2009). Not only will this reduce the effectiveness of the medication, but it will also allow for learning to occur, making the fear in that setting more advanced. For cases which will require immediate chemical restraint, it is best to create a plan to administer the injection upon entrance to the hospital or, in some cases, the parking lot. Allowing the pet to wait in the lobby will likely increase agitation and arousal and lower the effectiveness of the medication. Typically, injectable forms of sedation/anesthesia administered intramuscularly are the most effective means of rendering a fear-aggressive or highly fearful patient safe to handle. The clinician should use sound medical judgment to determine appropriate dosages and drugs based on age, temperament, and degree of health/disease. Once you have made your drug selection, you must now make a plan for how to administer it. Some patients will tolerate a quick injection while eating food during a gentle, but secure, collar hold. Others require more creativity and finesse and can be dangerous if not done correctly. See Chapter 22 for recommendations on safely administering chemical restraint to dogs and cats.

Once the injection has been administered, tools to block visual and auditory stimuli, such as the ThunderCap (Thunderworks, Durham, NC, USA) over the eyes and cotton balls in the ears, will help maintain the animal on an even plane of sedation. Keep these animals in a quiet area, rather than the open treatment room, as this is more conducive to a full sedation response. The plane of sedation you are trying to accomplish is one where no physical restraint is needed, and the animal cannot remember the interaction and create or further a fear of handling. For patients that show mild to moderate fearful or fearfully aggressive behavior in a veterinary clinic setting, PVPs may be enough. You should also plan to prescribe PVPs for animals that will undergo injectable forms of chemical restraint so that lower doses of injectable medications can be utilized and to block fear and associated learning from the startle/discomfort of the injection. See Chapter 22 for detailed protocols for pre-visit pharmaceuticals and injectable chemical restraint.

Handling Tools

Animal handling tools are designed to expedite veterinary procedures and increase handler and patient safety, which, in turn, reduces patient stress, reduces staff stress, and increases client satisfaction. The key to successfully integrating handling tools into veterinary practice is using them *correctly*, using them *often*, and using them *early*. Handling tools are most helpful if integrated early into the handling plan. Clients should be encouraged to expose their pet to these tools, including food for counterconditioning, at home, away from the presence of noxious stimuli, so that the tools do not become predictors of stressful events.

Canine Handling Tools

Muzzles

The "sleeve" style of muzzle fits tightly over the nose and mouth, holding the mouth closed (Figure 11.15). The pros of this type are that the muzzle can be placed quickly if it is the stiffer, leather type and the animal can lick food from the open front of the muzzle. Cons are that the muzzle prevents the dog from panting and should only be worn for brief procedures as the patient may overheat if they wear the muzzle for more than a few minutes. This is especially true for highly agitated patients whose body temperatures are already elevated above the normal range. Furthermore, the dog can still bite with the exposed incisors. Soft canvas types collapse and are difficult to place safely on a dog already fearful enough to display aggressive behavior during an emergency placement. The "basket" style of muzzle is an open plastic or metal cage or basket which encloses the entire nose and mouth (Figure 11.16). The pros of this type are that the muzzle allows for some level of panting, making it safer to be worn for longer procedures (and when a dog is housed in a hospital kennel), and that food can easily be smeared along the inside of the muzzle, encouraging the dog to place its nose into the muzzle without a struggle (Figure 11.17).

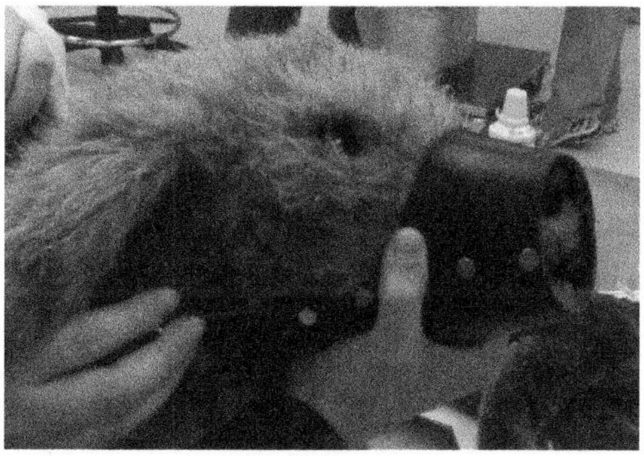

Figure 11.15 A leather sleeve-style muzzle keeps a dog's mouth closed, limiting the ability to pant. Dogs should not wear this type of muzzle for more than three to five minutes, as they cannot adequately regulate their body temperature and may overheat. *Source:* Meghan E. Herron.

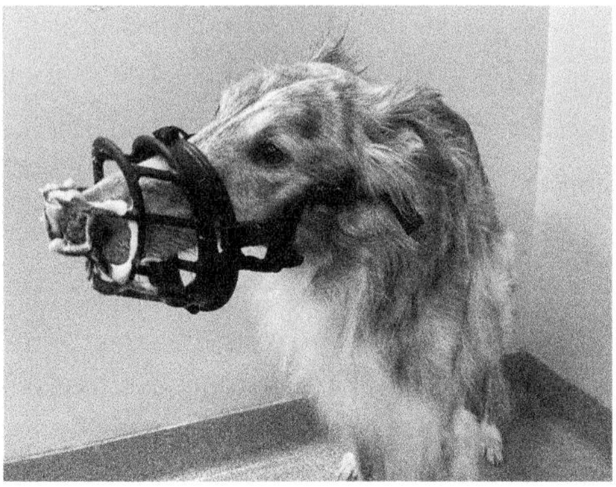

Figure 11.16 A basket-style muzzle allows more room for a dog to pant and better regulate body temperature. *Source:* Meghan E. Herron.

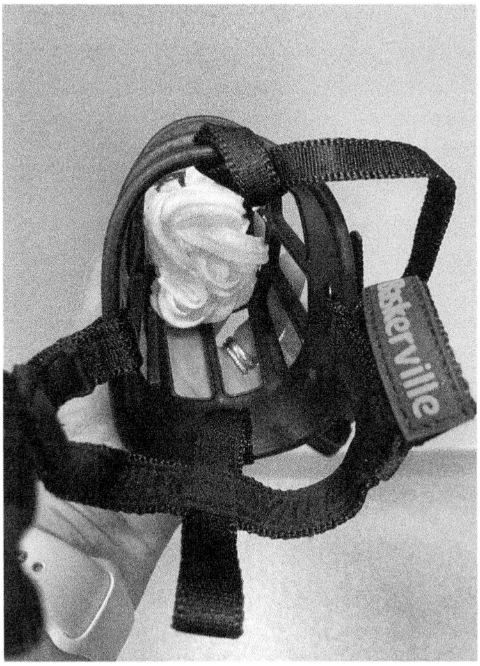

Figure 11.17 The basket-style muzzle serves as a vehicle for food delivery, both to encourage the dog to investigate the muzzle and for continued counterconditioning while the dog wears the muzzle. *Source:* Meghan E. Herron.

Goals of using a muzzle include:

1) Using less physical restraint
2) Allowing for continuous feeding of the patient
3) Safely administering chemical restraint

The muzzle is *not* intended to allow you to use maximal restraint, many handlers, or to continue to do painful or socially invasive procedures. In ideal cases, when the procedure is not essential, you can send a client home with a muzzle and training advice. This allows the dog to safely walk into the clinic wearing it comfortably. Another option is to have the client muzzle the dog in the clinic or the car (if safe to do) at the time of the visit. Be aware that you are liable for a client's injury from their own pet during a medical appointment. See Box 11.5 for guidelines on determining when it is safe and appropriate for a client to place a muzzle on their own dog in your clinic or hospital. You can also train your staff to perform desensitization and counterconditioning for muzzle placement so that the dog will willingly place their nose into the muzzle after a few minutes of training. This technique is more successful when the dog is naïve to the muzzle and has little to no previous negative interactions when wearing a muzzle. When that is not safe or feasible, you can consider a quick scoop of the muzzle (with food inside when safe and appropriate). Proper placement of the muzzle in this manner should start with the handler standing to the side of the dog, facing the same direction. The handler should then place the muzzle on from behind and from the side, scooping the muzzle under the chin of the dog, rather than over the head (Figure 11.18). It may help to prevent the dog from backing up as the muzzle is placed, using a wall or a person. Be quick and deliberate, as there may not be multiple opportunities for placement once the animal realizes the intention of the handler.

Lastly, an advanced technique is "drive-by" muzzling. This method requires skilled handlers and should be practiced with docile dogs before ever attempting on a dog with known fear or aggression. This method requires three people: one person to hold the muzzle to the side of the dog, another to hold the leash and walk on the opposite shoulder of the dog, and a third person to walk just behind the dog. The

Box 11.5

Guidelines on determining when and if it is safe and appropriate for a client to place a muzzle on their own dog in your clinic or hospital (Herron and Shreyer 2014). Keep in mind you are liable for any client injuries sustained in your practice, even if it is from their own pet.

- Ask whether the dog has any history of family-directed aggression (e.g. ask whether the dog has ever growled, nipped, snapped, or bitten them, even once, when it was approached at rest, had its mouth or face handled, or its food bowl or toys were handled).
- Ask what the clients think about placing a muzzle on the dog. Do they feel comfortable? Are they safe or capable?
- Describe how you would like the client to place the muzzle on the dog, and make sure they do not have any questions or concerns before proceeding.
- Supervise the client's placement of the muzzle as well as the patient's body language, and if you sense a problem, you can ask the client to stop.
- Pay attention to the client's nonverbal communication signs when asking these questions, and if you sense that they are uncomfortable despite their verbal consent, it may be best not to proceed with having them muzzle the dog.

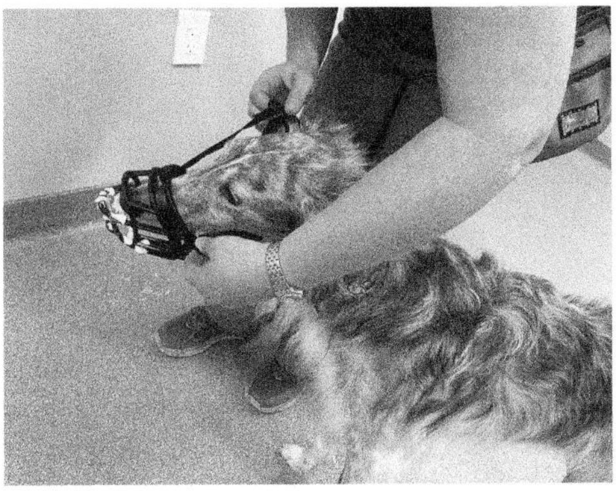

Figure 11.18 A basket muzzle filled with food is quickly scooped onto the dog from the side while the handler faces the same direction as the dog. *Source:* Meghan E. Herron.

person holding the muzzle coordinates movement and counts "1-2-3." At the count of 3, the muzzle-holding handler scoops the muzzle onto the dog in one quick movement. The leash holder then grasps the muzzle, holding it in place while the muzzle holder fastens the straps. At the same time, the handler in the back uses their legs to prevent backward movement, which might allow the dog to back out of the muzzle. You definitely only get one chance with this one, and chemical restraint should be immediately administered once the dog is muzzled. See the online materials for a video example of this technique. Chapter 22 discussed alternative strategies for administering intramuscular injections of chemical restraint when a dog cannot safely be muzzled.

Helping Clients Feel Comfortable Using a Muzzle on Their Dog

Many clients struggle when the idea of a muzzle is broached. Using empathy and judgment-free statements will help you gain buy-in. For example:

"Mr. Jones, Steve is painful and he is also fearful here – the pain is probably making him have a harder time than usual. Many dogs are fearful at the vet, just like us at the dentist, so it's not surprising. Steve doesn't want us to hold him to examine him – that kind of restraint is hard and scary for him. To be able to look at his leg and recheck his heart, I'll need to place a muzzle. The nice thing for him is a muzzle lets me use less

restraint, so in the end will hopefully make this easier for him. In fact, training him to wear a muzzle happily can actually make all vet visits easier for him. We have a handout that explains what I mean and why it can be so helpful. Remember, the muzzle doesn't mean he's bad or mean – he's just painful or scared or doesn't understand what we want..."

Dog Appeasing Pheromones (DAP), (ADAPTIL®; ThunderEase®)

This synthetic pheromone product is available in a spray, body heat-activated collar, and plug-in diffusers (Figure 11.3). DAP is an analog of the appeasing pheromone produced by a nursing bitch immediately after she whelps puppies. The natural pheromones are emitted from the sebaceous glands in the inter-mammary sulcus, and serve as a signal of food, comfort and safety for the puppies. DAP has been shown clinically to have a calming effect on puppies and adult dogs in a veterinary setting (Kim et al. 2010; Siracusa et al. 2010, Mills et al. 2006). The spray can be applied to a bandana that can then be placed on the dog upon arrival or applied to a towel and placed on the exam table. Always supervise dogs wearing bandanas to prevent entanglement or ingestion. Never spray directly on a dog, and be sure to allow a brief time for an application to "air out" prior to placing the bandana on a dog. Diffusers can be plugged into outlets in exam rooms, treatment areas, and kennel areas where dogs are housed. In facilities with frequent air exchange, you may need to replace the cartridges more frequently than with home use. Another product, ZENIDOG® (Virbac, FortWorth, TX), has more recently come on the market and one study shows it has similar efficacy to ADAPTIL® in calming dogs (Nicolas et al. 2022). For clinics where electrical outlets may be limited, this gel-based, nonelectrical diffuser may be a viable alternative option.

ThunderCap (ThunderWorks, Durham, NC, USA)

This cap is a sort of "blindfold" made of soft, semi-opaque fabric that covers the dog's eyes to limit the intake of visual stimuli, thereby reducing stress associated with the anticipation of procedures (Figure 11.19a). When dogs do not witness the events prior to the procedure, the chances are much greater they will remain calm. It is helpful for dogs with aggression issues associated with the sight of unfamiliar dogs or people when moving them from the car to the lobby, through the treatment area, or from one part of the hospital to another. Hospitalized dogs with dog aggression issues can wear this cap when confined to

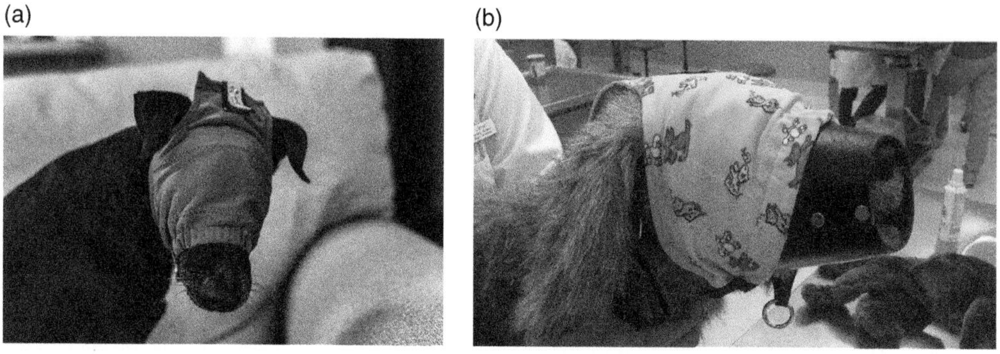

Figure 11.19 The ThunderCap reduces visual input that might increase FAS. It can be used alone (a) or in addition to a muzzle (b). *Source:* ThruZLens Photography/Zach Judy (a), Meghan E. Herron (b).

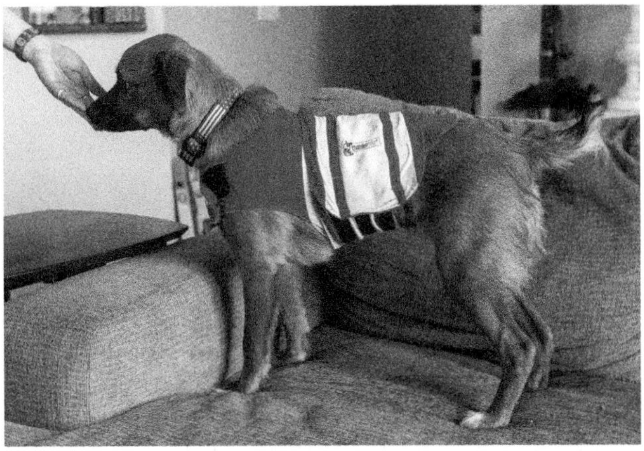

Figure 11.20 A Thundershirt can be calming for many dogs from the firm, balanced pressure it provides. *Source:* ThruZLens Photography / Zach Judy.

prevent agitation from the sight of other passing or hospitalized dogs, as long as they are supervised while wearing it. This does not serve as a muzzle, although it can be placed over or under a muzzle (Figure 11.19b) and is best used after the clients have acclimated the dog to wearing it through counterconditioning at home.

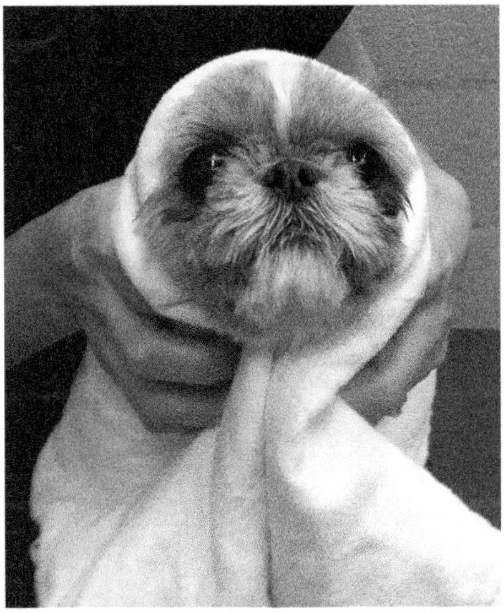

Figure 11.21 Towel restraint of a small dog. *Source:* Meghan E. Herron.

Thundershirt (ThunderWorks, Durham, NC, USA)

This tool is a body wrap that swaddles the dog, providing firm, balanced pressure around the chest and torso (Figure 11.20). Design is based on evidence that evenly applied pressure on the body may reduce anxiety and fear (Cottam et al. 2013, Grandin 1992). For dogs who are calmed by this pressure, the shirt can be applied prior to entering the veterinary clinic and/or applied before the exam begins.

Towel Restraint

For dogs who cannot be muzzled due to brachycephalic conformation or intense fear of the muzzle created by prior misuse, towels can be used to provide control of the head (Figure 11.21) (Yin 2009). To restrict head movement a towel can be rolled and wrapped around the neck and chest like a brace and held tightly. The towel should be thick and pressure applied evenly from just below the chin down to the chest (Figure 11.22) (Yin 2009). Prevent dogs from backing out of this type of head restraint by positioning your body behind them (Yin 2009). Apply just enough pressure to restrict movement and not restrict breathing (Yin 2009). Some small dogs can be wrapped in a towel "burrito" as you would wrap a cat.

Elizabethan Collar Restraint

For dogs who cannot be muzzled due to brachycephalic conformation or intense fear of the muzzle, Elizabethan collars can be used to provide some control of the head (Figure 11.23) (Yin 2009). The authors have found that for toy breeds in particular, applying a Velcro® Elizabethan collar is far more efficient and safer than attempting to place (and buckle!) a tiny muzzle. If safe for the client to place the collar, it may be best to have them place it at home, prior to entering the clinic. The head can be controlled, using two hands behind the collar to grasp the neck and head firmly, but gently. An additional advantage of the Elizabethan collar is that it often provides a visual barrier so that the patient cannot see and anticipate portions of the procedure or examination.

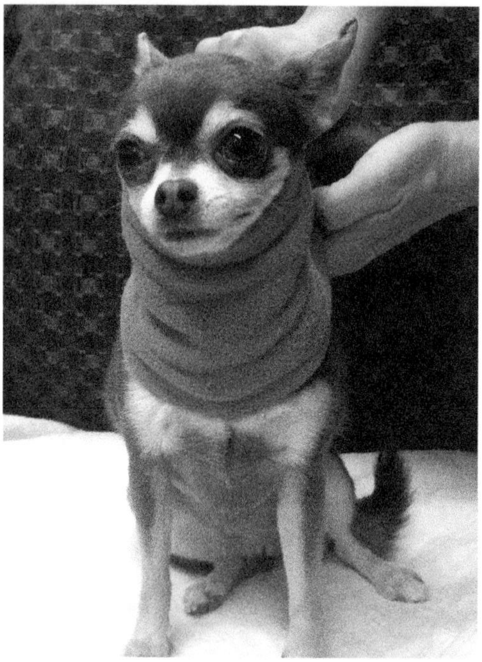

Figure 11.22 Head control with the use of a neck towel in a small dog. *Source:* Meghan E. Herron.

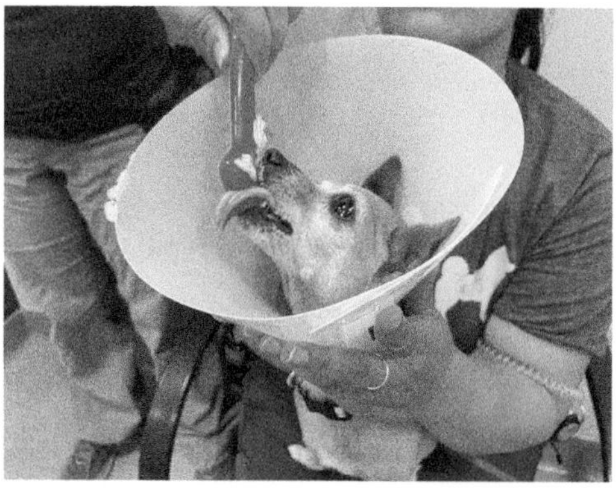

Figure 11.23 Use of an opaque, white Elizabethan collar for head restraint and for reducing visual stimuli in the peripheral visual fields. *Source:* Meghan E. Herron.

Feline Handling Tools

The Carrier

The cat's own carrier can be a valuable handling tool, especially for fearful cats. Carriers should be of the type that allows the cat to easily exit on its own or have a removable/movable top that allows the cat to remain in the bottom portion during examination (Figure 11.24) (Yin 2009). A towel can then be slid under

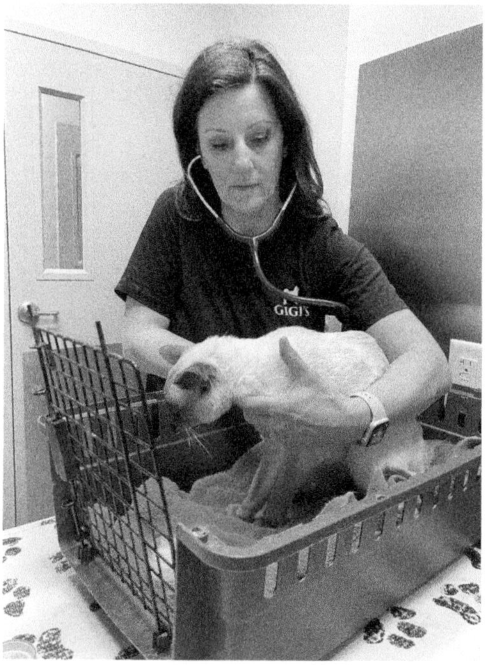

Figure 11.24 A cat is examined at the bottom of the carrier. This allows the cat to remain in the comfort of a familiar enclosure. Keeping the door on the carrier also prevents forward movement. *Source:* With permission from Aditi Czarnomski.

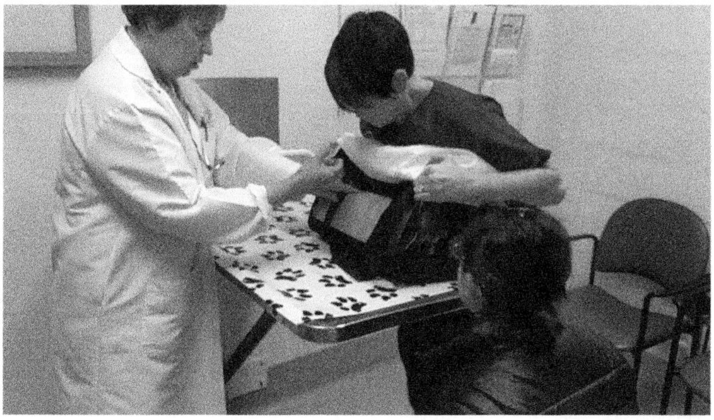

Figure 11.25 A cat that historically has a level 4–5 FAS during veterinary handling is given an IM injection of chemical restraint before coming out of the carrier. *Source:* With permission from Susan Barrett.

the top and over the cat as the top half of the carrier is slowly lifted and removed (Yin 2009). This method allows the cat to remain in a familiar area and tends to prevent fleeing as the sides of the carrier provide some sense of concealment. Soft sided carriers provide protective contact for handlers and are useful for cats in need of intramuscular injections for chemical restraint. In this case, the cat remains in the familiar carrier while the soft side is pressed up against the animal at the injection site (Figure 11.25 – also see online materials for video example). Allowing hospitalized cats to have their own carrier within their cage will also provide a sense of familiarity and stress relief. Keeping the familiar carrier within the cage has been shown to help hospitalized cats go back to eating sooner during recovery (Griffith et al. 2000). The carrier is a most effective tool for cats that have been conditioned to feel comfortable entering on their own and remaining calm in it during car travel. See Appendix B for a client handout on carrier training for cats.

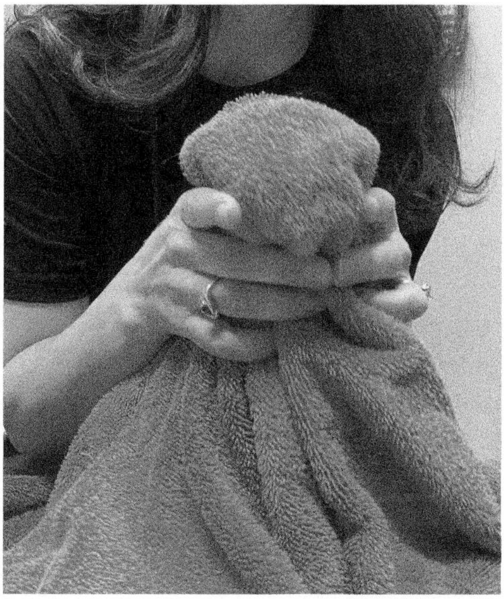

Figure 11.26 A cat is protected from visual stimuli and forward movement with a towel. Using the Low Stress Handling® techniques of ring hold and lateral support from the handler's forearms and dorsal support from the handler's chest prevents flailing and gives a sense of security. *Source:* With permission from Aditi Czarnomski.

Towels

Expertise in towel wrapping and restraint is an essential skill for safe and humane cat handling (Yin 2009). Head control and reduction of visual stimuli are the primary purposes of towels when handling cats (Yin 2009). For fleeing or fearful cats, often it is enough to place the towel over the head, then push the towel under to include the head and feet (Yin 2009). Any movement forward will be inhibited by the pressure of the towel, and many cats will then remain still. You can then achieve additional control by applying the Low Stress Handling® ring hold technique over top of the towel and creating an imaginary "box" around the patient with the forearms, abdomen, and chest (Figure 11.26) (Yin 2009). The clinician then has access to the rear end of the cat for auscultation, abdominal palpation, and medial saphenous venipuncture. For access to the head of the cat, or for cats that are stressed by having the head covered, Low Stress Handling® immobilization can be performed using a towel wrap (aka "half burrito wrap"). In this method, the cat is first placed on the center of the towel, and the front of the towel is pulled up around the neck to keep control of the head. Then, while holding the towel in place with one hand, the other hand is used to wrap the sides of the towel around the body of the cat (Yin 2009). Be sure that the wrap fits snuggly to provide firm, balanced lateral support (Yin 2009). This will prevent flailing and help the cat remain calm, while preventing scratching with the front or rear claws (Figure 11.27a–c).

(a) (b) (c)

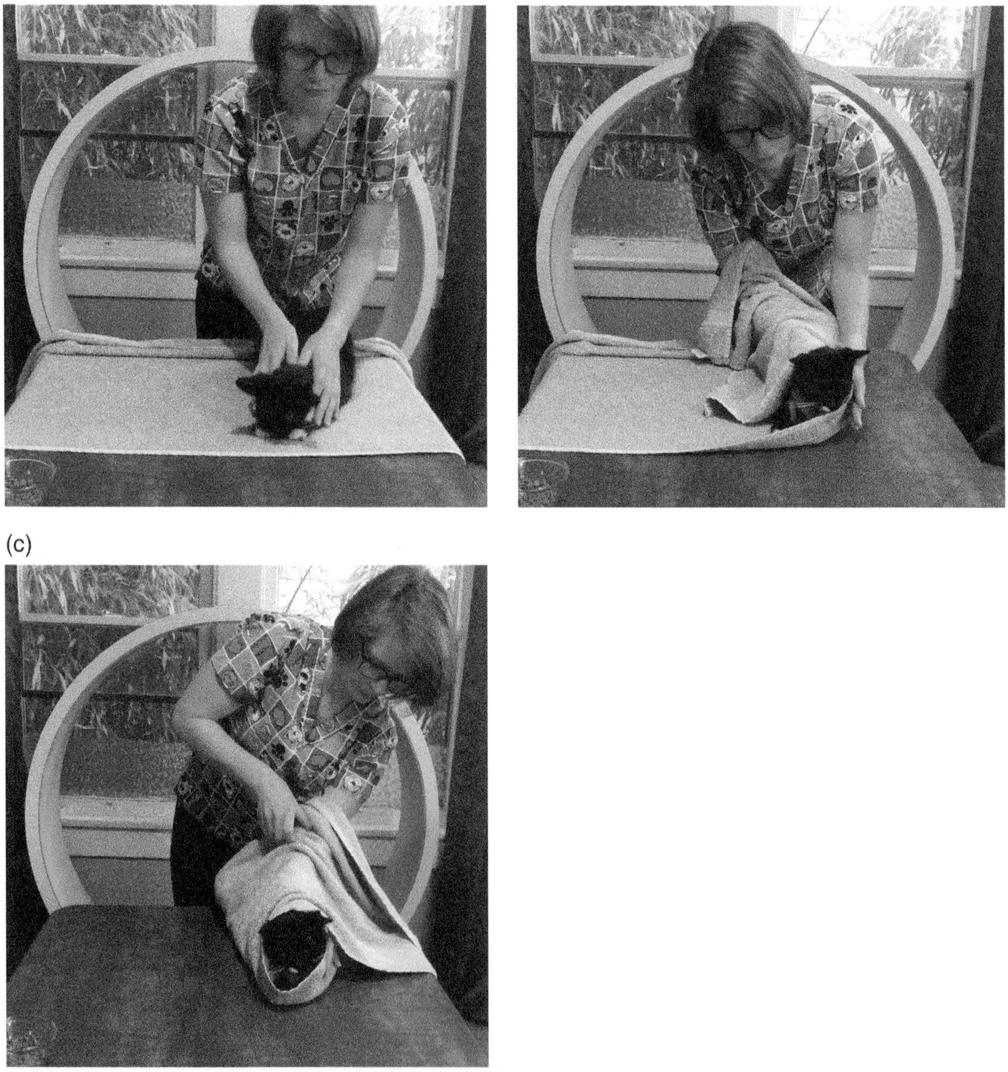

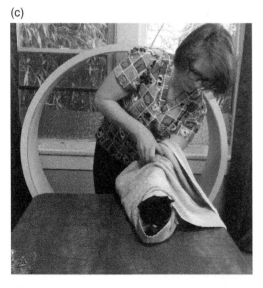

Figure 11.27 The handler demonstrates the Low Stress Handling® "half-burrito" wrap toweling method. First, the cat is placed off center onto a towel in dorsal recumbency (a). Next, the handler secures the left side of the cat's body by pulling the left flap of the towel tightly over the dorsum of the cat and then under (b), then pulling the right flap tightly over the dorsum and under the cat so the entire body is secured in the Low Stress Handling® "burrito" (c). A Low Stress Handling® "full burrito" wrap would pull the front of the towel over the cat's head before wrapping the sides. *Source:* With permission from Denise Johnson.

Feline Appeasing Pheromones (FELIWAY® Classic and Optimum)

FELIWAY® Classic and Optimum are available in a spray and plug-in diffuser. FELIWAY® Classic is an analogue of the facial pheromone released from the perioral gland of cats when cheek rubbing (bunting) on prominent objects, people, and other animals. Cats typically perform bunting behaviors when in an environment they perceive to be safe and comforting. FELIWAY® Optimum is a patented blend of pheromones known as the Feline Pheromone Complex, which provides an enhanced message of social confidence in the environment. Placing either of these synthetic pheromone products in the hospital environment may help cats eat faster (Griffith et al. 2000) and be more tractable with handling (Kronen et al. 2006). These pheromones may be useful in treating aggressive behavior between cats and reducing stress-related marking behaviors, suggesting a calming effect in general which is highly applicable to the veterinary clinic setting. Pheromones should not be directly sprayed onto the cat. Instead, spray the exam table towel, cage padding, and/or the inside of a cage cover or carrier, several minutes (ideally 20) before they come into contact with the cat. Often, a towel or blanket can be draped over half of the cage door to give the cat the ability to feel hidden as well as to hold a sprayed pheromone product.

EZ Nabber (Campbell Pet Company, Brush Prairie, WA, USA)

In this tool, mesh netting is tightly secured to a metal enclosure, which opens and closes manually to allow for capture and restraint of cats. It is especially helpful for feral or fear-aggressive cats who are fleeing or housed in a wall unit cage, as it puts a 2-foot distance between the handler's hands and the cat (Figure 11.28a–c) (Yin 2009). It is used to administer chemical restraint intramuscularly, as injections can easily be given through the mesh

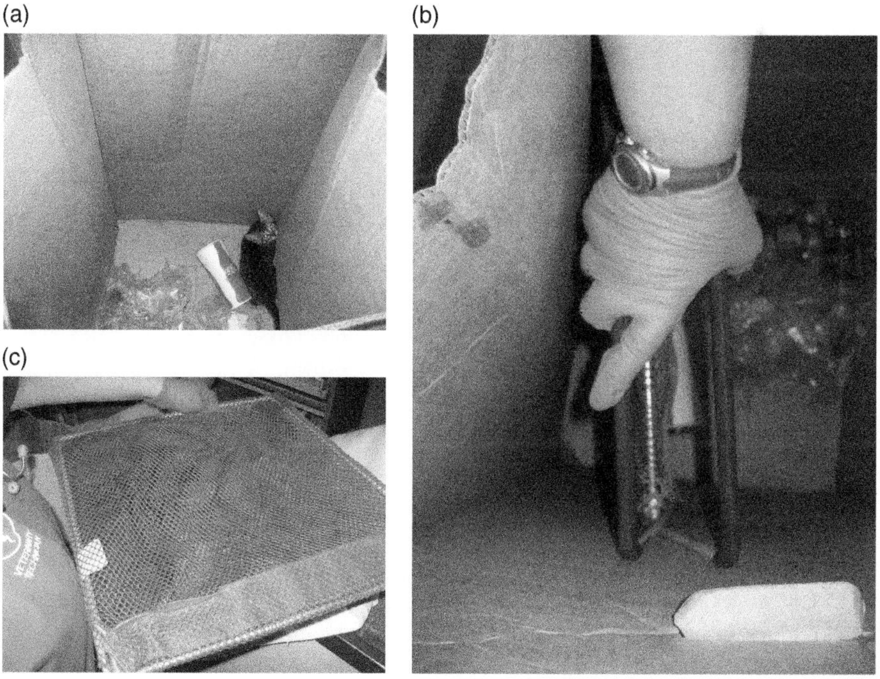

Figure 11.28 A fear-aggressive, feral kitten (a) was brought into an emergency clinic by a good Samaritan. A technician uses the EZ Nabber to retrieve the kitten (b) quickly and safely to administer an IM injection of chemical restraint while secured in the netting (c) and then immediately places the kitten into a hospital cage. *Source:* Meghan E. Herron.

netting. Cover the netting with a towel once the cat is captured to reduce visual exposure and stimuli which may exacerbate stress (Yin 2009). Release cats back into a carrier or cage immediately after administering chemical restraint so that time within the mesh is minimized.

Muzzles

In cats, muzzles are typically used to cover both the mouth and the eyes. This provides safety to the handler as well as minimizes visual stimuli that may be stressful for the cat. Soft, nylon muzzles are useful if visual stimulation blocking is the primary goal. Stiff leather or plastic cone-shaped muzzles are preferable for aggressive cats, as they are unable to bite through the tougher material. Place the muzzle from behind the head, using one swift motion to place the muzzle coming up from under the chin of the cat. One handler should place pressure on the muzzle, holding it in place, while a second handler secures the ties or Velcro® straps. A third handler may be needed to prevent the cat from backing out of the muzzle if the other handlers are unable to do so.

Conclusion

In conclusion, safe, effective, and humane handling of dogs and cats requires careful assessment of your patient's emotional state, your own words and actions, as well as the environment in which you both find yourselves. Considering how your patients perceive their surroundings and mitigating factors that may contribute to their FAS levels will go a long way toward improving patient welfare and client satisfaction. Keep your toolboxes full and readily at hand, and work together with your staff to make sure everyone is well-versed and rehearsed when it comes to using the tools and techniques associated with low-stress veterinary handling.

References

American Veterinary Medical Association Policy. (2022). Physical Restraint of Animals. https://www.avma.org/KB/Policies/Pages/Physical-Restraint-ofAnimals.aspx (accessed 14 February 2023).

Anthony, A., Ackerman, E., and Lloyd, J.A. (1959). Noise stress in laboratory rodents: I. Behavioral and endocrine responses of mice, rats, and guinea pigs. *J. Acoust. Soc. Am.* 31: 1437–1440.

August, J.R. (1988). Dog and cats bites. *J. Am. Vet. Med. Assoc.* 193: 1394–1398.

Bear, M.F., Conners, B.W., Paradiso, M.A. The chemical senses. In: Neuroscience: Exploring the Brain. 4. Philadelphia: Lippincott Williams & Wilkins; 2015. p. 278–90.

Bekoff, M. Scent marking by free ranging domestic dogs: olfactory and visual components. *Biol. Behav.* 1979;4:123–39.

Belew, A.M., Barlett, T., Brown, S.A. Evaluation of the white-coat effect in cats. *J. Vet. Intern. Med.* 1999;13:134–42.

Bowman, A., Dowell, F.J., Evans, N.P., and Scottish, S. (2017). The effect of different genres of music on the stress levels of kennelled dogs. *Physiol. Behav.* 171: 207–215.

Carlstead, K., Brown, J.L., and Strawn, W. (1993). Behavioral and physiological correlates of stress in laboratory cats. *Appl. Anim. Behav. Sci.* 38: 143–158.

Clinchy, M., Sheriff, M.J., and Zanette, L.Y. (2013). Predator-induced stress and the ecology of fear. *Funct. Ecol.* *27* (1): 56–65.

Coleman, G.J., Hemsworth, P.H., and Hay, M. (1998). Predicting stockperson behaviour towards pigs from attitudinal and job-related variables and empathy. *Appl. Anim. Behav. Sci.* *58* (1–2): 63–75.

Cottam, N., Dodman, N.H., and Ha, J.C. (2013). The effectiveness of the anxiety wrap in the treatment of canine thunderstorm phobia: an open-label trial. *J. Vet. Behav.* 8: 154–161.

Crouse, S.J., Atwill, E.R., Lagana, M. et al. (1995). Soft surfaces: a factor in feline psychological well-being. *Contemp. Top. Lab. Anim. Sci.* 34: 94–97.

Crowell-Davis, S.L. White coat syndrome: prevention and treatment. *Compend. Contin. Educ. Vet.* 2007;29:163–5.

Drobatz, K.J. and Smith, G. (2003). Risk factors for bite wounds inflicted on caregivers by dogs and cats in a veterinary teaching hospital. *J. Am. Vet. Med. Assoc.* 223: 312–316.

Grandin, T. (1992). Calming effects of deep touch pressure in patients with autistic disorder, college students, and animals. *J. Child. Adolesc. psychopharmacol.* 2: 63–72.

Griffith, C.A., Steigerwald, E.S., and Buffington, C.T. (2000). Effects of a synthetic facial pheromone on behavior of cats. *J. Am. Vet. Med. Assoc. 217* (8): 1154–1156.

Griffin, F.C., Mandese, W.W., Reynolds, P.S. et al. (2021). Evaluation of clinical examination location on stress in cats: a randomized crossover trial. *J. Feline Med. Surg. 23* (4): 364–369.

Grigg, E.K., Liu, S., Dempsey, D.G. et al. (2022). Assessing the relationship between emotional states of dogs and their human handlers, using simultaneous behavioral and cardiac measures. *Front. Vet. Sci.* 9: 897287.

Gunter, R. (1995). The absolute threshold for vision in the cat. *J. Physiol.* 114: 8–15.

Hawthorne, A.J., Loveridge, G.G., and Horrocks, L.J. (1995). The behavior of domestic cats in response to a variety of surface textures. *Proceedings of the 2nd International Conference on Environmental Enrichment* (ed. B. Holst), pp. 84–94. Copenhagen, (Denmark), CZ.

Hemsworth, P.H. (2003). Human-animal interactions in livestock production. *Appl. Anim. Behav. Sci.* 81: 185–198.

Hemsworth, P.H. and Coleman, G.J. (2010). Stockperson Behaviour and Animal Behaviour. In: *Human-Livestock Interactions: The Stockperson and the Productivity of Intensively Farmed Animals*, 103–119. CABI.

Herron, M.E., Shofer, F.S., Reisner, I.R. Survey of the use and outcome of confrontational and non-confrontational training methods in client-owned dogs showing undesired behaviors. *Appl. Anim. Behav. Sci.* 2009;117:47–54.

Herron, M.E. and Shreyer, T. (2014). The pet friendly vet practice: a guide for practitioners. *Vet. Clin. Small Anim. Prac.* 44: 451–481.

Jeyaretnam, J.H., Jones, H., and Phillips, M. (2000). Disease and injury among veterinarians. *Aust. Vet. J.* 78: 625–629.

Kim, Y.M., Lee, J.K., Abd el-aty, A.M. et al. (2010). Efficacy of dog-appeasing pheromone (DAP) for ameliorating separation-related behavioral signs in hospitalized dogs. *Can. Vet. J.* 1: 380–384.

Kogan, L.R., Schoenfeld-Tacher, R., and Simon, A.A. (2012). Behavioral effects of auditory stimulation on kenneled dogs. *J. Vet. Behav.* 7: 268–275.

Kronen, P.W., Ludders, J.W., Erb, H.N. et al. (2006). A synthetic fraction of feline facial pheromones calms but does not reduce struggling in cats before venous catheterization 1. *Vet. Anaesth. Analges. 33* (4): 258–265.

Kry, K. and Casey, R. (2007). The effect of hiding enrichment on stress levels and behavior of domestic cats (*Felis sylvestris catus*) in a shelter setting and the implications for adoption potential. *Anim. Welf.* 16: 375–383.

Mandese, W.W., Griffin, F.C., Reynolds, P.S. et al. (2021). Stress in client-owned dogs related to clinical exam location: a randomised crossover trial. *J. Small Anim. Prac. 62* (2): 82–88.

Mazur, J.E. (2016). Basic principle of classical conditioning. In: *Learning and Behavior*, 8e, 60–82. Upper Saddle River (NJ): Pearson Education.

Merola, I., Lazzaroni, M., Marshall-Pescini, S. et al. (2015). Social referencing and cat–human communication. *Anim. Cogn.* **18**: 639–648.

Merola, I., Prato-Previde, E., and Marshall-Pescini, S. (2012). Social referencing in dog-owner dyads. *Anim. Cogn.* **15**: 175–185.

Miller, P.E. and Murphy, C.J. (1995). Vision in dogs. *J. Am. Vet. Med. Assoc.* 207: 1623–1634.

Mills, D.S., Ramos, D., Estelles, M.G. et al. (2006). A triple blind placebo-controlled investigation into the assessment of the effect of dog appeasing pheromone (DAP) on anxiety related behaviour of problem dogs in the veterinary clinic. *Appl. Anim. Behav. Sci.* 98: 114–126.

Morgan, K.N., Tromborg, C.T. Sources of stress in captivity. *Appl. Anim. Behav. Sci.* 2007;102:262–302.

National Research Council (NRC) (2006). *Nutrient Requirements for Dogs and Cats.* Washington, DC: National Academy Press.

Nicolas, C.S., Espuña, G., Girardin, A. et al. (2022). Owner-perception of the effects of twolong-lasting dog-appeasing pheromone analog devices on situational stress in dogs. *Animals.* 12 (1): 122.

Pollard, J.C. and Littlejohn, R.P. (1994). Behavioural effects of light conditions on red deer in a holding pen. *Appl. Anim. Behav. Sci. 41* (1–2): 127–134.

Siracusa, C., Manteca, X., Cuenca, R., et al. Effect of a synthetic appeasing pheromone on behavioral, neuroendocrine, immune and acute-phase perioperative stress responses in dogs. *J. Am. Vet. Med. Assoc.* 2010;237:673–81.

Stella, J.L. and Croney, C.C., 2016. Environmental aspects of domestic cat care and management: implications for cat welfare. *Sci. World J., 2016.* https://doi.org/10.1155/2016/6296315.

Stellato, A.C., Dewey, C.E., Widowski, T.M., and Niel, L. (2020). Evaluation of associations between owner presence and indicators of fear in dogs during routine veterinary examinations. *J. Am. Vet. Med. Assoc. 257* (10): 1031–1040.

Stellato, A.C., Flint, H.E., Dewey, C.E. et al. (2021). Risk-factors associated with veterinary-related fear and aggression in owned domestic dogs. *Appl. Anim. Behav. Sci. 241*: 105374.

Stoddart, D.M. The Ecology of Vertebrate Olfaction. London: Chapman and Hall; 1980.

Takahashi, L.K., Nakashima, B.R., Hong, H.C. The smell of danger: a behavioral and neural analysis of predator odor-induced fear. *Neurosci. Biobehav. Rev.* 2005;29: 1157–67.

van Oostrom, H. and Knowles, T.G. (2018). The clinical efficacy of EMLA cream for intravenous catheter placement in client-owned dogs. *Vet. Anaesth. Analg. 45*: 604–608.

Veranič, P. and Jezernik, K. (2001). Succession of events in desquamation of superficial urothelial cells as a response to stress induced by prolonged constant illumination. *Tissue and Cell 33* (3): 280–285.

Volk, J.O., Thomas, J.G., Colleran, E.J., and Siren, C.W. (2014). Executive summary of phase 3 of the Bayer veterinary care usage study. *J. Am. Vet. Med. Assoc. 244* (7): 799–802.

Wagner, K.A., Gibbon, K.J., Strom, T.L. et al. (2006). Adverse effects of EMLA (lidocaine/prilocaine) cream and efficacy for the placement of jugular catheters in hospitalized cats. *J. Feline Med. Surg. 8*: 141–144.

Wells, D.L. (2006). Aromatherapy for travel-induced excitement in dogs. *J. Am. Vet. Med. Assoc.* 6: 964–967.

Yin, S. (2009). *Low Stress Handling, Restraint, and Behavior Modification of Dogs and Cats.* Davis, CA, Cattle Dog Publishing.

Part II

Clinical Concepts in Animal Behavior

12

Addressing Canine and Feline Behavior Problems in Clinical Practice

The Art of Behavior Triage

Traci Shreyer[1], *Susan Barrett*[2], *and Allison Shull*[3]

[1] *Purdue University, The Croney Research Group, West Lafayette, IN, USA*
[2] *VCA Morris Animal Hospital, Small Animal Clinical Private Practice, Lancaster, OH, USA*
[3] *ASPCA Cruelty and Recovery Center, Columbus, OH, USA*

Your 4:00 p.m. appointment is a new patient presenting for annual vaccinations, a two-year-old castrated male German Shorthaired Pointer named Roentgen. The family recently moved to town, and your technician hands you a sparse record from the previous veterinarian – puppy booster series, routine castration, a single episode of otitis externa after swimming. "He is a friendly guy, should be easy; no issues," she says over her shoulder as she takes his fecal sample to the treatment area for flotation. You are relieved to hear this since you have dinner reservations at 5:00 p.m. and this patient is your last case of the day. You poke your head around the corner. "Let's rock and roll – go ahead and draw up the Bordetella and Leptospirosis vaccines and I will get started on my exam."

Roentgen is, as promised, a model patient – wiggly and gregarious as you enter the examination room, greeting you excitedly with a wagging rear and relaxed eyes. He is already sniffing the treats in your hand, which you give to his mom after introducing yourself. You ask her to feed them to Roentgen one at a time to keep him focused as you perform your physical examination, and he is soft and unconcerned under your hands. Your technician joins you after setting up the fecal, and Roentgen continues to anticipate each treat without noticing his vaccinations or blood draw. Although your technician is in position for restraint if needed, Roentgen never stops eating and does not turn his head toward your needle pokes. You mentally congratulate yourself – this is how it is done!

The client has been chatting throughout the visit, but not about Roentgen since he is healthy. Life has been hectic with the move and the kids starting school; real estate prices are crazy; the farmers' market down the street has great produce. Your technician excuses herself to retrieve Roentgen's preventatives and you glance at the clock: 4:22 p.m. "What else can I do for you and Roentgen today?" you ask, to close the visit. Maybe we should try the stuffed mushroom appetizer this time, you think. The client hesitates a moment, then blurts, "I guess there is something." The image in your mind of the stuffed mushrooms pops like a cartoon balloon. She pets Roentgen softly and looks at him as she asks, more of him than of you, "How do we keep him from stealing all our stuff and biting us when we try to take it back?"

Introduction to Animal Behavior and Veterinary Behavioral Medicine, First Edition. Edited by Meghan E. Herron.

Companion website: www.wiley.com/go/introductiontoanimalbehavior

Introduction

If you are like most clinicians, you wish that your clients had reasonable expectations of how many concerns can be adequately addressed during the typical veterinary wellness visit. Not only do many clients present their pets with a long list of issues, but some of those issues fall into the "medical" category, while some fall into the "behavior" category (an area that gets less curriculum time for most clinicians in training). Even though many clinicians are less comfortable with behavioral components of clinical medicine, behavior problems are a common concern raised by clients during general practice visits. Surveys show that 72–90% of clients want some sort of help with their pet's behavior problems (Catanzaro 2001; Sherman and Serpell 2008). The reality is many general practice veterinarians do not feel equipped with adequate time or knowledge to effectively address their patients' behavior problems. The result is that many clinicians avoid the behavior piece of the puzzle entirely; a 2013 study showed that only 17% of client-reported behavior problems were indeed addressed by the veterinarian (Roshier and McBride 2013).

When clients cannot turn to the veterinarian for behavior advice, the results range from frustrating to tragic. Risky alternate sources such as the internet, TV personalities, or untrustworthy pet professionals may offer misinformation (often based on outdated methods) that are at best ineffective, or at worst, exacerbate the behavior issue and lead to fear or aggression. This chapter will empower you to effectively address behavior concerns during the typical veterinary appointment using a 5-step framework. You can give Roentgen's family a safety plan, and you can still have a good quality of life and enjoy those stuffed mushrooms! (See online materials for Chapter 12 for a full behavior triage example for Roentgen.)

The concept of triage is familiar to us in medical situations, particularly emergency medicine, and can be summarized as *the efficient assessment and addressing of an issue.* The term "triage" implies that the practitioner is not allotted adequate time to fully address the issue or its impacts on the family. This concept may be new to you when we discuss its application to behavioral medicine. Essentially, behavior triage recognizes that in a typical veterinary visit, behavior problems may be identified by you or mentioned by the client that are of a magnitude beyond your expertise or the time allotted during the visit. In practical "appointment" terms, this may look like:

- Rapid triage during a typical medical appointment.
- Full behavior triage appointment scheduled at a later date (for instance, if you offer to schedule more time to discuss Roentgen's resource guarding during a separate appointment with you).
- Immediate scheduling of the patient for a "full" behavior consultation, where detailed diagnosis and treatment information will be shared (this may be within your practice if behavioral medicine is an area of interest/expertise or referral to an academically trained behavior service). The nature of these appointments is such that they are lengthy. If the client chooses this route, you will provide the client "triage"-sized information to help while awaiting the full appointment.

Some behavior problems warrant immediate intervention by the veterinary team whether or not time has been appropriately allotted (Martin et al. 2014). Examples are immediate risk of injury to the pet, humans, or other animals, risk of severe damage to the home or possessions of the family, and risk of impending relinquishment of the pet or euthanasia. Urgent triage can be performed using the principles in this book, and most often these patients will require referral to an academically trained behaviorist. In such cases, boarding the pet at the veterinary facility may be needed to give the owner some relief.

The Importance of Communication

> **Four Core Communication Skills (Shaw 2006)**
>
> - **Open-ended questions** – Encouraging the person to elaborate without shaping or focusing the content, e.g. "How is McGyver doing today?"
> - **Empathetic statements** – Appreciate another person's predicament or feelings and communicate that understanding back to the client in a supportive manner, e.g. "Seeing Roger and Emma fight must have been really scary!"
> - **Reflective listening** – Reflecting back in your own words the content or feelings behind the person's message, e.g. "So you mentioned that Michelle urinated in your bed last night and you are frustrated with her spitefulness."
> - **Nonverbal communication** – Behavioral signals excluding verbal content; 80% of communication, e.g. eye rolls, arms crossed, flushing of face or chest.

You might guess that the combination of a topic outside the clinician's comfort zone, plus a topic that may be embarrassing or emotional for the client, can make for an awkward exchange. It is no surprise that the authors have found that the foundation of efficient and effective behavior triage is solid communication. Just as some clients may stigmatize mental health issues in humans, they may extrapolate such views to their pets and avoid admitting or discussing behavior concerns. As with any sensitive topic, it becomes even more critical to rely on four core communication skills (Shaw 2006) – open-ended questions, empathy, reflective listening, and nonverbal communication (see box). These skills help build and maintain rapport with the client, and later help you deliver management information that is critical for effective triage. In addition, the authors have found that immediate and nonjudgmental normalizing is the most powerful tool in our toolbox for enhancing rapport with the client during these difficult conversations. In the case of Roentgen, or with any behavioral concern, we might respond initially with, "Oh, I'm sorry to hear that he [insert behavior concern here]. Lots of dogs do, and it can be a big concern for any family."

Imagine that your open-ended question about the behavior of Jeannie, a 12-year-old Miniature Poodle, reveals that she snapped at the client's granddaughter last week. You now must triage an important behavior concern as well as address Jeannie's medical issues. Attempting to do both may give neither adequate attention without putting you seriously behind schedule or, worse, opening you up to ethical concerns or legal liability. The authors would suggest an approach like this:

"Mrs. Mitchell, I hear that you are concerned about Jeannie snapping at your grandchild and you have every right to be – that is scary! You came in today for Jeannie's vaccines, anal sacs, itchy skin and heartworm test, but I'd really like to discuss the snapping especially if your granddaughter will be at your house again soon. Please help me set our priorities today. We can discuss Jeannie's new concerning behavior today and get everything else done at another appointment on Thursday. How does that sound to you?"

This approach shows that you are willing and able to discuss the problem and invite the client to prioritize their goals for the appointment. Even if they do not schedule the behavior discussion now, they will feel safe to engage you if the concern rises in priority.

When we acknowledge that clients may hesitate to discuss behavior, we realize how critical it becomes to use a combination of open-ended screening questions and careful interpretation of verbal "red flags" (See online materials for Chapter 12 for details) to paint an accurate picture of the patient's behavioral wellness. Fear or aggression toward people or other animals can be overt and easy to identify in the clinic setting, but other issues such as resource guarding in the home, destructive behaviors when left alone, or house-soiling issues may only be apparent through dialogue with the client. Just because the patient seems behaviorally appropriate in front of you does not preclude including at least one open-ended question during each visit to elicit behavioral concerns at home – "it sounds like Roentgen has been feeling well physically; tell me how his behavior has been" or "tell me how he is getting along with the family." Asking such questions at the start of the visit (or utilizing the brief behavioral assessment screening tool we will show you below) can elicit concerns earlier in the appointment and give you extra time for your behavior triage and medical workup.

The Five Steps of Behavior Triage

The key to successful behavior triage is realizing that you do *not* need to make a firm behavioral diagnosis, even though you may suspect what the final diagnosis might be. The focus of behavioral triage is the recognition of the problem and level of client concern, assessment of risk to the patient or other people or animals, and the rule out of medical issues that may be contributing to the behavior. Additionally, willingness to discuss the problem with the family and to attempt some intervention in the form of prevention, stress reduction, and enrichment will let the client know that you are interested and willing to help with the problem. Your goal is to keep things safe and prevent escalation of the problem until you make a plan to fully address the issue (either yourself or through referral).

The behavior triage process is one that we have condensed down to steps that any general practitioner can easily perform within the confines of a typical outpatient appointment with the support of the entire veterinary team.

The steps we propose are:

History
Medical Rule Outs
Safety Advice
Stress Reduction
Recommended Referral

Step 1 – Taking a History

History taking is the same process we use for every appointment. Use the following steps for taking a history when performing a triage of behavioral complaints. Note that a more detailed behavioral history will be collected to make a diagnosis and plan later during the full behavior consultation.

- List client complaint(s)
- Ask for phenotypic descriptions
- Make a problem list
- Ask client to rank them
- Engage the client in active choices
- Set realistic expectations

The Four Habits Model (Adams and Frankel 2007)

- Invest in the beginning
  - Create rapport quickly
  - Elicit the full spectrum of concerns
  - Plan the visit
- Elicit the client's perspective
  - Ask for client's ideas
  - Elicit specific requests
  - Explore the impact on the patient/client's life
- Demonstrate empathy
  - Be open to client's emotions
  - Make at least one empathic statement
  - Convey empathy nonverbally
  - Be aware of your own reactions
- Invest in the end
  - Deliver diagnostic information
  - Provide education
  - Involve client in making decisions
  - Complete the visit

Building trust during this process is crucial. Medical interviewing is the foundation of medical care and is the clinician's most important activity (Frankel and Stein 2001). The four habits approach, paired with the four core communication skills (see Box 12.4) will help you establish and maintain your client's trust.

How Do We Gather All of this Information in a Timely Manner?

To help quickly obtain the behavioral concerns, we propose the use of behavior wellness assessments (see Figures 12.1 and 12.2) that clients can complete at home prior to or at the start of the appointment. This survey can be

The Ohio State University Veterinary Medical Center

Canine Behavioral Wellness Assessment

1. Does your dog ever urinate or defecate outside accepted areas? ☐ Yes ☐ No
2. Does your dog damage or destroy items or furniture? ☐ Yes ☐ No
3. Does your dog have any problems with other dogs or pets?
   Inside your house ☐ Yes ☐ No
   Outside your house ☐ Yes ☐ No
4. Does your dog ever growl, lip-lift, lunge, nip, snap at, scratch, bite or attack people? ☐ Yes ☐ No
   If "YES" check all that apply ☐ Family ☐ Strangers ☐ Vet
5. Does your dog ever display unruly behaviors? ☐ Yes ☐ No
   (jumping up, begging, stealing food, pulling on leash, etc.)
6. Does your dog ever appear scared (trembling, hiding, whining) of things? ☐ Yes ☐ No
   (thunderstorms, strangers, men, other dogs, etc.)
   If "YES", what? ______________________
7. Does your dog play too rough (leaving bite or scratch marks)? ☐ Yes ☐ No
   If "YES" check all that apply ☐ Humans ☐ Dogs
8. Has there been any recent change in your dog's behavior, activity or disposition? ☐ Yes ☐ No
9. Do you have any other concerns about your dog's behavior?
   ____
   ____
   ____
   ____

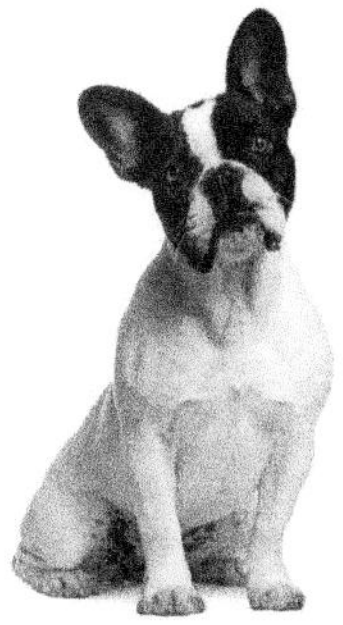

Developed by T. Shreyer with support of the Kenneth A. Scott Charitable Trust

THE OHIO STATE UNIVERSITY
VETERINARY MEDICAL CENTER

Veterinary Medical Center—Community Practice
601 Vernon L. Tharp St.
Columbus, OH 43210 **614-292-6661**
vet.osu.edu/communitypractice

Figure 12.1 Canine behavioral wellness assessment.

The Ohio State University Veterinary Medical Center

Feline Behavioral Wellness Assessment

1. Does your cat ever urinate or defecate outside the box? ☐ Yes ☐ No
2. Does your cat spray? ☐ Yes ☐ No
   (ex. backs up to a wall kneads his/her feet while sprays urine onto the surface)
3. Does your cat ever hiss, swat, growl, nip, or bite people? ☐ Yes ☐ No
   If "YES" check all that apply ☐ Family ☐ Strangers
4. Does your cat chew, scratch or destroy things in your home? ☐ Yes ☐ No
5. Does your cat have any problems with other cats or pets in your home? ☐ Yes ☐ No
6. Has there been any change in your cat's behavior, activity, or disposition? ☐ Yes ☐ No
7. Does your cat play too rough? ☐ Yes ☐ No
   If "YES" check all that apply ☐ Humans ☐ Animals
8. Can we provide any further information about your cat's behavior? ____________________

____

____

____

____

____

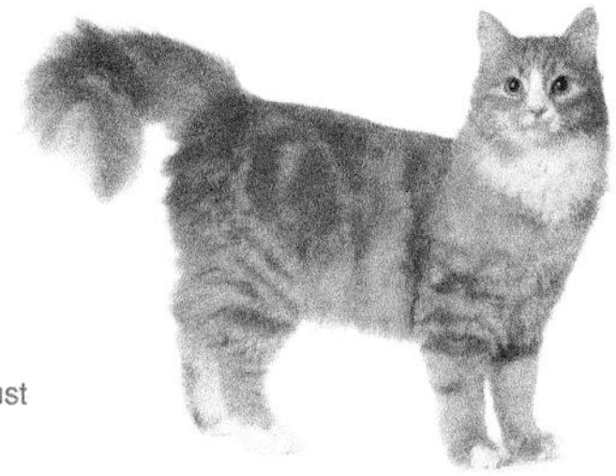

Adapted From, "Feline Behavior Guidelines" AAFP
Developed by T. Shreyer with support of the Kenneth A. Scott Charitable Trust

THE OHIO STATE UNIVERSITY
VETERINARY MEDICAL CENTER

Veterinary Medical Center—Community Practice
601 Vernon L. Tharp St.
Columbus, OH 43210 **614-292-6661**
vet.osu.edu/communitypractice

Figure 12.2 Feline behavioral wellness assessment.

screened for problems that may warrant further discussion during the appointment. Reviewing such surveys before or at the beginning of the appointment can help prevent surprises at the conclusion of the visit when your hand is on the door. You do not want to run out of the precious time needed to collect samples for the medical rule outs, or to perform the triage process. Because animals with other behavioral problems are more likely to behave aggressively at the veterinary hospital (Appleby et al. 2002), the wellness screens can also assist you in triaging the handling of the patient and improving safety for the entire team. Typical red flag phrases used by the client can also assist in identifying areas that may be of concern (see online materials for Chapter 12 for common "red flag" client phrases and how to interpret them).

Now that I have this information, what questions do I ask to be most effective and efficient?

ABCs of a Behavioral History

Many clinicians struggle with managing the information in a behavioral history and efficiently funneling it down into useful components. Behavior can be simplified by breaking it down into 3 pieces – the antecedent(s), the behavior, and the consequence(s). This is based on a large body of scientific theory and research beginning with the work of BF Skinner's theory on operant conditioning, followed by Lovaas, Bijou, and others' work in *applied behavior analysis*. See Figures 12.3 and 12.4 for a pictorial depiction of the ABCs of a behavioral history.

Identify the Antecedent

The antecedents are what happens right before the target behavior. These are also sometimes called "triggers." Triggers may be sights, sounds, sensations, scents – anything that can cause a reaction in the pet. Understanding the triggers will generate your safety and avoidance advice. It is important to gather all scenarios in which the behavior has occurred, including location, time of day, response-eliciting stimuli, and the target in cases of aggression. Many clients report initially that the behavior is unpredictable because they are unaware of these patterns or of all the triggers/antecedents until they are prompted and guided through this process. It is important to realize these responses occur even if the trigger is not actually life-threatening or the client does not perceive the trigger as problematic.

Describe the Behavior

The behavior in this scenario is the client's complaint or the behavior that you, as the clinician, have targeted as problematic. A clear picture of the exact behavior(s) exhibited will allow you to utilize the triage process more effectively. Start by identifying what the target behavior looks like. It is critical to get a **phenotypical description** (see Box 12.1) of the behavior versus simply the client's opinion about why the behavior occurs, the pet's

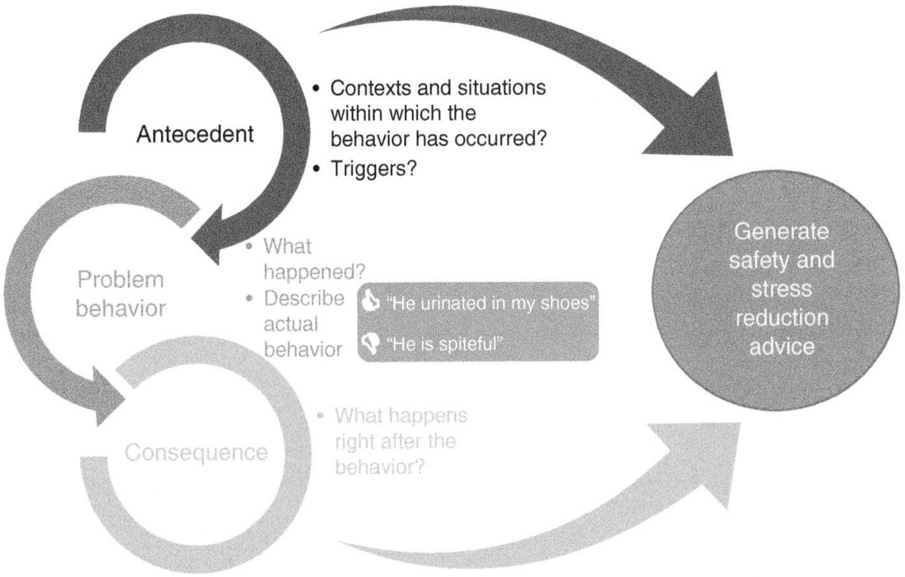

Figure 12.3 Collecting a behavior triage history.

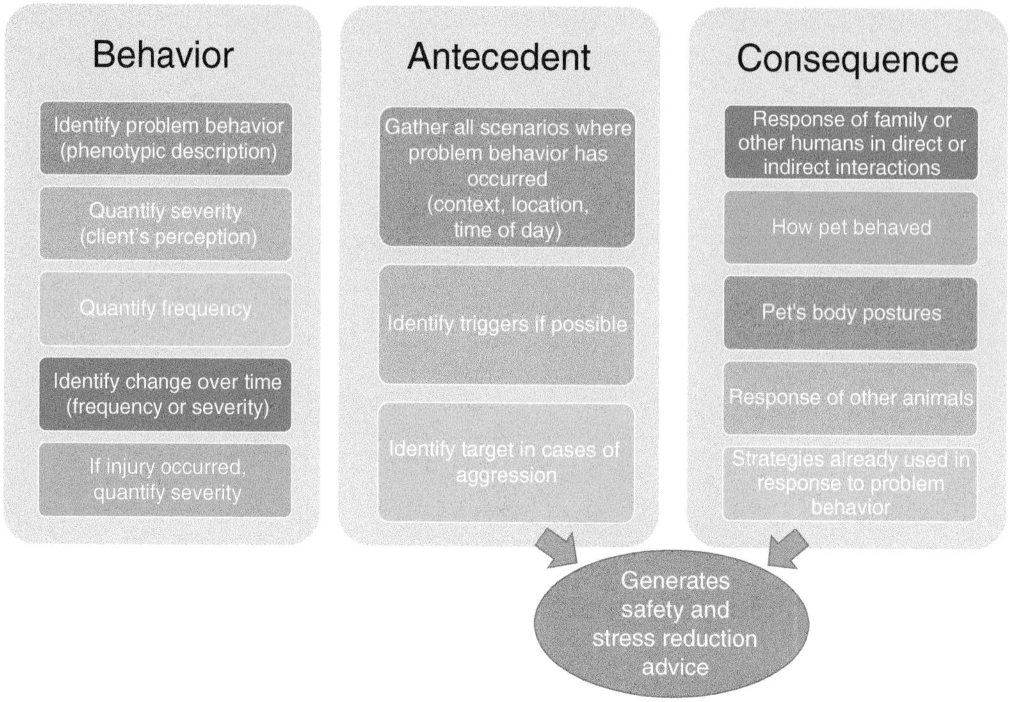

Figure 12.4 A pictorial representation of the ABCs and how they inform the triage process.

Box 12.1 Phenotypic descriptions versus opinion

Phenotypic description – Statements of verifiable fact. Examples: "His eyes are brown" or "Spike urinated in my shoes".

Opinion – Statements of feelings, attitudes, or beliefs. They are neither true nor false. Examples: "His eyes are pretty" or "Spike is spiteful."

Communication tip:
While encouraging descriptive accounts is key, we err when we default to discounting information that does not gel with our science (e.g. when the client is wrong). We must listen for clues to how the client views the problem. Even if incorrect, it allows us to know how best to calibrate our response in a way that the client can hear.

For the sake of relationship building, we may not need or want to correct the information. Its value will be in screening for emotional content, or for barriers that may impact adherence to the treatment plan.

In some cases, the client's "wrongness" is significant enough that it needs to be corrected or we risk having the pet harmed, e.g. if the "wrongness" is "I need to punish my cat every time he pees on the carpet." Circling back to the topic of correction versus responding immediately to the client's share is most effective when this is needed.

perceived motivation for performing the behavior, or the pet's suspected emotional state while performing the behavior. Perceptions and emotions influence the client's language and descriptions of their pet's behaviors, which can significantly reduce the accuracy, and exponentially increase collection time and the entire visit duration.

Determine the Consequence

The consequence(s) occurs just after the behavior. This "what happened next?" applies to both the behaviors (including body language) of the patient and any people or other animals involved in the specific scenario. Although we do want to know about client responses to their pet's behavior, the term consequence is not synonymous with punishment here - assuming so will limit the collection of important information. Consequences will affect your safety and stress reduction advice and may also give you indications about how this behavior pattern is being reinforced or maintained, and guide any direct recommendations. Discussion regarding the consequences often reveals behaviors that the client will need to discontinue for safety and success. Trust and rapport must be built *throughout* the history-taking process and will facilitate the ease by which the delivery of these recommendations is given. The "consequence" portion is explored last for this reason.

Although not collected in this order, remembering the ABCs will help you quickly identify the important components of the behavior sequence needed to generate safety advice, create a list of recommendations for short-term stress reduction, and effectively triage the level of intervention required for the case. Most often, we identify a problem behavior first, then try to identify triggers for it. Figure 12.3 summarizes typical flow and important areas to explore in behavioral triage history taking.

Trigger Stacking and Threshold

Case Study – Trigger Stacking

Bruiser is fearful during storms, displays aggression toward dogs he sees on walks, and has been diagnosed with separation anxiety. He has never shown any human-directed aggression. Bruiser's family left him home alone for several hours. During this time there was a significant thunderstorm. Upon return, Bruiser was happy to see his family and greeted everyone, including the visiting grandchild. Soon after the neighbor's dog ran into Bruiser's yard barking. The visiting toddler joined Bruiser at the window to see what the barking was all about. Bruiser bit the child on the cheek, seemingly without warning. The multiple stressful events prior to the bite pushed Bruiser closer and closer to the threshold. When the child approached, this seemingly small stressor depleted his coping ability, and for the first time, he reached the threshold for aggression to a human.

When a trigger (antecedent) for behaviors associated with arousal, anxiety, or fear occurs, the physiologic response is an increase of stress hormones in the body – the fight or flight response. The time required for these hormones to return to baseline is highly variable and depends on the animal, the stressor, and many other factors (Moberg 2000). It may take hours for these hormones to return to normal levels. The ability of the individual pet to cope with a trigger impacts the intensity of the response to that trigger. If the pet remains below threshold, the client may not observe an untoward behavioral response in the pet. In other words, while a trigger may cause a stress response, the patient that is able to cope remains "below threshold," and the client does not observe a behavior they perceive as problematic.

Trigger stacking occurs when multiple stressful events occur in a short period of time. Each stressful event causes an increase in stress, and the body does not have time to return stress hormones to baseline. Each event brings the pet closer to its threshold for performing the problematic behavior. The client may see only the last trigger as the one that sent the pet over threshold and caused an unwanted behavior. For example, a dog that "bit the child with no warning" may actually have been experiencing multiple triggers leading up to the event. This is important to delve into so that appropriate safety advice can be generated.

Some patients live with chronic stress or illness and, therefore, live close to the threshold of what might trigger an aggressive or panicked response. In these patients, seemingly small stressors can cause what the client perceives as exaggerated responses to antecedents. Identifying the source of chronic stress or illness becomes as important as identifying the triggers that preceded the over-threshold behavior.

Client and Patient Red Flags in Behavioral History

While the behavioral wellness form (Figures 12.1 and 12.2) is a means to identify "red flags," there may be additional clues that your patient's behavioral wellness is compromised. Client language choice and specific patient behavior(s) inside or outside the hospital environment also yield clues.

Some ways of describing the pet may be "red flags" inviting exploration. For example, a client may tell you their pet has "been abused." This is a common description that may indicate improper socialization or fears and phobias, whether or not the pet was actually abused. Explore this further by asking the client "Tell me more about that."

Similarly, behaviors observed in the hospital may also signal to the professional that a problem may be brewing outside the hospital environment. For example, a patient that shows aggression with handling may have other fears that deserve investigation. You can investigate this further with questions like "How has he done with other veterinary visits?" or "Tell me about his comfort level with strangers" or "How does he do with nail trims at home?" See the online materials for Chapter 12 for patient "red flags" and how to interpret/explore them further.

A Special Note About Puppies and Kittens (Red Flag)

Puppies and kittens who exhibit lack of affiliative (friendly) behavior or show fear of new environments and people deserve special attention. Puppies and kittens should be joyful, soft, wiggly, and they should be engaging with people, objects, and the environment. They should not hide under chairs nor separate themselves from you and your staff. The urgency for intervention intensifies when these behaviors are associated with puppies and kittens seen during sequential wellness and vaccination appointments (e.g. under 20 weeks of age). Godbout et al. (2007) used puppy behaviors such as active avoidance, locomotion, panting, and vocalization to easily identify these statistical outliers. We consider these patients "red flag" patients that warrant behavioral intervention quickly. See Chapters 6 (Puppies) and 7 (Kittens) for a review of developmental stages that play a role in both the emergence of problem behaviors and effective interventions, as data also indicates that these fearful behavior patterns predict similar risky patterns in adult dogs (Godbout and Frank 2011). These young patients are at higher risk for future relinquishment or worse - behavioral euthanasia. Interventions are needed to support the protective client bond with that animal and prevent its formation from being blocked or broken due to client frustration and unmet expectations about living with the pet (Martin et al. 2014). The authors consider these patients to be "behavioral emergencies." Immediate effective intervention is needed.

Step 2 – Medical Rule Outs

Behavior problems often have a basis in a medical condition and, conversely, a medical problem may be a result of a behavior disorder. It is a fallacy to consider medical and behavior problems separately – we do this here solely for ease of explanation. As veterinarians, we use the medical model, a scientific process involving observation, description, and differentiation, which moves from recognizing and treating symptoms to identifying disease etiologies and developing specific treatments (Shah and Mountain 2007). The familiar DAMNIT

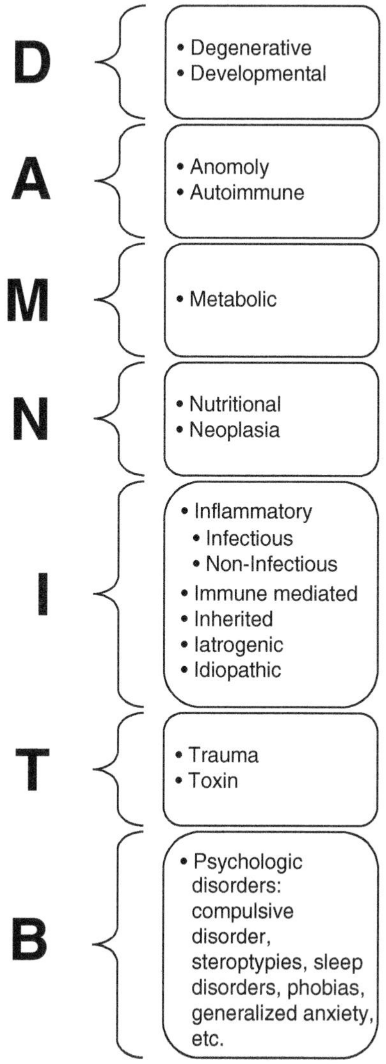

D
• Degenerative
• Developmental
A
• Anomoly
• Autoimmune
M
• Metabolic
N
• Nutritional
• Neoplasia
I
• Inflammatory
• Infectious
• Non-Infectious
• Immune mediated
• Inherited
• Iatrogenic
• Idiopathic
T
• Trauma
• Toxin
B
• Psychologic disorders: compulsive disorder, steroptypies, sleep disorders, phobias, generalized anxiety, etc.

Figure 12.5 The DAMNIT-B scheme for differential diagnoses of presenting behavioral problems as a means of establishing a list of medical rule outs.

scheme (Figure 12.5) can be used with the recognition that behavioral and medical comorbidities are frequently and intimately linked (Figure 12.6). Landsburg et al describe a DAMNIT-B scheme, which includes "Brain" to include common behavioral complaints (Landsberg et al. 2013).

Medical problems often contribute to behavior concerns. The concept of trigger stacking applies in this situation, as illness or pain can decrease the patient's ability to cope with stressors. Dogs and cats who are painful or sick may show increased aggression towards humans or other animals or have increased sensitivities to people, objects, and situations they fear. Cognitive decline or other aging problems (decreased vision, decreased hearing) can present as increased aggression, decreased affiliative behavior, and nocturnal wakefulness. Hyperthyroidism in cats can present as aggression and inappropriate elimination. The authors have diagnosed several patients presenting for multiple GI foreign bodies with hyperadrenocorticism with no other clinical pathologic abnormalities. Lick granulomas may have a basis in a skin disease that causes pruritus, which provokes licking that eventually becomes self-soothing. All of these examples show the intertwining of medical and behavioral pathologies.

If a pet presents with an acute change in behavior, it is the authors' experience that one must delve diligently into a hunt for underlying medical conditions. Acute behavior changes, particularly after social maturity has passed, often have a basis in a medical condition, particularly in the absence of a major change in the pet's environment. The collection of a complete history is important to finding clues that the behavior truly is new. Ruling out medical problems generally requires a thorough history, physical exam, minimum database (see Box 12.2), orthopedic and neurologic evaluations, +/− any indicated imaging or other diagnostic testing (e.g. further endocrine testing) (Horwitz and Pike 2014). This will also serve as a baseline for any needed pharmacologic intervention.

Step 3 – Safety Advice

Cases where there is a risk that the patient may injure themselves or others may require you to address at least prevention/safety advice to identify and avoid all previously known triggers for the behavior. Share and document your concerns with the client, even if the client does not identify this as high priority.

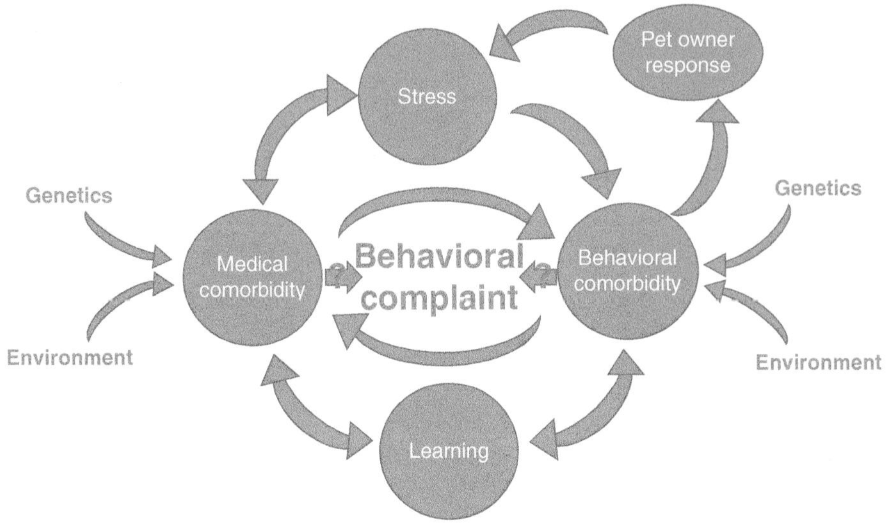

Figure 12.6 Behavioral and medical diagnoses are not mutually exclusive and are frequently and intimately linked.

Box 12.2 Minimum diagnostic database for behavior triage. Adapted from Horwitz and Pike 2014

Physical examination
Basic neurologic and orthopedic assessment
CBC
Chemistry panel
Total T4*
Urinalysis

* If total T4 is low, also run Free T4 by ED and TSH

The goal of the safety advice is to keep the pet and people from getting hurt, as well as to prevent the patient's ability to practice the unwanted behavior. The more times a behavior is rehearsed, the more likely it is to be performed again. Safety advice does not replace a behavior treatment plan, nor does it require a diagnosis.

When giving safety advice:

- Be specific
- Address known issues
- Address likely issues
- Chart

Safety advice is generated from the ABCs you identified in the history. You may need to be creative and engage the client in practical solutions for their family – the more feasible the plan, the higher the probability of success. Let us consider a dog who becomes destructive and injures themselves when left alone. The safety advice for this pet is "don't leave them alone until a behavior consultation for a full behavior plan can be done". Ways to accomplish this may include hiring a pet sitter, taking the dog to a well-run daycare, rotating work schedules, or any other creative solution. You might gain help from a medical standpoint by prescribing "crisis buster" medications as part of the safety plan. It is not up to you to solve this problem for the client within the confines of the triage – your job is to suggest safety steps that are doable for their family and to guide them in the goals of the safety plan. Do not underestimate your clients' creativity or commitment! One client built a separate room adjacent to their home (complete with a separate fenced yard) to solve their family's dog-to-dog aggression issue. Client engagement in the process may bring forward excellent solutions that you did not anticipate, so do not neglect to partner with them in finding solutions.

The more difficult it is for the client to accomplish or implement safety advice, the more urgent a full behavior consultation becomes.

Ask the client for help and feedback: "Where are we going to fail?" "What have I missed?" "Tell me where you see a problem with our plan so we can adjust it if we need." Keep in mind safety advice may not be successful if the pet cannot tolerate it – stress reduction is an essential simultaneous step with safety.

In cases of aggression, or where pets or people are being injured, safety advice may need to be given even if the time is not available for a full behavior triage. Documentation of your discussions in the medical record is extremely important in these cases.

Step 4 – Stress Reduction

Stress is the imbalance between environmental demand and response capability (McGrath 1970), or the inability to cope with an environment. Two main types of stress exist: normal or "good" stress and distress or "negative" stress (overload). Distressed animals often respond with one of the four F's - flight, fight, (Cannon 1929), freeze, or fidget (Gray 1988). Fear, arousal, and anxiety are the gas in the engine of most problems. The reduction of distress supports welfare of the patient, improves the patient's tolerance of prescribed management strategies, and, therefore, also increases the client's adherence to an agreed-upon safety plan. A multimodal approach is most effective. Collaborate with the client on how to implement all the stress reduction strategies that the case allows. Reduction strategies generally fall into the following categories:

- Environmental enrichment
- Exercise
- Pheromone therapy
- Elimination of stressful interactions between the client and the pet
- +/− "Crisis buster" medication

Environmental Enrichment

Environmental enrichment is the improvement in biological functioning of animals as a result of modifying their environment (Newberry 1995) and is accomplished through additions to the environment that are safe and perceived as positive by the patient. Environmental enrichment can be organized into five categories: social, nutritional, occupational, sensory, and physical (See online materials for Chapter 12 for full description and examples). Enrichment programs promote behavioral wellness and mitigate distress through consistency, predictability, and promoting an animal's sense of control over the environment and themselves. Effective environmental enrichment programs increase environmental complexity and normal species-typical behavior, facilitate normal temporal patterns of behavior, reduce abnormal and problem behavior, and help animals cope with stressors (Shepherdson 1994).

Tailor enrichment activities to each patient's presenting problem behavior, individual preferences, living environment, and level of practicality for caretakers. Considering the context of reported problem behaviors and how each individual pet responds uniquely to stress will also help clarify which environmental enrichment practices are likely to be most impactful. Select enrichment activities that encourage pets to perform natural behaviors such as social interactions, exploring and interacting with the environment, and chewing. For example, food puzzles can stimulate appetitive behaviors, increase diversity of behavior, and decrease the frequency of barking (Schipper et al. 2008).

Begin by first providing enrichment activities during calm relaxed periods (e.g. not associated with presenting problematic behavior). This will aid in general stress reduction, ensure the patient both knows how to use the enrichment and is comfortable doing so and does not inadvertently make an association between a new enrichment activity and negative emotional state associated with situations surrounding the problem behavior. Next, you may advise the client to implement targeted enrichment activities offered just prior to and during situations associated with the problematic behavior. Rotate enrichment activities and items frequently (Pullen et al. 2012). Enrichment is only valuable if it matters to the pet. An item or activity is not enriching if the patient does not use it, is afraid of it, or is bored with it.

After implementation of environmental enrichment, utilize continued monitoring of body language and behavior to ensure the pet is enjoying the experience, evaluate if the practices are effective and when it is time to rotate enrichment tools. As recommended by the American Veterinary Society of Animal Behavior (2021), all training activities should be implemented using the most effective and humane, scientific, evidence-based methods of force-free, positive reinforcement training. Lastly, encourage caretakers to strictly supervise first interactions with enrichment activities to ensure safety. It is critical to monitor pets until sure how they will use and engage with the enrichment tools, particularly toys and chews, to ensure the pet will not break off pieces that are sharp or can be swallowed.

Exercise

While proper exercise certainly has physical health benefits for dogs and cats, it likely has behavioral ones as well. While the data is extremely limited in dogs and virtually nonexistent in cats, there is ample literature on other mammals, from rodents to humans, that allows us to infer that exercise can be an effective tool in managing their behavioral health. For example, voluntary exercise has been shown to produce anxiolytic and antidepressant effects in mice (Duman et al. 2008). Physical activity interventions have a large academic evidence base for adults (men and women), and a growing one for adolescents and children (Carney and Firth 2021). Exercise is recommended as an adjunctive piece in the mental health care of people with diagnoses ranging from anxiety disorders to depression (e.g. major, pre/postpartum) and schizophrenia (Ashdown-Franks et al. 2019). Tiira and Lohi (2015) found a correlation between dogs' caregiver-reported daily amount of exercise and canine anxieties (e.g. noise sensitivities and separation anxiety).

Begin by advising clients on appropriate exercise intensity levels for their pets, time limitations, and examples of specific activity opportunities to ensure that they are safe for the individual patient. Then ensure that the specific activities do not contradict other behavioral avoidance advice. For example, dog play may provide both social and exercise opportunities, but dogs displaying aggression toward unfamiliar dogs certainly do not belong at the dog park. They may, however, be able to play with dogs from the household in a secure private area protected from other dogs. Cat families may need extra help identifying types of play that encourage gross movement and exercise for their pets. Some experts recommend utilizing a cat's "prey preference" (Dickman and Newsome 2015) if it is known. For example, if a cat shows hunting behavior directed at birds (feather toys), mice (fur-covered toys, balls, or pompoms), lizards (streamers or ribbons), or insects (laser pointer), it may inform what types of play activities a cat is most likely to engage in. Some cats may be encouraged to chase toys such as feathers or ribbons on a stick. Incorporating steps, climbing, or jumping up and over furniture can add aerobic activity to these common play activities. Caretakers of cats that like to chase after balls can create an opportunity for speed and continued play by placing ping-pong balls in a dry bathtub or teaching the cat to fetch.

Pheromone Therapy

Synthetic pheromone therapy (refer to Chapter 4 for a review of natural pheromones and their functions) can be used to modulate emotional states. In our clinical experience, pheromone therapy is a useful tool in both the prevention and reduction of feline and canine stress and is particularly effective when combined with other evidence-based behavior management and modification strategies. While there are some conflicting opinions, adjunctive pheromone therapy is easy for clients to implement, has no known side effects, and is a very practical, safe recommendation (Landsburg et al. 2013).

An analog of the F3 fraction of the feline facial pheromone, which is currently sold under the name FELIWAY Classic®, can reduce urine marking (Frank et al. 1999; Mills and Mills 2001; Mills and White 2000; Pageat 1997; White and Mills 1997) and signs of stress in cats traveling (Gaultier et al. 1998), ease the stress related to new environments (Pageat and Tessier 1997), including those associated with the veterinary hospital (Griffith et al. 2000) and handling (Kronen et al. 2006; Pereira et al. 2015), as well as reduce clinical signs of Feline Idiopathic Cystitis (Gunn-Moore and Cameron 2004), a syndrome strongly associated with stress. An analog of feline appeasing pheromone, marketed as FELIWAY Multicat®, reduced aggression in housemate cats when used along with behavior modification techniques (DePorter et al. 2019). A newer product, FELIWAY Optimum®, includes a feline pheromone complex that addresses multiple stress-related behaviors including urine marking, destructive scratching, social, nonsocial and situational fears, and inter-cat conflict (De Jaeger et al. 2021).

ADAPTIL®, now sold as ThunderEase®, includes a synthetic maternal pheromone (dog appeasing pheromone), and has been used to reduce stress during travel (Gaultier and Pageat 2003), in rescue and sheltered dogs (Osella et al. 2015; Tod et al. 2005), in dogs with separation anxiety (Gaultier et al. 2005; Kim et al. 2010) and noise phobia (Landsberg et al. 2015; Levine and Mills 2008; Sheppard and Mills 2003), to improve cat-dog interactions (Prior and Mills 2020), to reduce fear of handling and the hospital environment (Mills et al. 2006; Siracusa et al. 2010), to ease the stress associated with a puppy's transition from its dam and litter into a new home environment (Gaultier et al. 2009; Taylor and Mills 2007) and exposures during the socialization phase (Denenberg and Landsberg 2008). Another product, ZENIDOG® (Virbac, Fort Worth, TX), has more recently come on the market and one study shows it has similar efficacy to ADAPTIL® in calming dogs in their homes (Nicolas et al. 2022). For homes where electrical outlets may be limited, this gel-based, nonelectrical diffuser may be a viable pheromone therapy option.

Stop Stressful Interactions

Discontinuation of punishment or other inconsistent, stressful, negative interactions between the caretaker(s) and the patient is critical. Any strategies that utilize techniques that are perceived as aversive *by the pet* can be problematic, particularly with sensitive animals. Physical correction or punishment is always discouraged as it may exacerbate the problem, create fear between caregiver and pet, increase anxiety, and even lead to aggression (Herron et al. 2009). It may also blunt important signals of behavioral intent, making it more difficult for clients to predict impending aggression and reducing safety.

Behavior modification strategies should remain focused on least invasive minimally aversive (LIMA) techniques (Lindsay 2005), such as positive reinforcement and negative punishment (see Chapter 5). These techniques come with fewer risks of "side effects" or unintended consequences such as classically conditioned negative emotional responses. Clients may have attempted aversive strategies to stop or discourage specific pet behavior. In many sensitive animals, what may seem to be a "low-level" correction such as scolding or startling with sound or water can produce the same complications as "high-level" corrections such as shock in more tolerant animals. Interactions that caretakers *intend* to be positive, yet the pet's behavioral signals indicate that they are not, must also be discontinued (e.g. rough play, social interactions, or approach of fearful animals, and interactions with their own species to whom they are fearful). Consistent, predictable interactions are key. To illustrate how critical this is, livestock work has shown that while positive interactions are ideal, surprisingly even consistent negative interactions with handlers create less animal distress than those that include a mix of both positive and negative interactions (Hemsworth et al. 1987). In the author's experience, some of the most distressed and dangerous patients are those with caretakers whose responses to their pet's behavior vacillates wildly between extremely permissive and punitive responses.

Finally, requesting that a client discontinue a pattern of behavior with their animal can be difficult. Success requires careful and effective communication, and great care should be taken to accomplish that. Disappointment surrounding the loss of the "pet they imagined" or the ability to interact with their animal in a manner that they themselves find rewarding can play a role. Inadvertently eliciting shame surrounding being wrong or having engaged in a pattern of behaviors that have unintentionally harmed the pet they love can also contribute to increased resistance to receiving these recommendations.

Crisis Buster Medication

Incorporating medications into the patient's plan is often needed for safety and stress reduction to be successful. "Event" medications such as clonidine, gabapentin, trazodone, and certain benzodiazepines can be used individually or in combination to quickly decrease fear and anxiety in the right patient. See Chapter 21 for more information on pharmacologic interventions, including immediate-acting medications to provide crisis relief for animals awaiting a full behavior evaluation and plan. We often refer to these immediate-acting medications as "crisis busters" when communicating with clients, because their effects can be seen the day that they are given (e.g. differentiating them from those that require daily administration for up to four to six weeks to take full effect). This immediate relief impacts the patient, their caretakers, and your plan's success.

These medications can make the use of other stress reduction strategies more successful, maximizing their full benefit. Reduction of patient distress decreases their psychological suffering and the likelihood of injury to themselves or others. It also increases the patient's ability to tolerate critical management and safety advice (e.g. confinement and separation from humans or pets in the family).

When help is not provided to blunt negative responses to management strategies, clients are unlikely to follow your safety advice, increasing risks. They may also become increasingly frustrated and consider relinquishment or euthanasia before a full behavior consult can be attained. On occasion, we will also start longer-acting medications at the time of triage (e.g. selective serotonin reuptake inhibitors), particularly when the wait time for referral to an academically trained behaviorist is long. Need help getting started? Veterinary behaviorists frequently offer "vet-to-vet" consultations regarding psychotropic medications, particularly for patients scheduled and waiting to be seen.

Step 5 – Recommended Referral

While your more complicated and/or dangerous behavior cases should be referred to an academically trained behaviorist immediately, many others can be referred to other resources, including trainers, handouts, and basic wellness education. Figure 12.7 illustrates the preferred interventions for behavior problems based on severity. Many behaviors that clients may ask you about are undesired yet normal behaviors, such as dogs who jump on strangers, dig holes in the backyard, and chew on items, and cats who scratch furniture or jump on counters. Animals are highly driven to perform species-typical behaviors, and it is important to ensure that appropriate outlets for these behaviors are provided. You can utilize the help of handouts and qualified trainers to help with behavioral wellness-related concerns. This is represented in Figure 12.7. in green, below the blue line.

Animals with more severe problems and those involving abnormal behavior (Figure 12.7 above the blue line) will need additional intervention from you or a behavior professional. Significant fearful, repetitive/

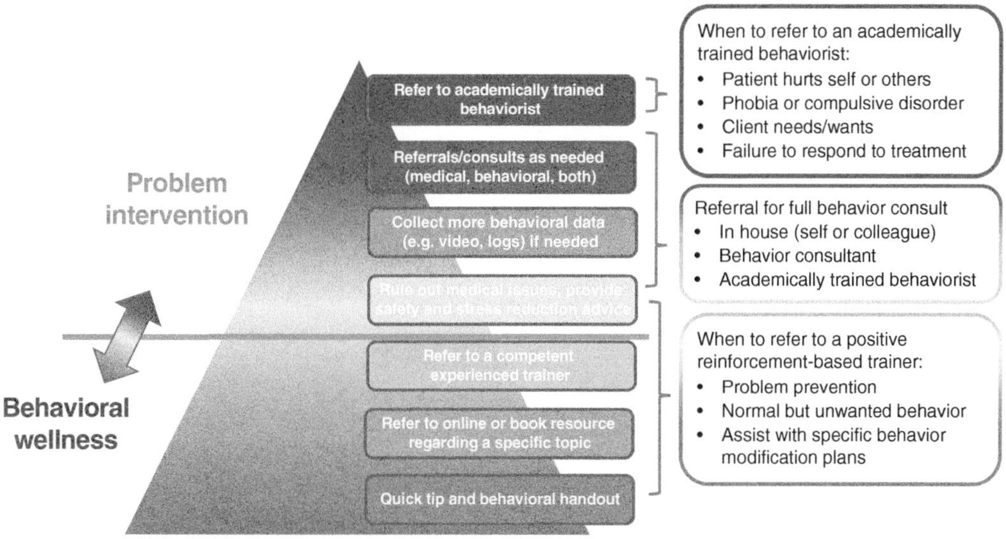

Figure 12.7 The behavior triage pyramid gives an overview of how to handle and refer behavior cases.

compulsive, and aggressive behaviors often require more than training. While training of specific behaviors will likely be a part of a behavior modification program, it will fall short of addressing these issues alone. In fact, anxious or fearful pets likely will not be able to effectively learn unless the underlying cause of their objectionable behaviors is identified and treated appropriately. Effective referral to humane, evidence-based resources for intervention must also be appropriately tailored to the type of presenting behavior. For example, a referral to an academically trained behaviorist may be overkill for litter box training a new kitten, and most certainly a handout or quick exam room tip from the veterinary care team is a dangerously inappropriate referral resource for a dog that recently went through a plate glass window during a storm or for one who bit a small child.

Who Are Behavior Professionals?

Evidence based strategies are as critical in behavioral interventions as they are in medical ones. Trained behavior professionals are an important part of the extended veterinary team and are vital to the success of many of the challenging behavior problems faced every day in general practice.

The types of professionals are:

1) Professional trainers – Teach key skills to animals and provide tools and information to clients promote behavioral and overall wellness. They are also used to help implement a behaviorist's behavior modification plan. Refer to a trainer for normal but undesirable or unruly behaviors or for basic training of skills (Hanmerle et al. 2015).
   ►Certifications to look for: KPA CTP, CPDT (See Appendix).
2) Behavior Consultants – Help identify what is causing the problem, develop an intervention plan to change the problem behavior, and help the caregivers learn how to execute that plan (Miller 2016).
   ►Certifications to look for: CTC, IAABC.
3) Academically trained behaviorists – These specialists are specifically trained to treat problem behaviors. Referral to these specialists is recommended for patients who hurt others (animal or human), hurt themselves, have profound phobias, or have multiple problems. Aggression, particularly pets who inflict serious injuries, should always be referred to an academically

trained behaviorist. Referral is also indicated if the patient fails to respond to your initial therapy or your client requests it (Hanmerle et al. 2015).

- ►Applied animal behaviorists (MA, MS, or Ph.D.) – Certification will be CAAB or ACAAB, and have a master's or Ph.D. related to applied animal behavior.
- ►Veterinary Behaviorists – Veterinarians who have done additional training and achieved board certification in veterinary behavior. Certification will be DACVB.

4) Veterinary technicians with specialty certification in behavior – Certification will be RVT-VTS (Behavior), and many will have other certifications such as those associated with professional trainers and consultants.

If an academically trained behaviorist is not available in your area, remote consultations may be available, or look for a DVM/VMD with a special interest in or *practice limited* to behavior.

Resources for Finding Behavior Professionals

- AVSAB Humane Dog Training Position Statement https://avsab.ftlbcdn.net/wp-content/uploads/2021/08/AVSAB-Humane-Dog-Training-Position-Statement-2021.pdf
- AAHA Behavior Guidelines – Choosing a Team https://www.aaha.org/aaha-guidelines/behavior-management/assembling-a-team/
- Fear Free Happy Homes Finding a Qualified Trainer or Behavior Consultant https://www.fearfreehappyhomes.com/kit/behavior-problem-solving/download/19169/?fbclid=IwAR0tJZ5v49MnMnSHTPvGJqSebnt3L67jq-BkGvYm2HZajM5UBD_wRA2gOOQ
- Team Tool: Help veterinary clients find a dog trainer in 4 easy steps (Lisa Radosta, DVM, DACVB) https://www.dvm360.com/view/team-tool-help-veterinary-clients-find-dog-trainer-4-easy-steps

There is an overlap between these professionals – experienced and skilled trainers can help identify when further referral is needed. Consultants can often assist with less complex problems and will also help you and your client identify when referral to an academically trained behaviorist is needed. If medications are needed, only a licensed veterinarian and/or veterinary behaviorist can prescribe.

Finding a Behavior Professional

The behavior professional field is largely unregulated and difficult for both veterinary professionals and clients to navigate. Poor advice may not only block success but cause harm by escalating or creating new problems to add to the complaint list (Hanmerle et al. 2015). Care should be taken that your clients are referred to a professional practicing humane, science-based techniques (Hanmerle et al. 2015). Based on current scientific evidence, the American Veterinary Society of Animal Behavior recommends that only reward-based training methods be used for all dog training, including the treatment of behavior problems (AVSAB 2021).

There are many credentialing organizations, although lack of regulation means that there is no legal educational requirement or credentialing that is required to call oneself a trainer, behavior consultant, or behaviorist. Literally anyone can use these terms. Credentials do not guarantee the methods used will be appropriate for your clients. This means that you must research your behavior partners carefully before making a referral.

Carefully consider your training and behavior consultant partnerships via the following steps:

1) Identify certifications (Appendix) – Does the certification match with the services offered?
2) Identify membership in organizations that promote non-aversive LIMA (least intrusive minimal aversive) methods, for example, Pet Professional Guild and Fear Free®.
3) Visit the professional's website – Look for certifications and training philosophy including the use of "buzzwords" (see

Box 12.3) and red flags (see Box 12.4). Look at the pictures and videos – Assess body language of the animals in the images and look for choke, shock, or prong collars.

Box 12.3 "Buzzwords" to avoid in training and behavior consulting

- Balanced – Generally refers to trainers who use both reward-based and aversive training methods. "Balanced" interactions are known to be the most stress-provoking in livestock.
- Dominance – Use of dominance in training and consulting is outdated (see AVSAB Dominance Position Statement: https://avsab.ftlbcdn.net/wp-content/uploads/2019/01/Dominance_Position_Statement-download.pdf).
- Pack leader, alpha, respect, "pack heals the dog," leadership – May indicate use of outdated dominance theory.
- Guarantee – No behavior professional should guarantee results.

Box 12.4 Behavior professional red flags

AVSAB and AAHA recommend changing professionals if any of the following are observed:

- Prong or choke collars
- Shock collars sometimes known as "e-collars" or electronic collars
- Collar jerks or yanks
- Use of dominance methods, e.g. "alpha rolls" or "dominance downs"
- Use of other intimidation such as yelling, staring, squirting bottles, shaker noise cans, compressed air
- Forcing fearful dogs to stay in class
- Having a high student-to-teacher ratio

4) Read testimonials and social media (look for use of shock collars or other aversive methods).
5) Ask questions:
   Does the professional attend continuing education regularly or is it required by their certification?
   Does the professional have liability insurance?
   What training philosophy/methods does the professional use? For example, you can ask, "Under which situations do you use pinch, choke, and shock collars?" The trainer should answer that they never do (Radosta 2019).
6) Visit and watch a training session (class or private if allowed) – There is a demand for non-aversive methods, and some will say they use only positive reinforcement when they actually use aversive methods. The pets and the people should look comfortable and like they are having a good time. It is never acceptable for a consultant to be shaming or derogatory with a client when teaching them to help their pet.
7) Remember that only veterinarians can legally recommend/prescribe medications. While you want trainers/nonveterinary behavior professionals to refer dogs back to you who may need assistance from anxiety-relieving medications, it is inappropriate for them to recommend specific medications or to adjust doses.
8) Check references.

Self-Referrals and Cases you Feel Comfortable Seeing

As a general practitioner, you may have an interest in behavior cases, as so many of our clients ask for this help. If so, continuing education will be critical in building your knowledge base about the diagnosis and treatment of behavior problems. The behavior cases you may wish to see will vary with your interest, opportunities for training and continuing education, and possibly even with experience with your own pets. For example, if you have managed your own pet with separation anxiety, you may feel well-equipped to treat this type of case in your general practice. Other examples are inappropriate elimination, noise phobias, digging, and unruly behavior. You may even feel comfortable managing inter-cat aggression problems. In general, the authors recommend referral for aggression and patients that have failed to respond to your initial therapy.

Setting Up the Behavior-focused Visit

As mentioned in the introduction, you may see behavior cases in three main circumstances:

1) Brief triage – A triage performed within the confines of a medical appointment; generally needs to be followed by either a full triage appointment and/or referral.
2) Full triage – Generally a standalone appointment to perform the steps in this chapter more completely, with the intention of referral for diagnosis and treatment if needed.
3) Full behavior consult – For the practitioner with an interest in behavior, you may see a behavior problem with the plan of diagnosing and making a behavior modification plan for the pet.

The brief triage is in response to a significant concern presented during a medical appointment, where you feel there is danger to the pet, humans, or other animals, and the client has elected to focus on the medical concerns. This abbreviated triage generally consists of identifying triggers, consequences, and generating as much safety advice as possible. For example, for a pet that growled at a child, safety advice is that the dog should have no contact with children until a full triage or referral can be accomplished. The authors engage the clients to think of other triggers to avoid, and also briefly discuss safe haven (e.g. a safe space that includes all important resources for the pet and enrichment) and stress reduction for the pet.

A full triage, as discussed above, may be within confines of another traditional visit, or scheduled separately. It is the authors' experience that an effective behavior triage appointment may take more time than an average general practice appointment, and we recommend scheduling an hour to start. In addition, many patients presenting with behavior problems may need triage for handling (see Chapters 11 and 22). The whole veterinary team is crucial to success in identifying the concern and scheduling the appointments appropriately. During a full triage appointment, if patient demeanor allows, collect your minimum database (Box 12.2). You will need to make time for adequate documentation, as clear instructions are needed. Use handouts whenever possible. Documentation of your recommendations is crucial, as there may be liability if your instructions are not followed, particularly in aggression cases. The follow-up to this appointment will be referral (handouts, trainer, self-referral, or behavior professional). The fee structure should take into consideration several factors, including the practice's current exam fees, space, and personnel resources utilized, as well as time to prepare and deliver your recommendations. Keep in mind that your medical rule out process is likely to generate additional revenue which may help justify the extended examination time.

A full behavior consult involves the triage process history, medical rule outs, followed by a behavioral diagnosis and discussion of the management of the problem, including safety advice and stress reduction strategies, as well as the substantial addition of a full behavior modification plan and follow up to ensure needed adjustments to the plan can be made. You may choose to limit the types of cases seen to those with which you have experience, e.g. separation anxiety, inappropriate elimination, and noise phobias. Referral is always recommended when the pet is injuring themselves or others, when there are multiple problems, or the patient has not responded to initial therapy. We would recommend starting with an hour-long appointment (base this on your needs), with scheduled follow up appointments (these could be via telemedicine if needed). The consult fee should be higher than a regular general practice appointment or a triage appointment, as continuing education is generally needed to effectively see these types of appointments and greater time is often invested in preparation, delivery, and follow-up.

Behavior Professional Certifications

Certification	Title	Certifying organization	Notes
		Academically trained behaviorists	
DACVB	Diplomate of the American College of Veterinary Behaviorists	American College of Veterinary Behaviorists	Veterinarians with advanced training in behavior
ACAAB	Associate Certified Applied Animal Behaviorist	Animal Behavior Society	Academically trained applied animal behaviorists (MS, PhD)
CAAB	Certified Applied Animal Behaviorist		
RVT-VTS (Behavior)		Academy of Veterinary Behavior Technicians	Registered Veterinary Technician with advanced training in behavior
CCAB	Certificated Clinical Animal Behaviorist	Association for the Study of Animal Behavior	UK Certification
		Consultants and trainers	
CTC	Certificate in Training and Counseling	The Academy for Dog Trainers	+R
ABCDT	Animal Behavior College Certified Dog Trainer	Animal Behavior College	LIMA
CDT	Certified Dog Trainer	Association of Animal Behavior Professionals (AABP)	
CDBT	Certified Dog Behavior Technologist		
CPBT	Certified Parrot Behavior Technologist		
CCBT	Certified Cat Behavior Technologist		
CABT	Certified Animal Behavior Technologist		
CCA-CDT	Certified Dog Trainer	Canine Club Academy	Appears to be +R
CCDT	CATCH Certified Dog Trainer	CATCH Canine Trainers Academy	Based on CPDT and APDT standards
CDBC	Certified Dog Behavior Consultant	IAABC	LIMA
CCBC	Certified Cat Behavior Consultant		
CHBC	Certified Horse Behavior Consultant		
CPBC	Consultant Parrot Behavior Consultant		
CABC	Consultant Animal Behavior Consultant		
ACDBC	Associate Certified Dog Behavior Consultant		
IAABC-ADT	Accredited Dog Trainer		
SBA	Shelter Behavior Associate		
CSB-D	Certified in Shelter Behavior – Dog		
CSB-C	Certified in Shelter Behavior – Cat		
CSBS	Certified Shelter Behavior Specialist		

(Continued)

Certification	Title	Certifying organization	Notes
CPDT-KA	Certified Professional Dog Trainer – Knowledge Assessed	Certification Council for Professional Dog Trainers® (CCPDT)	APDT LIMA
CPDT-KSA	Certified Professional Dog Trainer – Knowledge and Skills Assessed		
CBCC-KA	Certified Behavior Consultant Canine – Knowledge Assessed		
Cert CBST	Canine Behavior Sciences and Technology Certificate	Companion Animal Sciences Institute	Appears to be +R
Cert CF	Canine Fitness Certificate		
Cert CN	Canine Nutrition Certificate		
Cert DDC	Dog Daycare Certificate		
Cert DT	Dog Training Certificate		
Cert FBST	Feline Behavior Sciences and Technology Certificate		
Cert PBST	Parrot Behavior Sciences and Technology Certificate		
Cert PDTST	Professional Dog Training Science and Technology Certificate		
Cert SRW	Shelter and Rescue Work Certificate		
Dip ABT	Diploma in Animal Behavior Technology		
Dip CBST	Diploma in Canine Behavior Science and Technology		
DIP CCBT	Diploma of Canine Counseling and Behavior Training		
Dip FBST	Diploma of Feline Behavior Science and Technology		
Dip PBST	Diploma in Parrot Behavior Science and Technology		
CTDI	Certified Trick Dog Instructor	Do More with Your Dog!	Appears to be +R
CTBC	Certified Training and Behavior Consultant	Dog Training Internship Academy	Appears to be +R
CDW	Certified Dog Walker	Previously Dogtec, now DogBiz	Appears to be +R
CBATI	Certified Behavior Adjustment Training Instructors	Grisha Stewart, MA, CPDT-KA, KPACTP	+R
KPA CTP	Karen Pryor Academy Certified Training Partner	Karen Pryor Academy	+R
PMCT	Pat Miller Certified Trainer	Peaceable Paws, Pat Miller, CBCC-KA, CPDT-KA	+R
VSA-CDT	Victoria Stilwell Academy Certified Dog Trainer	Victoria Stillwell Academy	+R
VSPDT	Victoria Stilwell Positively Dog Trainer		
AKC CGC	American Kennel Club Good Citizen Evaluator	American Kennel Club (AKC)	
CDT	Certified Dog Trainer	Various Organizations	Check with trainer
IACP-CDT	Certified Dog Trainer	International Association of Dog Trainers	NOT LIMA
IACP-CDTA	Certified Dog Trainer Advanced		
NADOI	Certified by NADOI	National Association of Dog Obedience Instructors (NADOI)	NOT LIMA

Other Important Certifying Organizations

Fear Free® – www.fearfreepets.com – provides online education to professionals (veterinarians, veterinary technicians, behavior consultants, trainers, groomers, pet sitters, boarding kennels, and shelters). Fear Free® Certified Professionals and Practices have taken knowledge-based assessment in recognition of and implementation of strategies that reduce pet fear, anxiety, and stress.

Pet Professional Guild – www.petprofessionalguild.com – To be in any way affiliated with the Pet Professional Guild all members must adhere to a strict code of conduct. Pet Professional Guild members understand Force-Free to mean: No shock, No pain, No choke, No fear, No physical force and No compulsion-based methods are ever employed to train or care for a pet.

References

Adams, C.L. and Frankel, R.M. (2007). It may be a dog's life but the relationship with her owners is also key to her health and well being: communication in veterinary medicine. *Vet. Clin. North America: Small Anim. Pract.* 37 (1): 1–17.

Appleby, D., Bradshaw, J., and Casey, R. (2002). Relationship between aggressive and avoidance behaviour by dogs and their experience in the first six months of life. *Vet. Rec.* 150 (14): 434–438.

Ashdown-Franks, G., Sabiston, C.M., and Stubbs, B. (2019). The evidence for physical activity in the management of major mental illnesses: a concise overview to inform busy clinicians' practice and guide policy. *Curr. Opin. Psychiatry* 32 (5): 375–380.

American Veterinary Society of Animal Behavior (AVSAB) (2021). AVSAB position statement on humane dog training. s.l. https://AVSAB.org (accessed 25 February 2024).

Cannon, W.B. (1929). *Bodily Changes in Pain, Hunger, Fear, and Rage: An Account of Recent Research into the Function of Emotional Excitement*, 2e. New York: Appleton-Century-Crofts.

Carney, R. and Firth, J. (2021). Exercise interventions in child and adolescent mental health care: an overview of the evidence and recommendations for implementation. *JCPP Adv.* 1 (4): e12031.

Catanzaro, T.E. (2001). *Promoting the Human-Animal Bond in Veterinary Practice*, 1e. Ames, IA: Iowa State University Press.

De Jaeger, X., Meppiel, L., Endersby, S., and Sparkes, A.H. (2021). An initial open-label study of a novel pheromone complex for use in cats. *Open J. Vet. Med.* 11 (3): 105–116.

Denenberg, S. and Landsberg, G.M. (2008). Effects of dog appeasing pheromone (D.A.P.®) on anxiety and fear in puppies during training and on long-term socialisation. *J. Am. Vet. Med. Assoc.* 233: 1874–1882.

DePorter, T., Bledsoe, D., Beck, A., and Ollivier, E. (2019). Evaluation of the efficacy of an appeasing pheromone diffuser product vs placebo for management of feline aggression in multi-cat households: a pilot study. *J. Feline Med. Surg.* 21 (4): 293–305.

Dickman, C.R. and Newsome, T.M. (2015). Individual hunting behaviour and prey specialisation in the house cat *Felis catus*: implications for conservation and management. *Appl. Anim. Behav. Sci.* 173: 76–87.

Duman, C.H., Schlesinger, L., Russell, D.S., and Duman, R.S. (2008). Voluntary exercise produces antidepressant and anxiolytic behavioral effects in mice. *Brain Res.* 1199: 148–158.

Frank, D., Erd, H.N., and Houpt, K.A. (1999). Urine spraying in cats: presence of concurrent disease and effects of a pheromone treatment. *Appl. Anim. Behav. Sci.* 61: 263–272.

Frankel, R.M. and Stein, T. (2001). Getting the most out of the clinical encounter: the four habits model. *J. Med. Pract. Manage.: MPM* 16 (4): 184–191.

Gaultier, E., Bonnafous, L., Bougrat, L. et al. (2005). Comparison of the efficacy of a synthetic dog appeasing pheromone with clomipramine for the treatment of separation-related disorders in dogs. *Vet. Rec.* 156: 533–538.

Gaultier, E., Bonnafous, L., Vienet-Lagué, D. et al. (2009). Efficacy of dog appeasing pheromone in reducing behaviours associated with fear of unfamiliar people and new surroundings in newly adopted puppies. *Vet. Rec.* 164: 708–714.

Gaultier, E. and Pageat, P. (2003). Effects of a synthetic dog appeasing pheromone (D.A.P.®) on behaviour problems during transport. In *Proceedings of the 4th International Behavior Meeting* (ed. Seksel K., Perry G., Mills D.), pp. 33–35 Caloundra, Australia, Posta Graduate Foundation in Veterinary Sciences, Sidney.

Gaultier, E., Pageat, P., and Tessier, Y. (1998). *Effect of a Feline Facial Pheromone Analogue (Feliway®) on Manifestations of Stress in Cats During Transport*, 198. Clermont-Ferrand, France: INRA.

Godbout, M. and Frank, D. (2011). Persistence of puppy behaviors and signs of anxiety during adulthood. *J. Vet. Behav.* 6 (1): 92.

Godbout, M., Palestrini, C., Beauchamp, G., and Frank, D. (2007). Puppy behavior at the veterinary clinic: a pilot study. *J. Vet. Behav.: Clin. Appl. Res.* 2: 26–135.

Gray, J.A. (1988). *The Psychology of Fear and Stress*, 2e. Cambridge: University Press.

Griffith, C.A., Steigerwald, E.S., and Buffington, C.A. (2000). Effects of a synthetic facial pheromone on behaviour of cats. *J. Am. Vet. Med. Assoc.* 217: 1154–1156.

Gunn-Moore, D.A. and Cameron, M.E. (2004). A pilot study using synthetic feline facial pheromone for the management of feline idiopathic cystitis. *J. Feline Med. Surg.* 6 (3): 133–138.

Hanmerle, M., Horst, C., Levine, E. et al. (2015). 2015 AAHA canine and feline behavior guidelines. *J. Am. Anim. Hosp. Assoc.* 51 (4): 205–221.

Hemsworth, P.H., Barnett, J.L., and Hansen, C. (1987). The influence of inconsistent handling by humans on the behaviour, growth and corticosteroids of young pigs. *Appl. Anim. Behav. Sci.* 17 (3–4): 245–252.

Herron, M.E., Shofer, F.S., and Reisner, I.R. (2009). Survey of the use and outcome of confrontational and non-confrontational training methods in client-owned dogs showing undesired behaviors. *Appl. Anim. Behav. Sci.* 117 (1–2): 47–54.

Horwitz, D.F. and Pike, A.L. (2014). Common sense behavior modification: a guide for practitioners. *Vet. Clin. North America, Small Anim. Pract.* 44 (3): 401–426.

Kim, Y.M., Lee, J.K., Abd El-aty, A.M. et al. (2010). Efficacy of dog-appeasing pheromone (DAP) for ameliorating separation-related behavioral signs in hospitalized dogs. *Canadian Vet. J. = La revue veterinaire canadienne* 51 (4): 380–384.

Kronen, P.W., Ludders, J.W., and Erb, H.N. (2006). A synthetic fraction of feline facial pheromones calms but does not reduce struggling in cats before venous catheterisation. *Vet. Anaesth. Analg.* 33: 258–265.

Landsberg, G., Hunthausen, W., and Ackerman, L. (2013). *Behavior Problems of the Dog and Cat*, 3e. New York: Saunders Elsevier.

Landsberg, G.M., Beck, A., Lopez, A. et al. (2015). Dog-appeasing pheromone collars reduce sound-induced fear and anxiety in beagle dogs: a placebo-controlled study. *Vet. Rec.* 177: 260.

Landsburg, G., Hunthausen, W., and Ackerman, L. (2013). Phermone therapy. In: *Behavior Problems of the Dog and Cat*, 3e, 144–145. New York: Saunders Elsevier.

Levine, E.D. and Mills, D.S. (2008). Long-term follow up of the efficacy of a behavioural treatment programme for dogs with firework fears. *Vet. Rec.* 162: 657–659.

Lindsay, S. (2005). *Handbook of Applied Dog Behavior and Training: Procedures and Protocols.* Ames, IA: Blackwell Publishing.

Martin, K., Martin, D., and Shaw, J.K. (2014). Small animal behavior triage: a guide for practitioners. *Vet. Clin. North America: Small Anim. Pract.* 44 (3): 379–399.

McGrath, J.E. (1970). *Social and Psychologial Factors in Stress.* New York: Holt, Rhinehart & Winston.

Miller, J. (2016). Animal behavior consulting 101 part 1: what is an animal behavior consultant? https://iaabc.org/articles/animal-behavior-consulting-101-part-1-what-is-an-animal-behavior-consultant (accessed 06 November 2021).

Mills, D.S. and Mills, C.B. (2001). Evaluation of a novel method for delivering a synthetic analogue of feline facial pheromone to control urine spraying by cats. *Vet. Rec.* 149: 197–199.

Mills, D.S., Ramos, D., Estelles, M.G., and Hargrave, C. (2006). A triple-blind placebo-controlled investigation into the assessment of the effect of dog appeasing pheromone on anxiety related behaviour of problem dogs in the veterinary clinic. *Appl. Anim. Behav. Sci.* 98: 114–126.

Mills, D.S. and White, J.C. (2000). Long-term follow-up of the effect of a pheromone therapy on feline spraying behaviour. *Vet. Rec.* 147: 746–747.

Moberg, G.P. (2000). Biological response to stress. In: *The Biology of Animal Stress* (ed. G.P. Moberg and J.A. Mench), 1–21. Walllingford, UK: CABI Publishing.

Newberry, R.C. (1995). Environmental enrichment: increasing the biological relevance of captive environments. *Appl. Anim. Behav. Sci.* 44 (2): 229–243.

Nicolas, C.S., Espuña, G., Girardin, A. et al. (2022). Owner-perception of the effects of two long-lasting dog-appeasing pheromone analog devices on situational stress in dogs. *Animals 12* (1): 122.

Osella, M.C., Bergamasco, L., Beck, A., and Gazzano, A. (2015). Adaptive mechanisms in dogs adopted from shelters: a behavioural assessment of the use of a synthetic analogue of the canine appeasing pheromone. *Dog Behav.* 1 (2): 1–12.

Pageat, P. (1997). Experimental evaluation of the efficacy of a synthetic analogue of cats' facial pheromones in inhibiting urine marking of sexual origin in adult tomcats. *J. Vet. Pharmacol. Therapy* 20: 169.

Pageat, P. and Tessier, Y. (1997). Usefulness of the F3 synthetic pheromone, Feliway®, in preventing behaviour problems in cats during holidays. *Proceedings of the First International Conference on Veterinary Behavioural Medicine*, p. 231, Birmingham, England (1–2 April 1997). Potters Bar, Herts: Universities Federation for Animal Welfare.

Pereira, J.S., Fragoso, S., Beck, A. et al. (2015). Improving the feline veterinary consultation: the usefulness of Feliway® spray in reducing cats' stress. *J. Feline Med. Surg.* 18 (12): 959–964.

Prior, M.R. and Mills, D.S. (2020). Cats vs. dogs: the efficacy of Feliway Friends™ and Adaptil™ products in multispecies homes. *Front. Vet. Sci.* 7: 399.

Pullen, A.J., Merrill, R.J., and Bradshaw, J.W. (2012). Habituation and dishabituation during object play in kennel-housed dogs. *Anim. Cognit.* 15: 1143–1150.

Radosta, L. (2019). Team tool: help veterinary clients find a dog trainer in 4 easy steps. https://www.dvm360.com/view/team-tool-help-veterinary-clients-find-dog-trainer-4-easy-steps (accessed 06 November 2021).

Roshier, A.L. and McBride, E.A. (2013). Canine behaviour problems: discussions between veterinarians and dog owners during annual booster consultations. *Vet. Rec.* 172 (9): 235.

Schipper, L.L., Vinke, C.M., Schilder, M.B., and Spruijt, B.M. (2008). The effect of feeding enrichment toys on the behaviour of kennelled dogs (Canis familiaris). *Appl. Anim. Behav. Sci. 114* (1-2): 182–195.

Shah, P.J. and Mountain, D. (2007). The medical model is dead – long live the medical model. *British J. Psych.* 191 (5): 375–377.

Shaw, J.R. (2006). Four core communication skills of highly effective practitioners. *Vet. Clin. North America: Small Anim. Pract.* 36 (2): 385–396.

Shepherdson, D. (1994). The role of environmental enrichment in the captive breeding and reintroduction of endangered species. In: *Creative Conservation* (ed. P.J. Olney, G.M. Mace, and A.T. Feistner), 167–177. Dordrecht: Springer.

Sheppard, G. and Mills, D.S. (2003). Evaluation of dog appeasing pheromone as a potential treatment for dogs fearful of fireworks. *Vet. Rec.* 152: 432–436.

Sherman, B.L. and Serpell, J.A. (2008). Training veterinary students in animal behavior to preserve the human–animal bond. *J. Vet. Med. Educ.* 35 (4): 496–502.

Siracusa, C., Manteca, X., Cuenca, R. et al. (2010). Effect of a synthetic appeasing pheromone on behavioural, neuroendocrine, immune, and acute-phase perioperative stress responses in dogs. *J. Am. Vet. Med. Assoc.* 237: 673–681.

Taylor, K. and Mills, D.S. (2007). A placebo-controlled study to investigate the effect of dog appeasing pheromone and other environmental and management factors on the reports of disturbance and house soiling during the night in recently adopted puppies (*Canis familiaris*). *Appl. Anim. Behav. Sci.* 105: 358–368.

Tiira, K. and Lohi, H. (2015). Early life experiences and exercise associate. *PLoS ONE* 10 (11): e0141907.

Tod, E., Brander, D., and Warian, N. (2005). Efficacy of dog appeasing pheromone in reducing stress and fear related behaviour in shelter dogs. *Appl. Anim. Behav. Sci.* 93 (3-4): 295–308.

White, J.C. and Mills, D.S. (1997). Efficacy of synthetic feline facial pheromone (F3) analogue (Feliway®) for the treatment of chronic non-sexual urine spraying by the domestic cat. *Proceedings of the First International Conference on Veterinary Behavioural Medicine*, p. 242, Birmingham, England (1–2 April 1997).

13

Feline Elimination Disorders

Amy L. Pike

Animal Behavior Wellness Center, Fairfax, VA, USA

Introduction

Urination and defecation outside of the litter box, often termed "feline inappropriate elimination" (FIE), is still a top behavior problem among our feline patients, and it continues to be the number one reason people relinquish their cats to shelters (Patronek et al. 1996; Salman et al. 2000). It can be one of the most frustrating disorders for clinicians to treat because of the insidious chronic nature of the disease, often made worse with any lack of client compliance.

Many of the issues that families consider to be behavior problems in their feline companions arise from normal behavioral patterns and repertoires that the cat performs in a location or manner that is undesired by the humans in the home. Inappropriate elimination is one such behavior that often stems from normal ethological and behavioral needs and, as such, may be better termed feline *undesirable* elimination (FUE). Many, if not most, instances of elimination outside of a human-designated area may seem quite *appropriate* from the cat's point of view. Understanding normal elimination behavior in cats can help us elucidate the underpinning of each patient's elimination disorder and allows the clinician to change the behavior in a way that is acceptable both to the client and the feline(s).

Normal Elimination Behavior

Cleanliness of the nest is an important predator avoidance strategy. Mother cats (queens) maintain cleanliness of the nesting site by stimulating the kitten's urogenital reflex and then consuming any eliminations (Beaver 2003). This process continues until roughly six weeks of age, well after the kittens are mobile and even after they are able to voluntarily eliminate starting around three weeks of age (Rosenblatt 1971; Himwich 1970). Cats are certainly fastidious creatures by nature, a trait that also translates to their need for a pristine litter box.

Latrine habits and preferences are developed early in a kitten's life. Kittens innately begin to rake loose dirt and sand and spend more time in the litter box or latrine site, starting around four weeks of age (Beaver 2003). Once exploration of the litter box begins, elimination in that area and subsequent covering behavior of the eliminations begins shortly thereafter (Beaver 2003). The kittens will gain familiarity with the desirable elimination area and often develop their substrate preferences through observation of the queen (Beaver 2003). When cats develop substrate and location preferences as a result of learning from the queen, caretakers need to be aware of such preferences in order to offer the most hospitable site and substrate for that cat.

Introduction to Animal Behavior and Veterinary Behavioral Medicine, First Edition. Edited by Meghan E. Herron.

Companion website: www.wiley.com/go/introductiontoanimalbehavior

Toileting Behavior

Normal urination behavior for the purpose of toileting includes sniffing (Figure 13.1) and then digging in the substrate to create a well over which cats will then position their hind end. Most cats will then squat down as if sitting, with their haunches not touching the substrate and their tail held stiff and pointed straight back (Figure 13.2). When finished urinating, cats will cover their excrement. While covering will help cleanliness and odor control, the cat's keen sense of smell can still detect urine odor through the covering and cats are known to sniff covered urine sites (Turner et al. 2000). Normal urination occurs on average two to three times daily (Panaman 1981) and interestingly most of the time is performed in the morning versus the evening time.

Feces are deposited by cats roughly three times daily in the wild, but house cats may only defecate once or twice daily, depending on their diet (Panaman 1981; Jackson 1951). Cats will dig in the litter substrate prior to defecation, although not as much as before urination (Panaman 1981), and in the core territory, they will often cover the feces to maintain cleanliness and odor control (Liberg 1980). Cats are often seen sniffing their feces prior to burying them because the motor pattern of raking is initiated by the smell of the fecal material (Panaman 1981). Cats can be inhibited from using a latrine site or litter box by the presence of existing fecal odor which is another reason that litter boxes must be kept pristine at all times (Beaver 2003). Cats in the wild do not deposit feces all in one location but will deposit throughout the core territory, along hunting trails, and outside of their territory as well (Beaver 2003). The covering of the feces and dispersal of deposition locations both act as a form of highly effective parasite control (Beaver 2003).

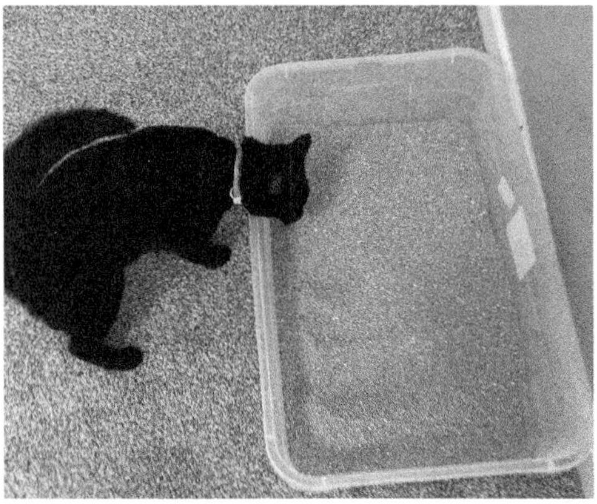

Figure 13.1 Cat's sniff the litter box substrate before digging and eliminating as part of a normal elimination behavioral pattern. *Source:* Photo credit: Meghan E. Herron.

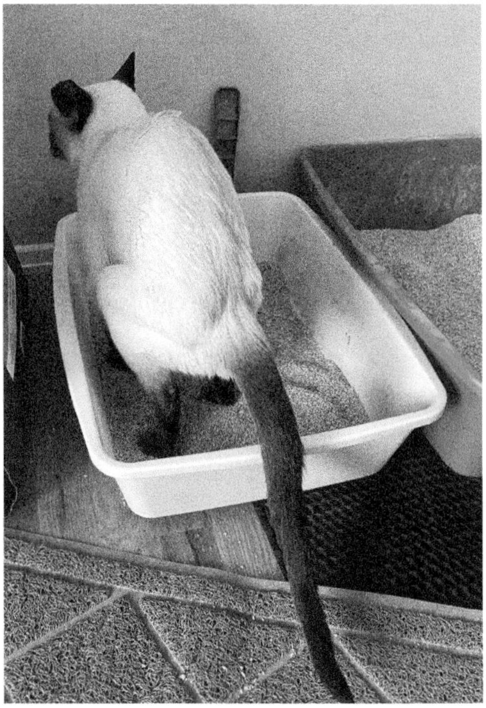

Figure 13.2 Normal toileting posture for a cat eliminating in a litter box. *Source:* With permission from Aditi Czarnomski.

Marking

Urine marking is typically a normal behavior and is one of many forms of marking that a cat will perform. Cats, especially intact males, will urine mark to denote territory boundaries and to provide themselves a sense of familiarity which not only reduces encounters with unfamiliar intruders but also provides them comfort within their roaming area (Dehasse 1997; Gosling 1982). Intact females will frequently mark during their heat cycles. These are examples of normal sexual marking. Urine marking is not limited to males or cats left unaltered and can be seen in approximately 10% of neutered males and 5% of spayed females (Hart and Barrett 1973), especially when their environment is overly stressful (Beaver 2003). We call this stress-related urine marking.

Cats that are urine marking can be distinguished from those eliminating for bladder emptying purposes based on the classic body posture, location of the urine deposits, and the amount of urine deposited. Marking involves the cat standing, with the tail held high and rigid, and the hind end pointed in the direction of the object to be marked (Figure 13.3). The tail will frequently quiver during the deposition process. Urine is most often deposited on territory boundaries or sites of social significance to the cat and is most frequently, but not always, found on vertical surfaces. Typically only a small amount of urine is deposited in droplets, leading to the commonly accepted term of urine spraying. Occasionally cats will spray large volumes of urine and some cats will even assume a marking posture when toileting in the litter box. Whether this unusual pattern is related to stress regarding litter box hygiene or a previously painful experience remains unstudied. We suspect there are a number of factors contributing to the development of these patterns, but likely involve both genetics and early life experiences.

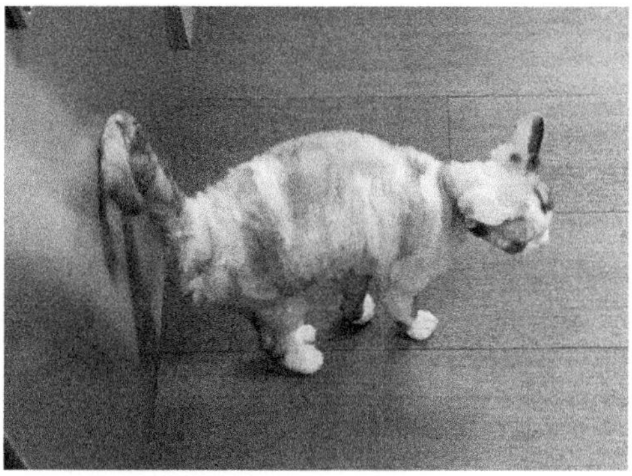

Figure 13.3 A cat stands with tail held high and rigid with her hind end pointed toward an object (dishwasher) she intends to mark with urine. *Source:* Amy Pike.

Keep in mind that there are always outliers to the typical urine marking presentation. Some cats may urine mark on horizontal surfaces (aka "squat mark"). This pattern may be challenging to distinguish from undesirable toileting behaviors, particularly if the urination is not witnessed. Two distinguishing characteristics of this pattern are that horizontal marking will (1) occur in or around socially significant items or locations and (2) not be associated with any digging or covering behaviors before or after urine deposition (Herron 2010). A genetic component to urine marking has been shown to exist (Halip et al. 1992) in certain lines of cats, a fact that breeders should know and report to families purchasing these kittens.

While **middening** (marking with feces) is often anecdotally considered a differential for defecation outside of the litterbox, experts believe that cats do not actually mark territory using fecal material (Beaver et al. 1989; Fox 1975; Gorman and Trowbridge 1989; Hart 1974). Cats may, however, mark with feces because of stress. The social significance of the location of fecal deposition may help differentiate between middening and simple bowel emptying.

Undesirable Toileting

As described above, toileting behaviors serve the purpose of emptying bladder and bowel and are associated with a squatting posture (Turner et al. 2000) (Figure 13.4). Toileting cats will typically display digging behaviors before and covering behaviors after eliminating, even if there is no substrate present to create a well or to cover (e.g. a cat toileting on carpet or a couch cushion will still go through the motions of digging and covering even though this substrate will not actually cover their eliminations). Most often this presents as a cat

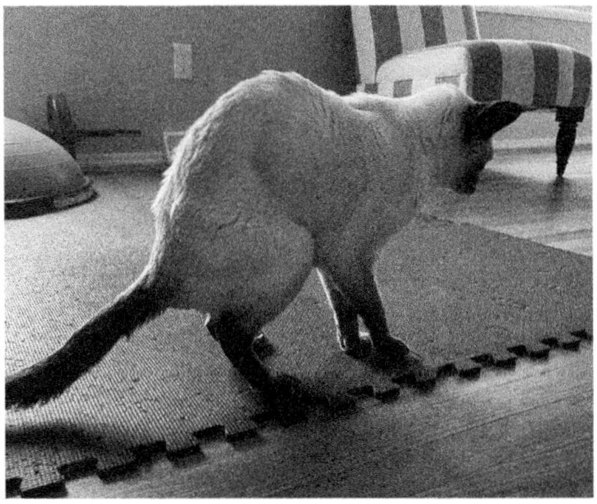

Figure 13.4 A cat toilets outside of the litter box. This is differentiated from marking behavior as there was scratching behavior prior to and covering behavior just after eliminating this classic squatting posture. *Source:* With permission from Aditi Czarnomski.

eliminating large volumes, as would be associated with a fully voided bladder or bowel, onto a horizontal surface. Toileting behaviors that occur outside of the litter box are often related to litter box management/hygiene as cats develop aversions to the available litter box options and preferences for those outside of the human-designated elimination area(s). Not uncommonly, cats develop an instant and powerful aversion to even the most hygienic of litter boxes because of a painful elimination episode. A single experience of painful elimination can be enough to create long-lasting litter box avoidance, even when the source of pain is resolved.

History Taking for Elimination Disorders

Taking a thorough history of the cat's housing environment, social relationships, and eliminative behavior is the first step in directing treatment. The history of the who, what, where, why, and how the cat is eliminating inappropriately will help guide the clinician to the root cause and successful treatment plan. An efficient means of collecting all of this information is having clients complete a behavioral history questionnaire (see online materials for Chapter 12).

Who-

Finding the actual culprit(s) of the inappropriate elimination may be more difficult than it seems on the surface. While the client may bring you the cat whom they assume is the culprit, this does not fully exclude other participants in a multi-cat household, nor does it guarantee the examined cat is not just a victim of circumstance. The client may have witnessed this cat eliminating outside of the litter box multiple times, but unless these are the only times the behavior has occurred, we cannot rule out other participants solely based on this theory. Clients may also assume incorrectly, perhaps based on historical undesirable toileting or marking episodes in this cat, the cat's anxious personality, or witnessing some investigative behavior of the inappropriate eliminations, but not the actual elimination itself.

There are many ways that we can determine the culprit(s), but none are without their flaws or pitfalls. In a multi-cat household, cats can be isolated to their own secluded space and litter boxes so that any eliminations can be definitively assigned. However, isolation in and of itself can be stressful, and thus cause a non-culprit to start eliminating inappropriately. Isolation of cats away from cats they are having conflict with can also diffuse a common underlying reason for not using the litter box and thus solve the issue while not determining the actual culprit. If defecation is the primary elimination of concern, nontoxic glitter or the shavings of wax crayons of different colors can be placed into canned cat food and fed to each individual in the home. The resulting feces will identify the culprit(s) based on the colors deposited in each elimination. If urination is the primary concern, the orange portion of six fluorescein stain strips can be torn off and placed into a gel capsule and fed to one of the cats, and over the next 24 hours, that cat's urine will glow the distinct apple green with a blacklight. Families need to be aware that this technique will stain whatever surface the urine is deposited on, and several weeks of giving the strips to every cat in the house may be needed to rule out the possibility of multiple participants.

It is also important to understand the social dynamics of who lives in the household, including all the animal and human members. While domestic felines are capable of being social, the natural ethology to live in matrilineal colonies may result in social conflict among unrelated females and males living in a household. Multi-cat households have also been shown to have a higher likelihood of urine marking and undesirable toileting than single-cat households (Barcelos et al. 2018). Sociability of the individual cat with conspecifics also lies on a spectrum with some being much more pro-social and willing to live with conspecifics than others. You should ask families in a multi-cat household if they see affiliative behaviors between the cats, including mutual allogrooming and resting in proximity to other cats. Alternatively, do they see obvious signs of conflict such as hissing, growling, or chasing (not in play) between any of the housemates or toward outdoor cats seen through a window or door? This can help determine if inter-cat conflict is a contributing factor.

Cats being a unique combination of both predator and prey species can make living with other animal species potentially problematic and stressful for the cat. This can be especially true when living with dogs with strong predatory tendencies. A clinician should not assume that they know all the animal members of the house as some clients may take certain pets to other veterinarians. This occurs for a variety of reasons: the rescue organization the pet was adopted from offered free or discounted care from a particular veterinary office; pets of other species go to a particular veterinary office; or perhaps the pet was rehomed from a friend or family member and the client chose to keep their care with their previous veterinary office to maintain continuity.

Pets living in busy households or those with small children may face more stress regularly. For many of these cats, successful resolution may require substantial environmental modifications, as well as medication. Therefore, knowing who lives in the house (even if moderately transient like the adult daughter's dog who comes over when she is out of town, or college-aged children and snow-birding grandparents who are there for months at a time) is relevant to diagnosing and treating the problem.

Other players in the equation include neighborhood animals that are not part of the patient's household. Outdoor animals, especially other cats, that do not live in this house but are either viewed or smelled by the indoor residents can create stress and conflict leading to FUE.

What-

The first step in identifying an appropriate treatment plan is characterizing the elimination patterns. Is it urine, feces, or both? If urine, does this seem like toileting, urine marking, or both? Traditionally, urine marking has been distinguished from undesirable toileting by the body posture, locations of eliminations, and covering behavior (or lack thereof) after elimination. A recent study showed the odds of making a urine marking diagnosis were higher when the patient was standing, when the urine was deposited on a vertical surface, when the urine was of a small or medium volume, and when the patient made no attempts to cover the elimination (Barcelos et al. 2018). However, the sensitivity and specificity of each criterion are not perfect, and clinicians will benefit from taking the entire history into account rather than relying on these four factors alone.

The other historical "what" information needed is: what type of litter box style is provided; what type of litter substrate is used; what types of cleaning products are used to clean the box; and what type of substrate is the elimination occurring on (if there is a consistent pattern). In addition, we need to know what types of interventions the caregiver has tried to correct this behavior and whether any of them improved or worsened the problem.

When-

The onset and timing of the undesirable elimination can help us narrow down our differential diagnoses. Any sudden change of behavior is medical until proven otherwise. However, if the onset is acute, but the timing is correlated with a change in the environment (such as the addition of a new cat, or a shift in the client's work schedule), then behavior etiologies may be the sole underlying cause. Even seemingly insignificant or small changes within the environment can be seen as significant and cause sickness behaviors like undesirable elimination to occur in cats (Stella et al. 2011), so clinicians and clients should not discount even the most minute possibility.

Where-

Identifying where the litter boxes are located can help determine if there are distinct locations or particular boxes that the patient is avoiding. The reasons for this avoidance can be multifactorial, including: the location has auditory (e.g. loud washing machine nearby), visual (e.g. too exposed to household members), tactile (e.g. located on a slippery or cold surface), or olfactory (e.g. lack of cleaning or too strong of cleaning chemicals used) sensory inputs that are aversive to the cat; the box itself is aversive to the cat because of the size, shape, accessibility or substrate used; or, the location and box are being blocked, either subtly or overtly, by a housemate.

Identifying where the undesirable eliminations are deposited can determine if there is a substrate or location preference. Knowing these preferences can help the clinician make the litter box more hospitable to the cat, including putting one in a preferred location and using a substrate for which the cat already shows a preference.

Having enough space and territory are key for minimizing stress for felines, especially in a multi-cat household and one where there is inter-cat conflict. Knowing where the cats each rest in relation to one another, where they eat and drink, and where they can be found for the majority of their day and night can help dictate environmental modification plans.

Why-

Knowing why this behavior is occurring in this particular patient allows clinicians to determine the differential diagnoses, appropriate diagnostics, the likelihood that a particular treatment will be successful, and what the prognosis for resolution of a particular case actually is. In addition, when clinicians and clients alike know these risk factors, we can improve early detection and implementation of prevention strategies. There are known risk factors for lower urinary tract diseases (LUTD), including the breed, age, sex, and spay-neuter status (Lekcharoensuk et al. 2001) (see Box 13.1). There are also known risk factors for development of feline interstitial cystitis (FIC), including being male, overweight, and purebred (Cameron et al. 2004).

The other "why" that must be answered is the "why are you now seeking treatment" question to the caregiver when the disorder has gone on for some time. In these cases, it is not until the clients reach a certain breaking point that they seek treatment. Understanding what this breaking point was can help determine prognosis for a resolution that is acceptable to the client (see Box 13.2).

How-

To better understand predispositions and underlying etiologies, we need to know how

Box 13.1 Risk factors for lower urinary tract diseases (LUTD)

Breed risk factor	Disease
Russian Blue, Himalayan, Persian	Urocystolithiasis
Abyssinian	Bacterial urinary tract infection
Manx, Persian	Congenital urinary tract defects
Manx	Urinary incontinence

Age risk factors	Disease
2–7 years old	Urethral plug, neurogenic disorders, congenital disorders, iatrogenic
4–10 years old	Idiopathic, urethral obstructions, urocystolithiasis
>10 years old	Urinary tract infection, neoplasia

Sex and spay/neuter status risk factors	Disease
Castrated male	Every cause of LUTD except UTI and incontinence
Spayed female	Urocystolithiasis, UTI, neoplasia
Intact female	LOWER RISK for all causes of LUTD except for neurogenic and iatrogenic

the family would describe their cat's personality. This can help us better understand if stress and a nervous personality are at play.

The litter box offerings, maintenance, and hygiene are important factors in FUE. How many separate litter boxes are offered to the cat? How often is the litter box scooped and cleaned of waste and how often is it completely dumped out and cleaned fully?

Knowing how often the cat uses the litter box for normal elimination and how often the caregiver is finding the undesirable elimination can not only determine the severity, but it can also help pinpoint the trigger for the problem.

Box 13.2 Every client has their own breaking point

During my residency, I was presented with a 17-year-old FS DSH that was urinating inappropriately out of the litterbox. The referring veterinarian had done a great job of ruling out any medical etiologies prior to referral. The cat had been urinating outside of the litter box on three specific locations on the carpet, showing a distinct location and substrate preference. Upon further questioning of the client, the cat had been urinating outside of the litter box since she was first adopted from the shelter. She had not attempted any treatment in the past and was simply living with the issue until this referral. When I asked the client why she was seeking treatment after almost 15 years of problematic behavior, her response was "We are getting new carpet next month." Needless to say, I gave her a fairly poor prognosis for full resolution in just a few weeks' time.

Ruling Out Medical Disorders

Whenever a clinician is presented with a behavior concern in a pet, they must rule out medical underpinnings first. This is especially important when the behavior is brand new, as the majority of acute elimination problems are likely to be medical in origin (Overall 2003). Anything that affects the urgency, frequency, or quantity of elimination can lead to elimination outside of the litter box. Common differentials for undesirable urination include a urinary tract infection, urinary calculi and plugs, renal disease, endocrinopathies, structural anomalies, or neoplasia of the urinary system (which thankfully is rare in cats) (Overall 2003). Common differentials for undesirable defecation include parasitic infections, bacterial overgrowth, constipation/obstipation, and structural anomalies or neoplasia of the gastrointestinal tract. In addition, anything that affects the cat's ability to access the box, including cognitive changes, osteoarthritis, or obesity, can also cause undesirable elimination (Overall 2003).

Your minimum database for diagnostics should include a complete physical exam, urinalysis, fecal floatation and smear, a complete blood count, and a biochemical profile +/− a total t4. Based on age, the results of your initial diagnostics, and other symptoms, additional diagnostics may include urine culture, full thyroid panel, abdominal ultrasound or radiographs, or spine and extremity radiographs.

Since behavior is a rule-out diagnosis, only when all medical disorders are ruled out and fully treated can we confidently move into diagnosing and treating a behavioral disorder. It is important to note that once a medical disorder is treated, the behavior may remain, due to a conditioned negative emotional response with the litter box or location, or a conditioned positive emotional response to the newly chosen substrate or location. Upon full resolution of the medical etiology, behavioral intervention will then still be needed.

Behavior Diagnoses for Undesirable Elimination

Litter Box Aversion

Aversion to the litter box can develop because of poor cleaning hygiene or from other unpleasant characteristics of the box. For example, covered litter boxes may trap odors and prevent the cat from having a safe vantage point for the approach of other animals during elimination, causing them to eliminate in a more open and safe area. Litter boxes that are too small, do not contain enough litter, or contain liners that are potentially aversive for cats with intact claws can also create an aversion to the elimination area. A common cause of litter box aversion is the experience of a painful elimination. Often these cats will defecate right next to the box as the litter box is in a desired location but the memory of the painful experience makes them reluctant to enter the actual box (Figure 13.5). Once the medical problem has resolved, the cat may still recall the unpleasant experience and, therefore, avoid the previously used litter box.

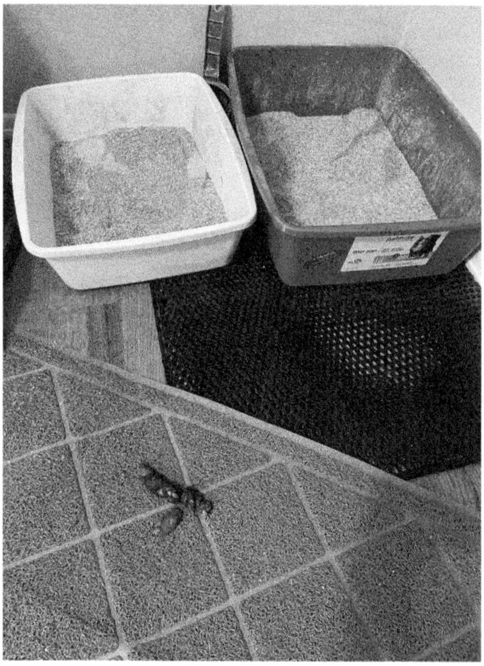

Figure 13.5 An older cat with osteoarthritis tends to defecate right next to the litter box as a result of pain experienced when squatting to defecate. *Source:* With permission from Aditi Czarnomski.

Substrate Aversion

Substrate aversions may develop as a result of scented litters (Horwitz 1997), such as aromatic pine or cedar shavings, or because of an unpleasant texture, such as large gravel or pellets. Signs of "dissatisfaction" with the litter box or substrate include a cat that investigates

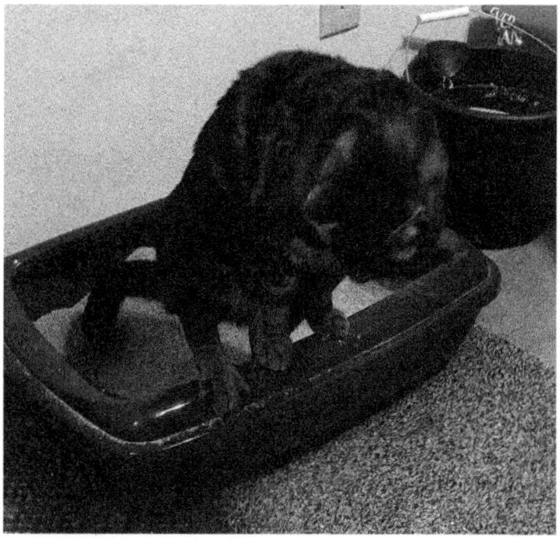

Figure 13.6 Cats that perch on the edge of the litter box to eliminate may be doing so in attempts to minimize contact with the litter. This posturing is commonly associated with a substrate aversion. *Source:* With permission from Katherine Pankratz.

and then avoids entering a box, avoids digging and circling or covering waste while in the box, scratches the surrounding wall or sides of the litter box rather than the litter, and perches on the sides of the box (Figure 13.6). In fact, cats with elimination problems spend less time digging in the litter and are less likely to cover their waste (Horwitz 1997).

Location Aversion

A location aversion can develop as the cat has an agonistic encounter with another household cat, is startled by loud noise or commotion, or has difficulty accessing the elimination area. This can be a problem with multiple cat households where social conflict may prevent some of the household cats from entering the designated elimination area. Geriatric cats may have difficulty accessing litter boxes that require the cat's ascending or descending a flight of stairs or hurtling gates or other obstacles which may have been set up to keep other animals or children from accessing the box. Litter box, substrate, and location aversions are not mutually exclusive and often there are multiple motivational diagnoses.

Substrate Preference

As the various aversions prevent cats from utilizing their designated elimination areas, preferences for alternative substrates often develop. For example, if the litter box is not scooped regularly and the cat chooses to eliminate on another clean substrate, it may develop a preference for the new, non-aversive material. Substrate preferences can develop with or without the presence of an aversion and are most commonly associated with a preference for soft, absorbable material, such as rugs, bedding, piles of clothing, and linens (Figure 13.7). Less common are cats that prefer open hard surfaces, such as wood or linoleum floors. Finally, cats with medical illnesses that may not have been able to reach the litter box may develop preferences for substrates on which they eliminated.

Location Preference

Location preferences may develop as a result of a cat's desire for privacy, need for a quiet area, or ability to access a specific location. Furthermore, cats are attracted to previously soiled areas and may be more likely to eliminate in a location where other cats have eliminated, or where they themselves have previously eliminated. Clients may attempt to relocate the litter box and find the cat prefers the previous location.

Anxiety Related Elimination

Each individual cat has a unique threshold for tolerating poor litter box management. Anxiety-provoking events and the presence of underlying stressors can change this threshold quickly. A cat who previously tolerated a dirty litter box or a difficult-to-access location may suddenly develop aversions or preferences with the addition of environmental stressors, such as new pets or people in the home, household renovations, or agonistic interactions with human or feline household members. Furthermore, cats with anxiety about new

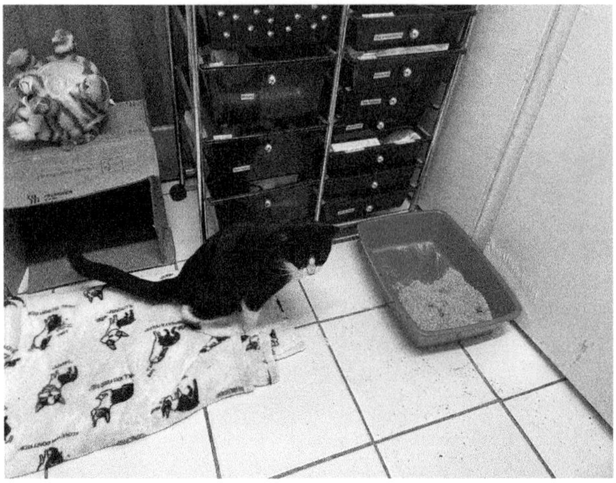

Figure 13.7 A cat urinates on a soft blanket next to his litter box. The cat may have a preference for eliminating on soft items as a result of the litterbox being untidy and too small.
Source: Photo credit: Meghan E. Herron.

household members or other household changes may be too nervous to venture to the location of their litter box. Cats may also toilet outside of the litter box as a result of separation distress (Schwartz 2002), either during the workday or after an extended absence. Although anxiety is more commonly associated with urine marking, it is equally important to recognize when anxiety is playing a role in undesirable toileting behaviors and to address accordingly.

Feline Interstitial Cystitis

Feline interstitial cystitis (FIC), also known as feline idiopathic cystitis, is essentially a medical and behavioral crossover diagnosis. FIC is diagnosed when inflammation of the bladder and urethra is clinically present but no physical etiology can be identified. The cat may show various combinations of clinical signs, including undesirable elimination, hematuria, pollakiuria, dysuria, and stranguria (Westropp and Buffington 2004). The disorder is a result of a complex interaction between the bladder, the nervous system, adrenal glands, and environment in which the cat lives (Buffington et al. 2002). It is important to remember that this is a systemic disorder *affecting* the lower urinary tract, and not a primary disorder *of* the lower urinary tract.

Clinical signs of FIC may not be limited to the lower urinary tract either and may include gastrointestinal, respiratory, dermatologic, central nervous system, cardiovascular, and immune system dysfunctions. When signs extend beyond the urinary system and tend to wax and wane in severity dependent upon stressful events, the term **Pandora Syndrome** is often used (Buffington 2011). It is the activation of the central neurohormonal stress response system that results in the conglomeration of clinical signs in the body.

Nonobstructive FIC will generally resolve on its own, with or without treatment, in about two to five days. That said, studies have shown close to 60% of FIC cases will recur (Kaul et al. 2020) with up to 80% recurrence in some studies (Defauw et al. 2011). Obstructive FIC is a medical emergency, and there are many medications and treatments that have been proven effective to address the urinary pathologies associated with an active flare-up (obstructive or nonobstructive). Such treatments are outside the scope of this chapter. We will instead focus on treatment options that can prevent both FIC and behavioral FUE.

Approach to Treatment

For urine marking cats, neutering is recommended and should resolve the problem for 90% of males and 95% of females (Hart and Barrett 1973). Offering a marking station in the locations already being used can provide a solution that may be more amenable for both human caretakers and cats. A marking station can be made by placing absorbable pads taped or pinned to the wall with a small "lip" on the floor to catch any urine drips. Alternatively, a litter box can be turned on its edge and placed with the inside bottom against the vertical surface with a small amount of litter placed on the side edge (that is now on the floor) to catch any drips. This allows the cat to perform the behavior in a spot that is not ruining the furniture, curtains, or walls. Limiting visual access to environmental triggers, such as outdoor cats, may also reduce marking. Other forms of marking behavior, such as scratch marking on desirable substrates, should be encouraged. The remaining basic treatment principles are universal for both undesirable marking and toileting behaviors and can work as an adjunct in treating medical elimination problems:

- Litter box management and hygiene
- Management of soiled areas
- Environmental modification
- Synthetic pheromones
- Anti-anxiety diets, supplements, and medications

Litter Box Management and Hygiene

Cats are normally fastidious creatures about their nest and latrine site. This means that the litter box must be kept as clean as possible to hold any appeal. This includes once to twice daily scooping of waste material, if not immediately after the material is deposited. Even if a cat smells its own waste in a box, it may be unwilling to use it for additional deposits. The entire box should be emptied, cleaned every one to three weeks with a product that does not leave a strong odor after being rinsed, and then refilled. The boxes themselves should be replaced every year as the smells can start to seep into the plastic over time, especially if the cat causes damage to the box with its claws during raking and covering behaviors.

The boxes used should be roughly 1.5–2.5 times the length of the cat from noise to tail. This tends to be larger than most commercially available litter boxes (Guy et al. 2014). Use of plastic storage bins makes for an appealing alternative (Figure 13.8).

Covered litter boxes may be acceptable, even preferred by some cats, especially when they are larger than other open box options in the home (Grigg et al. 2013; Villeneuve-Beugnet and Beugnet 2020). That said, covered boxes trap odors and their foul smells may be less noticeable to the caretakers and, therefore, less likely to be scooped/cleaned as often as necessary. Families will run into trouble with covered boxes when they do not maintain pristine cleanliness and/or when there are multiple cats in the home who may ambush one another when exiting the box. If a cat routinely deposits urine over the sides of the walls of the box because of not crouching down far enough to urinate, then a box with higher sides, such as a tall storage

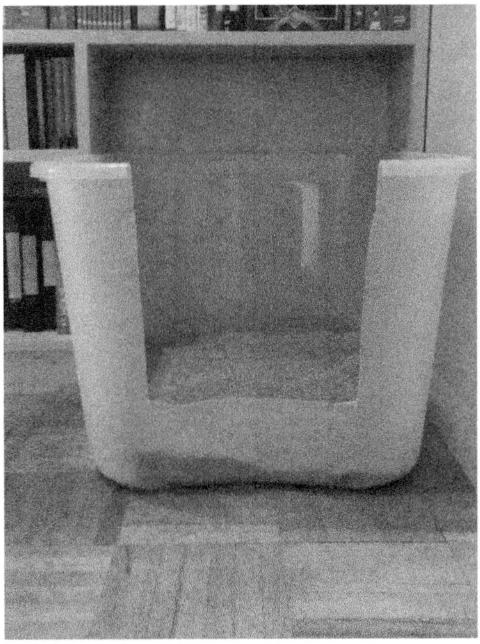

Figure 13.8 Plastic storage bins, appropriately modified for easy access, make great litter boxes. They are inexpensive, deep, large, and easy to clean. *Source:* With permission from Craig Zeichner.

tote, can be used with a small entrance cut out of one side. Motorized, self-cleaning litter boxes offer increased cleanliness, but may also become associated with aversive noise and movement, making them less appealing to many cats.

The box should be filled with litter at a depth of at least three inches so that the cat can readily dig a well and cover their eliminations as desired. Most veterinary behaviorists agree and one study confirmed that cats show a preference for clumping-clay litter (Villeneuve-Beugnet and Beugnet 2018). Another study showed a strong correlation between the use of unscented litter and a lower likelihood of undesirable elimination (Horwitz 1997). Hence, unscented, clumping-clay litters make the top of the recommended litter-type list. Reasons to avoid many commercially available litters are discussed in Box 13.3.

If there appears to be a specific preferred substrate a cat frequently uses *outside* of the box, often that same substrate can be provided *inside* of the box to increase appeal. An outdoor cat that is now housed indoors may use a box filled with mulch chips or sand. A cat that urinates on the bathroom rugs may use a litter box lined with a rubber-backed rug that can be rotated out with a new clean rug daily and thrown in the washing machine to clean. Caretakers can provide a "cafeteria" of litter boxes each with a different substrate option to identify what each cat prefers when given a choice.

Most clinicians have heard the concept of "N + 1"- the idea that households should have one more litter box than the number of cats living in the household. There are no studies that show this is the appropriate number of boxes, and many households that provide that many boxes still struggle with undesirable elimination. A better formula to follow might be to have enough boxes, located on all levels of the house, to allow each cat to access a box without encountering another cat. This may end up being more than N+1. Cats are likely to use boxes near areas (core areas) where they spend most of their time and may not find it appealing to traverse several flights of stairs to access a box in an area they rarely inhabit. The boxes should also be placed in locations that have multiple entrances and exits and not in small

Box 13.3 What is wrong with these litters?

While some cats prefer these nontraditional, yet commercially available litter substrates, most cats have an innate tendency to eliminate on fine, clumpable substrates. Clumping clay litters are more comfortable on their paws and are the most hygienic when scooped as they leave little waste behind.

Pelleted – These litters, while appealing to humans because they are low on dust, are large, awkward, and do not match a cat's natural preferences. Furthermore, feces can stick to pellets and cats may not be able to avoid stepping in them when attempting to cover eliminations.

Corn, wheat, or walnut-based – Cats avoid elimination in proximity to food stations. Some cats may see these food-based litters as such and avoid their use as a toilet. Even more concerning is that cats who ingest these materials are at a dangerous risk for intestinal blockage.

Non-clumping clay – This substrate cannot be scooped as readily as a clumping litter and will remain soiled until the contents are dumped and the substrate replaced.

Crystals – While some breeders prefer to use this litter in their catteries, the average domestic cat has likely never used this type of litter. Most brands contain large, rough crystals which do not fit the natural preference of cats and may be uncomfortable on their paws. Purebred cats with early experience using this litter type may be some of the few who prefer it.

Pine or cedar shavings – These substrates have powerful aromas which may cats find aversive. They also cannot be scooped as readily and will remain soiled until the contents are dumped and the substrate replaced.

corners where a cat could get trapped by another cat. If there is a location that is being used consistently for UE, a solution is often to just provide a box in that location.

Management of Soiled Areas

As cats are attracted to previously soiled areas and may be inclined to over-mark or use them for future toileting, proper cleaning is necessary. Although a variety of pet waste cleaning products exist, studies have shown that enzymatic cleaners are the most effective at reducing and preventing the return of urine odors (Beaver et al. 1989). If the problem is chronic, the underlying carpet pads and baseboards may need to be replaced in order to completely eliminate excrement odors (Figure 13.9a,b).

Once the areas have been treated, the cat's ability to resoil them should be managed. This can be accomplished by placing plastic or foil coverings on top of them. This creates both an unappealing tactile sensation when the cat walks in that area and an impenetrable barrier that prevents resoiling of the carpet. Blocking access to bedding and picking up throw rugs and laundry is also important for cats with a preference for soft substrates. Should the cat repeatedly soil a particular area despite these changes, it may be an indication of a location preference and a litter box should be placed in that exact location.

Multimodal Environmental Modification

The indoor-only environment, while an effective means to prevent infectious disease and injury, can be monotonous and stressful, and lead to undesirable expression of normal behaviors, including FUE, if the humans in the home are not proactive. Being proactive means providing outlets for normal, natural behaviors for which cats are highly motivated to perform BEFORE they become a problem. Multimodal environmental modification (MEMO) aims to enhance the individual's environment to reduce stress and relieve social pressure. MEMO alone has been shown to significantly reduce signs associated with lower urinary tract disease, fearfulness, nervousness, and clinical symptoms of the respiratory tract (Buffington et al. 2006). MEMO helps prevent recurrence of FIC and, when implemented proactively, could help prevent episodes before they begin (Buffington 2004).

(a)

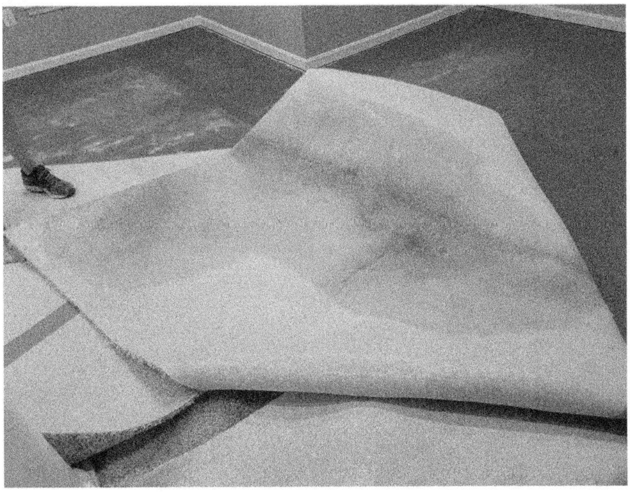

(b)

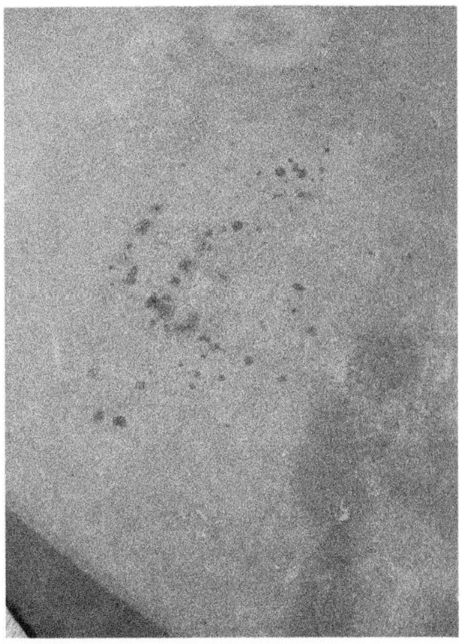

Figure 13.9 Chronic house soiling can lead to saturation of carpet padding (a) and cement subflooring (b), requiring replacement and/or extensive cleaning.

One essential component of MEMO is increasing the amount of *usable* territory. Providing enough quality space for each cat in the household can be difficult, especially for people living in an apartment or condo. If the family has an outdoor space, they could create a "catio" – an enclosed outdoor patio or balcony – which would allow safe outdoor access (Figure 13.10).

Within the home, vertical space options can substantially increase the amount of territory and provide cats high vantage points from which they can monitor for threats, such as other cats or dogs in the home. Other territory options include increasing hiding options based on each cat's preferences. Some cats like to hide underneath objects, while others may prefer to hide high up in a wall-mounted cubby. For homes with major inter-cat conflict, separate core areas or territories where each of the parties can be confined completely away from one another may be necessary either temporarily or permanently. Multi-cat households with agonistic interactions are more likely to struggle with urine marking, undesirable toileting, and FIC. Screening for inter-cat tension is a necessary step in diagnosing and treating FUE cases (Pryor et al. 2001; Jones et al. 1997). For more on inter-cat conflict, including diagnosing and appropriate treatment, see Chapter 14.

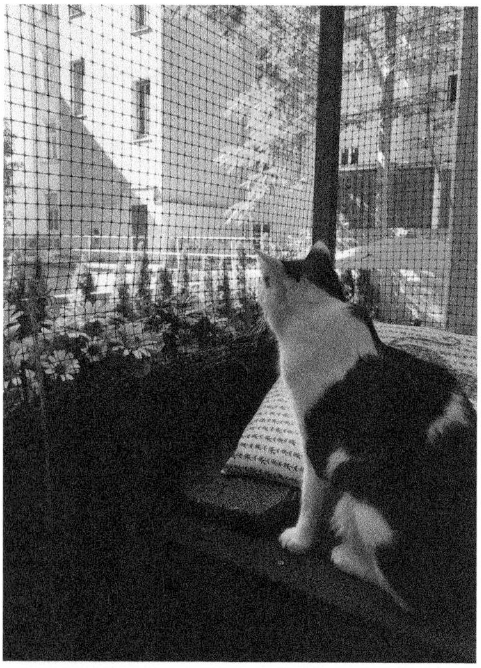

Figure 13.10 A balcony or patio can be enclosed with netting or fencing to create a "catio." This allows cats a safe outdoor space to enjoy fresh air, sunshine, and the sights and sounds of birds and other animals. *Source:* With permission from Kelly Ballantyne.

Providing a behaviorally rich environment is a key component of lower-stress life and reducing lower urinary tract signs for cats. This can include hunting and foraging opportunities with feeder toys, interactive play, as well as training using positive reinforcement. See Chapter 7 for greater detail on providing indoor environments that allow for ample hunting, chewing, scratching, and viewing.

More frequent and predictable interactions and avoidance of punishment techniques will strengthen the human-animal relationship. This means caregivers need to avoid verbal reprimands and squirting the cat with water, as well as the use of remote punishers like scat mats or compressed air even if a cat demonstrates FUE right in front of them. As difficult as showing restraint in these situations may be, the alternative leads to increased stress for the cat, a negative association getting established with the person that is administering the punishment, and worsening of FUE behaviors.

Synthetic Pheromones

Synthetic pheromones mimic the natural pheromones cats emit from certain body parts, such as their cheeks and mammary glands. Refer to Chapter 4 for a review of natural pheromones and how mammals detect, process, and utilize them for communication.

FELIWAY® Classic (Ceva Animal Health, Lenexa, KS) – This product mimics a fraction of the facial pheromone that cats deposit in their environment when they bunt (rub their cheeks on objects/people). Available in a spray and diffuser, it helps to relieve stress by helping the cat feel comfortable in unfamiliar or stressful environments, much like if they came upon previously self-marked locations in their home. The diffusers or spray should be used in core locations, such as around food, water, litter boxes, and resting spots, and in locations where the cat is urine marking. Studies suggest this product may help decrease urine marking, prevent urine marking, and decrease recurrence of FIC (Frank et al. 1999; Gunn-Moore and Cameron 2004; Pageat 1996; White 1997; Hunthausen 2000; Mills and White 2000; Ogata and Takeuchi 2001; Mills and Mills, 2001; Mills et al. 2011; Pageat 1997).

FELIWAY® Multi-cat (Ceva Animal Health, Lenexa, KS) – This product mimics the maternal appeasing pheromone that queens produce when nursing their kittens. It works in a similar fashion to ADAPTIL® (for dogs) in terms of being able to comfort and relax cats in stressful situations (including single-cat households or environments such as the veterinary office). Available in a diffuser only, this product should be placed in areas where cats spend a majority of their time. FELIWAY® Multi-cat helps reduce common signs of tension between cats at home, such as staring, fighting, chasing, and blocking (DePorter et al. 2014).

FELIWAY® Optimum (Ceva Animal Health, Lenexa, KS) – This product is a patented blend of pheromones known as the Feline Pheromone Complex, which provides an enhanced message of social confidence in the environment. In theory, this product could be used when the benefits described for the previous two products are desirable in the same location (Figure 13.11).

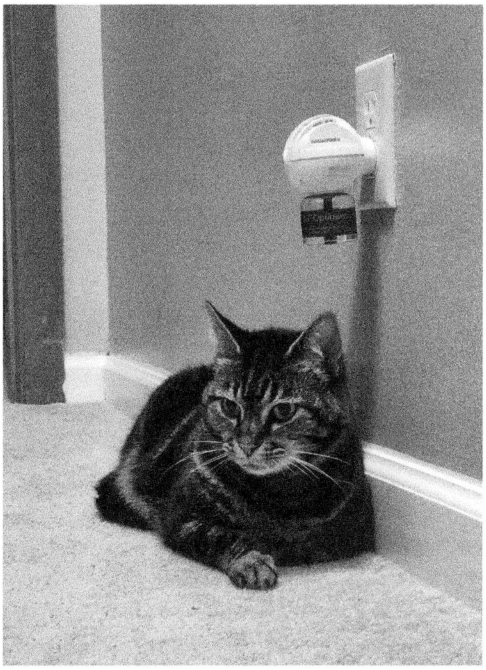

Figure 13.11 This cat routinely rests under the FELIWAY® Optimum diffuser in the hallway of the home – a location he rarely frequented prior to the diffuser being placed there. The synthetic Feline Pheromone Complex emitted from this diffuser is intended to promote relaxation and ease social tension between cats and seems to be working well for this particular cat. *Source:* Photo credit: Emma Walsh.

Diets, Supplements, and Medications

The goal of specialized diets, supplements, and medications is to support and help regulate the body's response to and improve its ability to cope with a stressful environment. Stress is an underlying component of FIC and many cases of FUE, making anxiolytic products a key component of intervention.

Anxitane® (Virbac, Westlake, TX) – This supplement is made of L-Theanine, an amino acid found in green tea which increases GABA concentrations, an inhibitory neurotransmitter, which dampens anxiety responses by stopping neural transmission and the excessive firing associated with anxiety. It can also increase serotonin and dopamine levels as well, making it well suited to help in a variety of different situational and global anxiety disorders. Anxitane® has been shown to reduce undesirable urination and defecation and other stress-related clinical signs in cats (Dramard et al. 2018).

Zylkene® (Vetoquinol, Fort Worth, TX) – This supplement contains alpha-casozepine which is a protein derived from milk. Alpha-casozepine binds to the benzodiazepine receptors in the brain, causing calm and relaxation without the sedation. Zylkene® has been shown to decrease anxiety in cats (Beata et al. 2007).

Purina Veterinary ProPlan Calming Care® (Nestle Purina Petcare, St. Louis, MO) – This supplement contains a proprietary probiotic, BL999, *Bifidobacterium longum*, which has been shown to improve stress responses in cats infected with Feline Herpes Virus 1 (Davis and McGowan 2021).

Royal Canin Calm® (Royal Canin, St. Charles, MO) – The Calm® diets contains alpha-casozepine and tryptophan, and are available as a single diet, a GI formulation, and with the S/O Index. Tryptophan is a precursor for serotonin, a neurotransmitter central to anxiety regulation. Alpha-casozepine binds to the benzodiazepine receptors in the brain, causing calm and relaxation without sedation. This diet was shown to be effective in reducing stress associated with being in a new environment (Landsberg et al. 2017), as well as increased blood tryptophan levels and decreased urinary cortisol in treated cats (Miyaji et al. 2015).

Hill's® Prescription Diet c/d Multicare Stress (Hill's, Topeka, KS) – This diet also contains alpha-casozepine and tryptophan in addition to the normal c/d formulation. This diet was shown to decrease recurrence of FIC (Naarden and Corbee 2020).

Anti-anxiety medications – Many psychotropic medications have been studied in the treatment of FUE in cats. The addition of such medication should be considered when non-pharmaceutical options have failed or when the ability to reduce household stressors is limited and/or when the cat's life or ability to remain in the home is in immediate jeopardy. In the latter two cases, medication should be prescribed simultaneously with litter box and other environmental modification strategies. See Chapter 21 for additional, detailed information.

Conclusion

Clinicians and families can work together to diagnose and treat feline elimination disorders. Understanding normal elimination behavior, taking a thorough history, and ruling out and treating any underlying medical disorders are key to developing a successful treatment plan. Due to the emotional and financial burden elimination disorders can take on human caregivers, regular follow-up is recommended. Keeping in close contact will help troubleshoot any snags in the treatment plan that should be remedied sooner rather than later.

References

Barcelos, A.M., McPeake, K., Affenzeller, N., and Mills, D.S. (2018). Common risk factors for urinary house soiling (periuria) in cats and its differentiation: the sensitivity and specificity of common diagnostic signs. *Front. Vet. Sci.* *5*: 108.

Beata, C., Beaumont-Graff, E., Coll, V. et al. (2007). Effect of alpha-casozepine (Zylkene) on anxiety in cats. *J. Vet. Behav.* *2* (2): 40–46.

Beaver, B.V., Terry, M.L., and LaSagna, C.L. (1989). Effectiveness of products in eliminating cat urine odors from carpet. *J. Am. Vet. Med. Assoc.* *194* (11): 1589–1591.

Beaver, B.V. (2003). Feline eliminative disorders. In: *Feline Behavior: A Guide for Veterinarians*, 247–273. St. Louis, MO: Saunders.

Buffington, C.T., Teng, B., and Somogyi, G.T. (2002). Norepinephrine content and adrenoceptor function in the bladder of cats with feline interstitial cystitis. *J. Urol.* *167* (4): 1876–1880.

Buffington, C.T. (2004). Comorbidity of interstitial cystitis with other unexplained clinical conditions. *J. Urol.* *172* (4): 1242–1248.

Buffington, C.T., Westropp, J.L., Chew, D.J., and Bolus, R.R. (2006). Clinical evaluation of multimodal environmental modification (MEMO) in the management of cats with idiopathic cystitis. *J. Feline Med. Surg. 8* (4): 261–268.

Buffington, C.T. (2011). Idiopathic cystitis in domestic cats—beyond the lower urinary tract. *J. Vet. Intern. Med. 25* (4): 784–796.

Cameron, M.E., Casey, R.A., Bradshaw, J.W.S. et al. (2004). A study of environmental and behavioural factors that may be associated with feline idiopathic cystitis. *J. Small Anim. Pract. 45* (3): 144–147.

Davis, H. and McGowan, R. (2021). Effect of *Bifidobacterium longum* 999 supplementation on stress associated findings in cats with FHV-1 infection. *American College of Veterinary Internal Medicine (ACVIM) Forum 2021 Proceedings* vmeeting.

Defauw, P.A., Van de Maele, I., Duchateau, L. et al. (2011). Risk factors and clinical presentation of cats with feline idiopathic cystitis. *J. Feline Med. Surg. 13* (12): 967–975.

Dehasse, J. (1997). Feline urine spraying. *Appl. Anim. Behav. Sci. 52* (3–4): 365–371.

DePorter, T., Lopez, A., and Ollivier, E. (2014). Evaluation of the efficacy of a new pheromone product versus placebo in the management of feline aggression in multi-cat households. *Proceedings of the American College of Veterinary Behaviorists and the American Veterinary Society of Animal Behavior 2014 Veterinary Symposium.*

Dramard, V., Kern, L., Hofmans, J. et al. (2018). Effect of l-theanine tablets in reducing stress-related emotional signs in cats: an open-label field study. *Ir. Vet. J. 71* (1): 1–7.

Fox, M.W. (1975). The Behavior of Cats. In: *The Behaviour of Domestic Animals* (ed. J.P. Signoret, B.A. Baldwin, D. Fraser, and E.S.E. Hafez), 295–329. London: *Bailliere, Tindall and Cox.*

Frank, D.F., Erb, H.N., and Houpt, K.A. (1999). Urine spraying in cats: presence of concurrent disease and effects of a pheromone treatment. *Appl. Anim. Behav. Sci. 61* (3): 263–272.

Gorman, M.L. and Trowbridge, B.J. (1989). The role of odor in the social lives of carnivores. In: *Carnivore Behavior, Ecology, and Evolution* (ed. J.L. Gittleman), 57–88. Boston, MA: Springer.

Gosling, L.M. (1982). A reassessment of the function of scent marking in territories. *Z. Tierpsychol. 60* (2): 89–118.

Grigg, E.K., Pick, L., and Nibblett, B. (2013). Litter box preference in domestic cats: covered versus uncovered. *J. Feline Med. Surg. 15* (4): 280–284.

Gunn-Moore, D.A. and Cameron, M.E. (2004). A pilot study using synthetic feline facial pheromone for the management of feline idiopathic cystitis. *J. Feline Med. Surg. 6* (3): 133–138.

Guy, N.C., Hopson, M., and Vanderstichel, R. (2014). Litterbox size preference in domestic cats (*Felis catus*). *J. Vet. Behav. 9* (2): 78–82.

Halip, J.W., Luescher, U.A., and Mckeown, D.B. (1992). Inappropriate Elimination in Cats. I. *Feline Practice (USA) 20* (4): 1–24.

Hart, B. and Barrett, R.E. (1973). Effects of castration on fighting, roaming, and urine spraying in adult male cats. *J. Am. Vet. Med. Assoc. 163* (3): 290–292.

Hart, B. (1974). Normal behavior and behavioral problems associated with sexual function, urination, and defecation. *Vet. Clin. North Am. 4* (3): 589–606.

Herron, M.E. (2010). Advances in understanding and treatment of feline inappropriate elimination. *Topics in Companion Anim. Med. 25* (4): 195–202.

Himwich, W.A. (1970). Reflex development and behavioral organization. In: *Developmental Neurobiology*. Springfield, IL: Thomas.

Horwitz, D.F. (1997). Behavioral and environmental factors associated with elimination behavior problems in cats: a retrospective study. *Appl. Anim. Behav. Sci. 52* (1–2): 129–137.

Hunthausen, W. (2000). Evaluating a feline facial pheromone analogue to control urine spraying. *Vet. Med.* 95 (2): 151–154.

Jackson, W.B. (1951). Food habits of Baltimore, Maryland, cats in relation to rat populations. *J. Mammal.* *32* (4): 458–461.

Jones, B.R., Sanson, R.L., and Morris, R.S. (1997). Elucidating the risk factors of feline lower urinary tract disease. *N. Z. Vet. J.* *45* (3): 100–108.

Kaul, E., Hartmann, K., Reese, S., and Dorsch, R. (2020). Recurrence rate and long-term course of cats with feline lower urinary tract disease. *J. Feline Med. Surg.* *22* (6): 544–556.

Landsberg, G., Milgram, B., Mougeot, I. et al. (2017). Therapeutic effects of an alpha-casozepine and L-tryptophan supplemented diet on fear and anxiety in the cat. *J. Feline Med. Surg.* *19* (6): 594–602.

Lekcharoensuk, C., Osborne, C.A., and Lulich, J.P. (2001). Epidemiologic study of risk factors for lower urinary tract diseases in cats. *J. Am. Vet. Med. Assoc.* *218* (9): 1429–1435.

Liberg, O. (1980). Spacing patterns in a population of rural free roaming domestic cats. *Oikos* 35 (3): 336–349.

Mills, D.S. and White, J.C. (2000). Long-term follow up of the effect of a pheromone therapy on feline spraying behaviour. *Vet. Rec.* *147* (26): 746–747.

Mills, D.S. and Mills, C.B. (2001). Evaluation of a novel method for delivering a synthetic analogue of feline facial pheromone to control urine spraying by cats. *Vet. Rec.* *149* (7): 197–199.

Mills, D.S., Redgate, S.E., and Landsberg, G.M. (2011). A meta-analysis of studies of treatments for feline urine spraying. *PloS One* *6* (4): e18448.

Miyaji, K., Kato, M., Ohtani, N., and Ohta, M. (2015). Experimental verification of the effects on normal domestic cats by feeding prescription diet for decreasing stress. *J. Appl. Anim. Welf. Sci.* *18* (4): 355–362.

Naarden, B. and Corbee, R.J. (2020). The effect of a therapeutic urinary stress diet on the short-term or recurrence of feline idiopathic cystitis. *Vet. Med. Sci.* *6* (1): 32–38.

Ogata, N. and Takeuchi, Y. (2001). Clinical trial of a feline pheromone analogue for feline urine marking. *J. Vet. Med. Sci.* *63* (2): 157–161.

Overall, K.L. (2003). Medical differentials with potential behavioral manifestations. *Vet. Clin.: Small Anim. Pract.* *33* (2): 213–229.

Pageat, P. (1996). Functions and use of the facial pheromones in the treatment of urine marking in the cat: interest of a structural analogue. *Proceedings and Abstracts of the XXI Congress of the World Small Animal Veterinary Association* WSAVA, pp. 197–198.

Pageat, P. (1997). Experimental evaluation of the efficacy of a synthetic analogue of cats' facial pheromones (Feliway) in inhibiting urine marking of sexual origin in adult tom-cats. *J. Vet. Pharmacol. Ther. (United Kingdom) 28*: 1055–1063.

Panaman, R. (1981). Behaviour and ecology of free-ranging female farm cats (*Felis catus* L.). *Z. Tierpsychol.* *56* (1): 59–73.

Patronek, G.J., Glickman, L.T., Beck, A.M. et al. (1996). Risk factors for relinquishment of cats to an animal shelter. *J. Am. Vet. Med. Assoc.* *209* (3): 582–588.

Pryor, P.A., Hart, B.L., Bain, M.J., and Cliff, K.D. (2001). Causes of urine marking in cats and effects of environmental management on frequency of marking. *J. Am. Vet. Med. Assoc.* *219* (12): 1709–1713.

Rosenblatt, J.S. (1971). Suckling and home orientation in the kitten: a comparative developmental study. In: *The Biopsychology of Development* (ed. E. Tobach, L.R. Aronson, and E. Shaw), 345–410. Academic Press.

Salman, M.D., Hutchison, J., Ruch-Gallie, R. et al. (2000). Behavioral reasons for relinquishment of dogs and cats to 12 shelters. *J. Appl. Anim. Welf. Sci.* *3* (2): 93–106.

Schwartz, S. (2002). Separation anxiety syndrome in cats: 136 cases (1991–2000). *J. Am. Vet. Med. Assoc.* *220* (7): 1028–1033.

Stella, J.L., Lord, L.K., and Buffington, C.T. (2011). Sickness behaviors in response to unusual external events in healthy cats and cats with feline interstitial cystitis. *J. Am. Vet. Med. Assoc.* *238* (1): 67–73.

Turner, D.C., Bateson, P., and Bateson, P.P.G. (ed.) (2000). *The Domestic Cat: The Biology of its Behaviour*. Cambridge University Press.

Villeneuve-Beugnet, V. and Beugnet, F. (2018). Field assessment of cats' litter box substrate preferences. *J. Vet. Behav.* *25*: 65–70.

Villeneuve-Beugnet, V. and Beugnet, F. (2020). Field assessment in single-housed cats of litter box type (covered/uncovered) preferences for defecation. *J. Vet. Behav.* *36*: 65–69.

Westropp, J.L. and Buffington, C.T. (2004). Feline idiopathic cystitis: current understanding of pathophysiology and management. *Vet. Clin.: Small Anim. Pract.* *34* (4): 1043–1055.

White, J.C. (1997). Efficacy of synthetic facial pheromone (F3) analogue (Feliway) for the treatment of chronic non-sexual urine spraying by the domestic cat. *Proceedings of the First Conference on Veterinary Behavioural Medicine*. Universities Federation for Animal Welfare.

14

Feline Aggression

Carlo Siracusa

University of Pennsylvania, Department of Clinical Sciences and Advanced Medicine, School of Veterinary Medicine, Philadelphia, PA, USA

Introduction

With a prevalence between 15 and 50% of the population studied, feline aggression is a less frequent complaint than other presentations like problematic elimination and scratching. Yet it remains a relevant cause of relinquishment and euthanasia (Albuquerque and Soares 2019; Bamberger and Houpt 2006; Casey et al. 2009; Souza-Dantas et al. 2009; Fatjó et al. 2006; Ramos and Mills 2009; Scarlett et al. 1999; Wassink-van der Schot et al. 2016). Aggression can be directed to people, other cats, or other animals (often dogs).

Neurophysiology of Aggression

From a neurophysiological standpoint, two types of aggression can be distinguished: affective (emotional) and predatory. **Affective aggression** is associated with strong emotions and is characterized by a high degree of sympathetic nervous system activation, vocalizations, and threat displays, with the goal of threatening harm to the individual perceived as a potential danger. The goal of predatory behavior is instead to kill and eat a prey. Predatory displays are characterized by a lower degree of sympathetic nervous system activation and fewer vocalizations and threat displays than those seen with affective aggression – the predator does not want to be noticed by the prey. Affective and predatory aggression are controlled by different neuronal pathways and different regions of the hypothalamus (medial for affective aggression, and lateral for predatory aggression). Early studies to differentiate these two types of aggression were actually conducted in laboratory cats and then applied to different species (Carlson and Birkett 2017). In this chapter, we will refer to affective aggression as *aggression*, and to predatory aggression as *predatory behavior*.

Aggression is hierarchically controlled by different regions of the brain and is initiated by various pathways which activate the stress response. The stress response is the biological response activated when an animal perceives a threat or challenge. The activation of this response can result, among other biological processes, in four different behavior displays: aggression (fight), escape (flight), tonic immobility (freeze), and displacement (fidget) (Carlson and Birkett 2017). Based on their personality, individuals will tend to respond to threats with consistent behavior responses in similar contexts (coping strategy). Whether an

Introduction to Animal Behavior and Veterinary Behavioral Medicine, First Edition. Edited by Meghan E. Herron.

Companion website: www.wiley.com/go/introductiontoanimalbehavior

individual perceiving a threat will respond aggressively or not is determined by an analysis of the sensory stimuli perceived, which give information on the status of the environment, and their comparison with previous experiences. In some cases, if after repetition cats learn that freezing is not an effective coping strategy for threat avoidance, they may change strategies to one of fight or aggression. The neurotransmitter serotonin (5 HT) is known to modulate the emotional response and the display of aggressive behavior, with lower level of serotonin promoting a more risky and impulsive response to a perceived threat (Reisner et al. 1996; León et al. 2012; Bear et al. 2016; Carlson and Birkett 2017). This research suggests that animals with abnormal 5 HT regulation may not modulate emotions well and, therefore, be more apt to reach for an aggressive strategy even toward more benign threats.

Aggression As a Normal Social Behavior of Cats

From an ecological and ethological perspective, aggression is a normal behavior. Aggressive displays are often made of threats rather than harmful behaviors, and their goal is to avoid a direct physical confrontation that may result in lethal injuries. Fighting is rarely the first choice for a healthy animal, because it is dangerous and highly energy-consuming. One of its main functions is to defend and distribute access to valuable but limited resources (e.g. food, safe spaces) among individuals and to protect oneself against injuries by others. Aggression, together with affiliative, pro-social behavior, helps to maintain stability within a social group. While **affiliative behaviors** are used to increase proximity among individuals of a social group, aggressive behaviors are used to keep or increase distance between individuals of a group. Outside of a social group, aggression helps to defend the territory and the resources in it (Bradshaw et al. 2012; Bradshaw and Cameron-Beaumont 2014; Bradshaw and Hall 1999; Brown and Bradshaw 2014; Macdonald et al. 2000; Nelson and Kriegsfeld 2018).

The social behavior of the domestic cat, *Felis silvestris catus*, is greatly influenced by the environment in which the feline lives, as cats are able to live both in groups and as solitary individuals. This adaptability derives from the relatively recent domestication, which occurred about 12,000 years ago (Driscoll et al. 2007) and made the solitary wild cat, *Felis silvestris spp*, a non-obligate social animal (e.g. able to share its territory when abundant resources are available). The diet of *Felis silvestris spp* consists of small prey that is consumed individually, but domestication has provided circumstances where large quantities of food are concentrated in small areas that can attract and sustain numerous cats. For example, garbage disposal areas representing a valuable and reliable source of food are easily accessible to cats in cities and suburbs. They also attract small rodents as do grain storage areas in farms. Nevertheless, it is important to keep in mind that cats are phylogenetically a solitary species that has adapted to share its habitat with humans and other cats under specific environmental conditions created by human intervention. Given the relatively short history of social animals, cats do not have sophisticated communicative skills but can form social groups called **colonies** that are based on a matrilineal composition. As discussed in Chapter 3, females often live together and cooperate in rearing each other's offspring and defending the colony from intruders (Bradshaw et al. 2012; Crowell-Davis et al. 2004; Macdonald et al. 2000; Natoli et al. 2001; Serpell 2014; Turner 2014).

In an unrestricted environment, colonies are spontaneously formed by related cats, who retain the ability to remain or leave the group. Based on this premise, household groups of domestic cats and people living in confinement do not represent a colony, but rather a social group artificially created by humans. Cats living in a household environment have often been "forced" to live with other animals and humans, without the ability to choose whether they want to join or leave the social group. These constraints may make it more difficult for some cats to peacefully manage social interactions and avoid aggressive interactions. This distinction between feline colonies and household groups is relevant to understanding and treating cat behavioral problems caused by social dysfunction (Bernstein and Friedmann 2014; Siracusa 2016a).

Many obligate social species, including the wolf and the African wild dog, regulate the interactions within their social unit by establishing a **linear hierarchy** social organization (Boitani et al. 2016; Bonanni and Cafazzo 2014; Macdonald and Carr 2016). Aggressive and affiliative interactions among domestic cats of the same colony have been studied, but a well-defined linear hierarchical structure has not been identified. Nevertheless, social stability within the group is achieved through displays of affiliative behaviors like allogrooming and allorubbing, avoidance of dangerous aggressive interactions through deference and ritualization, and maintenance of a safe interindividual distance. These strategies are enhanced if individuals also have the ability to keep a safe distance between them which is pivotal to create harmony in groups of household cats (Bernstein and Friedmann 2014; Bradshaw et al. 2012, pp.142–160; Crowell-Davis et al. 2004; Macdonald et al. 2000; Natoli et al. 2001; Siracusa 2016a; Turner 2014).

Spatial organization in feral cats is regulated by the abundance and density of food. Cat population has the highest density in environments where the latter is high, e.g. in urban areas; while in areas where the food is abundant but clumped, e.g. farms and rural environments, the cat population has a lower density (Liberg et al. 2000). In the domestic environment food is usually abundant, so cats can live in a relatively crowded environment. However, when food or other resources are not adequately distributed in the household, cats may be unable to regulate their distance so as to prevent **agonistic** interactions. Most of the time, cats prefer to keep some interindividual distance and to be out of each other's sight (Barry and Crowell-Davis 1999; Broom and Fraser 2007). When keeping safe interindividual distances is not doable, conflicts among the cats of a group may arise. In order to prevent conflicts, each cat should have all the resources (food and water, resting places, litters, toys, and so on) available in the area of the heaviest regular use within the home range, e.g. the core area (Bernstein and Friedmann 2014; Bernstein and Strack 1996).

Mutual affiliative behaviors are important to strengthen and confirm the social bond between two individuals and likely serve to maintain the specific common scent of the group. Allogrooming, allorubbing, nose-touch/sniff and prolonged proximity (e.g. lying together) are common affiliative behaviors. Affiliative behaviors are more likely to be mutually displayed by **preferred associates**, e.g. cats in a colony or household group that spend more time together than would be expected by chance. A preferred association can exist between two males (Figure 14.1), two females, or a male and a female and tend to persist over time even if the colony organization is disrupted (Crowell-Davis et al. 2004). Although adult cats play with each other,

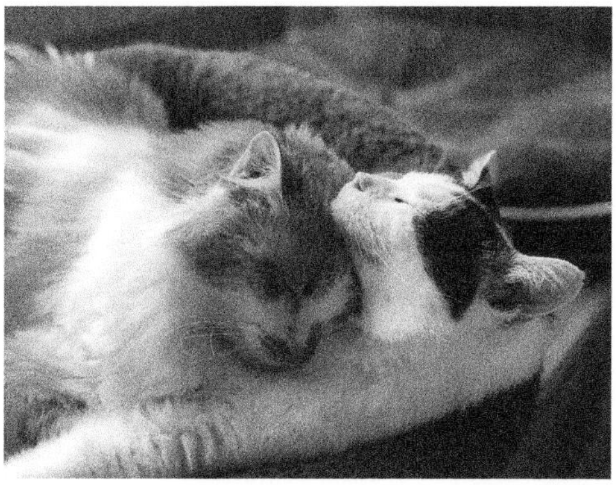

Figure 14.1 These two cats have been friends for life and engage in the close, physical contact often seen between preferred associates. *Source:* With permission from Abra Foster.

playing does not have the same relevance in strengthening social bonds between cats as it does in obligated social species (e.g. dogs). Social play is prevalent in kittens and peaks at 12–14 weeks, but playing with objects, which simulates predatory behavior, is still common in adult cats (Bateson 2014).

Because most cats living in groups spend most of their time out of each other's sight, safe havens that allow cats to retreat and hide should be provided within the core area (Heath 2009; Siracusa 2016a,b). There are exceptions to this, as preferred associates spend more time in proximity, when compared to some individuals that need to consistently keep a safe distance from each other in order to avoid agonistic interactions (Crowell-Davis et al. 2004). Littermates spend more time in close proximity and groom each other more frequently than unrelated cats, probably due to their early socialization and long-term coexistence (Bradshaw and Hall 1999).

Agonistic interactions are meant to increase the distance between two individuals. They can be very subtle and may not be displayed as overt aggressive behavior (behavior that threatens to or cause body injuries). Most agonistic interactions are in fact meant to prevent the escalation of a conflict to overt aggression, which may cause injuries and be life-threatening for the individuals involved. Deference is, for example, one of the mechanisms described in cat colonies to avoid aggressive interactions (Crowell-Davis et al. 2004) in which one cat would walk away, for example, from a resource, when a potentially threatening individual is approaching. When these mildly agonistic interactions fail, for example, if the threatened individual cannot walk away, overt aggression can ensue. Based on this mechanism, we can distinguish a gradient of agonistic behaviors from low to high aggressiveness:

- Low aggressiveness: avoidance/deference
- Medium aggressiveness: growling, hissing, spitting, swatting (threatening to scratch)
- High aggressiveness: yowling/screaming, lunging, scratching, biting

When Cat Aggression Becomes a Behavior Problem

All cats use agonistic interactions with low, medium, or even high aggressiveness as part of their normal behavior repertoire to protect valuable resources and for personal safety. This agonistic behavior is usually ritualized and unlikely to cause severe injuries. As an example, male unneutered cats can display very aggressive threats like yowling or screaming during conflicts over territory of access to females (Turner 2014). Often these very intense threats will result in one of the two individuals deferring before the conflict escalates to severe biting and scratching.

However, the intensity and/or frequency of aggression can sometimes escalate and lead to dangerous interactions. This can happen when a cat sends agonistic signals to which the receiver does not respond as expected, e.g. increasing its distance. As a non-obligate social species that spends most of its time at a distance from other individuals (Barry and Crowell-Davis 1999; Crowell-Davis et al. 2004), the domestic cat is likely to encounter these aggressive interactions as it usually shares a confined space in close contact with other cats and humans. In such context, aggressive encounters can happen accidentally even when none of the individuals interacting is displaying an abnormal behavior. Two cats that are usually able to prevent aggressive interactions by keeping a safe interindividual distance may find themselves unexpectedly in a smaller environment, for example, in the kitchen at feeding time. Similarly, a child may approach a cat that is hiding under the bed and that, therefore, cannot easily walk away. This aggression can usually be addressed with changes in the environment and simple behavior modification; one can make sure that the two cats of the example are always able to keep a safe interindividual distance by feeding them in separate rooms.

Some cats, however, have poorer social skills than others. These cats may repeatedly stalk and chase away a cat living with them, even when the latter did not show any threatening behavior (at least initially, as most cats respond with fear-based aggression to these repeated attacks). This lack of social skills should be expected in a non-obligate species like the domestic cat, which has started to live in close groups only after their recent domestication and only when the right conditions ensue. Because this aggressive behavior can be considered normal in cats, it may be very difficult if not impossible to correct.

When Cat Aggression Becomes Abnormal

Even in a species with a narrower range of overt social behavior cues like the domestic cat, not all aggression should be considered normal or expected. Consider for example a situation in which a cat perceives an incidental short stare from another cat or a human as a threatening behavior and responds with very intense aggression like lunging, scratching, and biting. This behavior may be the result of an underlying dysregulation in the stress response that modulates negative emotions like fear, frustration, and anxiety. The consequence being excessive arousal, which causes severe aggressive responses to benign interactions and threats of mild-to-moderate intensity. Abnormalities in brain chemistry or lesions in the brain areas that control aggressive behavior, lower concentrations of central 5 HT, or high concentration of norepinephrine or dopamine have been associated with increased aggression (Amat et al. 2013; Bear et al. 2016; Carlson and Birkett 2017; Reisner et al. 1996). This dysregulation usually requires professional help from a veterinary behaviorist, who should determine the source of the abnormal behavior (primary behavior disease versus physical disease) and determine appropriate treatment including psychotropic medication if indicated.

Based on these premises, we will define pathological aggression in the domestic cat as a display of aggressive behavior characterized by a disproportionately intense response (growling, hissing, spitting, swatting, yowling/screaming, lunging, scratching, and biting) to a benign interaction or to a mild-to-moderate trigger; and/or by the inability of the cat to easily return to a basal level of arousal once the perceived threatening stimulus is removed; and/or by the inability to respond appropriately to environmental stimuli (including training via operant conditioning) secondary to the excessive arousal.

Because all affective aggression is invariably caused by an activation of the stress response, whether normal or pathological (Bear et al. 2016), one should classify aggression based on a well-differentiated underlying neurophysiology/pathology. In this chapter, we will classify cat aggression based primarily on the body language display and motivation, and secondarily on the context in which the aggression occurs.

Physical Disease and Aggression

The link between physical illness and behavior changes is of great interest in behavioral medicine, and physical disease should always be considered among our differential diagnoses. Contrary to what is often believed, there are no clear boundaries between physical and behavioral illness. Physical disease causes behavior changes, and affective behavior changes regulated by the stress response can cause physical disease. The reciprocal link between behavior and the inflammatory and immune response has been extensively documented in the scientific literature, and it is known to be influenced by the host microbiome (Dantzer et al. 2008; Foster and McVey Neufeld 2013; Siracusa 2016b). Activation of proinflammatory cytokines induces a depressed state (sickness), which helps the individual to cope with the disease (e.g. an infection by exogenous pathogens) that triggers the inflammatory response. Circulating proinflammatory cytokines can enter the brain, where they have a direct inflammatory action and stimulate the production of other pro-inflammatory cytokines and prostaglandins. Although this inflammatory response does not produce tissue damage, it induces a negative behavioral change. Circulating pro-inflammatory cells also exercise their action on the brain indirectly through neuronal pathways, for example, activating a vagal response (Dantzer et al. 2008). The endogenous microorganisms constituting the intestinal microbiome may influence the behavior of their animal hosts through a similar action. The microbiota is capable of modulating the stress response via the hypothalamo–pituitary–adrenal (HPA)-axis, or directly through vagal neuronal stimulation and cytokine action (Foster and McVey Neufeld 2013).

For this intricate relationship between behavior and the immune response, inflammatory disease can cause behavior changes including aggression in cats (Stelow 2020). One of the most studied examples of disease reflecting the intersection between body, inflammation, and behavior is feline interstitial cystitis (FIC) (Buffington and Bain 2020; see also Chapter 13). At the origin of FIC is an alteration of the permeability of the bladder epithelium and its protective mucous barrier of glycosaminoglycans (GAGs) and glycoproteins caused by an activation of the stress response, and an increased sympathetic response associated with a local increase of CRF-related peptide signaling (Buffington 2011; Forrester and Towell 2015). Although FIC is commonly associated with house soiling, increased irritability and aggression are also possible due to the increased stress and inflammation and to the pain and discomfort associated with the condition.

In general, all diseases with an inflammatory component can be associated with increased irritability and aggression. This is the case of metabolic diseases like hyperthyroidism and gastroenteritis, allergic disease like dermatosis, and infectious disease like Feline Infectious Peritonitis (Stelow 2020). Chronic inflammatory skin and gastrointestinal conditions also alter the microbiota, further affecting the immune response and the behavior of an animal.

Pain (e.g. osteoarthritis, trauma, otitis, neuropathic pain, neoplasia, etc.) is another fascinating example of the interaction between physical and the behavioral mechanisms to determine a pathological state. This condition is in fact a psychophysical phenomenon in which the perception of a peripheral physical nociceptive stimulus is elaborated centrally by the same brain regions that control the stress response, ultimately generating an affective (emotional) response to pain (Wiese 2014). Behavioral changes including aggression are in fact considered the most reliable to detect acute and chronic pain in cats and dogs (Reid et al. 2018). Moreover, the presence of pain is of particular relevance because of the possible association between touching/handling a cat and triggering pain; the animal may therefore learn that interacting with other individuals is a potential source of pain (**classical conditioning**) and may display defensive pain-related aggression.

Pathologies that alter a cat's perception and/or proprioception, e.g. neurological, sensory, and cognitive problems, should also be investigated as possible causes of or contributing factors to aggression.

For a list of physical pathologies associated with behavior, changes, and aggression, see Table 14.1.

In conclusion, the work-up to approach aggression in cats must always include a thorough review of the medical history, a complete physical examination, a complete blood cell count (CBC), a chemistry panel including thyroid hormones in patients at risk for hyperthyroidism, and other diagnostics like radiographic or ultrasound imaging when indicated.

Classification of Cat Aggression

In the clinical setting, we can classify aggression based on its motivation, its context, and the body language displayed by the animal (De

Table 14.1 Physical disease associated with aggression.

Degenerative	Sensory decline, cognitive decline
Developmental	Lissencephaly, hydrocephalus
Metabolic	Hepatic or uremic encephalopathy, hyperthyroidism
Neoplastic	Intracranial neoplasia, pain-inducing neoplasia
Neurologic	Psychomotor or partial seizure, peripheral neuropathy
Nutritional	Thiamine, taurine, or tryptophan deficiency
Infectious	Rabies, pseudorabies, toxoplasmosis, Neospora caninum, FIV, FIP
Inflammatory	Feline idiopathic cystitis, granulomatous meningioencephalitis, arthritis, skin allergies, chronic GI disease
Parasitic	Ischemic encephalopathy
Toxins	Lead, zinc, methylphenidate, or heavy metal toxicity
Traumatic	Brain injury, traumatic causes of pain, cerebral infarct
Vascular	Cerebral infarct

Source: Adapted from Stelow (2020).

Porter 2018a, Ley 2021). Motivation and context are often the best descriptors of dog aggression for its complexity (Siracusa 2021). Conversely, cats tend to show very similar displays of aggressive behavior whether it is directed toward people, other cats, or other animals. Keep in mind that many offensive aggressive behaviors are silent and, thus, frequently missed by the human family members. Conversely, loud, dramatic displays of fear-related aggression are easily apparent and what are most frequently reported as the main aggression problem between two cats. In the author's experience, the most salient characteristic to differentiate these displays of

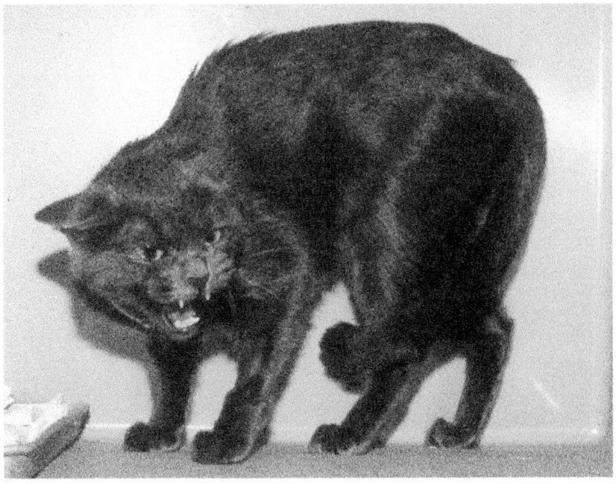

Figure 14.2 This cat is displaying fear aggression with an arched back, piloerection, and open mouth vocalizations. *Source:* With permission from Dr. Sharon Crowell-Davis.

aggression is the body posture, and not just vocalizations, of the cat observed.

Defensive or fear-related aggression: Growling, hissing, spitting, swatting, yowling/screaming, lunging, scratching, and/or biting or attempting to bite in response to a perceived threat from a familiar or unfamiliar person, familiar or unfamiliar animal. The body can be low on the ground, in dorsal recumbency (rolling over), crouched if the animal is cornered; or with an arched back and piloerection if the animal has the possibility of escape (Figure 14.2). The ears are flattened and the pupils dilated. This aggression tends to be overt and noticeable by human family members.

Offensive aggression: Following, stalking, running after, spitting, yowling/screaming, lunging, scratching, and/or biting or attempting to bite a familiar or unfamiliar person, familiar or unfamiliar animal. The body is kept at a neutral height and not lowered or arched. The ears can be forward or rotated laterally and the pupils may or may not be dilated. Attempting to chase an individual away from the territory (often described as *territorial aggression*) and experiencing *frustration* (when an expected outcome does not happen) are among the contexts in which cats display aggression with an offensive posture. A cat displaying offensive aggression can appear

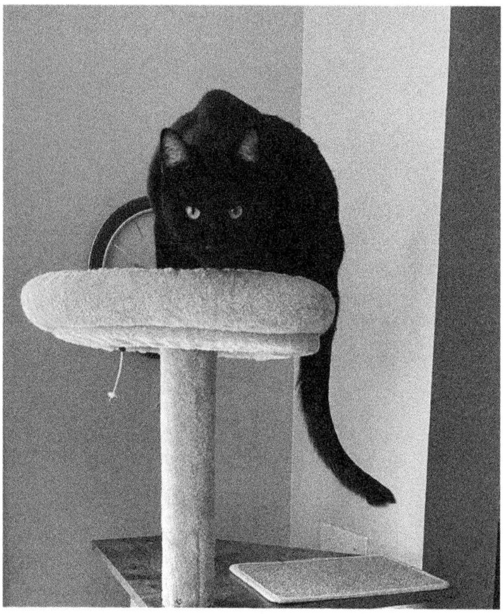

Figure 14.3 A cat shows confident, silent, offensive body posture toward another cat in the home to keep the other cat away from his coveted perch. *Source:* Meghan E. Herron.

remarkably collected and silent (Figure 14.3), particularly at the beginning of the interaction and when the behavior is displayed toward a familiar individual, such as another cat in the household. One might call these "covert" behaviors as they are often below the radar of naive human observers.

Redirected aggression: Both defensive and offensive aggression are characterized by a high degree of sympathetic nervous system activation, physical and emotional arousal, and can be redirected. A cat can redirect aggression toward an individual close by if the primary target of the aggressive behavior is not immediately accessible, or if the aggression is caused by an intangible environmental stimulus like an intense and/or sudden noise. Aggression manifested when physical disease significantly contributes to decreasing the threshold of reactivity of a cat is often defined as *irritable aggression* and can be redirected. Amat et al. (2008) observed that, in most situations, cats adopt a defensive body posture immediately before displaying redirected aggression.

General Guidelines for the Treatment of Aggression

The treatment of affective aggression includes three components, regardless of the specific target and context:

1) Safety and management: Creating a safe environment through strict preventive measures.
2) Environmental modification: Modifying the existing environment to minimize the perception of threats and challenges that would activate the stress response.
3) Behavior modification: Using classical and operant conditioning to make daily interactions more predictable and to improve the communication between the caregiver and the animal. This will, among other benefits, enable the caregiver to redirect the attention of the cat in situations at risk for aggression.

All these interventions will ultimately result in increased perception of control over the environment and, therefore, reduced activation of the stress response and improved welfare (Notari, 2009).

Safety and Management

Establishing a safe environment must always be the first step in the treatment of affective aggression. All the other components of the treatment may take some time to be implemented and give appreciable results, while safety can be implemented immediately by establishing and following clear and specific rules. Once the caregiver is able to operate in safety, environmental and behavior modification can be gradually implemented. Safety rules may need to be particularly strict at the beginning of the treatment, when the behavior modification (and the medication, if used) may not have yet reached its full effectiveness.

For example, if a cat is presented for lunging at, scratching, and biting people in the household, a rigorous confinement of the animal away from people may be necessary at the beginning of the treatment. Within this safe context, the veterinarian and the caregiver can then work on a treatment plan, including further changes in the environment and in the way that people interact with the cat and start medication if indicated. Creating a safe environment will drastically minimize the exposure of the cat to the stimuli that are perceived as a threat or challenge and will consequently promote desensitization to these stimuli. The environmental and behavior modification will then provide the caregiver of the cat with the tools to implement a controlled exposure to the threatening stimuli. This will in turn increase the cat's perception of safety and will promote less aroused and aggressive behavior. Once the environmental and behavior modifications have been well established, the safety rules can be reassessed and, if appropriate, less strict rules can be put in place.

Environmental Modification

Changes in the environment should be implemented with two main goals in mind:

1) Facilitating the enforcement of the safety rules established.
2) Increasing the control that the cat has over his environment to reduce distress and emotional arousal.

When enforcing safety, the use of physical barriers is often necessary to prevent interactions that may potentially lead to aggression. For example, the cat may need to be kept temporarily behind closed doors or in a large dog crate to prevent possible affective aggression (Figure 14.4).

All cats should be provided with core areas and safe havens around the house where they can remain undisturbed and can retreat when feeling overstimulated or unsafe (Figure 14.5). To minimize social conflicts, cats should be able to avoid interactions with other cats as they access their resources. Due to the variability of sociality between individual cats, some individuals may need an exclusive core area in

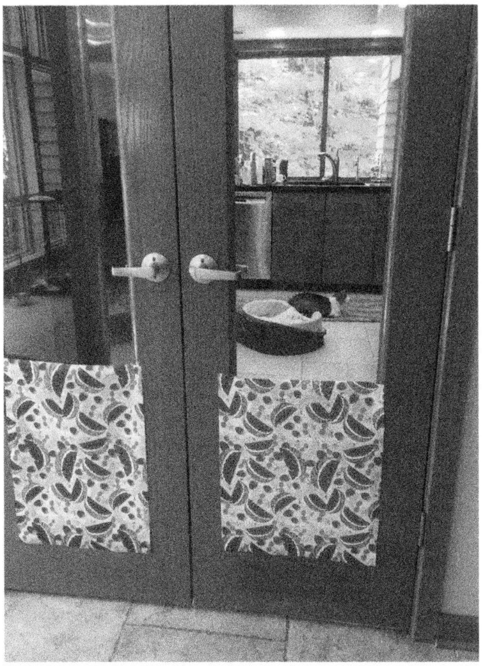

Figure 14.4 Part of safety and management often includes keeping a physical and visual barrier between cats to prevent affective aggression between them. *Source:* With permission from Peggy Kaplan.

which they can find refuge far enough from other cats, while others may tolerate overlap of their core areas. However, the interindividual distance is variable for each cat and depends on the quality of the relationship and interaction that two cats in the same group have. Vertical spaces can be useful to maintain individual distances and prevent aggressive interactions. Cats escaping from an aggressive interaction may prefer hiding places rather than elevated spaces (Barry and Crowell-Davis 1999).

Safe places can be represented by hiding spaces, for example under furniture; vertical spaces located at a higher level, for instance on top of kitchen cabinets; or confined spaces behind solid barriers, like behind a closed door with a collar or microchip-activated cat door. This will allow the cats the possibility to respond to the increased arousal and distress by enacting an escape-type response rather

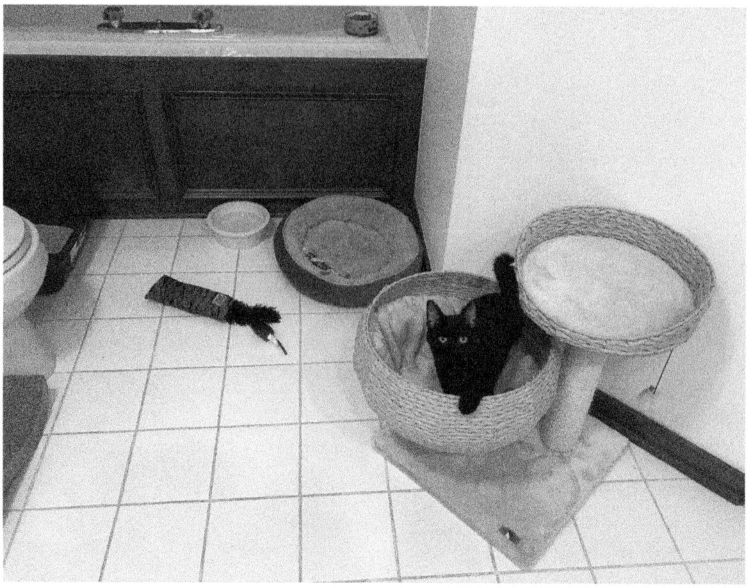

Figure 14.5 Cats sharing a home should have multiple core areas or safe-havens, such as this one, where food, water, scratching posts, latrine, and resting places can be easily accessed without altercations with other cats. *Source:* Meghan E. Herron.

than an aggression-type response. Aside from necessary and controlled interactions (e.g. a veterinary visit), cats should never be forced to have interactions that are not safe and enjoyable for them and may escalate to aggression. This is particularly important for cats with a history of aggression and for interactions between cats and small children.

Although less frequently used in cats than in dogs, handling and containment tools can be helpful to minimize the chance of an aggressive interaction. For example, choosing the right carrier can facilitate handling in one of the contexts in which cats are more likely to show aggressive behavior, e.g. vet visits. For this purpose, solid cat carriers in which the top can be easily taken apart from the bottom can facilitate a minimal-stress handling veterinary visit (Cannon and Rodan 2016; See Appendix B for information on carrier training). The use of a rigid cat muzzle or a soft cap can help prevent bites from cats that are particularly anxious. While muzzle training for cats is not usually promoted, cats that require frequent invasive veterinary procedures may be desensitized to wearing a muzzle or soft cap using counterconditioning with high-value food. Leashes and harnesses can be useful during reintroduction protocols of aggressive cats, when they tolerate them without increased stress.

Behavior Modification

As described in Chapter 5, cats respond to both behavior modification via **classical** and **operant conditioning**. Simple associations created via classical conditioning can be very helpful to handle a cat or redirect their attention. For example, cats tend to associate sounds preceding high-value food with the food itself. These sounds can therefore be used to redirect the cat's attention and promote a positive mood state in a context in which aggression may ensue. Cats can also learn positive associations via operant conditioning and then respond to specific stimuli in a very consistent and predictable way. A cat that has a positive association with being groomed and is consistently groomed in the same room, e.g. the bathroom, can learn to "go to your room" if this verbal cue is consistently preceding the grooming sequence. This verbal cue could then be used to send the cat to the bathroom if we need to confine him there to prevent an aggressive interaction, as long as the behavior of the cat is consistently paired with a positive outcome.

The main goals of behavior modification are improving the communication between cats and their caregivers and increasing the predictability and control in a potentially stressful context that may trigger aggression. In order to accomplish these goals, behavior modification should be focused, first, on establishing consistent and predictable interactions between the cat and the caregiver and, second, on providing the cat with directions to increase control over the environment. When excessive arousal does not allow the cat to "think" through a safe coping strategy, it is the caregiver's responsibility to "explain" to the cat how to safely handle a potentially challenging situation. For example, if a cat appears to be increasingly distressed by the presence of another cat with whom there is a history of aggression, the caregiver can redirect the former cat's attention and establish a channel of communication through the use of operant conditioning (e.g. asking the cat to "touch" the fingers), while moving away from the potential threat. In order to be able to do this in a critical context, a consistent response to the specific verbal cue should be taught via operant conditioning by repeating the exercise multiple times in a quiet environment.

When using behavior modification with an aggressive (or, more in general, overly aroused) cat, it is important to keep in mind that the level of distress that animals are experiencing will influence their ability to respond to our cues. In general, highly aroused and distressed cats are less responsive to operant conditioning and their ability to perform voluntarily may be impaired due to the activation of the limbic system that contrasts the activity of the reward system (Mills 2009; Notari 2009). The use of classical conditioning may still be effective when the cat is not responding to operant conditioning due to excessive arousal/distress. In these cases, exposing the cat to a "positive opposite," e.g. a high-value treat, may "flip the switch" from the aggressive sequence to one of food seeking.

Punishment of aggressive behavior, even verbal, must be avoided, as it is likely to intensify the undesired behavior and trigger an aggressive attack, create a negative association with the other individuals, and hinder progress.

Using Psychoactive Medication to Treat Affective Aggression

Most cases of affective aggression can be treated and managed using the three-component approach described above (safety + environmental modification + behavior modification). Some cases, however, may benefit from the use of psychoactive medication. When the aggression is recurrent, characterized by a high degree of emotional arousal and impulsivity, and/or does not respond well to environmental and behavior modification, the use of medication may help. The goal of drug treatment is to reduce excessive arousal and impulsivity and, therefore, to facilitate behavior modification.

No medication is labeled for the treatment of aggression by the competent agencies in the USA and Europe. Because of the role played by serotonin in regulating anxiety and aggression (Amat et al. 2013; Bear et al. 2016; Carlson and Birkett 2017; Reisner et al. 1996), serotonergic drugs, in particular selective serotonin reuptake inhibitors (SSRIs) and tricyclic antidepressants (TCAs) are used in the treatment of feline aggression (De Porter 2018a). There is no specific dosage or frequency of administration used for aggression problems, and the general indications about the use of these drugs should be followed (see Chapter 21). It is important to make the client aware that the use of medication does not eliminate aggression and the risk that an injury may still occur. For this reason, medication must be considered a complement to the overall treatment of aggression. Strict safety strategies, environmental and behavior modification will still represent the core components of the treatment for feline aggression. SSRIs and TCAs, as well as many other psychotropic drugs, have the potential to cause a paradoxical increase in arousal and aggression (Siracusa and Horwitz 2018). The treatment should be immediately discontinued if aggression worsens and a different medication should be chosen.

Psychoactive drugs with a mild or moderate sedative action are often used during minimal-stress handling of cats during veterinary visits. A single dose of gabapentin 100 mg or trazodone 50 mg administered before transportation to the veterinarian is often effective in reducing stress during veterinary visits (Stevens et al. 2016; Van Haaften et al. 2017).

Cat Aggression Directed to People

Cat aggression can be directed to familiar and unfamiliar people. We will here define familiar people as the individuals that consistently live in the same household and who, therefore, belong to the cat's stable social group. Conversely, we define unfamiliar people as the individuals that do not live in the same household and do not belong to the cat's stable social group. The group of unfamiliar people is not a homogeneous group and may include people that are complete strangers to a cat and people with whom a cat has regular interactions. This difference in the frequency of contact can influence the affiliative and agonistic interactions that a cat shows toward specific unfamiliar individuals. However, the lack of stable, frequent, and consistent contact happening within the cat's home range characterizes all these interactions to different degrees. Cat aggression to people is diagnosed in about 13–14% of cats presented to referral behavior clinics (Bamberger and Houpt 2006; Wassink-van der Schot et al. 2016) and has been reported to be the third most common behavioral reason for relinquishment of cats, after aggression between household cats and inappropriate elimination (Casey et al. 2009). Aggression directed to familiar people is the most commonly reported form of aggression to humans and can be defensive or offensive (Bamberger and Houpt 2006; Palacio et al. 2007; Wassink-van der Schot et al. 2016).

Fear-related aggression – Defensive or fear-related aggression is by far the most frequently observed (Palacio et al. 2007). Cats may develop fear of familiar people for a variety of reasons, including accidental or intentional startling, socially invasive or painful physical handling, and verbal and/or physical punishment. As described above body postures associated with fear are telltale for this diagnosis.

Frustration-related aggression – Frustration can be caused by many daily interactions with people of the household; for example, when an interaction is abruptly interrupted and a cat is still emotionally aroused or when an expected meal is delayed.

Territorial aggression – Offensive aggression directed toward unfamiliar people entering the cat's home territory or safe space is considered to be territorial in nature. Offensive aggression to familiar people in the context of territorial aggression is rare. In the author's experience, it is displayed with a purely offensive behavior (chasing away, lunging, scratching, and biting) when familiar people approach the territory or core area of the cat, usually corresponding to the area in which the cat has been confined due to his aggressive behavior.

Petting-induced aggression – One of the most typical contexts in which a cat can show aggression to people is prolonged petting (De Porter 2018b; Ley 2021). This is not always the case when people physically interact with cats. When people pet cats longer than they can tolerate or in an inappropriate area of the body, for example, the flanks or the abdomen, cats respond with quick bites and scratches. Most often this aggression looks offensive. Fear, anxiety, stress, and physical disease can make a cat more irritable and decrease its threshold of reactivity. In particular, diseases that cause hyperesthesia or pain can make a cat extremely sensitive to tactile stimulation (Siracusa and Landsberg 2020; De Porter 2018b).

Specific Treatment Recommendations for Physiological Aggression Directed to People

Most cat aggression to people can be considered physiological (think normal, but nuisance) and is due to inappropriate management or handling from humans, as is often then case in petting-induced aggression and fear-related aggression. Another typical context is represented by the aggression secondary to frustration that cats experience when they are not fed following a schedule typical of the species. In feral or semi-feral conditions cats eat multiple small preys (12–20) throughout the 24-hour day (Bradshaw et al. 2012; Turner 2014). This meal frequency is difficult if not impossible to reproduce in a typical household, where cats are fed less frequently and not always with a consistent schedule. These conditions can generate a significant amount of anxiety and frustration, especially when the expected time of a meal approaches, that can trigger undesired behaviors like aggression or inappropriate elimination.

These forms of physiological aggression can be often addressed by educating the client on the social behavior and environmental needs of cats (Crowell-Davis et al. 2004; Rochlitz 2005; Rochlitz 2014), with the goal to provide every cat with adequate abundance and distribution of resources, frequent small meals, appropriate and safe interindividual distance, and tolerable physical interactions. Specifically for petting-induced aggression, limits on physical touching are necessary. Physical contact during affiliative behavior among cats is typically short and limited to the head and neck areas (Siracusa 2016a). There is no standard amount of physical contact that a cat can tolerate and there are major differences among individuals. Moreover, an individual cat may not tolerate the same amount of physical interaction in all contexts.

Verbal cues taught via operant conditioning can be useful to redirect a cat's focus and change his mood state from negative to positive when early signs of fear, anxiety, or stress are detected. In cases of physiological aggression, the prognosis is favorable and most cats will be able to live safely and comfortably with the people in and around their household. Psychoactive medication is not necessary in the treatment of physiological aggression, but the use of synthetic pheromone therapy can encourage the perception of the household as safe (Mills et al. 2013).

Specific Treatment Recommendations for Pathological Aggression Directed to People

Some cat aggression to people is pathological. This aggression is characterized by emotional dysregulation and hyper-reactivity to stimuli, which trigger excessive emotional and physical arousal with severe signs of fear, anxiety, and stress. In these cases, a cat responds with intense aggression to mild stimuli that may not be perceived as threatening by people involved in the interaction. For the latter reason and because of the underlying emotional dysregulation, this aggression may be difficult to control with environmental management, behavior modification, and client education. In these cases, psychoactive drug treatment is often necessary to control the underlying emotional dysregulation.

Changes in the interaction between cats and people in the household, including separation and confinement, are usually the first step to take in the treatment of pathological cat aggression to people. In general, interaction should be limited to times when the cat is receptive and shows affiliative behaviors like head bumping and nose touching. Even in this case, the interaction and physical contact must be very brief. Physical contact may need to be avoided altogether with a history of severe biting and/or scratching, at least during the first 6–12 weeks of treatment. Separation and confinement to a safe haven can be more or less strict and prolonged, depending on the extent and severity of the aggression. For example, if a cat is reactive to common or subtle movements of people in the household, strict confinement to a safe haven may be necessary throughout the day. The cat could be allowed some supervised time outside of the safe haven when the person targeted by the aggression is sitting calmly and another person is present to redirect or remove the cat if necessary. This period of separation and confinement will provide time to implement safe changes to the household environment, behavior modification, and to allow the psychoactive drug treatment to reach a steady effect.

Several safe vantage and hiding spots can be created in designated areas around the house like elevated platforms on cat tress and shelves, cave-type beds, or underneath furniture. When allowed outside the confinement area, the cat can be encouraged to spend time in these spots by placing some favorite high-value food in them to create a positive association via classical conditioning. A "go to" cue to direct the cat to these areas can be taught via operant condition. When in his safe spots, cats must be left undisturbed.

Feeding devices and toys that allow the cat to perform a normal hunting + play + feeding behavior should be made available (see Chapter 7 for further information on setting up an environment for success). Both classical and operant conditioning techniques can be used for the cat to create a positive association with people. For example, a person approaching the cat can announce their name with a calm voice and then gently toss a high-value treat toward the cat (classical conditioning), or the cat can be asked to "touch" the hand of the person (Figure 14.6) and then be rewarded (operant conditioning). These techniques are more effective in cases of defensive fear-related aggression than in cases of offensive aggression. Physical interaction should be promoted only when necessary and it can be done in safe conditions. If a cat is aggressive to occasional guests only when touched, for example, physical contact can simply be avoided.

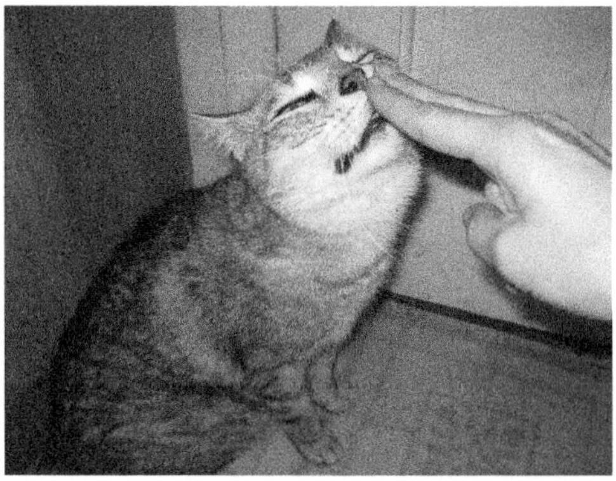

Figure 14.6 Cats can be taught to touch an outstretched finger or object on cue. Because the training to put this behavior on cue involves positive reinforcement, the cat also develops a positive emotional association with the person training it through classical conditioning. *Source:* Meghan E. Herron.

A cat must not be approached while showing aggression, when possible. Moving away from the cat is often the safest option. When handling is necessary, the hands and body of the handler must be adequately protected. Barriers and tools to deter the cat in case of aggression must be easily reachable around the house. Thick, large towels to throw on the aggressive cat or large cardboard panels to push the cat away are a few examples. Strong deterrents like water or high-pressure canned air should be used only when absolutely necessary for the immediate safety of people, as their use may cause further sensitization and result in a worsening of the fear and/or aggression. Serotonergic drugs, SSRIs and TCAs, in particular, are usually the first choice to treat cat aggression directed to people when a hyperactivation of the stress response with emotional dysregulation is identified. The use of analgesic or anti-inflammatory drugs is indicated when pain or paresthesia are suspected contributing factors (De Porter 2018a; Siracusa and Horwitz 2018).

Misdirected Play Behaviors

Although not truly a form of aggression, **misdirected play** is a frequent cause of bites and scratches directed toward people (Berger 2016; Palacio et al. 2007). Play behavior is a ritualized display of predatory-like sequences and is mostly directed to objects in adult cats (Siracusa 2016a). However, the lack of sufficient environmental enrichment or an inappropriate physical interaction initiated by humans can lead to severe scratches and bites. The prevention of injuries from misdirected play can be achieved by providing appropriate outlets to display object-play behavior, which is a normal behavior that cats need to perform. Food-enhanced toys and interactive feeding devices, interactive toys that mimic the behavior of natural prey, soft-toys with catnip or silver vine, must be part of a feline welfare-friendly household. See Chapter 7 to learn more about meeting cats' environmental and behavioral needs. Interactive play sessions with people must mimic predatory behavior (e.g. using a teaser wand toy) and be short (3–5 minutes) but repeated multiple times throughout the day. These play sessions will have to culminate in a consummatory phase that will end the prey-like sequence. This can be achieved by tossing a few high-value treats before removing the interactive toy. Failing to terminate the sequence with a consummatory phase may result in redirection of the cat's emotional and physical arousal toward the handler. Inappropriate play interactions may even trigger affective aggression if a cat becomes frustrated when the person walks away during an aroused interaction, or fearful when the person punishes the animal that plays rough. For the latter reason, playing with hands or feet must always be avoided, even with kittens.

Aggression Between Cats

Aggression between cats can be observed within the same household or with outdoor cats and can have an offensive or defensive display. Together with aggression to familiar people, aggression between household cats is among the most frequently reported contexts of aggression in cats in behavior clinics (Amat et al. 2008; Bamberger and Houpt 2006; Wassink-van der Schot et al. 2016). Interestingly, aggression is a far less common and less relevant in free-roaming cats of the same colony (Frank 2016), suggesting that indoor confinement may contribute to aggression between cats of the same social group. This is likely due to the fact that outdoor cats can freely join or leave a group and consistently keep a safe interindividual distance, while indoor cats cannot. Conflicting information has been produced on whether granting outdoor access to household cats influences the occurrence of aggressive behaviors (Frank 2016; Heidenberger 1997; Levine et al. 2005). Introducing a new cat in a stable household group triggered aggression in about half of the cases studied by Levine et al. (2005), and in about one-third of these cases the aggression continued for several months after the introduction. If scratching or biting occurred during the initial encounter, the aggression was more likely to last longer. When considering a sample of the general population of cats living in pairs, males are no more aggressive than females (Barry and Crowell-Davis 1999). Among a sample of cats referred for behavioral problems, males were more likely to be the aggressor than females, but the aggression was no more likely to be directed toward males than females (Lindell et al. 1997). This might mean that aggression displayed by a male cat can be more intense and more likely to be reported as a clinical problem. Protection of resources does not appear to be a primary cause for aggression, but the lack of interindividual distance when accessing clumped resources may trigger aggression when cats are

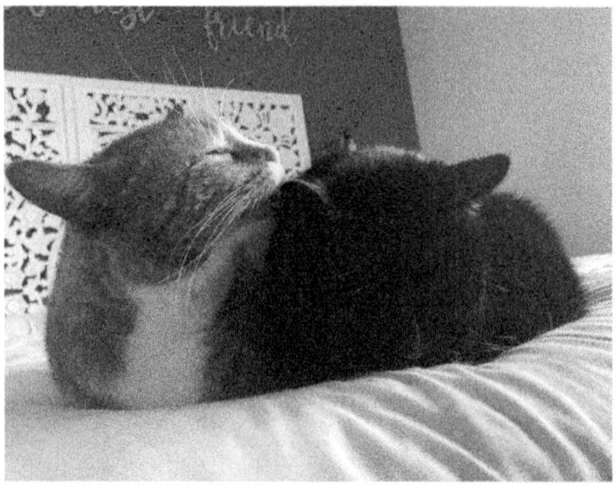

Figure 14.7 Two cats enjoy each other's close company and engage in allogrooming.
Source: Photo credit: Elaine McCarthy.

eating from a common food source (Barry and Crowell-Davis 1999; Bernstein and Strack 1996).

There is a negative correlation between the time that cats have spent living together and the frequency of aggressive interactions, e.g. cats that have lived together longer are less likely to show aggression to each other (Barry and Crowell-Davis 1999). Related cats are more likely to show affiliative behaviors like being in physical contact and allogrooming (Figure 14.7) than unrelated cats (Bradshaw and Hall 1999; Crowell-Davis et al. 2004). Therefore, acquiring two related kittens or two related adults that have lived together may minimize the risk of aggression between them. Introduction of a new cat in a multiple-cat household can be a trigger for aggression between cats living together, and their behavior during the first encounter may be determinant for their future relationship (Levine et al. 2005). In order to prevent aggression in a multiple cat household it is extremely important to introduce a new cat gradually.

Aggression Between Household Cats can have a Defensive or Offensive Display

Fear-related aggression – Defensive (fear-related) aggression is often seen immediately when a new cat is introduced to a new household, from either the resident or the new cat. Defensive aggression can also be the response of a cat to offensive or defensive aggression shown by another cat.

Territorial aggression – Offensive aggression between household cats can also be seen when a new cat is introduced, but usually has a later onset and develops progressively. In the author's experience, an example is represented by the introduction of a young cat in a household with an older resident cat. In this situation, the younger individual may progressively start to stalk and chase away the older cat, often pouncing on the back and biting the neck of the older cat. In response, the older cat will show defensive aggression. This context is often described as territorial aggression between household cats. Sometimes cats will also use offensive aggression to defend their access to resources like valuable resting spots, food, and toys.

Redirected aggression – Redirected aggression is not an unusual trigger of long-lasting conflicts between household cats. It can be caused by an environmental trigger that generates fear like loud noises, or frustration like an unreachable prey; and by offensive or defensive aggression toward another animal. For example, an indoor cat may see a stray outdoor cat from a window and become highly fearful and/or have high sympathetic nervous system arousal. Should another familiar cat bump into the highly aroused cat, he may fall recipient to redirected fear or territorial aggression. The sight of the recipient cat may then trigger the exact same fear response as the outdoor animal did, even days to weeks later, creating havoc in their relationship and household.

Specific Treatment Recommendations for Aggression Between Cats

The treatment and prognosis of aggression between household cats is influenced by the display and motivation of the aggression, and by whether the aggression is physiological or pathological. Offensive territorial aggression is an expected behavior that can be considered part of the normal repertoire of the domestic cat, which is a non-obligate social species. For this reason, this form of aggression can be *managed* with environmental and behavioral modification but not resolved. Conversely, defensive aggression has often a fair to good prognosis and responds well to desensitization and counterconditioning used to reduce the fear of the perceived threat. The presence of the emotional dysregulation typical of pathological aggression complicates the response to the treatment and the prognosis.

As seen for aggression directed to people, separation and confinement are typically the first step of our treatment plan. Each cat must be provided with a safe haven that includes the core needs and resources and be confined to it when at risk of being involved in an aggressive interaction. Depending on the context and severity of the aggression, separation and confinement may be more or less strict. For example, if a cat showing offensive aggression responds well to the human family members trying to redirect his attention using verbal cues and treats (operant conditioning), they may remain out with other cats when the humans in the household can actively supervise their interactions. Very fearful cats that are often the target of aggressive attacks will benefit from stricter confinement in a space that they perceive as safe. In the author's experience, interactions involving offensive territorial aggression are likely to require some degree of separation and confinement in the long-term.

In case of fear-related aggression, reintroduction of the animals following an 8–12-week separation period while implementing behavior modification (e.g. working on recalls and redirection cues) and, when indicated, drug treatment can be successful. The first step of the introduction will involve exposure of the cats to each other's smell. This can be achieved by rotating the cats in a common area different from the respective core areas, or allowing the cats to sniff each other through a barrier, e.g. through the base of a closed door. High-value treats can be dispensed to the cats at the opposite sides of the barrier, to create a positive association via classical conditioning. However, regular meals should not be dispensed to the cats at both sides of the barrier, as cats are solitary hunters and eaters and may be distressed by the presence of other cats when eating. Once the cats seem to be comfortable with the changes in their environment, a step forward can be made in the introduction protocol. Hissing, spitting, attempting to lunge toward, bite, or scratch the other cat, stiffening of the body with prolonged staring, or active avoidance of the other cat, are all signs that the cats are not comfortable one with each other. If cats seem to be comfortable with step one of the introduction protocol, a screen that allows visual contact can then be used. Only when the cats are comfortable enough with this situation, can the transparent barrier be removed and the introduction completed. It is important to make sure that all cats are aware that the barrier is being removed, before they have the chance to meet the cat that was separated from them, to avoid them being caught by surprise and startled. We must inform the caregivers at the beginning of the treatment that the introduction protocol may not be completed, and that some degree of separation between the cats may always be necessary. See the online materials for Chapter 14 for information on introducing and reintroducing cats.

An environment that provides for the physical and behavioral needs of the cat is essential to promote species-typical behavior, decrease stress and improve welfare, and, therefore, decrease the chance that affective aggression may occur (See Chapter 7) (Rochlitz 2014). If the presence of outdoor cats or other animals is a trigger of redirected aggression to household cats, opaque contact paper or window film can be placed on windows to block outdoor visual stimuli (Figure 14.8) and household background white noises can be used to muffle outdoor acoustic stimuli (e.g. vocalizations). Deterrents like water sprinklers or high-pressure canned air spray may be positioned around the perimeter of the house to

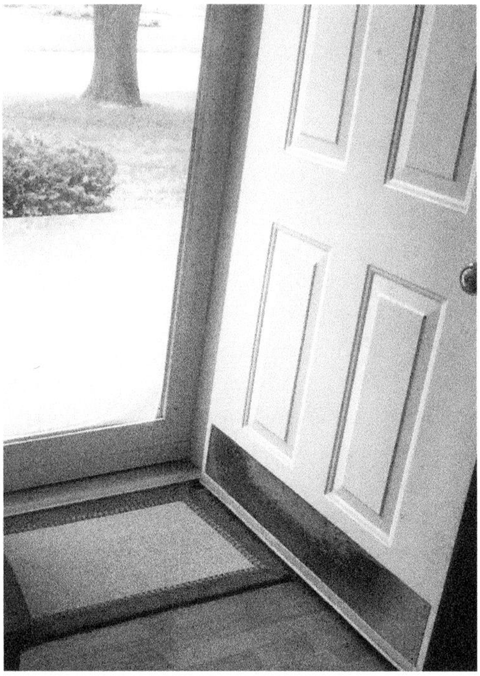

Figure 14.8 A rice paper patterned window film clings to the bottom portion of a storm door, preventing visual access to outdoor cats that might trigger an aggressive event for the cats inside the home. *Source:* Meghan E. Herron.

discourage the presence of outdoor animals. The exterior of entry points to the house must be accurately cleaned with detergents to eliminate possible odors and pheromones deposited by other animals.

Safety protocols should be implemented to minimize the possibility that injuries may occur to the cats during an aggressive interaction or to the people attempting to interrupt them. As seen before, aggressive cats should not be handled unprotected; thick blankets, towels, or cardboard panels can be used in this situation. Water or high-pressure canned air can be used to separate cats during a dangerous fight, only when strictly necessary. Redirection using a positively conditioned sound (via classical or operant conditioning) should always be tried first.

Drug treatment with serotonergic drugs, SSRIs or TCAs, can be used when intense fear, stress, or anxiety are identified as a contributing factor to aggression between cats. See Chapter 21 for classes, doses, and uses of psychoactive drugs.

In conclusion, we have seen how aggressive interactions are part of the normal behavior repertoire of the domestic cat and, for a non-obligate social species like this, should be expected to some degree in certain contexts. Educating cat caregivers on social behavior, creating a welfare-friendly environment, and working on behavior modification to enhance communication and predictability are keys to managing aggression. However, we have also seen how some cats are so highly arousable and impulsive that they respond to low-intensity triggers with extreme aggression. In this case, long-term separation or confinement and the use of psychoactive medication should be considered among our treatment options.

References

Albuquerque, N. and Soares, G. (2019). Epidemiology of domestic cat behavioral problems in the city of Porto Alegre/Brazil: a survey of small animal veterinary practitioners. *Ciência Rural* 49 (10): 90147.

Amat, M., Manteca, X., Brech, S. et al. (2008). Evaluation of inciting causes, alternative targets, and risk factors associated with redirected aggression in cats. *J. Am. Vet. Med. Assoc.* 233 (4): 586–589.

Amat, M., Le Brech, S., Camps, T. et al. (2013). Differences in serotonin serum concentration between aggressive English cocker spaniels and aggressive dogs of other breeds. *J. Vet. Behav.* 8 (1): 19–25.

Bamberger, M. and Houpt, K. (2006). Signalment factors, comorbidity, and trends in behavior diagnoses in cats: 736 cases (1991–2001). *J. Am. Vet. Med. Assoc.* 229 (10): 1602–1606.

Barry, K. and Crowell-Davis, S. (1999). Gender differences in the social behavior of the neutered indoor-only domestic cat. *Appl. Anim. Behav. Sci.* 64 (3): 193–211.

Bear, M., Connors, B., and Siracusa, C. (2016). Brain mechanisms of emotion. In: *Neuroscience*, 4e, 615–643. Philadelphia: Walters Kluwer.

Bernstein, P. and Friedmann, E. (2014). Social behavior of domestic cats in the human home. In: *The Domestic Cat: The Biology of Its Behavior*, 3e (ed. D. Turner and P. Bateson), 71–82. Cambridge, UK: Cambridge University Press.

Bernstein, P. and Strack, M. (1996). A game of cat and house: spatial patterns and behavior of 14 domestic cats (*Felis catus*) in the home. *Anthrozoös* 9 (1): 25–39.

Bateson, P. (2014). Behavioral development in the cat. In: *The Domestic Cat: The Biology of Its Behavior*, 3e (ed. D. Turner and P. Bateson), 11–26. Cambridge, UK: Cambridge University Press.

Berger, J.M. (2016). Feline aggression toward people. In: *August's Consultations in Feline Internal Medicine*, vol. 7 (ed. S. Hetts), 911–918. St. Louis, MO: Elsevier.

Boitani, L., Francisci, F., Ciucci, P., and Andreoli, G. (2016). The ecology and behavior of feral dogs: a case study from central Italy. In: *The Domestic Dog: Its Evolution, Behavior and Interactions with People*, 2e (ed. J. Serpell), 342–368. Cambridge, UK: Cambridge University Press.

Bonanni, R. and Cafazzo, S. (2014). The social organization of a population of free-ranging dogs in a suburban area of Rome: a reassessment of the effects of domestication on dogs' behavior. In: *The Social Dog; Behavior and Cognition* (ed. J. Kaminski and S. Marshall-Pescini), 63–104. San Diego, CA: Academic Press.

Bradshaw, J. and Cameron-Beaumont, C. (2014). The signaling repertoire of the domestic cat and its undomesticated relatives. In: *The Domestic Cat: The Biology of Its Behavior*, 3e (ed. D. Turner and P. Bateson), 67–93. Cambridge, UK: Cambridge University Press.

Bradshaw, J., Casey, R., and Brown, S. (2012). *The Behaviour of the Domestic Cat*, pp.1–15, 128–141, 142–160. Wallingford: CABI.

Bradshaw, J. and Hall, S. (1999). Affiliative behaviour of related and unrelated pairs of cats in catteries: a preliminary report. *Appl. Anim. Behav. Sci.* 63 (3): 251–255.

Broom, D. and Fraser, A. (2007). *Domestic Animal Behaviour and Welfare*, 4e, 73–76. Wallingford, UK: CABI.

Brown, S.L. and Bradshaw, J.W.S. (2014). Communication in the domestic cat: within- and between-species. In: *The Domestic Cat: The Biology of Its Behavior*, 3e (ed. D. Turner and P. Bateson), 37–62. Cambridge, UK: Cambridge University Press.

Buffington, C. (2011). Idiopathic cystitis in domestic cats-beyond the lower urinary tract. *J. Vet. Intern. Med.* 25 (4): 784–796.

Buffington, C. and Bain, M. (2020). Stress and feline health. *Vet. Clin. N. Am. Small Anim. Pract.* 50 (4): 653–662.

Cannon, M. and Rodan, I. (2016). The cat in the veterinary practice. In: *Feline Behavioral Health and Welfare* (ed. I. Rodan and S. Heath), 102–111. St. Luis, MO: Elsevier.

Carlson, N. and Birkett, M. (2017). *Physiology of Behavior*, 12e, 344–379. Essex. UK: Pearson.

Casey, R., Vandenbussche, S., Bradshaw, J., and Roberts, M. (2009). Reasons for relinquishment and return of domestic cats (*Felis Silvestris Catus*) to rescue shelters in the UK. *Anthrozoös* 22 (4): 347–358.

Crowell-Davis, S., Curtis, T., and Knowles, R. (2004). Social organization in the cat: a modern understanding. *J. Feline Med. Surg.* 6 (1): 19–28.

Dantzer, R., O'Connor, J., Freund, G. et al. (2008). From inflammation to sickness and depression: when the immune system subjugates the brain. *Nat. Rev. Neurosci.* 9 (1): 46–56.

De Porter, T. (2018a). Aggression/feline: classification, overview, and prognosis. In: *Blackwell's Five-Minute Veterinary Consult Canine and Feline Behavior*, 2e (ed. D. Horwitz), 145–158. Hoboken, NJ: Wiley Blackwell.

De Porter, T. (2018b). Aggression/feline: petting induced. In: *Blackwell's Five-Minute Veterinary Consult Canine and Feline Behavior*, 2e (ed. D. Horwitz), 199–210. Hoboken, NJ: Wiley Blackwell.

Driscoll, C., Menotti-Raymond, M., Roca, A. et al. (2007). The near eastern origin of cat domestication. *Science* 317 (5837): 519–523.

Fatjó, J., Ruiz-de-la-Torre, J.L., and Manteca, X. (2006). The epidemiology of behavioural problems in dogs and cats: a survey of veterinary practitioners. *Anim. Welf.* 15 (2): 179–185.

Forrester, S. and Towell, T. (2015). Feline idiopathic cystitis. *Vet. Clin. N. Am. Small Anim. Pract.* 45 (4): 783–806.

Foster, J. and McVey Neufeld, K. (2013). Gut–brain axis: how the microbiome influences anxiety and depression. *Trends Neurosci.* 36 (5): 305–312.

Frank, D. (2016). Intercat aggression. In: *August's Consultations in Feline Internal Medicine*, vol. 7 (ed. S. Hetts), 919–929. St. Louis, MO: Elsevier.

Heath, S. (2009). Aggression in cats. In: *BSAVA Manual of Canine and Feline Behavioral Medicine*, 2e (ed. D. Horwitz and D. Mills), 223–235. Gloucester, UK: British Small Animal Veterinary Association.

Heidenberger, E. (1997). Housing conditions and behavioural problems of indoor cats as assessed by their owners. *Appl. Anim. Behav. Sci.* 52 (3-4): 345–364.

León, M., Rosado, B., García-Belenguer, S. et al. (2012). Assessment of serotonin in serum, plasma, and platelets of aggressive dogs. *J. Vet. Behav.* 7 (6): 348–352.

Levine, E., Perry, P., Scarlett, J., and Houpt, K. (2005). Intercat aggression in households following the introduction of a new cat. *Appl. Anim. Behav. Sci.* 90 (3-4): 325–336.

Ley, J. (2021). Aggression – cats. In: *Small Animal Veterinary Psychiatry* (ed. S. Denenberg), 180–190. Boston, MA: CABI.

Liberg, O., Sandell, M., Pointer, D., and Natoli, E. (2000). Density, spatial organization and reproductive tactics in the domestic cat and other felids. In: *The Domestic Cat: The Biology of Its Behavior*, 2e (ed. D. Turner and P. Bateson), 119–150. Cambridge, UK: Cambridge University Press.

Lindell, E., Erb, H., and Houpt, K. (1997). Intercat aggression: a retrospective study examining types of aggression, sexes of fighting pairs, and effectiveness of treatment. *Appl. Anim. Behav. Sci.* 55 (1-2): 153–162.

Macdonald, D.W. and Carr, G.M. (2016). Variation in dog society: between resource dispersion and social flux. In: *The Domestic Dog: Its Evolution, Behavior and Interactions with People*, 2e (ed. J. Serpell), 319–341. Cambridge, UK: Cambridge University Press.

Macdonald, D.W., Yamaguchi, N., and Kery, G. (2000). Group living in the domestic cat: its sociobiology and epidemiology. In: *The Domestic Cat: The Biology of Its Behavior*, 2e (ed. D. Turner and P. Bateson), 95–118. Cambridge, UK: Cambridge University Press.

Mills, D.S. (2009). Training and learning protocols. In: *BSAVA Manual of Canine and Feline Behavioural Medicine*, 2e (ed. D.F. Horwitz and D.S. Mills), 49–64. Gloucester: British Small Animal Veterinary Association.

Mills, D., Braem Dube, M., and Zulch, H. (2013). *Stress and Pheromonatheraphy in Small Animal Clinical Behavior*, 225–241. Ames, Iowa: Wiley Blackwell.

Natoli, E., Baggio. A., and Pontier, D. (2001). Male and female agonistic and affiliative relationships in a social group of farm cats (Felis catus L.), *Behav. Process.* 53 (1–2): 137–143.

Nelson, R. and Kriegsfeld, L. (2018). *An Introduction to Behavioral Endocrinology*, 5e. New York, NY: Oxford University Press.

Notari, L. (2009). Stress in veterinary behavioral medicine. In: *BSAVA Manual of Canine and Feline Behavioural Medicine*, 2e (ed. D.F. Horwitz and D.S. Mills), 136–145. Gloucester: British Small Animal Veterinary Association.

Palacio, J., León-Artozqui, M., Pastor-Villalba, E. et al. (2007). Incidence of and risk factors for cat bites: a first step in prevention and treatment of feline aggression. *J. Feline Med. Surg.* 9 (3): 188–195.

Ramos, D. and Mills, D. (2009). Human directed aggression in Brazilian domestic cats: owner reported prevalence, contexts and risk factors. *J. Feline Med. Surg.* 11 (10): 835–841.

Reid, J., Nolan, A., and Scott, E. (2018). Measuring pain in dogs and cats using structured behavioural observation. *Vet. J.* 236: 72–79.

Reisner, I., Mann, J., Stanley, M. et al. (1996). Comparison of cerebrospinal fluid monoamine metabolite levels in dominant-aggressive and non-aggressive dogs. *Brain Res.* 714 (1-2): 57–64.

Rochlitz, I. (2005). A review of the housing requirements of domestic cats (*Felis silvestris catus*) kept in the home. *Appl. Anim. Behav. Sci.* 93 (1-2): 97–109.

Rochlitz, I. (2014). Feline welfare issues. In: *The Domestic Cat: The Biology of Its Behavior*, 2e (ed. D. Turner and P. Bateson), 131–154. Cambridge, UK: Cambridge University Press.

Scarlett, J., Salman, M., New, J. Jr., and Kass, P. (1999). Reasons for relinquishment of companion animals in U.S. animal shelters: selected health and personal issues. *J. Appl. Anim. Welf. Sci.* 2 (1): 41–57.

Serpell, J. (2014). Domestication and history of the cat. In: *The Domestic Cat: The Biology of Its Behavior*, 3e (ed. D. Turner and P. Bateson), 83–100. Cambridge, UK: Cambridge University Press.

Siracusa, C. (2016a). Creating harmony in multiple cat households. In: *August's Consultations in Feline Internal Medicine*, vol. 7 (ed. S. Hetts), 931–940. St. Louis, MO: Elsevier.

Siracusa, C. (2016b). Treatments affecting dog behaviour: something to be aware of. *Vet. Rec.* 179 (18): 460–461.

Siracusa, C. (2021). Aggression – dogs. In: *Small Animal Veterinary Psychiatry* (ed. S. Denenberg), 191–206. Boston, MA: CABI.

Siracusa, C. and Horwitz, D.F. (2018). Psychopharmacology. In: *Blackwell's Five-Minute Veterinary Consult Canine and Feline Behavior*, 2e (ed. D. Horwitz), 961–974. Hoboken, NJ: Wiley Blackwell.

Siracusa, C. and Landsberg, G. (2020). Psychogenic diseases. In: *Feline Dermatology* (ed. C. Noli and S. Colombo), 567–582. Cham, Switzerland: Springer Nature Switzerland.

Souza-Dantas, L.M., Soares, G.M., d'Almeida, J.M., and Paixão, R.L. (2009). Epidemiology of domestic cat behavioral and welfare issues: a survey of Brazilian referral animal hospitals in 2009. *Intern. J. Appl. Res. Vet. Med.* 7: 130–137.

Stelow, E. (2020). Behavior as an illness indicator. *Vet. Clin. N. Am. Small Anim. Pract.* 50 (4): 695–706.

Stevens, B., Frantz, E., Orlando, J. et al. (2016). Efficacy of a single dose of trazodone hydrochloride given to cats prior to veterinary visits to reduce signs of transport- and examination-related anxiety. *J. Am. Vet. Med. Assoc.* 249 (2): 202–207.

Turner, D.C. (2014). Social organization and behavioral ecology of free-ranging domestic cats. In: *The Domestic Cat: The Biology of Its Behavior*, 3e (ed. D. Turner and P. Bateson), 63–70. Cambridge, UK: Cambridge University Press.

van Haaften, K., Forsythe, L., Stelow, E., and Bain, M. (2017). Effects of a single preappointment dose of gabapentin on signs of stress in cats during transportation and veterinary examination. *J. Am. Vet. Med. Assoc.* 251 (10): 1175–1181.

Wassink-van der Schot, A., Day, C., Morton, J. et al. (2016). Risk factors for behavior problems in cats presented to an Australian companion animal behavior clinic. *J. Vet. Behav.* 14: 34–40.

Wiese, A. (2014). Assessing pain: pain behaviors. In: *Handbook of Veterinary Pain Management*, 3e (ed. J. Gaynor and W. Muir), 67–97. St. Luois: MO: Elsevier Health Sciences.

15

Canine Aggression

Gabrielle Carter

Royal Society for the Prevention of Cruelty to Animals Victoria, Burwood East, VIC, Australia

Introduction

Dog aggression is a serious public safety concern – both for people and other companion animals. Sadly, it is also the most common behavioral reason for death in dogs under three years of age (Yu et al. 2021). This puts the family veterinarian in an essential role in understanding, preventing, and knowing how to manage aggression in dogs. Such knowledge is crucial to maintaining a healthy human–animal bond and ensuring the welfare of the community and of the dogs themselves.

Believe it or not, aggression is a normal behavior, with obvious adaptive advantages. Aggressive behavior provided the domestic dog's ancestor an evolutionary advantage for maintaining access to essential resources and mates, and defense against threats. Through the process of domestication (see Chapter 2), docility and the propensity for tameness have been strongly selected for by humans and are heritable traits. That said, it is still not uncommon for dogs to use aggression when they perceive that their resources or they themselves are being threatened. It is estimated that 40% of dogs have growled at household members, 20% of them having growled or snapped over food, and 15% have bitten a household member (Guy et al. 2001). This means that for every seven dogs you see in practice, one is likely to have bitten the hand that feeds them.

What is Aggression?

Aggression is a distance-increasing signal that encompasses a suite of behaviors involving threats and/or causing physical or emotional harm. It is a complex behavior, often resulting from a culmination of multiple environmental, genetic, and learning factors. The motivations underlying aggression can vary greatly, both within an individual and between dogs. Most commonly, the motivation is to avoid or end an unpleasant (e.g., fear-inducing, irritating, or frustrating) or undesirable (e.g., having food taken away) event. The triggers for and contexts in which aggression is displayed are numerous and specific to the individual. Internal states related to disease, pain, hormonal status, and levels of arousal influence the expression of aggression.

Aggression versus Predatory Behavior

Whilst predatory behavior has the intent to harm, it is notably different in many ways from socially positioned and affective aggressions.

Introduction to Animal Behavior and Veterinary Behavioral Medicine, First Edition. Edited by Meghan E. Herron.

Companion website: www.wiley.com/go/introductiontoanimalbehavior

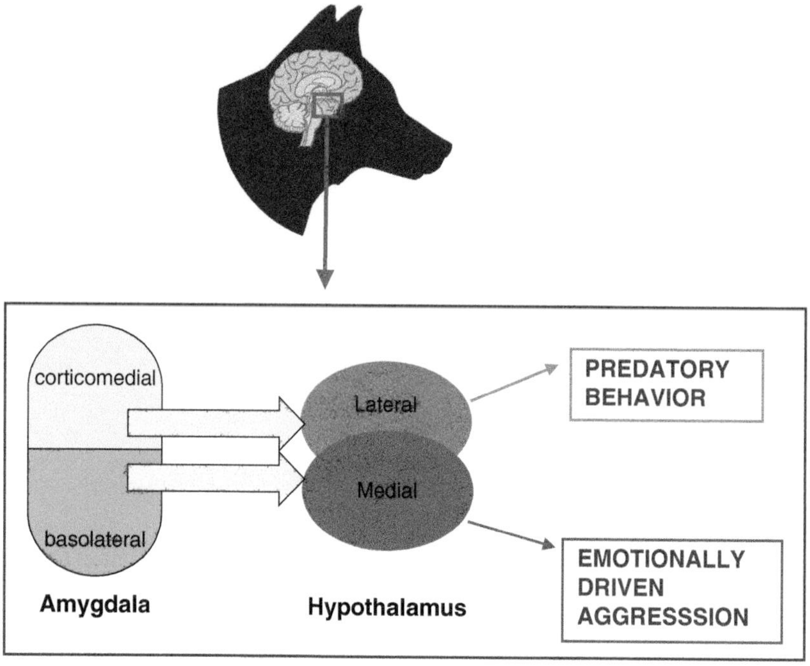

Figure 15.1 Different pathways for control of predatory behavior and emotionally driven aggression. Predatory behavior is controlled by the lateral hypothalamus, whilst emotionally driven aggression follows a different route starting in the ventrolateral hypothalamus. Lesions in the corticomedial amygdala increase predatory aggression, whilst stimulation of the basolateral amygdala produces emotionally driven aggression. Given the very different behavioral presentations, it is not surprising to learn that predatory aggression and emotionally driven aggression are controlled by different circuitry in the brain.

A primary difference is that predatory behavior has the intention of decreasing distance between predator and prey. As discussed in Chapter 14, we prefer to use the term predatory behavior rather than predatory aggression. It differs not only in behavioral presentation but is regulated by a different neurophysiological pathway (Figure 15.1).

Predatory behavior is characterized by a quiet attack and a distinct sequence of behavior, comprising see, orientate, stare, stalk, chase, grab bite, kill bite/shake, dissect, and consume. Attack is commonly directed to the neck, forelimbs, and shoulders, resulting in fractures to the forelimbs, crushing injuries to the throat, and tears to the skin and muscles of the neck and chest. Stimuli include fast movements, cries, and screams. Targets are prey species, such as cats, rabbits, and birds, and potentially young children, elderly humans, and other dogs.

Predatory behavior occurs without threat or warning, and the intent is to kill. In a full predatory attack, there is no graded response, and the dog may show little inhibition. The dog's focus is intense, and arousal can become high, making it extremely difficult to distract the dog. It is an instinctual behavior and differs markedly from socially motivated aggressions associated with emotional states such as anger, fear, anxiety, and frustration. Importantly, predatory behavior is highly rewarding. As an evolutionary strategy, deriving pleasure from behaviors that ultimately help the animal obtain food makes a lot of sense. However, this characteristic of predatory behavior, along with a strong genetic basis, makes treatment challenging. Calling the dog back for a bit of roast chicken is unlikely to compete with the innate reward of the predatory experience. Dogs can learn to inhibit the instinctual drive, especially when pursuit is not possible (e.g., on leash), and may appear "cured." However, treatment to curb instinctual behavior often shows limited success. Predatory attacks are dangerous and treatment unreliable, making management an essential recommendation for dogs displaying predatory behavior.

The Body Language of Aggression

Aggression is characterized by threatening or "warning" behaviors like growling, barking, and baring teeth, and "attack" behaviors like lunging, snapping, and biting – both with the intention of *increasing* distance between the aggressor and their perceived threat. Displays of aggression are generally exhibited in an escalating sequence and are accompanied or preceded by threatening (e.g. standing over, staring) or defensive, fear-based (e.g. ears being pulled back, and the tail held down) postures. Recognition of early warning signs allows handlers to take action to avoid escalation and injury (Figure 15.2).

The body language associated with aggression helps to distinguish between defensive and offensive aggression, suggesting insight into the dog's emotional status.

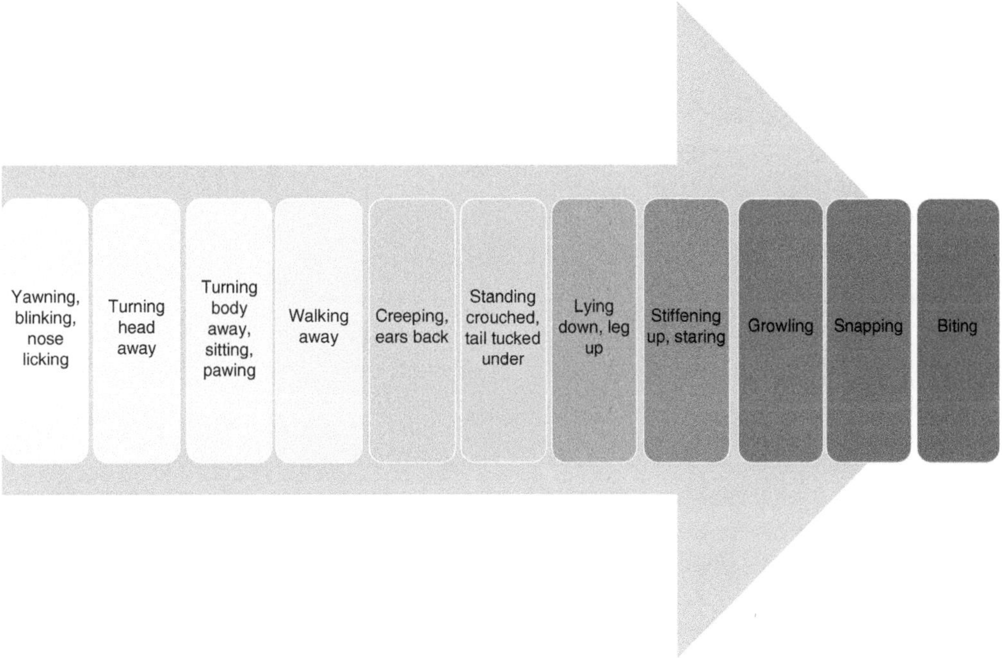

Figure 15.2 Behavior associated with escalation of fear-based aggression. As discussed in Chapter 11, aggression is a strategy dogs may utilize when escape and/or avoidance do not seem feasible and/or have failed in previous similar situations. Early signs of fear, anxiety, and stress (FAS) are also outlined in Chapter 11 and here we illustrate how early signs can progress to biting – sometimes with time and repeated interactions, and in some cases within a singular interaction. Early signs of FAS are shown in the first four yellow boxes. As FAS increases, the dog then starts to show nonthreatening behavior in an attempt to appease the perceived threat, indicated by the orange boxes. As the body starts to stiffen and the dog gives hard stares, the behavior is moving towards aggression. Finally, in the red boxes, we see growling and snapping as warnings of ensuing aggression, followed by behavior designed to harm – biting. Identifying the potential for escalation enables action to be taken early on, to avert threatening or harmful behaviors.

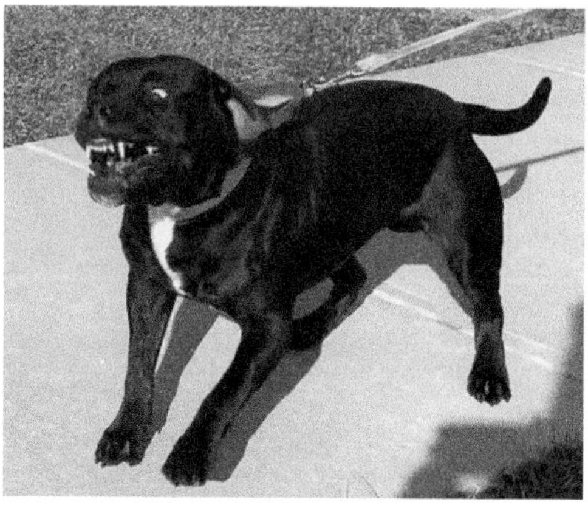

Figure 15.3 A defensively aggressive dog has his ears back, tail down, weight shifted towards the back, and is showing a full mouth display of teeth. *Source:* Meghan E. Herron.

Defensive Aggression

Defensive aggression is characterized by body language conveying fear. Presentations include a lowered body, leaning away or retreating, ears back and low, and a wide open mouth displaying all the teeth (Figure 15.3). Biting often takes the form of lunge-bite-retreat.

Offensive Aggression

Offensive aggression takes on a more confident presentation where the dog will be standing tall with the head up, maybe leaning and/or moving forward, with tail raised, and a vertical retraction of the lips, displaying the incisors and canines only (Figure 15.4). This type of aggression may be seen in territorial displays, hierarchal displays between dogs, maternal aggression cases, and in fear-based aggression that has been well-rehearsed (see Box 15.1). The more often fearful dogs rehearse aggressive behavior and learn that it is an effective means to increase distance from what threatens them, the more confident they become in using it. Over time the body language shifts from defensive to offensive. The root motivation, however, may still be fear.

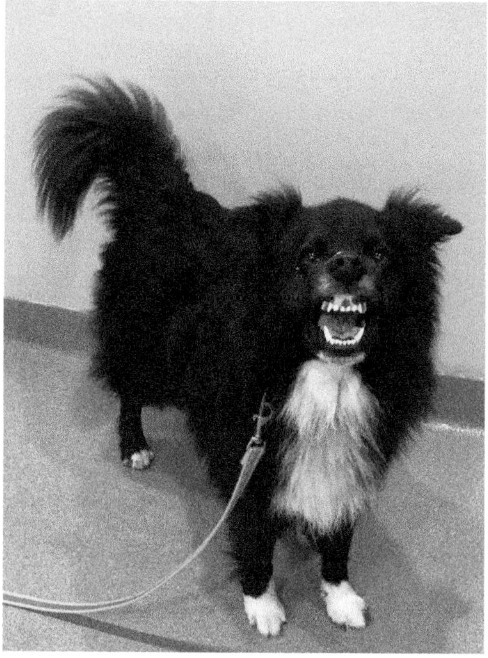

Figure 15.4 An offensively aggressive dog has his head and tail erect, a direct hard stare, and bares mostly the front teeth. *Source:* Meghan E. Herron.

A Mixed Bag

Dogs may present with a combination of these forms or move between these presentations, suggesting mixed emotions and changes over time and context. Consider the dog that barks confidently at the door when the doorbell rings, but shows a more defensive behavior, backing away, growling, and barking with lowered body and ears back when the visitor enters the home, and then as the visitor turns their back to walk away, the dog rushes forward and nips them on the heels or rear end. This would suggest initial confidence behind the barrier of the door – *perhaps this display will prevent them from entering?* The behavior then shifts to a more defensive posture as the visitor crosses the threshold of the doorway – here the dog may not feel safe enough to use aggression when closely confronted inside the home. Avoidance and defensive threats seem safer now. As the visitor turns their back though, the

Box 15.1 Case study of a one-year-old German Shepherd dog with offensive aggression

A one-year-old, female spayed, German Shepherd dog is presented with offensive aggression towards unfamiliar dogs. Video footage shows her barking at a small dog on leash, about 50 feet away. The small dog is sniffing and pays no attention to the German Shepherd. The patient is standing tall, leaning forward, with tail raised stiffly, ears erect and pointing forward, the head is held high, she is staring directly at the small dog, and there is general muscle tension in the face and body, along with piloerection along the spine. She looks very threatening and is pulling towards the small dog. Her history reveals that she was very shy in puppy classes and spent the first three weeks under the client's chair. She eventually came out and moved around the room and sniffed other dogs but did not play. Over the next few months, she would hide behind the client's legs when encountering other dogs on walks. This progressed to standing next to the client and growling. By 10 months of age, she would growl, bark, and lunge at passing dogs. Despite the presentation of offensively aggressive body language, the history reveals that motivation for the behavior is based on fear. This fear will need to be addressed to change her behavior.

dog gets just enough of a confidence boost to move forward more offensively and bite.

Additionally, a fearful emotional state results in rapid and persistent learning. In this state, if the dog learns that their aggression is successful in relieving their fear (e.g. the person/dog goes away), they are likely to use aggression in the same context in the future. Repeated successful use of this aggressive strategy reinforces the behavior, and the dog may use aggression preemptively to avoid scary encounters. In this scenario, the dog may show more confident body language, as they are not yet threatened (see Box 15.1).

Factors that Influence Aggression

Fear, Anxiety, and Pain

Fear is the most common motivation for aggressive behavior in dogs. Fearful dogs present a higher risk of aggression towards people (Flint et al. 2017; Guy et al. 2001) and dogs (Haverbeke et al. 2009; Arata et al. 2014), whilst social dogs are generally less fearful and less aggressive (Asp et al. 2015). Dogs showing aggression often have comorbid diagnoses of anxiety (Bamberger and Houpt 2006) or fear (Fatjo et al. 2007). It is important when evaluating dogs with aggression to carefully assess for signs of fear and anxiety, both through observation and history taking. When in a highly threatened state, the main behavioral responses are flight, fight, freeze, or display displacement behaviors (fidget). If flight is prevented (e.g. cornered, restrained, tethered, or on leash) then "fight" becomes more likely.

Not all fearful dogs show aggression, with some nearly always choosing the flight option. Why some fearful dogs rarely if ever resort to aggression when threatened may relate to genetics. That said, other more immediate health and experiential factors can lead to a sudden change in strategy.

The threshold for aggression may be much lower in an anxious dog than it would be for a non-anxious dog (Figure 15.5a). For example, a dog with fear aggression toward strangers may be triggered to aggress when an unfamiliar visitor reaches to pet them, whereas a dog with fear aggression *and* generalized anxiety might be triggered to bite when an unfamiliar person simply enters the house.

In a similar manner, pain or the anticipation of pain can lower the threshold for aggression (Figure 15.5b). Arthritis, ear infections, dental disease, pathology of the gastrointestinal tract, and other disease conditions may result in pain

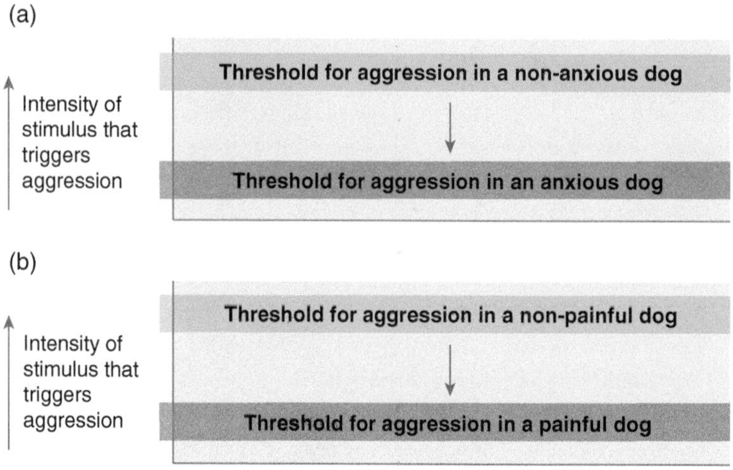

Figure 15.5 Effects of anxiety (a) and pain/discomfort (b) on the threshold of aggression in dogs. Anxiety, pain, and/or discomfort can all lower the threshold for an aggressive response. What might not trigger an aggressive response in a non-anxious, non-painful dog could certainly trigger aggression in one in a physically or mentally uncomfortable state. *Source:* Meghan E. Herron.

when dogs play or are handled, provoking an aggressive response. Other medical pathologies, which may not cause significant pain, but rather malaise and discomfort, can also increase irritability – defined as a lowered threshold for aggression. Aggression in dogs has also been correlated with gut health and microbiome status. Gut microbial composition has been shown to vary between dogs with and without intraspecific aggression (Kirchoff et al. 2019). These associations require further investigation before we can conclude a causative relationship but highlight the relationship between health status and aggression. A full medical examination is warranted in all cases of aggression (where possible) to rule out any painful and/or medical contributing conditions.

Arousal and Aggression

States of high emotional arousal, for example, anger, frustration, or even play, may increase the possibility of aggression, along with focusing attention, increasing the perception of threat, and reducing behavioral inhibition (Rayment et al. 2015). When highly excited, even social dogs if frightened or threatened are likely to "act first and think later." That is, we see more reflexive behavior and less cognitive thought. Combine high arousal with fear and anxiety and the risk of aggression is high. For example, when the doorbell rings and arousal is high, two dogs bouncing off each other in a narrow hallway as they race to the front door is a classic scenario resulting in an aggressive interaction.

Breed and Aggression

Breed differences in the prevalence and severity of household member-directed, stranger-directed, and dog-directed aggression have been identified (Duffy et al. 2008), and a genetic basis for these differing categories of aggression is suggested. Breed differences have also been potentially correlated with defensive (fear-based) and offensive aggressions, with different breeds showing aggression having different fear scores (Duffy et al. 2008).

Whilst breed differences in behavior are real, genetic variation within breeds is also relevant. That is, some individuals in the breed may have a high tendency to display aggressive behaviors and others a much lower tendency, and selective breeding to reduce the trait can alter the breed's overall aggressiveness within a few generations

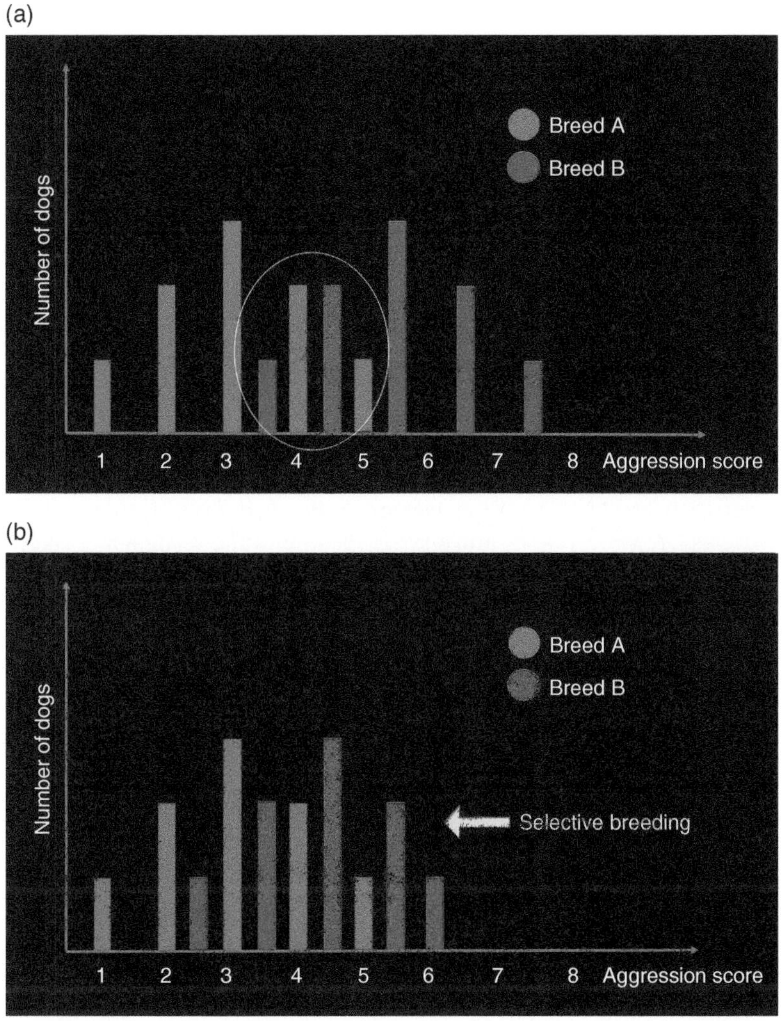

Figure 15.6 Selective breeding theoretical model shows how breeds can vary in characteristics such as aggression over time. Note that in graph (a) there is a distinct difference in aggression scores between Breed A (blue) and Breed B (red), with Breed B having higher aggression scores overall. Not all Breed B dogs have high aggression scores and there is some overlap between the two breeds as indicated by the columns circled in white. Graph (b) shows that by selectively breeding only those Breed B (red) individuals who have lower aggression scores, breeders can alter the aggression profile of Breed B so that it becomes similar to the aggression profile of Breed A within a few generations.

(Van Der Velden et al. 1976) (Figure 15.6). The upshot is that breed characteristics change over time and that the genetic pool in one part of the world may differ from that in another. For instance, Dachshunds in Australia may have a different propensity towards aggression than Dachshunds in Germany as a result of different breeding pedigrees. Similarly, Dachshunds in Australia in 1990 may have been more or less aggressive than Dachshunds in 2022. It is therefore spurious to make absolute breed assumptions regarding aggressive predisposition. If we are looking for the genetic basis of behavior within breeds, we may find that particular bloodlines are involved (Van Den Berg et al. 2003; Reisner and Houpt 2005), and that a particular trait is not necessarily inherent in the breed as a whole.

The genetic impact on aggression most likely results from the interaction of many genes and subsequently there will be variation in motivation, regulation, and expression between individuals. Add to this the interaction between genes and environmental influences and the pathways leading to aggressive behavior become infinite. Two dogs may present with the same behavior, but the pathway to get there may be very different. From a practical, clinical perspective this means each dog presenting with aggression must be assessed on an individual basis, to tailor a treatment plan and determine prognosis, rather than leaning on breed-specific characterizations.

Whist genetics influence the probability of a behavior, it is genetics interacting with the physical environment, learning, and social relationships that determine the behavioral outcome. For example, low levels of sociability have been associated with higher levels of stranger and child-directed aggression (Kaneko et al. 2013; Dodman et al. 2018). Sociability is influenced by genetics but is also highly dependent on social learning, especially early in life. The environment and learning experiences can be manipulated to provide strategies to reduce the expression of aggression.

Age and Aggression

Aggressive behavior in dogs often starts as dogs approach social maturity (refer to Chapter 6 for more details). In most behaviorists' experience, clients tend to seek help for the first time for aggressive behavior in dogs between eight months and three years of age. While most aggression may have an adolescent or adult-onset, young puppies (under 14 weeks of age) can present with serious aggression, but this is uncommon. Many clients may ask if the aggressive behavior is something their dog will "grow out of." Unfortunately, aggression is something that, if left to its natural course, will worsen with time and rehearsal of the behavior. Dogs may outgrow their puppy energy and rowdiness as they mature, but aggression is a completely separate entity from energy or manners. Interestingly, one study identified that dogs that suffered an illness during the first 16 weeks of life were more likely to have a high aggression score as adults (Podberscek and Serpell 1997).

Sex and Aggression

Hormonal status can impact the propensity to display aggression. Maternal aggression is one example, and there is some evidence that pseudopregnancy may also increase the propensity to use aggression (Borchelt 1983). However, controversy reigns around the relative propensity of male and female dogs to exhibit aggressive behavior and the effects of gonadectomy.

There is a marked lack of consistency in the literature regarding the association between sex, neuter status, and an aggression diagnosis. There is no consistent research to support the concept that in general male dogs are more aggressive than female dogs (Scandurra et al. 2018). In the category of intraspecific aggression, some studies conclude that males are more likely to fight, especially with other male dogs (Roll and Unshelm 1997), whilst others have found no sex differences.

Environment and Aggression

Ultimately, the nature of behavior is to be adaptable. Behavior needs to change in relation to environmental conditions to ensure positive outcomes for individuals over their lifetime. The important message here is that behavior changes and it does so in response to environmental changes and learning. To fully understand the development of behavior problems, we need to understand the impact of the environment, and, likewise, environmental management is extremely important in the treatment of aggression.

Environmental factors including where and how the dog is housed have been associated with increased risk of aggression. Dogs obtained from pet stores and/or born and raised in high-volume commercial breeding establishments have a higher propensity to display aggression towards people and other dogs. They are also more likely to have increased fear in response to strangers, children, other dogs, non-social stimuli, and being taken on walks (McMillan 2017; Appleby et al. 2002). Hsu and Sun (2010) reported increased risk of household member-directed aggression in dogs kept outside the house, and higher risk of aggression towards unfamiliar people in dogs living in rural areas and in houses with yard space. Irritability can also increase in response to environmental factors like loud and sustained noises. Dogs with a high aggression score are more likely to react to loud or high-pitched noises (Podberscek and Serpell 1997).

Confinement and restraint can intensify aggression. Dogs may show aggressive behavior in a cage or pen, or when on leash or tethered, but when released from confinement/restraint the aggression dissipates. Some dogs may display aggression towards unfamiliar people or dogs whilst on leash, but may not when off leash (see Box 15.2). The likely reason for this is that when restrained or confined, the option of flight has been removed, and so the "fight" option (aggression) becomes a more likely strategy when faced with a potentially threatening or scary situation. The confined/restrained dog is also more likely to feel vulnerable and experience a lack of control, increasing frustrative arousal and anxiety. Restrained dogs do not have the ability to use distance (and associated time) and space to try out behaviors like appeasement or friendly invitations such as play or assess how the intruder responds to their insecurity.

Learning and Aggression

The most apparent illustration of the impact of learning on aggression occurs when a specific event results in changed behavior. A man in a hat kicks the dog and the dog is now aggressive towards men in hats. However, more generalized learning is also impactful. For example, dogs that are appropriately socialized as puppies are less likely to exhibit aggression (Howell et al. 2015; Serpell and Jagoe 1995). There are reports of a reduced risk of aggression to unfamiliar people in dogs that have attended puppy classes (Casey et al. 2014). However, this finding is not consistent and may reflect different learning experiences. Poorly managed group classes and/or use of aversive training methods may increase aggressive behavior toward other dogs and people, rather than reduce it.

Box 15.2 Leash reactivity – What motivates this behavior and in general how can we change it?

Fearful dogs will often choose flight as a strategy to increase distance from the scary stimulus. When on leash, this option may be perceived as unavailable. Consequently, the fight response becomes more likely. It is not uncommon for dogs to only show aggression towards other dogs/people when on leash, and not when off leash. Off leash, these dogs can use the flight option, maintain a non-threatening distance from other dogs, and are able to express a greater range of appeasement behaviors, free from the restrictions of the leash. This creates a conundrum when we want to maintain control of the potentially aggressive dog, by keeping them on leash. The solution is to teach the dog that despite being on leash they can still "run away." When seeing other dogs, the owner does a U-turn and moves quickly in the other direction. In most cases, it is not long before the patient initiates the U-turn when seeing other dogs. The dog now has an acceptable coping strategy on leash, and we can start work on building confidence around social interactions with other dogs.

Propensity to use aggression is influenced by the nature of relationships with others. When social interaction results in a negative emotional experience (e.g. punishment, challenge over space, and important resources) the probability of aggression increases. The use of confrontational training techniques has been associated with a higher likelihood of aggression in dogs (Herron et al. 2009; Hus and Sun 2010). Additionally, as discussed in Chapter 11, there is an inherent miscommunication between dogs and people when conveying intent. For humans gazing directly at one another's face, leaning over, and hugging are often affectionate gestures, but for dogs, these same gestures (bending, leaning, reaching, hugging) are more likely to be interpreted as threats and result in some dogs responding aggressively.

Making an Aggression Diagnosis

Aggression in dogs is typically diagnosed based on the motivation for the behavior. Understanding the driving force behind aggression enables treatment focused on cause, rather than symptoms. Explaining the motivation for the dog's aggressive behavior helps families understand what may previously have been seen as unjustified behavior. Understanding can foster empathy and enable carers to make informed choices regarding management, with consideration of the dog's welfare. While there are multiple motivational diagnoses for aggression used in veterinary medicine, the vast majority boils down to a dog's perception that their personal safety and/or prized possessions are being threatened, making fear-related aggression and resource guarding some of the most commonly diagnosed conditions.

Step 1: Taking a History

The first step in diagnosing these conditions is taking a thorough and accurate history. As discussed in Chapter 12, a thorough history includes details regarding the physical environment, the events occurring just before and after the behavior in question, and details about the behavior itself. Specifically for aggression, we want to identify each trigger for aggression (what happened right before the behavior occurred), the target of the aggression (person, dog, both – familiar, unfamiliar, or both), and the level of aggression displayed (barking, growling, lunging, snapping, biting – level of injury, if any). An aggression screen in your history questionnaire is often helpful (Figure 15.7). When clients recount incidents of aggression, try to build a detailed screenplay of the event in your mind. Set the scene, see the activity of everyone in the picture, and envision the body language of the dog. Clients may not recognize important details that direct their understanding of the dog's aggression (see Box 15.3).

Step 2: Observation

If you are able to schedule a full behavior consultation, observation of the dog's behavior across a range of contexts, both during the consultation and from video footage of everyday interactions will be helpful. Such observation allows interpretation of the dog's body language and default reactions to triggers. Whilst history relies on the client's observation skills, this step allows you to objectively determine motivation and triggers and assess levels of underlying fear and anxiety. These will help confirm the motivation for aggression, triggers, and requirements for management and behavior modification.

Step 3: Medical Assessment and Rule Outs

Where possible, a full medical examination, including physical assessment, screening blood, and urine analysis, and where indicated imaging, is desirable to uncover underlying diseases that may increase irritability, or directly affect behavior. Refer to Chapter 12 for the

Interactions with household members

Please tell us if there is any aggression in the following circumstances to any members of your household. This may include growling, showing teeth, lunging, nipping, snapping, or biting. **Please fill in the chart with "Y" if there has been any aggression to any family member in each circumstance, "N" for no aggression, and N/A if the circumstance does not apply.**

Household members	Female adults	Male adults	Children	Specific person	Details
Petting or reaching for dog					
Hugging or kissing dog					
Bending over or staring at dog					
Bathing, grooming or towelling dog					
Disturbing dog when resting					
Pushing or calling dog off furniture					
Giving verbal or physical corrections					
Approach/interact when dog is eating					
Approach/interact when dog has bone or other chew item					
Putting on leash or collar					
Lifting dog					

Interactions with non-household members

Please tell us if there is any aggression in the following circumstances to any person who is not a member of your household. This may include growling, showing teeth, lunging, nipping, snapping, or biting. **Please fill in the chart with "Y" if there has been any aggression in each circumstance, "N" for no aggression, and N/A if the circumstance does not apply.**

Non-household members	Female adults	Male adults	Children	Specific person	Details
Petting or reaching towards dog					
Bending over or staring at dog					
Entering your house or yard					
Enter/exit any room in your home					
Passing when dog is on leash					
Passing when dog is in the car					
Interacting with dog on leash					
Interacting with dog away from home					
Putting on leash or collar					
Running, jogging, biking					

Figure 15.7 An aggression screen helps identify targets (dogs, people, households, and non-household members) and triggers (what situations provoke the aggression).

Interactions with other dogs

Please tell us if there is any aggression in the following circumstances to dogs. This may include growling, showing teeth, lunging, nipping, snapping, or biting. **Please fill in the chart with "Y" if there has been any aggression in each circumstance, "N" for no aggression, and N/A if the circumstance does not apply.**

Dog shows aggression towards	Companion dog in the household	Unfamiliar dog	Details
Carer gives attention to, or pets another dog			
Passing or seeing another dog on the street, whilst on leash			
Another dog entering your house or yard			
Another dog approaches or interacts when dog is eating, or near food			
Another dog approaches or interacts when dog has high value item			
Passing another dog when in the car			
Interacting with another dog when **on leash**			
Interacting with another dog when **off leash**			
When playing with another dog			

Figure 15.7 (Continued)

Box 15.3 Compare these two histories of the same aggressive incident

a) *The child was in the living room, playing on the floor. The dog entered the room and came over to where I was sitting on the couch, with the child at my feet on the floor, and the dog then bit the child.*
b) *Friends were visiting, and they were sitting on the couch opposite me. There was a coffee table between us. The child was playing on the floor at my feet. The dog entered the room and came to me. The child reached to pet her, and the dog went under the coffee table. The child reached to pet the dog again and the dog bit the child.*

The later history provides greater insight into the dog's motivation for aggression. A fear response indicated by initial withdrawal to a safer place under the table, and subsequently, a bite when flight was no longer an option suggest fear-based aggression. The presence of visitors and the child may represent unpredictability for this individual and this aspect warrants further investigation.

The dog that enters a room and walks up to a child and bites them, without provocation (history a), presents greater risk and carries a poorer prognosis, than a fear-aggressive dog that defaults to retreat, can be managed safely, and has a better prognosis for reducing aggression.

Obtaining a detailed and comprehensive history is imperative to inform management, treatment, prognosis, and outcome decisions.

Box 15.4 Can they not just make up their mind?

Many dogs may seem conflicted and/or wavering in their interactions with people and give confusing signals to the humans with whom they interact. For example, an individual dog may enjoy social interaction and be motivated to approach a visitor in a friendly manner, but they may also experience some anxiety about the outcome of interacting with the unfamiliar person. When the person reaches to pet the dog on the head, they experience fear and are motivated to withdraw. The associated high arousal and the limited ability to withdraw once they are close enough for the person to interact can result in growling, snapping, and biting. Clients will commonly describe the dog as a "Jekyll and Hyde," and report the dog approaching, seeking interaction, and then snapping. From the human's perspective, the aggression may appear completely unprovoked. These dogs can sometimes be "trickier" for clients to manage as their dogs seem to put themselves into the situation that triggers bites.

"Minimum Database" diagnostics for behavior problems.

After reviewing your history, assessing for medical contributions to behavior, and observing the dog in different contexts, you should be able to make a diagnosis based on the motivation for the behavior. Following is a list of differential diagnoses for aggressive behavior in dogs:

Fear-related aggression – Aggression in response to a perceived threat to a dog's personal safety. This type of aggression can take on a defensive or offensive form, depending on the context, previous learning, and other factors.

Resource guarding – Aggression in response to a perceived threat to food, items, and/or resources that are considered valuable to that individual dog. Anxious or fearful dogs that feel protected and secure in the proximity of a carer may show aggression if another individual (dog, person, or other animal) gets close or interacts with "their" person. The sense of safety provided by the carer has become a resource worth fighting for.

Conflict-related aggression – Aggression in response to a motivational conflict – generally an approach-withdrawal conflict. Body language is characterized by both approach (prosocial) and withdrawal (fear-based) behaviors, along with signs of anxiety like lip licking and yawning. Often appeasement behaviors are noted before and after the aggressive incident – loose, lowered body with low tail wag, dropped ears, and licking (see Box 15.4).

Conflict aggression is commonly directed towards a familiar human household member with whom the dog has a bond, but who either rationally or irrationally is perceived as a threat in certain contexts or circumstances. Carer-directed aggression has often been misinterpreted as dominance-related aggression. However, instead of seeing confident and assertive offensive aggression, more commonly we see conflict and approach-withdrawal behavior. There may be a history of punishment by the carer, which creates the conflicting motivations of care-seeking and fear. In these cases, it is inconsistency in interactions that underlies the conflict. Treatment focused on consistent and structured interactions that are rewarded goes a long way toward resolving this problem.

Territorial aggression – Aggression directed towards people or animals outside of the familiar household social group. It can occur in any area the dog perceives as its home base – crate, bed, house, yard, car, or even a frequented park. Signs of territorial aggression may begin to appear in the later part of the first year (Landsberg et al. 2003). It occurs equally in males and females and is not affected by neutering. Confining or restraining a dog may intensify territorial aggression.

In some cases, a fear component to territorial aggression is evident in the dog's body language. The dog may be barking and lunging at an "intruder" but at the same time backing away. The body may be low to the ground and the tail tucked. It has been suggested that more fearful individuals have a stronger need, than more confident dogs, for a "safe" place. This place of security becomes an important resource – one worth fighting to maintain.

Maternal aggression – Aggression directed towards people or animals when a bitch who is within weeks of whelping puppies perceives someone, or something, as a threat to her offspring. This type of aggression can be normal and is hormone-mediated.

Pain-related aggression – Aggression towards anyone or anything in response to pain or anticipation of pain during an interaction. This type of aggression can turn into fear-related aggression if dogs associate a certain person or context with the feeling of pain.

Irritable aggression – Pain and discomfort lowers the threshold for the intensity of a stimulus needed to trigger an aggressive response. For example, a dog may tolerate, even welcome, physical petting from family members, but on the day they are feeling nauseated or are having bowel discomfort, they growl and snap at someone who tries to pet them.

Episodic dyscontrol – A rare, seizure-based condition, that can result in aggressive outbursts directed at people, animals, or objects. Outbursts are characterized by pre-ictal mood changes and post-ictal lethargy and altered consciousness. Treatment with anticonvulsants is generally successful.

Social status aggression – Aggression directed at familiar dogs within the same household as a means of establishing which dog has preferential access to resources, including food, bones, resting places, and proximity to human family members. This most commonly occurs between dogs close in age as they approach social maturity.

Redirected aggression – Any of the above types of aggression can be redirected. In these cases, the recipient of the aggression is someone or something in proximity to the dog that is not the intended person or dog that motivated or triggered the behavior. For example, a dog with fear aggression towards other dogs on walks might redirect fear-related aggression when seeing an unfamiliar dog on the walk onto their housemate that is being walked next to them. The unfamiliar dog beyond the reach of the leash is the trigger and intended target, but the housemate dog is the recipient of the aggression simply due to proximity. Another common example is when a human household member attempts to soothe a dog who is barking at a delivery person outside the window and the dog bites the hand reaching for them. In both cases, the subject that was bitten was not the intended target, but rather in the wrong place at the wrong time. Due to the uninhibited nature of redirected aggression, it can result in severe injuries.

Aggression secondary to high arousal – Aggression characterized by the dog being in a high state of arousal and directed at other animals, humans, or items that generally do not trigger aggression. The high state of arousal may be associated with excitement, play, frustration, or startle. This may include generally sociable dogs that become highly excited at the arrival of visitors, aroused by cheers from a winning goal at a sporting event, or other sudden noises or commotions. It may be seen in dogs confined in a shelter when a person enters their pen and they become highly excited by the long-awaited social interaction. It may occur in high-arousal play with people or other dogs. The aggressor may have a generalized anxiety disorder or noise phobia as a comorbidity.

Socially facilitated aggression – Aggression on the part of a bystander dog who witnesses any of the above forms of aggression in another dog and is triggered to also aggress towards the target, even if they do not share the same motivation as the aggressor. Social facilitation can intensify territorial and other forms of aggression. If one dog is showing aggressive behavior, it is not uncommon for others to join in, intensifying the initiator's confidence and aggressiveness. This has important implications for management of territorial aggression, where controlling non-aggressive territorial behavior (e.g. running, barking, high arousal) of companion dogs in the household, will aid in reducing stimulus for the patient to develop aggression. Some of the most devastating, sometimes fatal, dog attacks have included some sort of social facilitation of aggression.

We can further classify aggression based on the target or recipient of the aggressive response, whether it be directed at humans, other dogs, or both. Identification of triggers and targets focuses the behavior modification plan and ensures the management plan keeps these specific targets out of harm's way.

Human-Directed Aggression

Human-directed aggression is the most common aggression complaint (Fatjo et al. 2007) and is generally defensive in presentation. In the majority of cases, the dog was known to the victim and incidents occurred in or around the home (Notari et al. 2020). Around half the bites occur when people are interacting with the dog – stroking, playing, restraining (Oxley et al. 2018). When bites to the face occur most commonly, the person is bending over the dog and have their face close to the dog's face (Rezac et al. 2015). A disproportionate number of bites are to children compared to the adult population, with the most common demographic being boys between the ages of five to nine (Shuler et al. 2008).

What About Dominance?

It has been purported that dogs' natural social structure is a dominance hierarchy. This is based on the idea that the distant ancestor of the dog, the wolf, forms a social dominance hierarchy and that dogs would also naturally do the same. This is problematic because (1) after 2000 years of domestication and selective breeding, dogs are quite different from wolves, and (2) wolves observed in the wild, as opposed to confined under research conditions, live in family groups. Given the basic social unit for humans is the family and that dogs have evolved to live with humans (and in recent times have been bred specifically for the purpose of companionship), it is more useful to view dogs as part of the family structure. In this model, there is no need to be "dominant" over resources or to maintain a hierarchical social structure, and instead, the focus moves to fostering a mutually beneficial, loving, caring human–animal relationship that underlies ethical pet ownership.

This is not to say that dogs will not fight for what they want or need, and individuals may be possessive over food, beds, toys, or even access to favored humans. It is, however, rare to find a dog that will show aggression over all resources and seek to control the behavior of all members of their social group. Indeed, this behavior could be regarded as pathological, akin to a megalomaniac. Instead, we more commonly observe one individual controlling access to food whilst another has first option to the preferred sleeping place. Instead of fighting, often these "rights" are established through appeasement behavior on the part of other individuals in the social group, preferring to relinquish control to avoid confrontation. These interactions can be easily understood outside the concept of dominance, and treatment based on possessive or protective motivations generally proves successful.

Aggression Directed Towards Other Dogs

Intraspecific aggression is directed towards members of the same species. In the case of dogs, this is aggression directed towards other dogs. Many of the same motivations underlying aggression towards humans can result in aggression towards other dogs – namely territorial, pain, fear, and conflict-related aggression and resource guarding.

Whilst both offensive and defensive aggression can be directed at humans and dogs, far more incidents of aggression toward dogs are offensive (Notari et al. 2020, Fatjo et al. 2007). The death rate in intraspecific aggression is higher than in dog-to-human aggression (Notari et al. 2020). Dogs that missed out on early socialization, and those not living with other dogs appear to have an increased risk of aggression towards unfamiliar dogs (Roll and Unshelm 1997).

Aggression Towards Dogs Within the Same Household

Not every dog wants the constant companionship of another dog in their home. Many dogs are able to meet and interact well with other dogs outside of their home but do not share their space or their resources well when forced to live with others. On the flip side, just because a dog initially shows aggression towards new or unfamiliar dogs, does not mean they are not capable of cohabitating happily after a well-managed, gradual introduction. There are few statistics that relate to which dogs might get along best in a home. Females in the same household are more likely to fight with one another than males or males and females housed together (Wrubel et al. 2011). Poor outcomes for reducing aggression between dogs in the same household have been associated with dogs of the same sex, a history of bites that broke the skin, and when the aggressor is triggered simply by the sight of the other dog (Feltes et al. 2020).

Fighting between females is often intense, uninhibited, and can result in severe injury. This problem can be difficult to resolve, despite neutering, psychoactive medications, and attempts at behavior modification. Aggression can be exacerbated during oestrus and pseudocyesis. Secure separation and management may be the safest option in some cases.

Onset of fighting may be associated with changes in the social structure, as one dog reaches social maturity (one to three years of age), or when a dog is added or removed from the household. The victim may come to use defensive aggression and often demonstrates avoidance behaviors, while the aggressor often takes on a more confident, offensive role. In the author's experience, it is nearly always the most anxious dog in the household that is the aggressor. It is postulated that these individuals have an increased need for control and predictability and achieve this in the social domain using aggression. These dogs tend to control access to high-value items, control space by guarding or displacing the other dog and routinely stare at the victim. Outright fighting may be initiated in tight spaces, such as doorways and hallways, where the victim enters the aggressor's personal space and has little opportunity to escape. Identifying triggers such as play, or other high arousal states (visitors at the front door), can aid in management. The welfare of the victim dog should also be considered as these dogs can become fearful, depressed, and reclusive.

General Principles of Treating Aggression Cases in Dogs

Management

Notice we did not say cure. Aggression in dogs requires safe management above all else. Recommendations must take into account the risk of injury to humans and pets in the home and the surrounding community. This risk assessment will involve consideration of the type and target of aggression, the potential injury the dog may cause, ability to house the dog safely, the physical and mental capabilities of people in the house, the likelihood of exposure to triggers, the ability to predict when aggression will arise, and to manage the dog when it does. Safe management strategies need to be put in place, including use of barriers, crates, confinement areas, muzzles, head collars, and harnesses.

Ensuring the handlers can recognize the signs of stress, fear, anxiety, and aggressive intent is essential before moving forward with any behavior modification plan. Review the canine body language information in Chapter 11 for an overview of fearful, defensively aggressive, and offensively aggressive body language.

Once you have established safe management strategies and tools that allow you to avoid/minimize triggers, you can work with the family to teach desirable, incompatible, and alternate behaviors to aggression, utilize counterconditioning and systematic desensitization to change the underlying emotion driving the behavior and address any anxiety that may be exacerbating the problem.

Identification and Avoidance of Triggers

Your verbal history and aggression screening questionnaire should allow you to work with the client to identify known triggers of the aggressive behavior. Next, you will want to coach the client on how to avoid each trigger. This helps prevent rehearsal of the aggressive behavior as a "successful" strategy and/or prevent the dog's response from escalating to a higher intensity/level of injury. As mentioned above, aggression tends to worsen with age and rehearsal, rather than improve.

If the dog shows aggression towards other dogs on walks, dog parks should be avoided, and the dog should be on leash and under effective adult control at all times in public. Walking dogs at times when, and in areas where, you are less likely to meet other dogs will reduce exposure to triggers. If a dog is seen at a distance likely to trigger an aggressive response, the client is instructed to immediately leave the area. If dogs in the same household are likely to fight over food or toys, each dog should be separated into a secure area, out of sight of the other dog, when given these items, and the items removed before the dogs are allowed to be together again. If the dog shows aggression when groomed and requires brushing or clipping, this should be conducted under sedation until behavior modification is successfully implemented. These management strategies will help avoid rehearsal, reinforcement, and escalation of aggression, as well as keep everyone safe.

Safety and Management Tools

Various equipment can be used to ensure the safety of people and other animals, enhance the handler's control of the dog in reactive situations, and provide the dog with a safe and secure place to alleviate fear and anxiety and reduce aggressive arousal.

Ensuring the home property is secure is often important. This involves making sure that people or other animals cannot enter the property without the family knowing and being able to manage the dog safely, and ensuring the dog cannot escape and pose a threat to the community. Fencing should be secure, and gates fitted with locks the dog and public cannot open. Safe areas to contain the dog such as a locked room or outdoor enclosure may be helpful if the dog shows aggression towards visitors. For some dogs, a baby gate fitted across a doorway may be sufficient to confine them. This can also provide security for the dog with fear aggression, knowing there is barrier between them and visitors.

Dog crates can also be used for safe confinement of some dogs. Dogs should be trained to accept crating by establishing a calm and secure association with the crate. Forcing a dog into confinement in the crate will likely increase fear and anxiety and aggressive arousal. Instead, with successful conditioning, the crate can be seen as a safe and secure place associated with relaxation.

Appropriately fitted muzzles can be used to ensure that if "things go wrong," no one gets hurt. Muzzles also have the advantage of signaling to other dog handlers to keep some distance. This can also be communicated through messaging on dog jackets, leads, and bandanas (Figure 15.8). Fitting a muzzle does not inherently mean that the dog can be allowed to freely roam in the house with visitors, or be let loose in the dog park. The dog can still experience fear, anxiety, and aggressive arousal

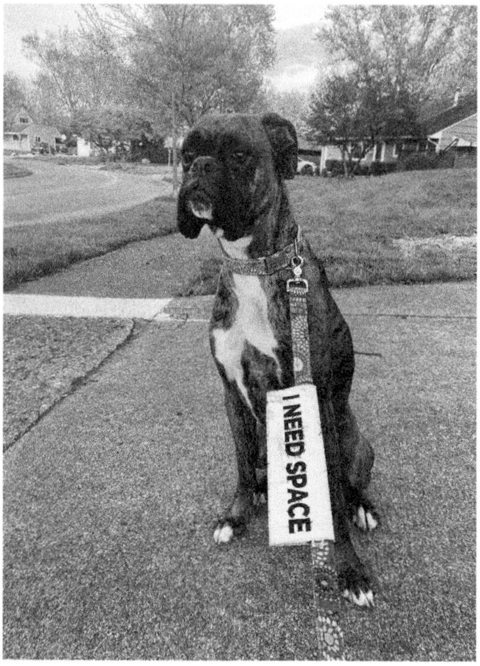

Figure 15.8 A dog with fear aggression and leash reactivity wears a message on a yellow leash cover which alerts passing people that he needs space. *Source:* With permission from Kelly Weimer.

whilst wearing the muzzle, and these are experiences we need to avoid, for the dog's welfare and to facilitate behavioral change. The dog should feel comfortable and relaxed wearing the muzzle – we do not want to add to their anxiety. The dog should be gradually conditioned to wearing the muzzle and a positive emotional association established.

There are various types of muzzles. Muzzles that hold the mouth closed should be avoided, as dogs regulate their temperature through panting and can easily become hyperthermic if unable to pant. Basket muzzles are recommended for this reason. In addition, basket muzzles allow dogs to drink (as long as the water bowl is deep enough to allow them to put both the muzzle and their mouth in the bowl) and for treats to be given. For dogs adept at pawing off the muzzle, some designs include a strap that starts at the top of the muzzle, runs up the center of the dog's face, and over the head to attach to the collar. There are also muzzles specifically designed for brachycephalic breeds. Custom made muzzles are also available to fit all head shapes and sizes.

Equipment to manage the dog's behavior safely and securely may also include harnesses and headcollars. If the dog is responsive to handling on a regular flat collar and leash (that is, without pulling excessively or choking) then other equipment may not be required. However, if the dog cannot be easily removed from a situation, is likely to pull the handler off-balance, or redirect aggression towards the handler, more control is needed. Front attach harnesses can offer more control by reducing pulling and enabling the handler to more easily turn the dog's body away from an inciting stimulus. This contrasts with back attach harnesses which may make pulling easier (think of sled dog harnesses).

Head collars can give the handler even more control over the dog's movement and can be helpful in preventing pulling and turning the dog's focus away from inciting stimuli (e.g. other dogs). However, they also need to be used humanely and if used incorrectly can cause unnecessary distress. It is important that they are fitted to ensure comfort and effectiveness and the handler is trained in using them correctly. Aversive experiences when encountering other dogs are likely to be counter-productive to relieving the underlying motivations of fear or anxiety.

The appropriate use of all equipment requires that it is fitted properly. Most equipment also requires that the dog is conditioned to feel relaxed and comfortable with its use. Veterinary technicians trained in behavior modification or professional trainers should assist caregivers in these processes.

Behavior Modification

The dog must be in a calm and focused state before commencing behavior modification. Whilst avoidance and management can help achieve an emotional state compatible with learning, medication to decrease anxiety may also be helpful before starting behavior modification. See Chapter 21 for information on the use of psychotropic medications to reduce fear, anxiety, and stress in dogs.

Teach Alternative Behaviors

Alternative, appropriate behaviors can be taught and rewarded in response to the stimulus for aggression (Box 15.5). The dog is provided with appropriate and successful options and encouraged to make nonaggressive choices. For example, dogs that bark and rush at visitors when the doorbell rings, can be taught to run to their crate for a high-value reward like liver treats when they hear the doorbell. For dogs that show aggression to visitors in the home, teach them to sit at a distance from the visitor where they receive tossed treats. This teaches them a nonscary way to interact with visitors, that has a positive outcome, removing conflict with these social interactions. In view of safety, these behaviors may be best taught whilst on leash and under control of an adult.

For dogs that show aggression towards people establishing a standard way of interaction can reduce stress associated with interactions. For example, if the dog learns that sitting when interacting with people always results in a positive and non-threatening outcome, then their anxiety is reduced. If the dog sits, and the unfamiliar person tosses them some treats and does not try to pet them, sitting for interactions is reinforced as a good behavioral strategy from the perspective of the socially anxious dog. It is a bit like "shaking hands" for people. Having a familiar, known, and predictable way of interacting that has a good (or neutral) outcome, reduces anxiety about how to engage with unfamiliar people.

Counterconditioning and Systematic Desensitization

Clients may be able to change the meaning of triggers through counterconditioning and systematic desensitization, but these strategies should only be attempted under the guidance of a behavior professional. Risks associated with managing the dog and implementing the behavior modification plan need to be clearly explained to all handlers.

In general, the aim of both counterconditioning and systematic desensitization is to reduce or eliminate the fear and anxiety underlying the dog's aggression. Remember that emotions are a big driver of behavior. Successful counterconditioning will change a negative emotional association with a particular stimulus or trigger for aggression, to a more positive emotional association (see Chapter 5 for a review). This is achieved by consistently pairing the trigger with a "good" outcome, e.g. treats. This association should be made every time the trigger occurs, irrespective of whether the dog responds with fear/anxiety/aggression or not.

Box 15.5 Teaching alternative behavior for aggression towards other dogs on walks

The first step in treatment is encouraging calm, focused, and non-reactive behavior, which often involves creating distance from the other dog. The handler directs the dog to do appropriate and desirable behavior that is rewarded. Commonly, this involves a fast U-turn and moving away from the trigger dog. The dog may then be directed to sit and look at handler. The reward of reduced fear by increasing distance from the trigger dog may be enough to reinforce the behavior but treats and praise can be added. Dogs with high arousal and anxiety may find it challenging to sit and look, and may do better if they can keep moving, or are allowed to explore the environment. Tossing treats in front of the dog and playing "find it" can help to provide the dog with a focus and maintain engagement. Fearful dogs may not take treats, and highly aroused dogs cannot focus, so both fear and arousal should be addressed prior to starting alternate behavior training.

For example, if the dog shows fear aggression towards visitors coming to the door, the caregiver can toss high-value treats to the dog every time a visitor appears at the door. When the visitor goes away the treats stop. That is, visitors predict treats. The association is NOT dependent on the dog's behavior, but rather the appearance of the trigger. This is a common area where caregivers make a mistake. The visitor comes to the door, they toss a handful of treats on the floor in front of the dog and the dog spends the next few moments picking up the treats and eating them. When all the treats are eaten, the dog looks up and barks at the visitor. The caregiver then starts tossing treats again. In this scenario, the treats have become dependent and associated with the dog barking and not with the presence of the visitor. To correct this the caregiver should focus on giving treats the whole time the visitor is present no matter how the dog behaves, and only stop when the visitor leaves. It does not matter whether the dog is eating treats, barking, or even walking away, if the visitor is present, they cause treats to rain down from the ceiling. The aim is that the dog now thinks visitors mean treats and they will "want" visitors to come to the door, rather than try and scare them away. Counterconditioning in this scenario is about building a positive emotional association with visitors.

Systematic desensitization the other hand tends to move a negative emotional association to a more neutral or non-significant association with the stimulus/trigger. This is achieved by exposing the dog to the trigger in a way that is not threatening and does not trigger fear or anxiety. Over time the intensity of the stimulus is increased, but only in a way and at a rate that ensures the dog remains calm and not fearful. For example, an unfamiliar person may be presented at a distance that allows the dog to remain calm and gradually the dog is walked closer (increasing the intensity of the stimulus) to the person. The rate at which the dog is moved closer is entirely dependent on the dog's response. You cannot move closer if the dog shows fear or anxiety. Only when a calm state is achieved can systematic desensitization be conducted. This requires that the handler is skilled in interpreting the body language of the dog. Successful systematic desensitization requires that a non-fear-inducing starting point is found and that the dog does not become fearful or anxious during the process. Remember, the aim is to establish a nonthreatening association with the stimulus, and that implementing systematic desensitization is entirely dependent on the dog's emotional reactions.

Avoid Using Positive Punishment

Punishment is not recommended in the treatment of aggression. First and foremost, it has the potential to increase the risk of injury. Confrontational training techniques result in aggressive responses from around 25% of dogs (Herron et al. 2009). The use of training that includes positive punishment increases the risk of aggression towards unfamiliar dogs (2.5 times more likely), and towards household dogs (3.8 times more likely) (Casey et al. 2014). Where positive punishment is used alone, or in combination with positive reinforcement, aggression scores are higher than when positive reinforcement is used as the sole training modality. There is no effect of breed, sex, or neuter status on the relationship between training methods and prevalence of aggression. Secondly, positive punishment has been linked to the development of fear-related problems (Blackwell et al. 2008). This is not surprising given the emotion underlying positive punishment is fear. In many cases, it is fear that is motivating the aggression being punished, and increasing fear is therefore contra-indicated. The fear generated by positive punishment also has the potential to generalize to other elements in the environment associated with the punishment. For example, a dog aggressive to unfamiliar dogs on the street may come to associate the presence of other dogs with fear of punishment (and not with its aggressive behavior). This is obviously counter-productive. Similarly, positive punishment can become associated with walks, the handler, or walking equipment, which now come to induce fear and potentially elicit aggression in more contexts. Thirdly, punishment is designed to suppress behavior, without addressing the motivation for the aggression. We want to treat the cause of the problem and not just the symptoms. If successful in eliminating the "symptoms," positive punishment may suppress warning signs like growling and snarling, with the result that dogs will skip this step in the future and progress to biting without warning. This makes for a more dangerous dog. When aggression occurs, it may be more intense and without warning. Additionally, without reinforcing alternative behavior, the dog may not perceive any option to use aggression.

Psychotropic Medications

Psychotropic medications can be lifesaving. When clients seek help for dogs showing aggression, there has often been a precipitating event, and the risk of a repeat incident needs to be addressed quickly. Medications that reduce anxiety and arousal can support faster and safer improvement. In cases of aggression, medication is always used in conjunction with a behavior modification and management plan. Without concurrent learning, improvement is likely to be limited and problems recur once medication is withdrawn.

Given the interplay of the multiple and varied factors leading to aggression, it is unlikely that any one medication will aid in reducing aggression in all individuals. The focus of medications can be to alleviate the fear and anxiety underlying the motivation to use aggression, to raise the threshold for what triggers an aggressive response, and to reduce arousal to a level at which the dog can learn and have a faster recovery when triggered. Not only can psychoactive medication help facilitate behavior modification, but it may also be indicated to improve the dog's quality of life. Both generalized and specific anxiety diagnoses may warrant the use of anti-anxiety medication. For example, a dog that displays fear aggression towards unfamiliar dogs, may experience significant anxiety on daily walks, to the point where they may not want to leave the house. This level of anxiety has a significant impact on the dog's welfare, and ability to live a "normal" life. If there is underlying pathology or a strong genetic component driving the aggression, long-term medication use may be required.

Many of the psychotropic medications used in the treatment of aggression, anxiety, and fear have the potential to worsen or disinhibit aggression. This means that where an animal may previously have inhibited aggression, there is potential for aggression to become disinhibited and thereby more frequent and/or severe. Additionally, if dogs are agitated as a side effect of a psychotropic medication, their threshold for aggression may be lowered. Fortunately, agitation and disinhibition are uncommon, however, it is important that clients are made aware of these possibilities, and dogs are managed safely (confined, avoid provocation) until the full individual effects of medications are known. It has also been postulated that relieving anxiety may make some individuals more confident in their use of aggression. However, in most cases, reducing anxiety and fear results in decreasing the need to use aggression. See Chapter 21 for a list and description of commonly used psychotropic medications in dogs.

Prognosis

Early Diagnosis, Treatment, and Management are Important in Achieving Good Outcomes

Factors including age of onset, duration, predictability, frequency, ability to control the dog safely, and owner compliance with treatment and management will inform prognosis. If there are underlying medical issues contributing to the behavior, then medical prognosis will affect behavioral prognosis. Reisner (1997) examined prognosis regarding positive and negative prognostic indicators. Positive prognostic indicators, in the case of human-directed aggression, include mild and inhibited aggression, aggression that is proportional to the intensity of the stimulus, predictable aggression in relation to both context and intensity, aggression that starts in socially mature dogs (>4 years), dogs with less than 18 kg body weight, households that do not include infants, toddlers, the infirm, or elderly, and caregivers who are willing and able to implement management and behavior modification and accept the risk of future aggression. Negative prognostic indicators (more likely to result in euthanasia as an outcome) include the opposite – aggression that is severe and poorly inhibited, aggression that is exaggerated in relation to the intensity of the stimulus, aggression that is unpredictable in either context or intensity, the dog is socially immature (<1 year), the dog weighs more than 18 kg, and the household includes infants, toddlers, the infirm, or the elderly, as well as caregivers who are reluctant or unable to implement management and behavior modification or accept risk of future aggression (Reisner 1997).

Other factors to consider include, but are not limited to:

1) frequency of exposure to risk situations/number of triggers.
2) the extent of warning signs, and latency to attack.
3) intensity of focus and ability to distract or redirect the dog.
4) the style of attack: are there multiple bites?, is the behavior predatory in nature?
5) comorbid behavior problems: is there a history of escaping?, is there significant anxiety affecting welfare?
6) access to a safe housing environment.
7) quality of life considerations.
8) ability of caregivers to recognize early warning signs.

Prognosis will also be affected by client expectations. For example, many people can teach their dogs to walk past unfamiliar dogs without an aggressive reaction. These dogs learn to avoid other dogs but do not necessarily develop skills for friendly interactions. Many clients are satisfied with this level of management and behavioral change and accept that their dog will not have "doggie friends."

Whilst many factors influence prognosis, the severity of injury plays a large role in determining prognosis. Serguson found that 71% of dogs reported for biting did not have additional bites reported, but if they did bite again, the severity of the bite was likely to be the same or more severe. Dogs who bit severely/repeatedly in the first aggressive incident were 1.7 times more likely to bite again (Serguson and Shabelansky 2022).

We must also ask how safe it is to work with and manage the dog. While there is no universally accepted bite severity description, many shelters and other animal behavior professionals will refer to the Dunbar bite scale (see Box 15.6). Practitioners sometimes give a more guarded prognosis and may lean towards strict management or euthanasia if the skin has been punctured (Bite level 3 and above). Level 4 and 5

Box 15.6 Bite assessment scale by Ian Dunbar, DVM, PhD, ranks the severity of a dog bite based on level of injury inflicted

Level 1 – Dog growls, lunges, snarls – no teeth touch skin.

Level 2 – Teeth touch skin but no puncture. May have red mark/minor bruise.

Level 3 – Punctures ½ the length of a canine tooth, one to four holes, single bite.

Level 4 – One to four holes from a single bite, one hole deeper than ½ the length of a canine tooth, dog clamped down and shook or slashed victim.

Level 5 – Multiple bites at level 4 or above. A concerted, repeated attack.

Level 6 – Any bite resulting in death of a human.

bites pose a significant risk to the community, and the outcome may be more guarded for dogs with this level of bite history.

Considerations for Rehoming/Relinquishing/Euthanasia

All dogs are capable of biting – period. Dog ownership always involves managing some level of risk, and individual clients will make different assessments of how much risk they can comfortably live with. The multiple factors discussed above under "Prognosis" will inform the outcome for the dog showing aggression. Assessing and weighing the impact of these factors is not an easy task. Whilst some criteria will clearly direct the assessor to specific outcomes (a dog with fear aggression towards children would be best situated in a home without children – for the benefit of the dog and children), other cases will be more equivocal. The decision to keep the dog will depend not only on the risk of physical and emotional trauma to people and other animals but also on the ability to safely house and manage the dog while maintaining an acceptable level of welfare. Busy households with multiple members, frequent visitors, and young children may find it impossible to safely contain a dog with aggression toward people.

Prognosis for improvement in behavior is therefore only one criterion influencing the dog's outcome. Consideration needs to also be given to the welfare of other animals and family members and environmental factors. Siracusa et al. reported dog-related factors increasing the risk of rehoming or euthanasia as "dogs with a heavier weight; mixed breed; aggression to familiar people over resources, resting places, or when groomed/medicated; aggression to unfamiliar people during interactions; a history of biting; and living in a family with children aged 13–17 years." Owner-related factors included the "use of punishment-based training and previous consultation with a non-veterinary behaviorist or trainer" (Siracusa et al. 2017).

The ability to redirect the dog when aggressively aroused is important. High arousal and intense focus make management more challenging and increase the risk of serious injury. Predatory behavior can be very dangerous and uninhibited as ultimately the intent is to kill.

Cases should be considered on an individual basis. Whilst large dogs can cause significantly more injury than smaller ones, if the large dog has only ever shown inhibited aggression like growling and air snaps, this may present less risk than a small dog that frequently punctures the skin, and/or directs bites towards the face. Increased frequency does not necessarily imply increased risk. If the aggression is highly predictable, it may be easily managed. For example, if the dog barks at the postman every day, but is restrained behind a fence, the risk is relatively low compared to a dog that is aggressive towards other dogs only once or twice a year but causes significant injury when it attacks. The lack of predictability makes the latter difficult to manage and there are limited opportunities to implement behavior modification strategies.

When to Consider Rehoming (or Relinquishment)?

Environmental factors are key in managing dogs with a history of aggression. Rehoming a dog diagnosed with mild fear aggression towards children may be moved to a home without children, assuming there is no community access or exposure to children. Likewise, dogs who do not share space and resources well with other dogs, but do not demonstrate major reactivity when encountering dogs in the community, may be rehomed as a single dog in the household. Human factors may also evoke consideration for rehoming. A frail, elderly person may not be able to safely manage a 30 kg dog with aggression towards joggers, whilst a stronger individual will be able to both control the dog and safely implement a behavior modification program. In households with cognitively impaired members consistency in interaction with, and safe management of, the dog may not be guaranteed. These challenges can be remedied through rehoming. There are few hard and fast rules, and each case needs to be assessed in view of the specific individual owner and dog parameters.

Rehoming should not be viewed as an "easy" solution, or a means to deflect responsibility. Most families want a safe pet, and unless safety and the dog's needs can be reliably met, rehoming can result in injury, distress to new caregivers, and welfare concerns for the dog. Sadly, dogs with aggression problems are also at risk for abuse as a consequence of their behavior. Rehoming should always occur with complete transparency of behavioral history, management, and treatment recommendations. Realistic expectations should be given, including a clear discussion of risk.

When to Consider Euthanasia?

Not all individuals have access to optimal solutions. Not all homes can provide the level of care and management required practically, financially, or emotionally. Living with high risk can be an extremely stressful experience for our clients. Injuries to people or dogs in the community can result in litigation and, in some cases, criminal charges. Financial and emotional hardship from lawsuits and the loss of homeowner's insurance are harsh realities for households harboring dogs with serious bite histories. Differing opinions around the most desirable outcomes can cause tension and friction within the household, straining family relationships. A desire not to pass this scenario on to another family can negate the option of rehoming. These considerations may push the decision towards euthanasia.

Whilst safety is always the first consideration, equally we need to consider the welfare of the dog. Unrelenting poor welfare may justify a decision for euthanasia. Persistent anxiety or fear, despite all attempts at relief, suggests poor welfare. Excessive confinement as a management strategy may also result in poor welfare. A dog contained in a locked pen to keep certain human or animal household members safe requires special effort to ensure its social, physical, and emotional needs are met.

Conclusion

As a normal adaptive behavior, aggression is unlikely to be eliminated from the behavioral repertoire of dogs. Living with dogs will always involve some level of risk, but the prevalence of aggression can be reduced through a combined approach of responsible breeding and awareness, manipulation of behavior, and management of the multitude of environmental influences that affect its expression. Sadly, as few as 10% of dogs euthanized for aggression had been referred to a behaviorist, and only around 3% had been prescribed pharmacological, nutraceutical, or pheromonal treatment (Boyd et al. 2018, Yu et al. 2021). As more and more veterinarians gain knowledge regarding the prevention, identification, and treatment of aggression in dogs, we can make an impact on some of these devastating statistics.

References

Appleby, D., Bradshaw, J., and Casey, R. (2002). Relationship between aggressive and avoidance behaviour by dogs and their experience in the first six months of life. *Vet. Rec.* 150 (14): 434–438.

Arata, S., Takeuchi, Y., Inoue, M., and Mori, Y. (2014). "Reactivity to stimuli" is a temperamental factor contributing to dog aggression. *PLoS ONE* 9: e100767.

Asp, H., Fiske, W., Nilsson, K., and Strandberg, E. (2015). Breed differences in everyday behaviour of dogs. *Appl. Anim. Behav. Sci.* 169: 69–77.

Bamberger, M. and Houpt, K. (2006). Signalment factors, comorbidity, and trends in behavior diagnoses in dogs: 1,644 cases (1991-2001). *J. Am. Vet. Med. Assoc.* 229 (10): 1591–1598.

Blackwell, E., Twells, C., Seawright, A., and Casey, R. (2008). The relationship between training methods and the occurrence of behavior problems, as reported by owners, in a population of domestic dogs. *J. Vet. Behav.* 3 (5): 207–217.

Borchelt, P. (1983). Aggressive behavior of dogs kept as companion animals: classification and influence of sex, reproductive status and breed. *Appl. Anim. Ethol.* 10: 45–61.

Boyd, C., Jarvis, S., McGreevy, P. et al. (2018). Mortality resulting from undesirable behaviours in dogs aged under three years attending primary-care veterinary practices in England. *Anim. Welf.* 27 (3): 251–262.

Casey, R., Loftus, B., Bolster, C. et al. (2014). Human directed aggression in domestic dogs (*canis familiaris*): occurrence in different contexts and risk factors. *Appl. Anim. Behav.* 152: 52–63.

Dodman, N., Brown, D., and Serpell, J. (2018). Associations between owner personality and psychological status and the prevalence of canine behavior problems. *PLoS ONE* 13: e0192846.

Duffy, D., Hsu, Y., and Serpell, J. (2008). Breed differences in canine aggression, 2008. *Appl. Anim. Behav. Sci.* 114: 441–460.

Fatjo, J., Amat, M., Mariotti, V. et al. (2007). Analysis of 1040 cases of canine aggression in a referral practice in Spain. *J. Vet. Behav.* 2 (5): 158–165.

Feltes, E., Stull, J., Herron, M., and Haug, L. (2020). Characteristics of intrahousehold interdog aggression and the dog and pair factors associated with a poor outcome. *J. Am. Vet. Med. Assoc.* 256 (3): 349–361.

Flint, H., Coe, J., Serpell, J. et al. (2017). Risk factors associated with stranger-directed aggression in domestic dogs. *Appl. Anim. Behav. Sci.* 197: 45–54.

Guy, N., Luescher, U., Dohoo, S. et al. (2001). Risk factors for dog bites to owners in a general veterinary caseload. *Appl. Anim. Behav. Sci.* 74 (1): 29–42.

Haverbeke, A., De Smet, A., Depiereux, E. et al. (2009). Assessing undesired aggression in military working dogs. *Appl. Anim. Behav. Sci.* 117: 55–62.

Herron, M., Shofer, F., and Reisner, I. (2009). Survey of the use and outcome of confrontational and non-confrontational training methods in client-owned dogs showing undesired behaviors. *Appl. Anim. Behav. Sci.* 117 (1–2): 47–54.

Howell, T., King, T., and Bennett, P. (2015). Puppy parties and beyond: the role of early age socialization practices on adult dog behavior. *Vet. Med. Res. Rep.* 6: 143–152.

Hsu, Y. and Sun, L. (2010). Factors associated with aggressive responses in pet dogs. *Appl. Anim. Behav. Sci.* 123: 108–123.

Kaneko, F., Arata, S., Takeuchi, Y., and Mori, Y. (2013). Analysis of association between behavioural traits and four types of aggression in *Shibu Inu*. *J. Vet. Med. Sci.* 75: 1297–1301.

Kirchoff, N., Udell, M., and Sharpton, T. (2019). The gut microbiome correlates with conspecific aggression in a small population of rescued dogs (*canis familiaris*). *Peer J.* 7 (6103): https://doi.org/10.7717/peerj.6103.

Landsberg, G., Hunthausen, W., and Ackerman, L. (2003). *Handbook of Behavior Problems of the Dog and Cat*, 408. Elsevier, Philadelphia: Saunders.

McMillan, F. (2017). Behavioral and psychological outcomes for dogs sold as puppies through pet stores and/or born in commercial breeding establishments: current knowledge and putative causes. *J. Vet. Behav.* 19: 14–26.

Notari, L., Cannas, S., Di Sotto, Y., and Palestrini, C. (2020). A retrospective analysis of dog-dog and dog-human cases of aggression in northern Italy. *Animals* 10 (9): 1662.

Oxley, J., Christley, R., and Westgarth, C. (2018). Contexts and consequences of dog bites incidents. *J. Vet. Behav.* 23: 33–39.

Podberscek, A. and Serpell, J. (1997). Environmental influences on the expression of aggressive behaviour in English Cocker Spaniels. *Appl. Anim. Behav. Sci.* 52: 215–227.

Rayment, D., De Groef, B., Peters, R., and Marston, L. (2015). Applied personality assessment in domestic dogs: limitations and caveats. *App. Anim. Behav. Sci* 163: 1–18.

Reisner, I. (1997). Assessment, management and prognosis of canine dominance-related aggression. *Vet. Clin. North America: Small Anim. Pract.* 27 (3): 479–495.

Reisner, I. and Houpt, K. (2005). National survey of owner-directed aggression in English Springer Spaniels. *J. Am. Vet. Med. Assoc.* 227 (10): 1594–1603.

Rezac, P., Rezac, K., and Slama, P. (2015). Human behaviour preceding dog bites to the face. *Vet. J.* 206 (3): 284–288.

Roll, A. and Unshelm, J. (1997). Aggressive conflicts amongst dogs and factors affecting them. *App. Anim. Behav. Sci.* 52 (3-4): 229–242.

Scandurra, A., Alterisio, A., Di Cosmo, A., and D'Aniello, B. (2018). Behavioral and perceptual differences between sexes in dogs: an overview. *Animals* 8 (9): 151.

Serguson, S. and Shabelansky, A. (2022). Exploring Factors Associated with Reoccurrence and Escalation of Dog Bites in Dogs with Animal Control Bite Reports *2022 Veterinary Behavior Symposium Proceedings*. American College of Veterinary Behaviorists, online recording June 22, 2022.

Serpell, J. and Jagoe, J. (1995). Early experience and the development of behaviour. In: *The Domestic Dog: Its Evolution, Behaviour and Interactions with People* (ed. J. Serpell), 79–102. Cambridge, UK: Cambridge University Press.

Shuler, C., DeBess, E., Lapidus, J., and Hedberg, K. (2008). Canine and human factors related to dog bite injuries. *JAVMA* 232 (4): 542–546.

Siracusa, C., Provoost, L., and Reisner, I. (2017). Dog and owner related risk factors for consideration of euthanasia or rehoming before a referral behavioral consultation and for euthanizing or rehoming the dog after the consultation. *J. Vet. Behav.* 22: 46–56.

Van Den Berg, L., Schilder, M., and Knol, B. (2003). Behavior genetics of canine aggression: behavioral phenotyping of golden retrievers by means of an aggression test. *Behav. Gen.* 33: 469–483.

Van Der Velden, N., De Weerd, T., Brooymans-Schallenberg, J., and Tielen, A. (1976). An abnormal behavioural trait in Bernese Mountain Dogs (*Berner Sennenhund*). *Tijdschr Diergeneesk* 101: 403–407.

Wrubel, K., Moon-Fanelli, A., Maranda, L., and Dodman, N. (2011). Interdog household aggression: 38 cases (2006-2007). *J. Am. Vet. Med. Assoc.* 238: 731–740.

Yu, Y., Wilson, B., Masters, S. et al. (2021). Mortality resulting from undesirable behaviours in dogs aged three years and under attending primary care veterinary practices in Australia. *Animals* 11 (2): 493.

16

Separation-Related Disorders in Dogs

Niwako Ogata

Purdue University, Department of Veterinary Clinical Sciences, College of Veterinary Medicine, West Lafayette, IN, USA

Introduction

Separation anxiety has been called by many different names because of its wide range of symptoms and causes. As the name implies, separation anxiety refers to pets that exhibit anxiety-related behaviors in the absence of their attachment figures, typically human family members. Theoretically, problematic behaviors are not included in this category if they are caused by reasons other than anxiety. However, accurately identifying the motivation or anxiety state of an animal when the human household members are away from home can be difficult. As a result, several terms to describe these behavioral problems are often used. In this chapter, we use the term "separation-related disorders" (SRD), which includes both separation anxiety and other separation-related behavioral problems.

SRD are the most studied behavior problem because of the heavy burden they place not only on pets but also on their family. In a recent large online survey of over 3,000 dog-owning households, fear- and anxiety-related behavior problems were present in approximately 26.2–44% of pet dogs, with separation anxiety being part of that range. Studies have reported SRD incidence of 13–18% (Dinwoodie et al. 2019; Tiira et al. 2016). In addition, when patients visiting behavioral clinics in North America were studied, separation anxiety accounted for 10–14% of all cases (Anderson et al. 2022; Bamberger and Houpt 2006). In one study, surveyed households with dogs reported a high incidence rate of nearly 50%, but only 13% of these cases were referred to professionals (Bradshaw et al. 2002), so the actual number of cases may be higher.

Nevertheless, the literature published to date does not necessarily present a unified view of SRD. A wide variety of etiologies exist, not all of which have been adequately identified despite this behavioral problem occurring only in a unique context (i.e. the owner's absence or perceived absence). In other words, the presenting signs of the problem and the response of affected dogs to common treatments vary widely. Thus, if the case does not respond positively to the first line of treatment from a primary veterinarian, it is likely to be a challenging case and may require prompt consideration for referral to a behavior specialist.

[Studies of SRD in cats have recently received more attention, and a recent feline owner survey-based study reported an incidence of 13.5% (de Souza Machado et al., 2020). Since the clinical manifestation of SRDs in cats is unlikely to cause to severe household destruction and/or noise complaints from concerned

Introduction to Animal Behavior and Veterinary Behavioral Medicine, First Edition. Edited by Meghan E. Herron.

Companion website: www.wiley.com/go/introductiontoanimalbehavior

neighbors, it is possible this number is actually higher.]

This chapter primarily focuses on SRD in dogs whose distress is triggered by the absence of people. In some cases, however, anxiety is triggered by the absence of only one specific person; in these cases, the presence of other people (other family members or a pet sitter) does not alleviate the anxiety. In a more typical presentation of separation anxiety, the symptoms are reduced by having any human present. Similarly, some dogs, although the minority, may exhibit anxious behavior in the absence of a specific cohabiting animal (generally of the same species), regardless of the presence of humans. This is oftentimes evident in related dogs that have not experienced life without their dam or sibling(s). Although it is possible to have some varieties of triggers in individual cases, the overall treatment plans are similar for each presentation.

Definitions and Variations on Separation-Related Disorders

Clinically, SRD can be divided into four major groups based on their presentation patterns – *normal separation-related behaviors, persistent SRD, intermittent SRD, and SRD associated with human sleep times.*

Normal Separation-Related Behaviors

These are dogs whose signs of distress are normal and expected and naturally resolve with a gradual introduction to the new home-alone routine.

Crying for protection and seeking attention are normal behaviors in puppies and adolescent dogs. When a puppy moves from its original home to a new family and is separated from their parents or siblings, it is normal for the puppy to be anxious and whine more in an unfamiliar place, when left alone, until it becomes used to the new family and environment.

Alternatively, adult or senior dogs who have never experienced environmental or major schedule changes but need to undergo it for the first time (for example, a move, going back to the office for work after a period of working from home, teenager moving away for college) may not cope well at the beginning. However, if the new environment, including a crate or exercise pen, or the new routine is gradually introduced over time and in standardized steps (see the treatment sections below), most dogs in this group become accustomed to it and the distress wanes.

Additionally, highly active young dogs can develop behavioral problems in the family's absence more due to frustration from being under-exercised or not being attended to, rather than anxiety. Management of these dogs is discussed later with treatment plans to provide physical and mental exercise.

Persistent Separation-Related Disorders

This diagnosis pertains to dogs adopted from shelters/rescues with an unknown background, who persist in showing separation-related problem behaviors despite a gradual introduction to the new environment and home-alone routine. This description also includes young dogs who have never recovered from the initial separation from mom and littermates. Signs in these dogs have persisted since puppyhood.

Shelter/Rescue Dog Persistent SRD

Some studies estimate that anywhere from 17–38% of dogs adopted from shelters or rescue centers have substantial SRD (Blackwell et al. 2016; Herron et al. 2014). When including mild to moderate forms of SRD, that number jumps closer to 90%, according to Bohland et al., 2023. Whether the SRD is a result of a traumatic separation and the resulting strong bonding with the new adoptive home, or simply a continuation of a problem that existed prior to the shelter stay remains to be seen. Dogs are social animals and generally prefer to spend time with other individuals, although having another dog in the home tends not to protect against the development of SRD in shelter and rescue dogs. While some adapt to the new routine fairly quickly, others demonstrate tremendous panic when left in their new home without their human companions. In many cases, the problem persists despite a gradual introduction to being left alone. If a dog's response to being left alone in an unfamiliar environment is uncertain, it is best to run a trial (for example, leaving for a short time to monitor the dog's response) prior to leaving alone for an extended period.

Juvenile Onset Persistent SRD

While it is normal and expected for a puppy to show initial distress when rehomed away from mom and littermates, some puppies do not recover despite a gradual transition and introduction to being alone. They bond closely with their human companions and persistently struggle in their absence. In addition, dogs that have been raised by the same family from puppyhood who were unable to practice the gradual transition to being alone mentioned above, due to certain circumstances (such as the dog's illness or injury) are included in this group.

Persistent Secondary SRD

Dogs who experience a frightening event in the home-alone environment, such as a home invasion or burglary, major storm, loud noise event, or housefire, may establish an association between being alone and the triggering event. These dogs will persist in showing SRD when left alone, even if the event never again occurs. On the flip side, secondary SRD may develop if the dog is repeatedly left alone and exposed to frightening events, such as repeated storms or local construction projects. This is when an *intermittent SRD* may transition to a *persistent SRD.*

Intermittent Separation-Related Disorders

Dogs may not exhibit problematic behavior every time they are alone. Commonly, in these cases, the behavior signs emerge suddenly, given the lack of earlier problems in the same environment.

Dogs in this group may tolerate being alone during routine absences (for example going to work on weekdays), but they react poorly to an unexpected absence (for example, going out to dinner on the weekend), where the period of absence may not be predictable to the dog. Family members may have to dress in work clothes in order to leave the house for unpredictable absences. Another clinical example is that dogs with *intermittent SRD* often tolerate being alone as long as they are left in an emotionally neutral environment, such as in a car, instead of the home where the dog has experienced distress when left alone.

For dogs with intermittent signs or irregular presentation of behavioral problems during the family's absence, another primary cause of behavioral symptoms, such as sound phobias or underlying medical conditions, are most likely. This is referred to as *secondary* SRD. These dogs do not react to the family's absence per se but to other fear or pain-provoking triggers that happen to occur simultaneously during their time alone. After that experience, the dog learns the association between the family's absence and the negative experience. For example, if a dog with storm phobia experiences a severe thunderstorm while the owner is away, it associates the absence of the owner with the thunderstorm. Some of these dogs show SRD only during thunderstorm season. However, when the experience of being alone during the thunderstorms is repeated, the dog's negative emotional association is solidified and then they persist in showing anxious behavior every time the family is away, regardless of the actual weather conditions. These latter cases are likely to be presented in the clinic as *persistent secondary SRD.* In some cases, dogs begin showing problematic behaviors during the family's absence without an apparent or obvious trigger. Once they have started to show the problem, they may continuously do so during any absence.

Without careful history taking, it is difficult to identify how such separation-related signs develop. If one only focuses on presenting behavior signs, the dog's clinical signs of being alone appear to be the same for the dogs with *normal, persistent*, and *intermittent SRD*. The differential diagnoses are discussed further in a later section.

Separation-Related Disorders Associated with Human Sleep Times

Problematic behavior signs mainly occur at night while the family is asleep. Old dogs that start to show SRD despite no environmental or schedule changes are also included in this group.

The clinical signs in this group are more specific, such as dogs anxiously pacing, being restless, and panting at night while the family is asleep. When these dogs are left alone in the daytime on a regular schedule, they may not always show signs of SRD. In other common clinical cases in this group, older dogs living in the same environment start to show SRD without obvious triggers. These older dogs become more nervous and anxious, even when the family is home. In many cases in this group, behavioral symptoms are triggered by underlying diseases.

[SIDEBAR: "I just cannot get to you!" Separation-related distress associated with a physical, but not visual or auditory, barrier between the family and pet is not uncommon in dogs. This behavior occurs when the family members are home or just outside the house, within sight and/or sound, but the dog is restricted from approaching them, due to some type of door, gate, or other barrier. This is a distinct problem from separation anxiety as it may or may not coincide with difficulty being home alone. These dogs will often settle if they have no auditory or visual signs that their human companions are within reach.]

Risk Factors

Age of Onset

The age of onset of SRD varies from puppies to older dogs, although there is a clinical tendency for normal separation-related behaviors to comprise younger dogs, while SRD associated with human sleep time contain older dogs.

Breed and Sex

There is no consensus on the predisposed breeds or sexes. Some studies have shown that neutering/spaying increases the occurrence of SRD (Flannigan and Dodman 2001; Storengen et al. 2014), while others have shown that intact dogs, especially males, have a higher occurrence (McGreevy and Masters 2008) or that spayed females have a lower incidence (Blackwell et al. 2016).

Anxiety disorders, including SRD, are influenced by many factors, and the full etiology of SRD has not been identified. A study that surveyed households with dogs found an association between insufficient early life experiences and anxiety disorders, including SRD. Furthermore, dogs receiving low-quality maternal care and less daily exercise had a higher incidence of anxiety disorders. That may partly explain the high prevalence of the clinical population in dogs from rescues and shelters (Tiira and Lohi 2015).

Common Signs

The most common signs of SRD are vocalization, destruction (Figure 16.1), and toileting (urination and defecation) in inappropriate places. These signs are commonly reported because they tend to leave behind evidence and may result in a significant psychological and financial burden for families (Figure 16.2). However, if a video camera is set up to observe

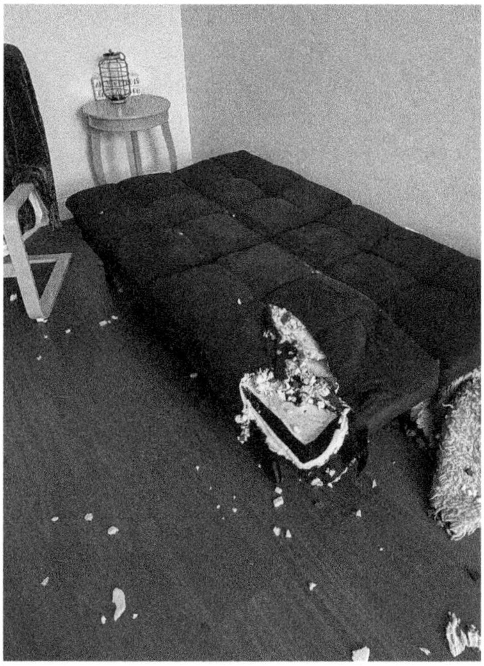

Figure 16.1 Dogs experiencing distress when home alone often cope by chewing/destroying household items as was done here on this futon. *Source:* Kristina Baucom.

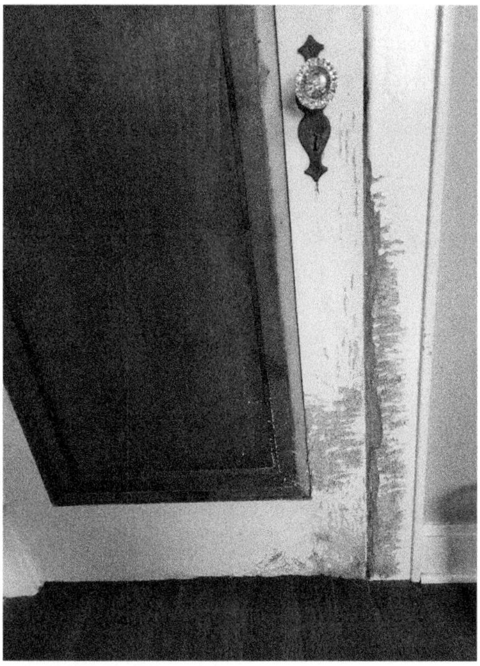

Figure 16.2 This door was destroyed when a dog was separated from the rest of the family, including the other dog to whom she was strongly bonded. The financial damage from this type of focused destruction can be substantial. *Source:* With permission from Rebecca King.

the dog's behavior, other behavior signs such as whining, drooling, pacing, panting, trembling, freezing, and scratching cages and doors without destroying them may also be identified. Additionally, a loss of appetite and depressive attitude in the family's absence are also observed. Many people report that their dog refuses to eat treats or play with food-stuffed puzzles during their absence but will eat them upon their return. It is critical for clinicians to seek resolution for *all* symptoms of SRD, rather than just those that cause problems due to complaints from neighbors or the financial cost related to damage to property. Many of these dogs experience extreme panic and engage in destructive chewing, particularly on items that contain the scents of family members. While undesirable, these behaviors are merely symptoms of that underlying emotion. These are not voluntary acts of spite or retaliation but rather attempts to cope with emotions that are beyond the dog's control. Each case is unique, and different dogs resort to different behaviors in their attempts to self-soothe. Some dogs may pace, vocalize excessively, urinate, and destroy any item they can find over the course of an hour, while others may simply urinate near the front door and then retreat to a corner and hunker down, trembling until their family returns. Thus, most dogs are exhausted at the end as they fail to cope in the given environment. Specific information identifying symptoms for further diagnosis and treatment plans is described in the following sections.

Strong Bond Between the Dogs and Human Family Members

The terms “excessive” or “hyper” attachment are often used to describe dogs with separation anxiety. These look like the “Velcro” dogs who never leave their person’s side, struggle to be shut out of a bedroom or bathroom, and hop up from a deep sleep to follow their preferred person from room to room. There is some disagreement about the correlation between attachment and separation anxiety as evidence suggests not all dogs with separation anxiety have excessive attachment problems (McGreevy and Masters 2008; Parthasarathy and Crowell-Davis 2006). Some researchers have called this “insecure” attachment rather than excessive attachment because in the studies these Velcro dogs did not focus on their person’s objects more than a stranger’s belongings when they were left alone in the experimental room. Moreover, they could not easily settle down upon reunion with their person. Thus, these researchers see the behaviors as insecure or ambivalent attachment instead of excessive or hyperattachment (Konok et al. 2011; Parthasarathy and Crowell-Davis 2006). In children and monkeys, these insecure attachment individuals are likely to develop anxiety disorders and more studies in dogs supported a similar view (de Assis et al. 2020).

Distress Surrounding Departures and Arrivals

Dogs who are anxious about family members moving from room to room at home will peak in their anxiety once it is evident that the family is preparing to leave the house. Specifically, the behavior signs mentioned above will be amplified and the vocalization or jumping up on people will intensify. In addition, some dogs confined to a certain area of the house such as bedroom, basement, or crate, resist going there, move reluctantly, or run away. Some dogs may growl or lunge at their caretaker when they are encouraged to move there.

When the family returns home, affected dogs may have difficulty calming down for several minutes following the reunion. They may be barking, whining, jumping up, unable to break focus on their person for several minutes. As noted above, it is also common for dogs to rush to eat the untouched treats and food from puzzle toys upon arrival. This indicates that the dog lost its appetite and curiosity in the absence of their person, which should be noted as a sign of anxiety in the home-alone environment.

Symptoms Occur Only When the Dog is Alone

Unless a family is capturing video footage, clinically reported symptoms of SRD are often biased toward those that leave evidence behind (including complaints from neighbors, the destruction of furniture, and elimination). Video recording is thus essential for diagnosing SRD and ruling out other potential etiologies for the behavior, particularly with destruction and elimination behaviors. When symptoms appear as the family prepares to leave the house, the likelihood of SRD is high. In typical SRD cases, the recorded videos show that immediately after the family leaves, the dog’s symptoms intensify, including crying, whining, scratching at the door, and sometimes self-injury. After that, the dog may calm down within a few minutes or repeat the same behavior for the rest of the absence. Some studies have shown that dogs are most distressed immediately after departure, while others have shown that behavior in response to anxiety and frustration caused by being left without a person occurs repeatedly at intervals of about 30 minutes (Lund and Jørgensen 1999). Studies have reported that some of these behaviors diminish over time (within approximately four hours) (Lund and Jørgensen 1999; Palestrini et al. 2010). However, leaving dogs until the behavior diminishes is not ideal because of the suffering they experience, as well as complaints from neighbors, and damage to property.

On occasion, dogs' outward signs of anxiety do not manifest until they have been alone for a prolonged period. For example, some dogs take time to engage, play with, and eat the food-stuffed puzzle toys and other enrichment left out for them at the time of departure. When they focus on these toys and treats, they seem to show minimal to no distress about being alone. Once the food is gone, though, they show anxiety-related behaviors, such as barking, pacing, scratching, or eliminating. Similarly, some dogs appear calm (i.e. no panting, pacing, or inappropriate toileting) for the first hour or two. They may or may not chew toys or treats. After that period, they suddenly start howling, as if calling for their family and howl repeatedly or intermittently until the family returns home. Many of these dogs can be left home successfully as long as the absence is brief. This is different from the more common presentation where a dog shows signs of anxiety for an absence of even a few minutes. These families often feel trapped in their homes as even the quickest of errands may mean destruction of their home and/or profound distress for their beloved pet.

Making a Definitive Diagnosis

Differential Diagnosis List

First, because problematic behavior has many overlapping motivations, it is common for some dogs to have more than one diagnosis for their behavioral problems. That said, it is important to rule out other diagnoses that may give the appearance of being related to separation distress but are in fact unrelated to being alone.

A) **Generalized anxiety disorder (GAD)**
A dog with generalized anxiety lives in a constant state of anticipation and seems unable to relax even in everyday life with their people right beside them. Although many dogs with this condition may have other specific anxiety-related problems such as SRD, there are many dogs with GAD whose behavior is unchanged when alone and many dogs with SRD who can be completely relaxed as long as a person is present.

B) **Fear of loud noises, including thunderstorms and fireworks**
As mentioned above, if a dog demonstrates intermittent signs of SRD, their trigger may not actually be being alone, but rather a noise event that occurs when they happen to be home alone. Screening for storm and noise fears is an essential part of the differentiating process, particularly when signs are intermittent, or started that way.

C) **Territorial aggression (TA)**
Dogs with TA may show destructive behavior around windows or doors where they view potential intruders. They also bark and may appear quite distressed. The manner of barking due to territorial aggression is different from SRD vocalizations. Audio or video recording would help to differentiate between the two.

D) **Insufficient housetraining**
A simple way to differentiate insufficient housetraining from SRD is to ask about house soiling patterns when the family is home with the dog, as well as how long their pet is alone when elimination occurs. It is also possible the dog has been harshly punished for eliminating in front of family members and without their presence it is now safe to eliminate indoors.

E) **Urine marking**
Urine marking has several potential motivations, including claiming territory, sexual status signaling, and excitement. They also mark out anxiety, which may only overlap with signs of SRD. Most of these dogs will have a history of urine marking in multiple contexts, not just when alone.

F) **Compulsive disorder (for example, self-injury)**
Compulsive disorder has several patterns, such as tail chasing or excessive licking. Usually, it is not associated with a particular context or trigger due to its compulsion,

although the stress of being alone may contextually exacerbate it.

G) **Underlying medical conditions**
Based on the clinical signs, possible medical conditions need to be screened out, especially if the onset is sudden or the dog is over seven years of age. In some cases, a definitive diagnostic exam may be required, such as suspicion of underlying pain.

H) **Cognitive dysfunction syndrome (primarily in older dogs)**
Brain aging impacts alterations in sensory processes, learning, and memory. This may contribute to increased anxiety in geriatric dogs. As a result, clinical signs of SRD are seen in older dogs, but the primary diagnosis is not SRD.

I) **Crate/confinement/barrier fear, anxiety, or frustration**
Some dogs have a specific fear of confinement (crate, wire cage, or small room) or merely a lack of experience and gradual exposure to it – both of which are unrelated to being alone. These dogs often do well with being left alone outside of the crate or confinement space. That said, dogs with separation distress when home alone often cope better and signs are minimized when given more space to pace and/or search for their people, making the crate or confinement merely an exacerbating factor (Figure 16.3). Video recording the dog alone for short periods, both when confined and when loose in a larger space, may be necessary to differentiate between the two.

J) **Destructive behaviors caused by boredom, exploration, or excess energy**
Chewing or tearing furniture and objects is commonly seen in young or active dogs left in a sterile environment. These behaviors also arise in dogs left alone without

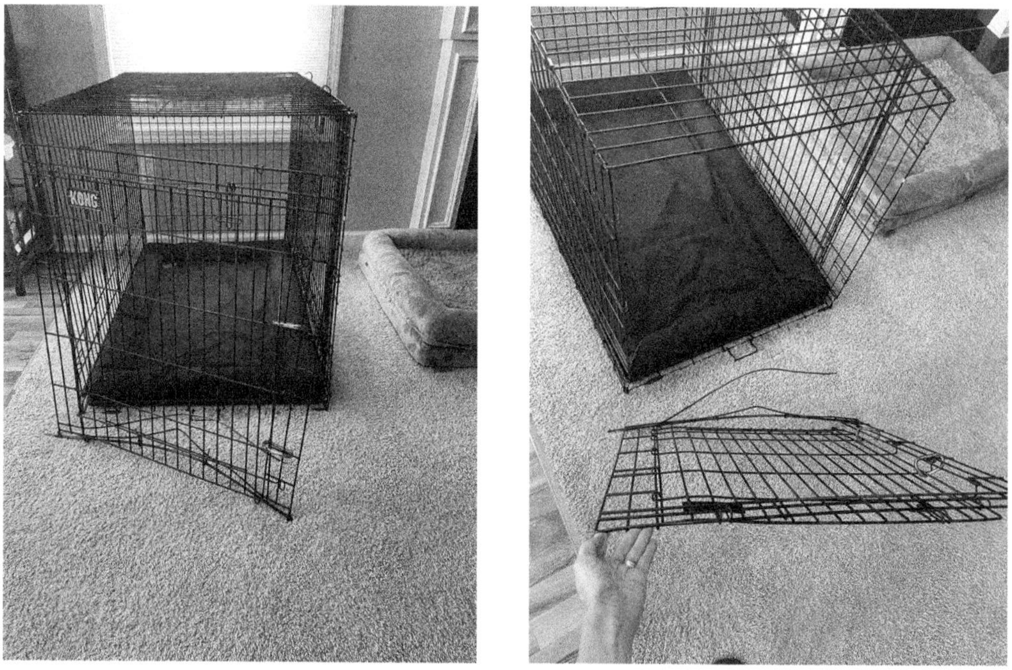

Figure 16.3 Whether a dog has a fear of confinement that is unrelated to SRD or if the confinement is exacerbating distress experienced when the dog is home alone, escape attempts from a crate like this can be the cause of serious injuries. *Source:* With permission from Patti Neyenhaus.

sufficient social and physical stimuli in their environment. Normal puppies and adolescent dogs will explore with their mouths and seek items to chew and destroy. If they have been punished for doing so in front of their human family members, they may simply feel it is safe to do so when no one is home. On video, these dogs will have playful, energetic body postures and show few signs of fear or distress.

Checkpoints to Differentiate Problems

Contexts of Incidents

SRD should be observed in the context of being alone or separated from the specific attachment figure. Separation anxiety is defined as an anxiety-related disorder in dogs whose signs are observed only in the family's absence or perceived absence (Horwitz 2000; Sherman and Mills 2008). Therefore, the first step in differentiating diagnoses is to identify the context in which behavioral problems occur. Carefully collecting history from clients should confirm the circumstance for most of the diagnoses listed above (A–H), as dogs with these conditions (A–H) show clinical signs that are not limited to being separated from their person.

Video Recording

The remaining two (I and J) are often misunderstood as separation anxiety because the contexts are frequently limited to situations when the attachment figure is absent. They are referred to as *other separation-related problems*. The key to differentiating these diagnoses is understanding what triggers these problems. Were they triggered by separation, confinement, boredom, or play? What is the emotional status of the dog? Has the dog's body language shown other demeanors such as frustration, boredom, or play? Without using video recordings, it is near impossible to differentiate them. When you are trying to differentiate between confinement anxiety and separation anxiety, it may help to video record the dog home alone crated as well as left to roam a larger area. Make sure the family removes dangerous and/or valuable items and stays nearby in case the dog begins to seriously damage household items.

Presence of Underlying Diseases

Some symptoms (for example, vomiting and diarrhea) are often misinterpreted as being stress-related; however, it is likely that underlying medical conditions have been overlooked. In some cases, the symptoms of the disease may become more apparent or worse in dogs in stressful environments. Therefore, a physical examination, bloodwork, and urinalysis are mandatory. If necessary, further definitive examinations such as diagnostic imaging or lab work can be added. As mentioned, especially for dogs in SRD associated with human sleep times, if the problem occurs irregularly, such as at night, it does not fit with other types of separation-related problems such as normal or persistent separation-related behaviors. Instead, differential behavioral- and medical-oriented diagnoses should be made.

Cognitive dysfunction syndrome (CDS) in older dogs is not uncommon, and some animals may have both cognitive dysfunction and underlying medical conditions. Common clinical signs of CDS, which can overlap with SRD, include disturbed sleep cycles, vocalization, and inappropriate elimination. When these signs are observed, the context of incidents as well as the presence or absence of other clinical signs of cognitive dysfunction may help rule it out. See the DISHAA screening questionnaire for CDS in the online materials for Chapter 23.

Approach to Treatment

Normal Separation-Related Behaviors

Dogs in this group may be puppies or adults with no prior experience being alone. Thus, teaching them how to cope with this new lifestyle is a mandatory step. The same protocol can be used as preventative advice for families expecting lifestyle changes in the near future.

Daily Exercise

Ensure young dogs receive daily physical exercise. Young healthy dogs are active and need to burn their energy through physical activity before you can expect to modify behavior. Maintaining a daily exercise routine will change their behavior and improve training overall. This is especially critical for dogs that show other separation-related problems triggered by boredom, exploration or play. Examples include brisk walking, jogging, or playing a fetch game.

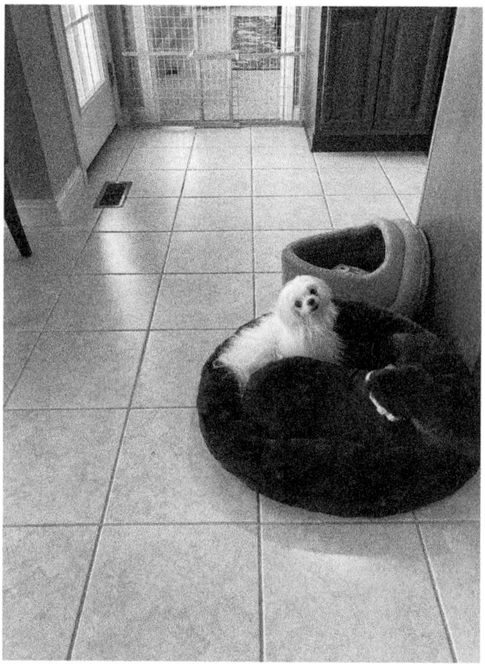

Figure 16.4 Two dogs enjoy time in a safe gated space in the kitchen where they have access to food, bed, water and enrichment when separated from the family. *Source:* Niwako Ogata.

Introducing a Safe, Designated Area Combined with Independence Training

It is important to introduce independence time gradually and at a time when the family is home. For a faster, easier transition to being alone, it may help to use a dog's favorite safe place as a designated area when it is independent of the family (Figure 16.4). If the dog is young and in the middle of house training, it is easier to confine them in a particular area (for example, kitchen or crate) when introducing independence time. If the dog is well-trained and does not chew furniture/walls in daily life, the family may want to use a certain area of the house, instead of crate, that the dog likes, such as the master bedroom, or basement.

This step needs to be gradually practiced, especially for dogs that are not used to being in confinement (for example, dogs with other separation-related problems).

1) Put the dog in the designated area for independence training and provide soft bedding, favorite toys, and food-dispensing puzzles to classically condition a positive emotional response to the setting of being alone.
2) The duration of the training can start in short increments, such as 15 minutes, or while the family performs a brief task or chore (for example, cooking, PC work, or taking a shower).
3) The physical distance from the dog gradually increases to the point where the person doing the training is out of sight.
4) Frequent practice per day over a short duration (from 15 minutes to 1 hour) is more productive than one-time practice for long hours of separation.
5) The duration and distance should not increase if the dog cannot settle in the safe place during this practice.
6) If the client reports no progress (i.e. cannot increase the distance and duration from the dog) after working on this for two weeks, it is possible that the dog's condition may have shifted to persistent SRD (Group 2).

Practice Departures with Counterconditioning

When dogs learn to stay in the designated area calmly and independently of the family, they can move to the actual departure training.

1) To start, additional and/or longer-lasting food puzzle items can be placed in the designated area to immediately capture the dog's attention. The family can then leave the home for 15–20 minutes as the dog engages in the food puzzles in the designated independence area.
2) As the dog becomes tolerant of alone time, the family can extend the time they are away from home by 15–20-minute increments. Eventually they can work up to leaving for a full 8-hour day if needed. Live video monitoring will help detect signs of distress. If the dog shows signs of panic (e.g. screaming, attempting to escape, hypersalivating), the humans should return home and start training again at a shorter increment.

Before and After Going Out

Although clients can talk to and interact with their dog when they leave and return, it is better to maintain a low-key interaction so that excitement and frustration are not inadvertently added.

Persistent SRD

Dogs from shelters/rescues with an unknown home alone history may not respond well to the above acclimation due to preexisting SRD prior to adoption. These dogs, as well as dogs with known SRD whose behaviors are refractory to the above training, may require additional intervention.

Consider Pharmacological Intervention

Because rehabilitation from SRDs involves both emotional conditioning and operant training, a multimodal treatment plan is recommended. Time restraints on traditional wellness appointments in a general practice leave insufficient time for comprehensive evaluation and treatment plans. These problems should be triaged as outlined in Chapter 12 and at minimum basic recommendations can be implemented before referring to a veterinary behaviorist or other behavior professional. Interestingly, the literature states that standard SRD behavior modification protocols, as opposed to advice tailored to the individual dog, still lead to improvement in more than half of the cases within two to three months (Blackwell et al. 2006; Cottam et al. 2008). An example of standard behavior modification protocols is outlined in online materials for Chapter 16.

Moreover, two FDA-approved medications (Clomicalm®, and Reconcile®) are available to treat separation anxiety in dogs. According to the results of clinical trials for these medications, the best outcome was observed when both medication and behavioral modification were implemented together (Sherman et al. 2007). The use of medication or behavior modification alone led to no significant difference in the clinical outcome, although medication on its own accelerated the reduction in some clinical signs (King et al. 2000; Landsberg et al. 2008; Sherman et al. 2007). Although having two FDA-approved medications available specifically for the treatment of separation anxiety is encouraging, it will take four to six weeks for either medication to reach the full clinical effects. Some dogs with persistent SRDs may show severe signs of anxiety; and waiting weeks for improvement may not be feasible. In these cases, adding a fast-acting event medication, such as trazodone, clonidine, gabapentin, or a benzodiazepine may be warranted at the beginning of the treatment period. See Chapter 21 for full details.

Summary

1) Avoid leaving the dog alone longer than they can tolerate, using a pet sitter, daycare, or arranging the family schedule to reduce the time of absence.
2) Be sure dogs are accustomed to the food-dispensing puzzle toys (and any other environmental changes) without being

associated with a departure for several days/weeks prior to departure training, otherwise, they will serve as departure cues which trigger anxiety, rather than serving as distraction or counterconditioning.

3) Begin one of the FDA-approved medications (Clomicalm® or Reconcile®) at the onset of treatment unless alternate medications are indicated (see Chapter 21).
4) If the symptoms are severe and if no alleviation is observed two to four weeks after the treatment, the dog should be referred to a behavior specialist.

Intermittent SRD and SRD Associated with Human Sleep Times

The dogs in these groups may show signs of SRD, but can be attributed to a secondary behavioral and/or medical diagnosis. Although the standardized treatment described for normal separation related behaviors is somewhat helpful to the dogs in these groups, treating the primary diagnosis is critical, and the overall treatment plan is often complex. Therefore, once the diagnosis of their primary condition is made, referral of such dogs to a relevant specialist is recommended.

Client Considerations

The treatment of behavioral problems differs from treatment of medical issues as most, if not all, treatment is carried out at home by family members. This means that while SRD are being treated, the client will have to tackle the problem daily for a long period, which can be stressful. As in the case of home care for other chronic diseases, a family's burden of living with dogs that have behavioral problems is substantial. If the prognosis is challenging, both dogs and their humans need continuous support. The family often feels blamed or judged due to their dog's behavior problems. Some clients may not know what to do or where to get help. A study showed that families living with pets with behavior problems feel the emotional burden of sadness, frustration, anger, guilt, and embarrassment, leading to social isolation. Further research shows that giving noncommittal or unclear advice to clients regarding a pet's behavior problem creates a feeling of frustration and/or negative emotional response (Roshier and McBride 2013). Thus, it is critical for clinicians to know how to appropriately differentiate and triage these problems, to provide appropriate treatments or guidance, and/or to refer to a specialist when problems are severe or out of the clinician's comfort zone or experience (Buller and Ballantyne 2020).

Concluding Remarks

1) Because the underlying cause and presentation of SRD vary greatly, the best results are obtained via multimodal treatment, including environmental and behavior modification and, in persistent cases, psychopharmacology.
2) Use caution not to overwhelm clients with an extensive treatment plan that may be challenging to implement (Takeuchi et al. 2000). Help set short-term, practical goals and refer to a specialist if more intense support that you can reasonably provide is needed.
3) If it is difficult to adjust the treatment plan based on the individual response and signs, it is appropriate to refer the dog to a specialist as soon as possible.
4) When implementing a behavior treatment plan, structured follow-up initiated by the veterinary team can help the owner's engagement, which can contribute to the perceived outcome (Radosta-Hunley et al. 2007).
5) Cases that show little response or worsen after the first-line treatment should be referred to a specialist.

References

Anderson, K.H., Yao, Y., Perry, P.J. et al. (2022). Case distribution, sources, and breeds of dogs presenting to a veterinary behavior clinic in the United States from 1997 to 2017. *Animals 12* (5): 576.

Bamberger, M. and Houpt, K.A. (2006). Signalment factors, comorbidity, and trends in behavior diagnoses in dogs: 1,644 cases (1991–2001). *J. Am. Vet. Med. Assoc. 229* (10): 1591–1601.

Blackwell, E., Casey, R.A., and Bradshaw, J.W. (2006). Controlled trial of behavioral therapy for separation-related disorders in dogs. *Vet. Rec.* 158: 551–554.

Blackwell, E., Casey, R.A., and Bradshaw, J.W. (2016). Efficacy of written behavioral advice for separation-related behavior problems in dogs newly adopted from a rehoming center. *J. Vet. Behav.: Clin. Appl. Res.* 12: 13–19.

Bohland, K.R., Lilly, M.L., Herron, M.E. et al. (2023). Shelter dog behavior after adoption: Using the C-BARQ to track dog behavior changes through the first six months after adoption. *Plos One 18* (8): e0289356.

Bradshaw, J.W., McPherson, J.A., Casey, R.A., and Larter, I.S. (2002). Aetiology of separation-related behaviour in domestic dogs. *Vet. Rec.* 151: 43–46.

Buller, K. and Ballantyne, K.C. (2020). Living with and loving a pet with behavioral problems: pet owners' experiences. *J. Vet. Behav.: Clin. Appl. Res.* 37: 41–47.

Cottam, N., Dodman, N.H., Moon-Fanelli, A.A., and Patronek, G.J. (2008). Comparison of remote versus in-person behavioral consultation for treatment of canine separation anxiety. *Appl. Anim. Welf. Sci.* 11: 28–41.

de Assis, L.S., Matos, R., Pike, T.W. et al. (2020). Developing diagnostic frameworks in veterinary behavioral medicine: disambiguating separation related problems in dogs. *Front. Vet. Sci.* 6: 499. https://doi.org/10.3389/fvets.2019.00499.

de Souza Machado, D., Oliveira, P.M.B., Machado, J.C. et al. (2020). Identification of separation-related problems in domestic cats: A questionnaire survey. *PLoS One 15* (4): e0230999.

Dinwoodie, I.R., Dwyer, B., Zottola, V. et al. (2019). Demographics and comorbidity of behavior problems in dogs. *J. Vet. Behav. : Clin. Appl. Res.* 32: 62–71.

Flannigan, G. and Dodman, N.H. (2001). Risk factors and behaviors associated with separation anxiety in dogs. *J. Am. Vet. Med. Assoc.* 219: 460–466.

Herron, M.E., Lord, L.K., and Husseini, S.E. (2014). Effects of preadoption counseling on the prevention of separation anxiety in newly adopted shelter dogs. *J. Vet. Behav. : Clin. Appl. Res.* 9: 13–21.

Horwitz, D.F. (2000). Diagnosis and treatment of canine separation anxiety and the use of clomipramine hydrochloride (Clomicalm). *J. Am. Anim. Hosp. Assoc.* 36: 107–109.

King, J.N., Simpson, B.S., Overall, K.L. et al. (2000). Treatment of separation anxiety in dogs with clomipramine: results from a prospective, parallel-group, multicenter clinical trial. *App. Anim. Behav. Sci.* 67: 255–275.

Konok, V., Dóka, S., and Miklósi, A. (2011). The behavior of the domestic dog (Canis familiaris) during separation from and reunion with the owner: a questionnaire and an experimental study. *App. Anim. Behav. Sci.* 135: 300–308.

Landsberg, G.M., Melese, P., Sherman, B.L. et al. (2008). Effectiveness of fluoxetine chewable tablets in the treatment of canine separation anxiety. *J. Vet. Behav.: Clin. Appl. Res.* 3: 12–19.

Lund, J.D. and Jørgensen, M.C. (1999). Behaviour patterns and time course of activity in dogs with separation problems. *App. Anim. Behav. Sci.* 63: 219–236.

McGreevy, P.D. and Masters, A.M. (2008). Risk factors for separation-related distress and feed-related aggression in dogs: additional findings from a survey of Australian dog owners. *App. Anim. Behav. Sci.* 109: 320–328.

Palestrini, C., Minero, M., Cannas, S. et al. (2010). Video analysis of dogs with separation-related behaviors. *Appl. Anim. Behav. Science* *124* (1-2): 61–67.

Parthasarathy, V. and Crowell-Davis, S.L. (2006). Relationship between attachment to owners and separation anxiety in pet dogs (*Canis lupus familiaris*). *J. Vet. Behav.: Clin. Appl. Res.* 1: 109–120.

Radosta-Hunley, R., Shofer, F., and Reisner, I. (2007). Comparison of 42 cases of canine fear-related aggression with structured clinician initiated follow-up and 25 cases with unstructured client initiated follow-up. *App. Anim. Behav. Sci.* 105: 330–341.

Roshier, A.L. and McBride, E.A. (2013). Veterinarians' perceptions of behaviour support in small-animal practice. *Vet. Rec.* *172* (10): 267–267.

Sherman, B.S., Landsberg, G.M., Reisner, I.R. et al. (2007). Effects of reconcile (fluoxetine) chewable tablets plus behavior management for canine separation anxiety. *Vet. Ther.* 8: 19–31.

Sherman, B.L. and Mills, D.S. (2008). Canine anxieties and phobias: an update on separation anxiety and noise aversions. *Vet. Clin. North Am.: Small. Anim. Pract.* 38: 1081–1106.

Storengen, L.M., Boge, S.C., Strøm, S.J. et al. (2014). A descriptive study of 215 dogs diagnosed with separation anxiety. *App. Anim. Behav. Sci.* 159: 82–89.

Takeuchi, Y., Houpt, K.A., and Scarlett, J.M. (2000). Evaluation of treatments for separation anxiety in dogs. *J. Am. Vet. Med. Assoc.* 217: 342–345.

Tiira, K. and Lohi, H. (2015). Early life experiences and exercise associate with canine anxieties. *PLoS ONE* 10 (11): e0141907.

Tiira, K., Sulkama, S., and Lohi, H. (2016). Prevalence, comorbidity, and behavioral variation in canine anxiety. *J. Vet. Behav. : Clin. Appl. Res.* 16: 36–44.

17

Equine Aggression

Jeannine Berger[1] *and Kathy Holcomb*[2]

[1] *Sacramento Veterinary Behavior Services, Vacaville, CA, USA*
[2] *University of California, Davis, School of Veterinary Medicine, Davis, CA, USA*

Introduction

Aggression, whether between horses or by horses toward humans, is one of the main issues that confront veterinarians who treat equine behavior problems. Because aggression can be dangerous and result in serious injuries (Grandin 1999), the caregivers are often in urgent need of help. As discussed in Chapters 14 and 15, the first step in evaluating aggressive behavior in animals is to determine if there is an underlying medical reason for the behavior. This involves a thorough physical examination and any warranted diagnostic assessments. Next, you can evaluate the type of aggression exhibited. This is done by establishing the motivation, trigger(s), and threshold leading to the problem behavior(s). The goal initially is to minimize incidents by avoiding the triggers, staying below the threshold to keep everyone safe, not aggravating the problem or having the horse practice the unwanted behavior, and then implementing a thoughtful behavior modification plan.

Aggression is a complex social behavior with multiple causes and has been defined as overt behavior with the intention of inflicting physical damage upon another individual (Moyer 1968). The horse, a social herbivore and prey species, is an animal that relies mainly on caution, speed, and agility for self-preservation. When faced with discomfort or perceived threat, given a choice, horses will most often move away. In most cases, aggressive behaviors in horses can be observed as self-defense. Flight is in most cases preferred to fight. However, if horses are unable to escape, they may defend themselves. Aggressive behavior can also be seen when the interests or needs of two or more individuals conflict, such as two stallions fighting for a mare. These conflicts are more likely to take place over limited, highly valued resources such as water, food, playmates, breeding mates, and shelter. Resource guarding, as can be seen in dogs, for example, is less common in the wild but can occur in domestic settings because caregivers tend to provide horses with limited resources: we determine the types, amounts, and scheduling of feed; caregivers choose companions; a single water source may serve multiple horses; space is restricted in most situations, which has shown to directly impact the amount and intensity of aggressive behaviors (Christensen et al. 2011; Fureix et al. 2012).

In most cases of conflict, horses engage in threat displays or ritualized fights that do not result in physical harm (Christensen et al. 2011). Behaviors in the agonistic ethogram of

Introduction to Animal Behavior and Veterinary Behavioral Medicine, First Edition. Edited by Meghan E. Herron.

Companion website: www.wiley.com/go/introductiontoanimalbehavior

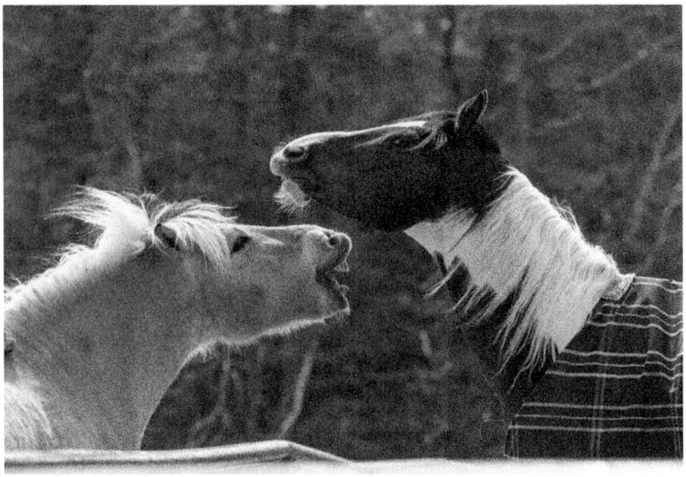

Figure 17.1 A horse offers a bite threat by retracting the lips to show teeth and gesturing the mouth toward another individual (horse, human, or any other potential threat) without making physical contact. If this warning is not heeded, further escalation of aggression is likely. *Source:* Photo credit: Dolores M. Harvey/Shutterstock.

horses (McDonnell 2003) can range from a mild head threat to more aggressive behaviors, including biting, kicking, circling, crowding, or even displacement. Head threats include pinned ears, head tossing with pinned ears, and a **bite threat** that deliberately makes no contact with the teeth (Figure 17.1). Raising and lowering a leg without force or aim may be a threat to kick or strike. Turning to present the rump to an opponent is a way to appear larger or can position the animal for a kick threat or kick. In some cases, merely resisting the commands from the handler may be considered a subtle form of aggression. If the other horse or a handler misses or ignores such threats, the conflict may escalate. Horses that have not been properly socialized with other horses at a young age, people without much experience around horses, and veterinarians that are focused on the medical area or condition are especially at risk for misinterpreting or missing such threats.

Horses are fast learners, and aggressive behaviors can also become conditioned or learned. That is, some horses can become sensitized to a particular threat or stimulus, and the behavior becomes a conditioned response of aggression toward another horse or the handler. For example, if horses are repeatedly exposed to a threat and cannot escape, they may then anticipate conflict and behave in an aggressive manner due to anxiety. Dangerous forms of aggression can develop if excessive force is applied repeatedly by a handler. Horses may become fearful and consequently develop signs of anxiety. They learn that "the best defense is a good offense" and may attack rather than flee or freeze. If this is a chronic situation, the warning signals may even be skipped altogether. The conditioned response can also happen toward another horse, for example, if the horse has unsupervised opportunities to practice the aggressive behavior toward another horse along a fence line for an extended period.

Aggression in horses can be categorized in several ways. Categories can be based on the source of the conflict as well as the target, the latter including aggression directed toward humans and aggression directed toward other horses or other animals. In some cases, subdividing these categories may be helpful.

Veterinarians frequently observe various types of aggression. Aggressive behavior of horses toward humans can be severe and dangerous, and a systematic approach is needed to avoid injury to horses and humans. Managing the environment, avoiding further aggression, and reestablishing a positive human–animal or animal–animal relationship is of utmost importance when addressing aggression in horses.

Categories of Aggression

Pain-induced Aggression

The first consideration when evaluating the cause of aggressive behavior is the possibility of discomfort or pain (Fureix et al. 2010; Gleerup and Lindegaard 2016; McDonnell 2005). A detailed history, complete physical and orthopedic exam should always be taken first with any type of aggression. Many veterinarians have had little training in pain recognition related to assessment of aggressive behavior changes, resisting commands, or even as a cause of changes in performance. The most recent advance in the recognition of subtle behavioral changes associated with pain is the investigation of facial expressions (Dyson et al. 2014; Gleerup and Lindegaard 2016; Mullard et al. 2017). Figure 17.2 shows examples of facial expressions associated with pain in a horse. Observation of the behavior in its normal context, either directly or from a video, is extremely helpful (McDonnell 2005). The level of pain tolerated by each animal differs; hence, how a horse reacts to pain may significantly differ from one horse to the next. Keep in mind that, as with people, the experience of pain is subjective and can increase irritability, lower the threshold for tolerance, lower performance and increase resistance, or even lead to aggression.

Pain-induced aggression develops directly out of experienced or expected pain and serves to eliminate, or attempt to eliminate, the source of pain. Lameness, injury, disease such as colic or neurologic processes (Macmillan 2013), management (Fureix et al. 2012; Hausberger et al. 2008), and some veterinary procedures

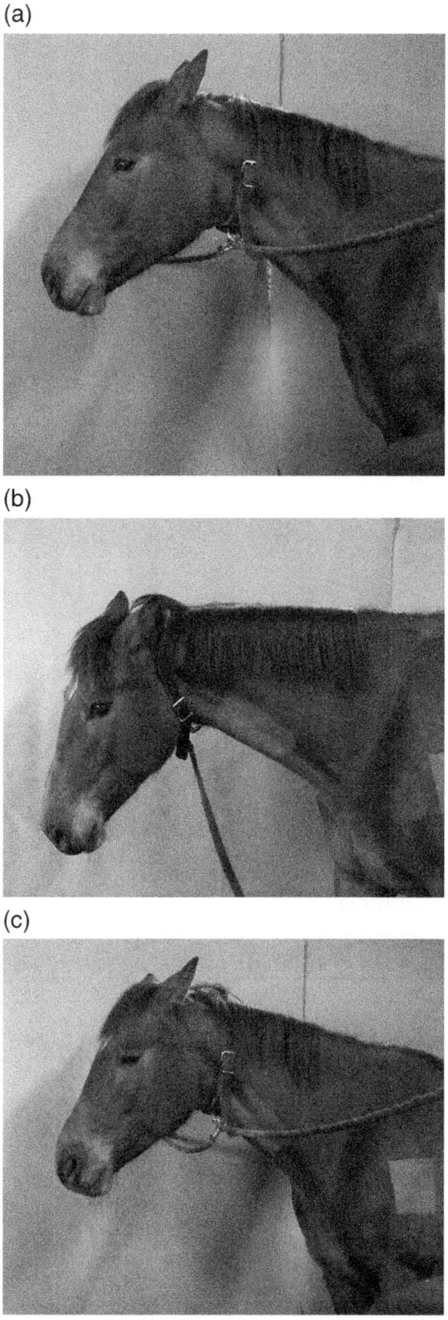

Figure 17.2 Illustration of the equine pain face in one horse (Gleerup et al. 2015): (a) the horse is relaxed; (b) the horse is in pain (somatic pain); (c) the horse is resting with semi-closed eyes; this horse rests with the ears backwards; however, the ears are additionally lowered when the horse is in pain. *Source:* Reproduced with permission from Dyson et al. 2014 / ELSEVIER.

are potential sources of pain. While an obvious cause of aggression is infliction of acute pain, research indicates that chronic discomfort or pain is an often-overlooked source of aggression as well (Fureix et al. 2010). Thus, for example, tack fit and rider/handler influence should be considered when localizing a source of pain or discomfort.

Even the most socialized and friendly horse may exhibit signs of aggression when in pain or being asked to perform when in pain. If a horse is in pain, generally uncomfortable or otherwise impaired, there may be increased risk or incidence for aggressive behavior. Distinguishing between chronic pain and irritable aggression may be difficult. That is why a detailed history and enhanced physical exam, including ophthalmic, orthopedic, and neurological evaluation, are always needed when assessing and diagnosing any form of aggression.

Conditioned response aggression can develop within this category, wherein the horse anticipates pain or a painful procedure because of a previous negative experience in a specific situation or procedure and displays aggression to avoid repeating a painful experience. Veterinary office aggression is recognized in small animals, and studies indicate that a great majority of dogs and cats show signs of fear in the veterinary office (Döring et al. 2009; Mariti et al. 2016; Mariti et al. 2015; Riemer et al. 2021). Horses are often examined in their home environment but can also develop fear or aggressive behavior in the context of veterinary visits due to sensitization by previous interactions experienced by the horse as negative, painful, or traumatic.

One of the author's (JBE) patients was a two-year-old Quarter Horse with severe aggression toward the handler for any type of veterinary exam or treatment but was otherwise a very social horse. As a young foal, this horse was very sick and required multiple injections, for which the foal had been held down physically by an increasing number of people until the foal was medically cured. The veterinary treatment was experienced as threatening, frightening, or just emotionally negative. Two years later, now bigger and stronger, the horse displayed severe signs of aggression to avoid any and all medical handling, anticipating a similar negative experience. Some horses can even learn from a negative or painful experience. Something minor, such as grooming over a painful area, could be enough to lead to anticipation and this type of aggression.

Treatment strategies for this type of aggression include:

- Eliminate the source of pain or discomfort. This often requires a medical diagnosis and specific treatment, such as for lameness or an ill-fitting saddle.
- Management: identify triggers and avoid any situation and handling that elicits pain or any aggressive behavior.
- Develop a proper pain protocol to alleviate the pain.
- Implement consistent positive and fear-free handling techniques to create new emotional responses.
- Use positive reinforcement training techniques to train new behavior responses.
- Implement a specifically designed desensitizing and counterconditioning behavior modification plan.
- Avoid all punitive and confrontational handling.

Social/Dominance-related/ Competitive Aggression

The horse, a social herbivore, is dependent on companions for safety, mutual comfort, grooming, and enhanced detection of food. As with other social animals, a stable group hierarchy is important for survival. Establishing status within a group is necessary to decrease aggression and injuries (Hartmann et al. 2009). If a hierarchy were not established and maintained, each horse would need to continually reaffirm their position, often by increasing levels of aggression. If the relationships are stable and the submissive animal defers to the more dominant animal without any threatening behavior, levels of aggression and consequent injuries are low. Constant changes to groups are challenging for horses (Christensen et al. 2011).

Dominance hierarchies in both feral and domesticated herds have been studied by many researchers (Berger 1977; Hartmann et al. 2017; Houpt and Keiper 1982; Houpt and Wolski 1980; Stanley et al. 2018). Observations of interactions between herd members have not been able to determine with any degree of certainty the correlation between physical characteristics and rank within the hierarchy itself, and rank order is not necessarily linear (Hartmann et al. 2017). However, horses appear to need direct contact in order to form dominance relationships. Furthermore, proximity alone does not cause horses to become **preferred associates** (Houpt 2005).

Treatment strategies for this type of aggression include:

- Management: identify triggers and avoid any situation that causes the aggression.
- Observe group dynamics to identify compatible horses.
- Remove any horse(s) that appear unable to settle into a hierarchy or continue to aggress other horses.
- Manage the environment to alleviate competition over resources. Offer enrichment by providing multiple locations of shelter, food, and water. Space out feed locations or utilize visual dividers to reduce conflict at feeding times. If multiple water sources are not practical, centrally place a single large source in the paddock; troughs in corners and along fence lines can be sites of congestion and conflict.
- Maintain stable groups as much as possible, although this can be challenging in boarding facilities where residents frequently change; hence, some facilities do not lend themselves for group housing.
- Paddock size appropriate for the number of horses allows lower-ranked horses to avoid potentially aggressive behavior from dominant group members. Block or round off corners to prevent one horse from trapping another.

Environmental management practices are often the key to treatment of this form of aggression in domestic settings. Where horses are kept in groups, you can facilitate peaceful establishment of dominance hierarchy by gradually introducing new horses. Start by first allowing interaction across a fence, or by pairing the new horse with a compatible established member of the group before having them join the full group. Joint trail rides can create positive, controlled interactions that can facilitate successful introductions. If it can be done safely, sometimes trailering horses together results in friendships.

A Note on Dominance:
Dominance is a relationship between members of the same species that is established by aggressive and submissive displays to determine who has priority access to resources such as food, resting spots, and mates. Dominance is not a personality trait nor a training method.

Territorial Aggression

Territorial aggression serves to keep others out of a particular area. A territory is an area that will be defended against any intruder. Compared to donkeys, horses are by nature not particularly territorial, and this form of aggression is seen rarely in the wild. Even examples of stallions chasing away an intruder are mainly due to defending the herd or a mare in heat, rather than the area itself. Similar to competitive aggression, this form of aggression may develop due to improper management of resources in domesticated settings. Other differentials like fear aggression, pain/irritable-related, or status-related aggression should be ruled out. Some horses become territorial about their stall and may show aggression to people who attempt to enter, such as stall cleaners and other handlers.

Treatment strategies for this type of aggression include:

- Management: identify trigger and avoid any situation that causes the aggression.
- Remove the horse from the area before entering the area; for example, remove the horse from the stall before cleaning the stall. If you cannot safely remove the horse, place the horse in a stall with a paddock where the two areas can be separated with a door or gate. One area should only be entered if the horse can be confined safely in the other part.
- A protected contact setting may be needed to safely implement a behavior modification plan (AVMA 2008).
- Move the horses to a new area as this may help to decrease "ownership" of one location.
- Offer enrichment and provide a larger space with multiple resources, such as water or feeding stations. For example, placing hay in all four corners of the paddock or stall may help to allow the horse to avoid conflict.

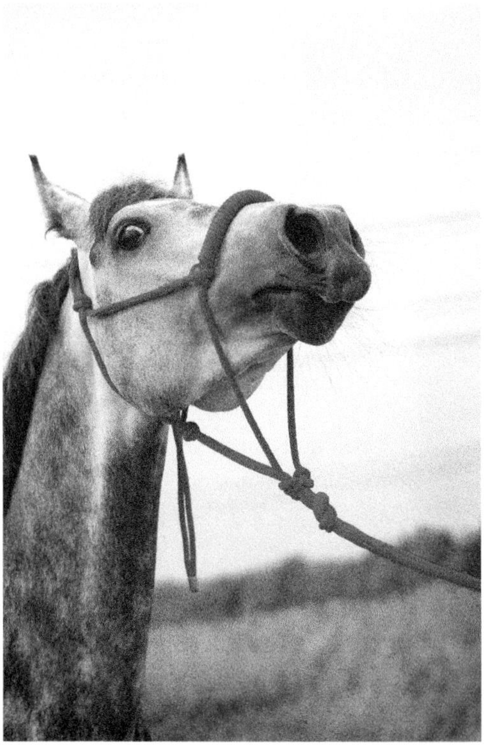

Figure 17.3 A fearful horse has his head held high with ears erect, eyes wide, and nostrils flared. An escalation to aggression will occur if the threat persists and escape is prevented. *Source:* Photo credit: mari_art / Adobe Stock

Fear-related Aggression

Fear is "an unpleasant often strong emotion caused by anticipation or awareness of danger," (Merriam-Webster Dictionary Online n.d.), an emotional response to ensure survival. As prey animals that evolved over the millennia, horses have a keen awareness of danger, speed, and an instantaneous response time to initiate flight from many of the real or perceived dangers they might encounter. However, if escape is not possible or fails, the animal may turn to aggression to fight for survival. Domestically, fear-related aggression can be a result of rough handling, punishment-based training methods, or previous exposure to negative experiences such as pain. During medical procedures and handling, this form of aggression is a very common type seen by veterinarians. Common triggers are injections or other mildly painful medical procedures, harsh handling, a new environment or handler, and any noises or threatening movements.

A fearful horse may appear very alert or hypervigilant, with the head held high and muscles tensed (Figure 17.3). A horse motivated by fear may act defensively by kicking a veterinarian, owner, or another horse, especially if the subtle behaviors and early warnings are missed or ignored. Because expressions of fear shown by body language can quickly escalate to violent attempts of escape or aggression, these behaviors need to be recognized and addressed early to keep horse and handler safe.

Treatment strategies for this type of aggression include:

- Management: identify triggers and avoid any situation that causes fear and aggression.

- Remove the fear eliciting trigger from the horse to a distance where the horse can remain calm.
- If you cannot remove the trigger, remove the horse from the fear eliciting environment to a distance where the horse can remain calm.
- Design a behavior modification plan using desensitization and counterconditioning to the specific triggers.
- Train better coping strategies using positive reinforcement techniques.
- Use humane tools to facilitate training.
- In some instances, psychotropic medications or supplements can be helpful (see Chapter 10).
- Offer enrichment: Mental and physical enrichment helps horses focus on a specific task and can reduce anxiety and fear. Use food enrichment with the goal of solving a problem and being mentally and physically engaged. Physical enrichment can be offered by teaching new skills using wooden logs or equine jumping equipment, such as poles, based on the horse's ability.

Maternal Aggression

Maternal aggression, characterized by protection of the offspring, is normal behavior facilitated by the post-parturient hormonal state, the physical presence of young, and usually decreases with time. The aggression may be directed toward people, other horses, or, in some pathological cases, toward the mare's own foal. Prevention is ideal, through positive interactions pre- and peri-partum as well as preventing unfamiliar people or other threats near the mare and foal during the first hours and days post-partum.

Treatment strategies for this type of aggression include:

- Management: avoid any situation that causes fear and aggression.
- Avoid contact with unfamiliar people or other animals, especially predators (dogs) and other horses, and minimize traffic in the barn.
- Handling should be minimal and positive (no punishment) by handlers with whom the horse is familiar and comfortable.
- Should the foal need to be treated medically, for safety reasons, a separate handler should control the mare. In severe cases, the mare should be placed behind a physical barrier where she will still be able to see her foal, or the mare may need to be sedated so the veterinarian can safely approach and treat the foal.
- Design and implement, step by step, a behavior modification plan using a desensitizing and counterconditioning protocol to approach the mare and foal.
- In some cases, psychotropic medication or supplements can be helpful (see Chapter 10).

Foal rejection is a type of maternal aggression directed toward the mare's own foal. These are more common in primiparous mares, and the Arabian breed seems to be more affected than any other breed (Juarbe-Diaz et al. 1998). In a medical setting, maternal rejection may occur with excessive disturbance, or if the odor or appearance of the foal is changed. Allowing the mare to have visual contact with the foal is useful if the foal must be separated from the mare or is too weak to suckle. Redirected aggression is also possible and needs to be considered as a differential diagnosis for foal rejection. For example, when a mare is aggressing toward another horse or a person, she might accidentally run over, bite, or kick her foal. Another differential when assessing foal rejection includes pain-induced aggression. The mare may be directly aggressive toward her own foal during a painful condition such as mastitis, from an injury to the udder, or general pain.

Three different types of foal rejection have been reported (Crowell-Davis and Houpt 1986).

Foal Directed Aggression

With Type 1 rejection, the mare accepts foal but does not allow suckling.

Treatment strategies for this type of aggression include:

- Management: identify triggers and avoid any situation that causes fear and aggression, and strictly supervise all mare–foal interactions to ensure they are positive for the safety of the foal and to prevent escalation of aggression.
- Desensitize and countercondition the mare to the foal, the foal approaching the mare, and the suckling process.
- Restrain the mare for several nursing sessions until she accepts the suckling process without any sign of avoidance or aggression.
- If the udder seems very firm or painful to the touch, milking the mare may help to relieve some pressure. If colostrum is milked out, you need to collect it and give to the foal within a few hours.
- If pain or discomfort of any kind is a contributing factor, implement an appropriate pain management plan immediately.

With Type 2 rejection, the mare tries to get away from the foal and may, in fact, be fearful of her own foal. In the process, the foal may get run over or hurt by the mare and be at risk for injury. The biggest risk, as for Type 1, is that the foal does not receive sufficient colostrum and nutrition.

Treatment strategies for this type of aggression include:

- Management: identify triggers and avoid any situation that causes fear and aggression. Strictly supervise all mare–foal interactions to ensure they are positive for the safety of the foal and to prevent escalation of aggression.
- Initially, the foal may have to be physically separated from the mare with a physical barrier to avoid the risk of injury. Ensure that the mare and foal can see, smell, and hear each other.
- In some cases, the foal may need to receive feeding from a bottle initially to ensure proper nutrition.
- Desensitize and countercondition the mare to the foal, the foal's presence, approach to the mare, and the suckling process itself. This will initially require restraint of the mare while feeding the mare grain at the same time. The foal should be handled by a separate person and brought to the mare gradually, in such small steps that the mare remains relaxed with no fearful or aggressive behavior observed.
- The mare should be restrained for several nursing sessions until she accepts the suckling process without any sign of avoidance or aggression.
- If the udder seems very firm or painful to the touch, milking the mare may help to relieve some pressure. If colostrum is milked out, you need to collect it and give to the foal within a few hours.
- If pain or discomfort of any kind is a contributing factor, implement an appropriate pain management plan immediately.
- The use of a tranquilizer or anti-anxiety medication or supplements could be considered.
- The presence of a dog or another horse has been suggested to stimulate the mare's maternal instinct to defend her foal and begin the bonding process. The thought is that maternal behavior kicks in with a threat against the foal. However, the authors think this approach could carry risk, causing the mare to injure the foal either through redirected aggression or by accident, running over the foal to attack the dog or other horse. This should only be considered in the presence of a skilled handler.

With Type 3 rejection, the mare tries to actively attack and bite the foal, usually at the neck or withers, and may shake, throw, or kick the foal in an attempt to kill it. This form is the most severe type of aberrant maternal behavior and, in most cases, requires immediate, permanent separation of mare and foal. The orphaned foal should be provided colostrum immediately to prevent hypoglycemia and provide critical immune support. If possible, introduce a lactating mare that lost her foal. Alternatively, some lactating mares will accept a second foal. Otherwise, providing a surrogate equine companion, and moving from bottle feeding to bucket feeding as soon as possible will help avoid inappropriate socialization and over-bonding with humans. The equine companion can be either a mare (ideally) or a gelding.

See the online materials for Chapter 17 for a case example of a mare with foal rejection.

Play Aggression

Why animals play has not fully been established, but we suspect play has many positive functions and allows mainly young animals to condition their body and "practice" for later in life situations (Oliveira et al. 2010). Therefore, play aggression could be considered normal behavior, especially when seen in young male horses. Keeping young horses in social group settings where play behavior can safely be practiced is helpful. Play aggression is a potential problem when directed toward humans or smaller animals. The play ethogram can include rearing up, biting, and kicking, which, when directed toward a human can be harmful. Punishment of this behavior is contraindicated, as horses may view the acts of punishment as play and encouragement of play. Thus, the behavior is inadvertently rewarded and may increase in intensity and frequency. People should be discouraged from playing any physical or chase games with a foal or young horse. Rather, they should engage in positive reinforcement training, teaching the horse desirable behaviors from a young age.

Treatment strategies for this type of aggression include:

- Management: identify triggers and avoid any interactions and situations that causes fear or aggression.
- Offer enrichment: Mental and physical enrichment helps horses focus on a specific task and can reduce anxiety and fear. Use food enrichment with the goal to solve a problem and be mentally and physically engaged. Physical enrichment can be offered by teaching new skills using wooden logs or equine jumping equipment, such as poles, based on the horse's ability. Offer the horse opportunities to engage in social, solitary, and object play.

Learned Aggression

Reminder: "Negative" in the term negative reinforcement does not mean "bad," but refers to **removal** of something as a consequence of a behavior.

Horses are generally quick learners. One way they learn is by negative reinforcement or removal reinforcement, a form of operant conditioning (see Chapter 5). That is, if pressure or something undesirable to the horse is present but is released or removed immediately upon occurrence of a behavior, the chance of that behavior occurring again increases.

This process of learning is commonly used to teach horses behaviors we would like them to perform. For example, a rider may apply a little pressure with the legs to the horse's sides, and when the horse starts walking, the leg pressure is immediately released. This teaches the horse that light leg pressure means to move forward. But suppose the horse is moving backwards when the leg pressure is accidentally released; the horse instead learns that leg pressure means to move backwards. Poor timing or poor understanding of this form of learning can obviously lead to problem behaviors, including aggression when horses are handled by unskilled people, or when the handling is too rough or confrontational. Most handlers will move away, as they should, to stay safe from a threatening horse, but this can consequently lead to learned aggression: the horse seeking to keep people away has just been rewarded for using aggressive behavior to achieve that distance. This is why all interactions with horses should ideally be positive, so that calm and desirable behaviors can be consistently rewarded. As mentioned above, this learning is a type of operant conditioning. Horses may also learn to show aggressive behavior by learning through classical conditioning, described in earlier chapters, and can happen when horses anticipate a negative emotional response and react in an aggressive manner.

Treatment strategies for this type of aggression include:

- Management: identify triggers and avoid any interactions and situations that cause aggression.
- Stop and regroup so a positive approach can be implemented to teach horses desirable behaviors with positive reinforcement.
- Use clicker training to consistently reward desired behaviors.
- Offer enrichment: Mental and physical enrichment helps horses focus on a specific task and can reduce anxiety and fear. Use food enrichment with the goal of solving a problem and being mentally and physically engaged. Physical enrichment can be offered by teaching new skills using wooden logs or equine jumping equipment such as poles based on the horse's ability.

Other Forms of Aggression

Mares in the Breeding Shed

Although males might show aggressive behavior more often, both at the inter- and intra-species level, due to the organizational effects of androgens on the brain, mares can be aggressive toward stallions when not in full estrous. Treatment includes ensuring that the mare is in full estrous before attempting breeding or by using artificial insemination.

Stallions in Breeding Shed

Stallions may refuse to stand for genital exam and washing *and* may charge the mare. Some stallions will wheel or kick out at the mare or the handler. Most of these problems arise from inadequate or improper handling. Treatment includes putting an efficient behavior modification strategy in place to train the stallion, using consistent handling by an experienced handler, and then providing training to the handlers on the home farm. For stallions who bite the mare with potentially too much force, physical management includes a muzzle or breeding bridle and a withers protector for the mare.

Intermale Aggression

Stallions may display aggression toward other male horses. The trigger may just be any evidence of another male horse, and the threshold can vary greatly. The ethogram is usually very ritualistic and includes posturing (Figure 17.4), vocalization, defecation, and behavior that may escalate to full attacks. In most cases, this type of aggression can be reduced by castration, as testosterone seems to be playing a significant role; however, this type of aggression can be seen in geldings as well. The timing of castration relative to the onset of aggressive behavior determines the reduction in aggression (Line et al. 1985).

Horse–Human Relationships:

Horse–human relationships are predominantly reflected by experiences and hence are conditioned responses rather than the often-repeated but false attribution to dominance behavior. Prevention of human-directed aggression consists of allowing horses to interact adequately with their conspecifics, especially during early development, and the proper teaching of ground skills using a non-confrontational approach. Using the dominance theory model during training is dangerous and has been shown, for example, to lead to increased aggression in canines (Herron et al. 2009). Successful equine handling skills require an understanding and proper application of learning theory, the equine ethogram, physiology, and behavior, as well as the desire and enjoyment of working

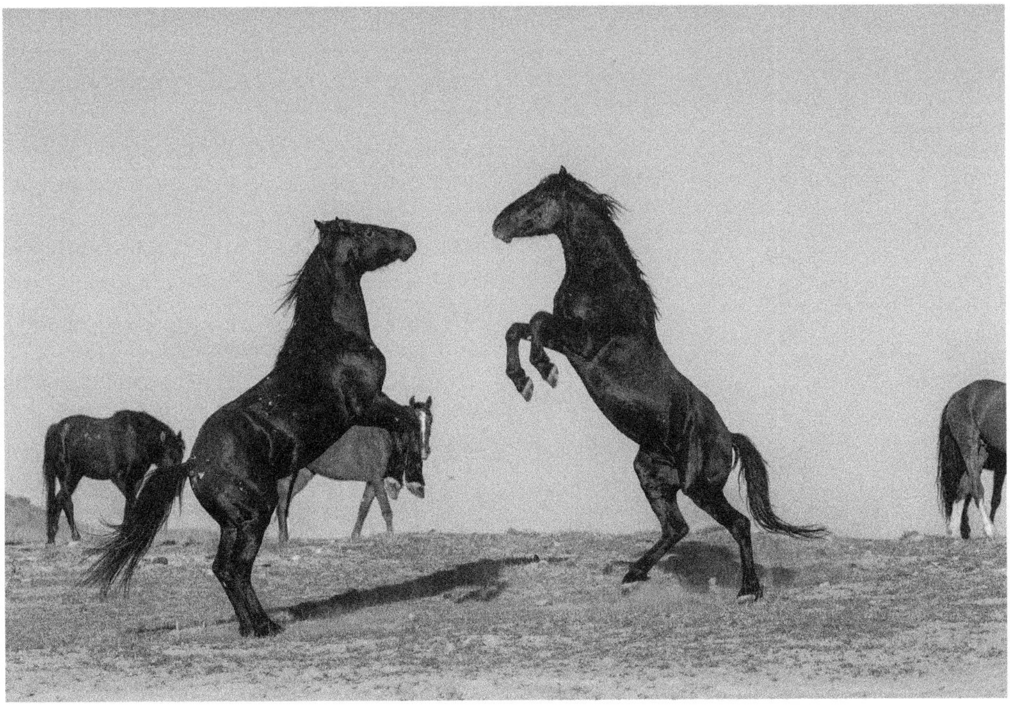

Figure 17.4 Intermale aggression. Stallions will posture with necks held high, ears back, sometimes circling, rearing, and kicking before engaging in an all-out fight. *Source:* Photo credit: natureguy/Adobe Stock

with a large prey-animal species. A desirable form of leadership with horses can be established with predictable positive outcomes for desired behaviors in a command-response-reward setting.

Diagnosis and Treatment Summary

When confronted with aggression problems during routine wellness visits in an equine practice, you may initially feel overwhelmed, even though you do not have the time or resources to adequately address them. As a general practitioner, you may be the first line of defense in getting help for this patient. That said, you *cannot* and *should not* attempt to resolve major aggression problems in a single wellness visit. What you *can* and *should* do is triage the situation by gathering a brief history, determining medical rule-outs, providing immediate safety and management and stress reduction advice, and then referring to an appropriate behavior professional (See Chapter 12 for a full description of the Behavior Triage). As you gain comfort and experience, you might consider seeing and treating these cases yourself in a separate, longer visit with the client and patient.

When you elect to assess and treat equine aggression cases, consider using the **Problem Oriented Veterinary Behavior Record** (POVBR) approach (Table 17.1), based on Weed's Problem Oriented Medical Record (POMR) (Weed 1968). Behavioral health documentation starts with creating a comprehensive problem list and reporting findings in a logical manner. This approach to behavior problems allows for a comprehensive treatment plan and leads to more positive outcomes. The POVBR described by Sung and Berger (2022) uses the same principles as those known in the POMR approach that practitioners are already familiar with. Behavior information observed,

Table 17.1 POVBR – The approach to behavior problems.

The POVBR approach for behavior problems	The Problem Oriented Veterinary Behavior Record is applied to behavioral health. It starts with creating a comprehensive problem list and documentation in a logical manner. This approach to behavior problems allows for a comprehensive treatment plan and leads to more positive outcomes.
The SOAP	
Subjective data	History: Every animal has a story – subjective data, history given by the owner, caretaker, or trainer
Objective data	Measurable information and observations; in person or by video – video can be helpful to avoid observer effect (Hawthorne Effect)
Assessment	Clinical impression and discussion of the problem(s); differential diagnosis, diagnosis, working diagnosis, and prognosis will be listed here
Plan of action	Outcome options, options, and resources for treatment, including management, type of behavior modification, enrichment and other recommended tools, medications and supplements, additional diagnostics needed, owner education, and follow-up plans

collected, and documented in a logical manner allows the practitioner to create a problem list, a management and treatment plan for any behavior related problems, not only in horses. The importance of creating a record for behavioral observations and problems is similar to any other medical problem. Behavior observations must be recorded in an objective and measurable way so they can be addressed and treated in a medical fashion. This is critical for decision-making and has value for tracking success and providing a prognosis.

Using the SOAP component of POVBR (Weed and Weed 2011)

Subjective (S): This is the subjective collection of data in the SOAP documentation. Taken by the veterinarian as the first step, it is a detailed history as provided by the owner, the caretaker, the trainer, or anybody that can provide information as it pertains to the problem behavior. History will include the horse's stabling environment, management, training, daily exercise and feeding schedule, use, number of people interacting with the horse, and so on. This document may contain lay terms, owner opinions, and owner "diagnosis." Any one or more of these can hold clues to the behavior.

Objective (O): Next, a thorough, objective physical exam is performed to identify or rule out any underlying medical disease or pain issues. This includes the basic TPR (Temperature, Pulse, and Respiration) and may include orthopedic, ophthalmic, dermatologic, and neurologic examinations. Detailed behavioral observations complete the exam, where the clinician describes all pertinent behaviors and the body language objectively, without making a diagnosis. Depending upon the behavior of interest, observations may take place at the clinic, on the farm, or from video recordings. McDonnell (McDonnell 2005) found that continuous recording of horses in their stalls over at least 24 hours can reveal behaviors and clues to behaviors that are not seen when people are present.

Assessment (A): Having completed the subjective and objective processes, the veterinarian then makes an assessment, ruling out the differential, drawing conclusions as to the motivation, and reaching a working diagnosis. At this stage, the questions asked are: What or who is causing or triggering the behavior? What does the body language look like? What is the possible motivation for the aggression? What is or are the triggers? Where is the threshold? What further medical workups or observations are needed? All these questions should be answered here.

Plan (P): Finally, the plan includes a prognosis, treatment plan, any client communication that is needed for education of the caregivers, the follow up plan, and possibly any outcome options. The treatment plan will in most cases include:

- Elements of safety and avoidance, first, to avoid further episodes of aggression and avoid any injuries to horses or humans.
- A training plan using a positive reinforcement approach to teach new behaviors that are incompatible with the unwanted or aggressive behaviors.
- Recommendations of humane training and management tools to set up the plan for success.
- A specific desensitizing and counterconditioning plan will be designed for most cases for the reintroduction of the specific triggers, creating a changed emotional response that does not elicit any aggression or fear.
- Supplements or medications to help the plan be successful.
- A follow-up plan is needed to track success and address setbacks. Owners need to be made aware that with any aggressive horse, lifelong management is needed.
- Although clients are often in need of urgent help with equine aggression, most aggressive behavior problems have taken some time to develop, and owners need to understand that it will take time and commitment to adhere to a well-designed plan to properly manage aggressive conditions.
- In some cases, humane euthanasia needs to be considered and/or discussed as an outcome option due to the risk of injuries.

What to Avoid When Addressing Aggression

Do Not

- Place the horse in the situation where they have displayed the aggressive behavior. Safety and avoidance are always the first steps in treatment.
- Fail to reinforce the wanted behavior. Be sure to remove pressure and add something good.
- Punish inappropriately: e.g. punish fear response.
- Repeat application of aversive stimuli regardless of response (nagging).
- Use poor timing by applying signals after the response.
- Fail to consider social needs.

Medication

Recent canine studies suggest that the neurotransmitter serotonin (5 HT) plays a role in modulation of aggression, with lower levels of a serotonin metabolite associated with aggressive dogs (Odore et al. 2020). These observations have led to the therapeutic use of selective serotonin reuptake inhibitors (SSRIs) with the aim to manipulate 5 HT concentrations in the synaptic cleft of aggressive dogs and many other species. There is little to no research studying the complex role played by the serotonergic system in the modulation of aggressive behaviors in horses, but fluoxetine has been described to alter behavior in horses successfully (Fontenot et al. 2021).

The main factor to consider in the choice of any psychotropic medication for horses is whether a short-term or long-term medication (or a combination of both) is beneficial to address anxiety-related or aggressive behavior problems. Many medications and supplements can be used, and the pros and cons must be weighed. The use of psychogenic medication in horses is very limited and prescribed only in specific situations. The size of the animal and the risk of using any medication which alters mentation or balance need to be considered when using drugs for a riding animal, and most medications are not allowed in competition.

In summary, medications should not be utilized without a comprehensive medical evaluation and without taking into account other non-behavioral effects.

References

AVMA (2008). *Welfare Implications of Elephant Training: Literature Review [Online].* American Veterinary Medical Association. Available at https://www.avma.org/resources-tools/literature-reviews/welfare-implications-elephant-training (Accessed 08 August 2022).

Berger, J. (1977). Organizational systems and dominance in feral horses in the Grand Canyon. *Behav. Ecol. Sociobiol.* 2: 131–146.

Sung, W. and Berger, J. (2022). Training and behavior modification for shelter cats. In: *Animal Behavior for Shelter Veterinarians and Staff*, 2e (ed. B.A. DiGangi, V.A. Cussen, P.J. Reid, and K.A. Collins), 445–475. Hoboken, NJ, Wiley.

Christensen, J.W., Søndergaard, E., Thodberg, K., and Halekoh, U. (2011). Effects of repeated regrouping on horse behaviour and injuries. *Appl. Anim. Behav. Sci.* 133: 199–206.

Crowell-Davis, S.L. and Houpt, K.A. (1986). Maternal behavior. *Vet. Clin. North America: Equine Pract.* 2: 557–571.

Döring, D., Roscher, A., Scheipl, F. et al. (2009). Fear-related behaviour of dogs in veterinary practice. *Vet. J.* 182: 38–43.

Dyson, S., Berger, J., Ellis, A., and Mullard, J. (2014). Can the presence of musculoskeletal pain be determined from the facial expressions of ridden horses (FEReq)? *J. Vet. Behav.: Clin. Appl. Res.* 19: 78–89.

Fontenot, R.L., Mochal-King, C.A., Sprinkle, S.B. et al. (2021). Retrospective evaluation of fluoxetine hydrochloride use in horses: 95 cases (2010–2019). *J. Equine Vet. Sci.* 97: 103340.

Fureix, C., Bourjade, M., Henry, S. et al. (2012). Exploring aggression regulation in managed groups of horses *Equus caballus*. *Appl. Anim. Behav. Sci.* 138: 216–228.

Fureix, C., Menguy, H., and Hausberger, M. (2010). Partners with bad temper: reject or cure? A study of chronic pain and aggression in horses. *PLOS ONE* 5: e12434.

Gleerup, K.B., Andersen, P.H., Munksgaard, L., and Forkman, B. (2015). Pain evaluation in dairy cattle. *App. Anim. Behav. Sci. 171*: 25–32.

Gleerup, K. and Lindegaard, C. (2016). Recognition and quantification of pain in horses: a tutorial review. *Equine Vet. Educ.* 28: 47–57.

Grandin, T. (1999). Safe handling of large animal. *Occup. Med.: State of the Art Rev.* 14: 195–212.

Hartmann, E., Christensen, J.W., and Keeling, L.J. (2009). Social interactions of unfamiliar horses during paired encounters: effect of pre-exposure on aggression level and so risk of injury. *Appl. Anim. Behav. Sci.* 121: 214–221.

Hartmann, E., Christensen, J.W., and McGreevy, P.D. (2017). Dominance and leadership: useful concepts in human-horse interactions? *J. Equine Vet. Sci.* 52: 1–9.

Hausberger, M., Roche, H., Henry, S., and Visser, E.K. (2008). A review of the human-horse relationship. *Appl. Anim. Behav. Sci.* 109: 1–24.

Herron, M.E., Shofer, F., and Reisner, I.R. (2009). Survey of the use and outcome of confrontational and non-confrontational training methods in client-owned dogs showing undesired behaviors. *Appl. Anim. Behav. Sci.* 117 (1–2): 47–54.

Houpt, K.A. (2005). *Domestic Animal Behavior for Veterinarians and Animal Scientists*, 4e. Ames, Iowa: Blackwell Publishing.

Houpt, K.A. and Keiper, R. (1982). The position of the stallion in the equine dominance hierarchy of feral and domestic ponies. *J. Anim. Sci.* 54: 945–950.

Houpt, K.A. and Wolski, T.R. (1980). Stability of equine hierarchies and the prevention of dominance related aggression. *Equine Vet. J.* 12: 15–18.

Juarbe-Diaz, S.V., Houpt, K.A., and Kusunose, R. (1998). Prevalence and characteristics of foal rejection in Arabian mares. *Equine Vet. J.* 30: 424–428.

Line, S., Hart, B., and Sanders, L. (1985). Effect of prepubertal versus postpubertal castration on sexual and aggressive behavior in male horses. *J. Am. Vet. Med. Assoc.* 186: 249–251.

Macmillan, K. (2013). Management of human-directed aggression in horses. *Proceedings Veterinary Behaviour Chapter, Science Week 2013*. QT Gold Coast: Australian and New Zealand College of Veterinary Scientists, 39.

Mariti, C., Bowen, J.E., Campa, S. et al. (2016). Guardians' perceptions of cats' welfare and behavior regarding visiting veterinary clinics. *J. Appl. Anim. Welf. Sci.* 19: 375–384.

Mariti, C., Raspanti, E., Zilocchi, M. et al. (2015). The assessment of dog welfare in the waiting room of a veterinary clinic. *Anim. Welf.* 24: 299–305.

McDonnell, S. (2003). *The Equid Ethogram: A Practical Field Guide to Horse Behavior.* Lexington, KY, Eclipse.

McDonnell, S. (2005). Is it psychological, physical, or both? In: *Proceedings of the 51st Annual Convention of the American Association of Equine Practitiners* (ed. T.D. Brokken), 231–238. Seattle, WA: AAEP.

Merriam Webster Dictionary. (n.d.) https://www.merriam-webster.com/dictionary/fear (Accessed 9 August 2022).

Moyer, K.E. (1968). Kinds of aggression and their physiological basis. *Commun. Behav. Biol.* 2: 65–87.

Mullard, J., Berger, J.M., Ellis, A.D., and Dyson, S. (2017). Development of an ethogram to describe facial expressions in ridden horses (FEReq). *J. Vet. Behav.* 18: 7–12.

Odore, R., Rendini, D., Badino, P. et al. (2020). Behavioral therapy and fluoxetine treatment in aggressive dogs: a case study. *Animals* 10: 832.

Oliveira, A.F.S., Rossi, A.O., Silva, L.F.R. et al. (2010). Play behaviour in nonhuman animals and the animal welfare issue. *J. Ethol.* 28: 1–5.

Riemer, S., Heritier, C., Windschnurer, I. et al. (2021). A review on mitigating fear and aggression in dogs and cats in a veterinary setting. *Animals* 11: 158.

Stanley, C.R., Mettke-Hofmann, C., Hager, R., and Shultz, S. (2018). Social stability in semiferal ponies: networks show interannual stability alongside seasonal flexibility. *Anim. Behav.* 136: 175–184.

Weed, L.L. (1968). Medical records that guide and teach. *N. Engl. J. Med.* 278: 593–600.

Weed, L.L. and Weed, L. (2011). *Medicine in Denial*, 167–169. Scotts Valley, CA: CreateSpace.

Further Reading

Beaver, B.V. (2019). *Equine Behavioral Medicine.* Academic Press.

Crowell-Davis, S.L. and Murray, T.F. (2006). *Veterinary Psychopharmacology*. Hoboken, NJ: Wiley. pp. 55, 98, 116–117, 141, 185, 191, 194–195, 197.

Houpt, K.A. (2005). *Domestic Animal Behavior for Veterinarians and Animal Scientists*, 4e, 37–57. Ames, Iowa: Blackwell Publishing.

McDonnell, S. (2003). *The Equid Ethogram: A Practical Field Guide to Horse Behavior.* Lexington, KY: Eclipse.

McGreevy, P. (2004). *Equine Behavior: A Guide for Veterinarians and Equine Scientists*, 119–164. London, New York: Saunders/Elsevier.

Yin, S.A. (2009). *Low Stress Handling, Restraint and Behavior Modification of Dogs & Cats: Techniques for Developing Patients Who Love Their Visits*, 55–76. Davis, CA: CattleDog Publishing.

18

Repetitive Behaviors in Companion Animals

Melissa Bain

University of California, Davis, School of Veterinary Medicine, Davis, CA, USA

Introduction

Repetitive behaviors are a sequence of movements often derived from normal behaviors (grooming, eating, and walking), performed seemingly out of context in a repetitive, exaggerated, ritualistic, and/or sustained manner. They can be classified according to their behavioral manifestation as one or more of the following:

- Locomotory: Behaviors that involve purposeful movement
- Hallucinatory: Behaviors that involve an apparent visual focus or fixation
- Oral: Behaviors that involve the mouth, lips, tongue, and/or ingestion
- Vocal: Behaviors involved in vocalization or auditory communication
- Aggressive: Behaviors that are threatening, either self-directed or toward inanimate or invisible targets

These types of behaviors are present in a vast array of manners and intensities in our companion animals. Some are intermittent, such as when a dog chases its tail when excited to eat its dinner, while others are more continuous, such as when the dog prefers to chase its tail instead of eating. Some popular social media videos are those of animals doing such behaviors. While they may be presented as humorous, when closely evaluated, it is apparent that a lot of these animals are in distress and/or experiencing anxiety.

Definitions and Motivating Factors

Repetitive disorder is the broad term comprised of different diagnoses. Common differential diagnoses for these behaviors include **displacement**, **compulsive**, **stereotypic**, and **attention-seeking**. Pathophysiologic causes must be taken into consideration before a more definitive diagnosis is made. Table 18.1 provides a summary of common behavioral diagnoses.

Clients frequently note that these behaviors interfere with normal daily activities of the pet. They often worsen over time, especially if an underlying stressor is not eliminated or if a family member plays an inadvertent role in reinforcing the behavior. It may be first exhibited in an acute conflict situation, which occurs when an animal appears to have difficulty in choosing which action it should take and may experience conflicting emotions, and has been shown to be correlated with aggressiveness (Sulkama 2022). The pet may then generalize to other situations, especially if the pet is exposed to prolonged or repeated conflict. Clients may be able to identify a specific

Introduction to Animal Behavior and Veterinary Behavioral Medicine, First Edition. Edited by Meghan E. Herron.

Companion website: www.wiley.com/go/introductiontoanimalbehavior

Table 18.1 Common behavioral differential diagnoses for repetitive behaviors.

Diagnosis	Definition	When it is displayed
Displacement behaviors	Behaviors performed out of context in relation to the situation. Often start when an external stressful event occurs.	In response to a stressful or triggering event, such as fear of unfamiliar people, other pets, loud noises, or when stressed about performing a particular behavior.
Compulsive behaviors	Regularly repeated behaviors that appear emancipated from their original context or trigger. There often is an underlying anxiety disorder.	In many different contexts, scenarios, and locations. Difficult to impossible to interrupt, often interfering with normal daily functioning.
Attention-seeking behaviors	Behaviors that an animal performs with the intention to gain attention or an interaction from someone. Attention could be something enjoyable (petting, getting a treat), or aversive (yelling, chasing).	Only when a person is present or might enter an area where the pet is. The attention given in response to these behaviors keeps them maintained.
Stereotypic behaviors	Repetitive, invariant behaviors without an apparent goal or purpose.	Generally occurs when the captive environment does not allow animals to perform the full range of species-typical behaviors.

stressful event (physical trauma or social stressors) that coincided with the onset of behavior. They have often attempted a variety of interventions, many of which can aggravate the problem, prior to seeking consultation.

Displacement Behaviors

Displacement behaviors are behavioral responses to an external stimulus, including, but not limited to, social conflict, frightening encounters, frustrating interactions, and other stressful events. The behaviors appear out of context in reference to the trigger. For example, a dog is frustrated that he cannot get closer to another dog on leash, so he spins in a tight circle. Spinning has nothing to do with gaining proximity to the other dog. It is displayed out of context as a means of displacing intense frustration. Another example would be a dog who continuously mounts other dogs in a dog park when nervous. While mounting is a normal, appropriate behavior during copulation, it is out of context for a neutered dog in this social setting. The mounting in this circumstance is a displacement of social anxiety and tension, as well as what are likely poorly developed intercanine social skills. Commonly, these triggers cause anxiety or overarousal, which precipitate the displacement behaviors (Bain and Fan 2012; Bain and Good 2015; Beaver 1994). Overgrooming, tail chasing, yawning, lip licking, and pacing are behaviors that are often described as displacement behaviors. Over time, they can transition into compulsive behaviors, especially if the behaviors become practiced or even inadvertently rewarded.

Often what is called a "compulsive" behavior in the literature is actually a displacement behavior, in that the behavior can be interrupted, often does not happen without a person present, and has an identifiable triggering event.

Compulsive Behaviors

To be considered compulsive, the behavioral pattern must be pronounced enough to exceed that necessary to meet the apparent goal, and/ or such that it interferes with the pet's normal functioning. They are fixed and independent of the environment, arise from an internally driven state, and consist of repetitive, relatively unvaried sequences of movements. In many cases, the behaviors derive from contextually normal maintenance behaviors (e.g. grooming, and hunting).

Compulsive behaviors often interfere with normal daily activities and functioning. The behaviors generally worsen over time and can start to occur in more contexts and with less provocation. They can arise from displacement behaviors if practiced and/or reinforced enough where they are emancipated from any original trigger or goal. Sometimes the client can identify a specific stressful event (physical trauma or social upheaval) that coincided with onset of a compulsive behavior. A physical insult can also incite a pet to direct its attention to that area, leading to compulsive behaviors. An example is clipping a front leg on a dog for a blood draw, leading to irritation and inflammation, then licking to relieve the irritation, and then transitioning to overlicking. This can also be brought about by atopy and inflammation. Genetic predispositions may also play a role, as Oriental-type breed cats have been reported to be overrepresented in orally-directed behaviors in some, but not all, studies (Bamberger and Houpt 2006; Bradshaw et al. 1997; Overall and Dunham 2002; Demontigny-Bédard et al. 2016; Wassink-van der Schot et al. 2016).

Compulsive behaviors represent the third most common reason for presentation to a veterinary behaviorist (Amat et al. 2009; Dodman et al. 2010; Seksel and Lindeman 1998). While these may present as primary diagnoses, they are often secondary to other diagnoses, such as generalized anxiety or separation anxiety. Sometimes the line is blurred with a comorbidity of anxiety; in focusing on only repetitive behaviors, one may not be addressing the pet in its entirety.

Obsessive-compulsive and related disorders (OCD) in humans are characterized by obsessions, thoughts, or urges, leading to compulsions, which are repetitive psychological or physical actions that are performed to alleviate the anxiety related to the obsessions one has. It is uncertain whether animals "obsess" or have thoughts or urges leading them to need to perform these behaviors. A current critical review article summarizes that, while behaviors are repetitive, there is no equivalency between human OCD and canine compulsive behaviors (Walsh 2020).

Attention-seeking Behaviors

These are behaviors for which an animal receives reinforcement from a person or, perhaps, another animal. Another term is "audience-affected behavior." A client may let a pet outside in response to spinning behavior or may feed the pet after it vocalizes repeatedly. Sometimes just making eye contact with a pet is enough of a reinforcement for the animal to continue to perform the behavior. Even something considered aversive, like a verbal reprimand, may be considered by the pet as reinforcing. A recent study demonstrated that owner-dog relationships may influence repetitive behaviors, such as with attention-seeking, and that changing how a person interacts with their dog can help reduce these behaviors (Hall et al. 2015).

Stereotypic Behaviors

These are repetitive, unvarying behavior patterns with no apparent goal or function. They are commonly displayed by long-term confined animals living in a barren environment. These behaviors are primarily identified in captive wildlife, production animals, and animals in laboratory settings, and rarely by domesticated pets, although this diagnostic term has been used in the past (Hewson et al. 1999; Mason 2006).

It is posited that the dopaminergic system is involved in perpetuating these behaviors. In a study of overeating in rats, it was noted that dopamine receptors were downregulated in obese rats. This downregulation was also correlated with compulsive food seeking in these rats, demonstrating that overconsumption of palatable food triggers addiction-like responses (Johnson and Kenny 2010). Related to this, certain medications, such as stimulants, are thought to induce stereotypies, as such drugs work via activation of the dopaminergic system (Longoni et al. 1991).

Specific Repetitive Behaviors

- Locomotory: spinning, tail chasing, pacing, freezing, and skin rippling
- Hallucinatory: shadow/light chasing, startling, and fly-snapping
- Oral: licking/chewing self or objects, air licking, flank sucking, fabric sucking, psychogenic alopecia, and **pica**
- Aggressive: self-directed aggression such as growling, biting at tail; aggressive behavior directed at inanimate objects

Locomotory

Spinning and Tail Chasing

These are common repetitive behaviors seen in dogs. Spinning can be thought of as a variant of tail chasing, where the dog spins rapidly in tight circles without apparent interest in the tail. Some studies suggest these behaviors occur at a higher rate in certain breeds, including Bull Terriers, German Shepherd Dogs, and Staffordshire Bull Terriers (Dodman et al. 1993). It has also been reported to be less likely seen in neutered females, and more likely to be seen in dogs that were reported to be shyer and be separated from their dam at an earlier age (Moon-Fanelli et al. 2011; Tiira et al. 2012). Medical conditions, such as impacted anal glands, neuropathy, or other underlying neurological conditions, should be considered for dogs displaying these behaviors.

Pacing

This behavior is not commonly seen in companion dogs but is reported in up to 93% of kenneled dogs when exposed to arousing stimuli (Protopopova 2016). When evaluating a dog for pacing, it should be noted which direction it chooses to pace, in order to help rule out an underlying neurological condition. A dog may also pace if it is unable to lie down comfortably due to an underlying painful condition.

Hind-end Checking

This behavior, reported to more likely be seen in Miniature Schnauzers, has been called a "compulsive disorder," in that they consistently perform this repetitively. Medical rule-outs must be considered, including potential neuromas or anal gland inflammation.

Freezing/Trancing

These behaviors, reported most commonly in Bull Terriers, consist of episodes of a slow-motion, trance-like gait, sometimes with components of pacing. They have been hypothesized to be a true compulsive disorder, partial complex seizures, a dermatological condition, or a gastrointestinal disorder (Lowrie et al. 2015).

Hallucinatory

Breed predispositions for many hallucinatory behaviors have been reported in herding breeds, such as Border Collies and German Shepherd Dogs, and those with intense focus and drive, such as terriers. Some dogs appear to be enjoying themselves, displaying play-like behaviors and tail wagging, during these episodes, while others appear anxious or frustrated that they cannot "catch" the fly or light. The pet is conscious during these episodes, and often can be distracted away.

Light or Shadow Chasing

This is when an animal tracks and chases lights and/or shadows. There may be a history of someone playing with a laser pointer or otherwise encouraging this behavior. A typical episode is an animal resting quietly and then focus onto a light or shadow around them.

Reflection Fixation

This is when an animal stares fixedly at a light or their reflection for prolonged periods. They seemingly get "stuck" and can be difficult to interrupt or redirect.

Chasing Imaginary "Prey"

Can be seen in breeds of dogs known for tracking/chasing small prey, such as Jack Russell Terriers. Vocalization, pouncing, and other behaviors often accompany this behavior.

Fly Snapping

In reality, this is air snapping, but it is displayed in a manner that makes it appear as though the animal is repeatedly trying to catch something in the air, such as a fly. Medical conditions, such as vitreous degeneration, gastrointestinal disorders, neurological conditions, and pain, need to be taken into consideration when presented with a dog performing this behavior (Bain and Fan 2012; Frank et al. 2012).

Skin Rippling (Feline Hyperesthesia Syndrome)

This has frequently been mentioned as a "compulsive disorder," in which a cat's skin ripples apparently without an inciting cause. However, a recent paper demonstrated that there must be a multidisciplinary diagnostic approach in diagnosing an underlying reason, now posited to be related to pain or other abnormal sensation (Amengual Batle et al. 2019).

Oral

Pica

This is defined as the ingestion of *non*food items. Siamese and American Domestic Shorthair cats are over-represented in those displaying abnormal ingestive behaviors (Bamberger and Houpt 2006; Bradshaw et al. 1997; Overall and Dunham 2002). Normal exploratory behavior should be ruled out; however, there is conflicting evidence on the relationship between age and repetitive behaviors, not pure exploratory behaviors (Bradshaw et al. 1997; Demontigny-Bédard et al. 2016). Interestingly, cats in this study that were fed *ad libitum* were less likely to display pica (Demontigny-Bédard et al. 2016).

Excessive Plant-eating

This is not considered pica unless it is extreme. Studies in dogs showed that those that did not appear ill before eating plants did not vomit, so plant-eating is not necessarily related to illness. Another conclusion from this study was that there was no relation between diet (raw, canned, or kibble) or anthelminthic treatment and plant eating (Sueda et al. 2008). While no peer-reviewed studies exist for cats, preliminary results demonstrate that the same holds true for cats eating plants excessively (Hart et al. 2019).

Fabric or Wool Sucking

This involves dogs and cats who lick, suck, or ingest fabrics, often those made of wool. Traditionally, this has been attributed to improper/premature weaning in cats and may be seen more frequently in Oriental-type breeds (Bamberger and Houpt 2006; Bradshaw et al. 1997; Overall and Dunham 2002; Demontigny-Bédard et al. 2016; Wassink-van der Schot et al. 2016). While licking and sucking behaviors themselves are fairly benign, one study did show a significant correlation between sucking fabric and ingesting fabric. Therefore, cats who are noted to suck on fabric should be closely monitored for potential ingestion and foreign body development (Demontigny-Bédard et al. 2016).

Flank-sucking

This is a unique, self-directed behavior that is over-represented in the Doberman Pinscher breed (Figure 18.1). In some cases, it can be a displacement behavior if the dog is not able to suckle on a piece of fabric (Moon-Fanelli et al. 2007). Recent research has identified a genetic link in which Dobermans exhibiting these behaviors had an identifiable

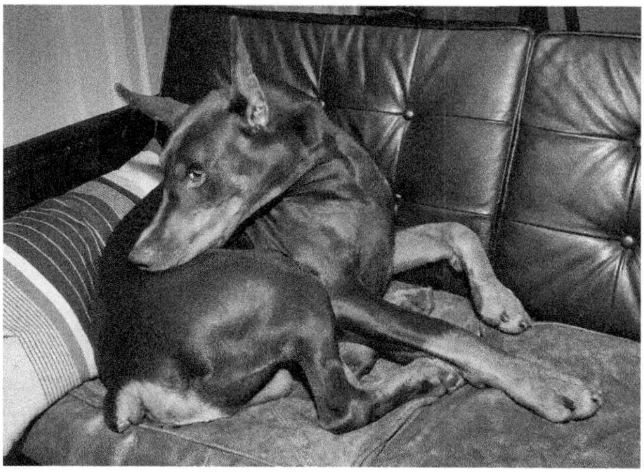

Figure 18.1 A Doberman Pinscher engages in self-directed flank sucking behavior. *Source:* With permission from Spencer Tull.

chromosomal link compared to unaffected dogs (Dodman et al. 2010; Ogata et al. 2013).

Excessive Licking

Licking can be self or object/surface-directed and can be a displacement behavior displayed when dogs are in anxiety-provoking situations. For example, a dog who is anxious about a new baby may lick them excessively, both as a means of investigation and to displace feelings of anxiety. Excessive licking that is not self-directed should be considered a sign of gastrointestinal discomfort until proven otherwise (Bécuwe-Bonnet et al. 2012). This holds true for both dogs and cats (Figure 18.2). Once physiological causes are identified, you can look for behavioral triggers.

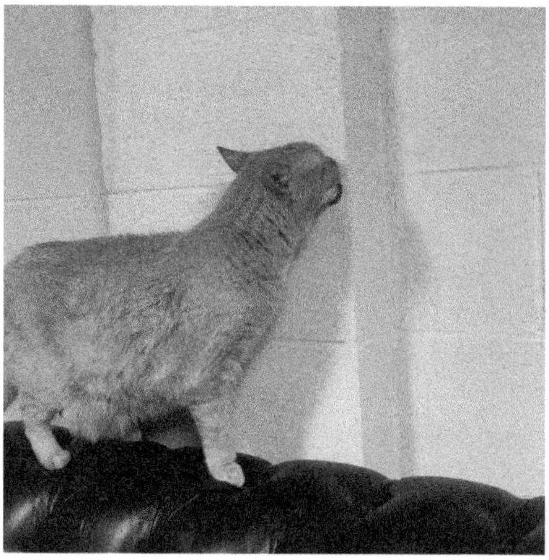

Figure 18.2 A cat with inflammatory bowel disease licks walls excessively when having flare-ups of gastrointestinal discomfort. *Source:* With permission from Denise Johnson.

Acral Lick Dermatitis

This is a syndrome whereby an animal excessively licks the dorsal aspects of the carpi, hocks, and/or digits, forming thick, hairless plaques (Figure 18.3). Inciting causes for **acral lick dermatitis** (ALD) commonly straddle both behavioral and physiological triggers (Shumaker 2019). The act of licking is both anxiety and pruritus-relieving, reinforcing the behavior for the alleviation of either ailment. The issue is more commonly reported in large-breed dogs, as well as Abyssinian and Siamese cats, and is often associated with an underlying medical condition (Denerolle et al. 2007; Young and Manning 1984).

Psychogenic Alopecia

Likely over-diagnosed, **psychogenic alopecia** is excessive self-directed licking which results in areas of hair loss (Figure 18.4). In most cases, this is a result of an underlying medical condition, such as dermatitis, gastrointestinal upset (abdomen-directed), or orthopedic pain (limb-specific). In rare cases, once physical

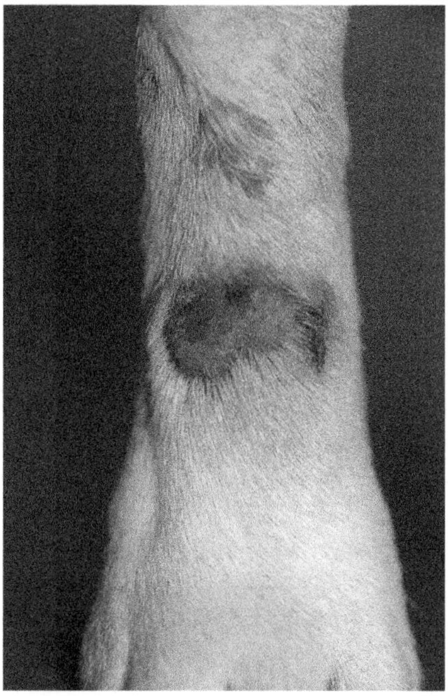

Figure 18.3 Acral lick granulomas form as a result of chronic, excessive licking and commonly have both behavioral and physiological triggers. *Source:* With permission from Lynette Cole.

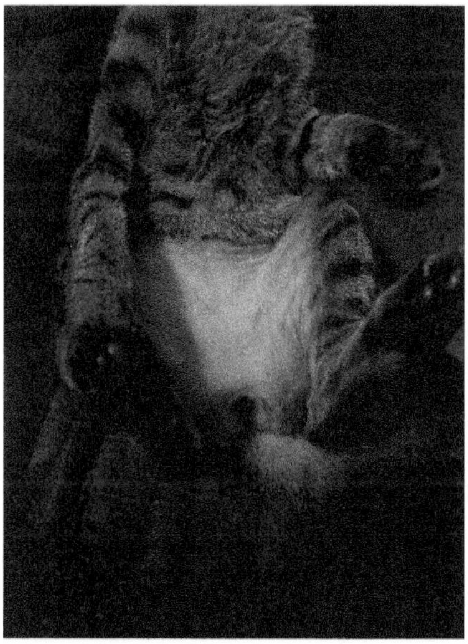

Figure 18.4 Psychogenic alopecia is a result of excessive self-directed licking. This diagnosis is made once all underlying medical etioloties have been ruled out. *Source:* With permission from Tiff McGregor.

etiologies have been ruled out, a psychogenic or compulsive motivation is identified, stemming from underlying stressors in the home environment. Research has shown that 90% of cats presenting with this condition have an underlying physiological problem, usually a dermatological condition (Waisglass et al. 2006; Santoro et al. 2021).

Physiological Differentials

As described with each behavior above, one should always consider underlying medical pathologies for pets displaying repetitive behaviors. An appropriate medical workup is suggested for these patients, starting with a minimum database of a physical exam, complete blood count, serum chemistry panel, fecal examination, and urinalysis. Advanced diagnostics are indicated based on baseline findings. Advanced imaging, starting with radiographs, of limbs or other areas of self-directed focus are indicated. In some cases, computed tomography (CT) and/or magnetic resonance imaging (MRI) may be necessary to rule in/out spinal cord or cauda equina pathologies triggering spinning, hind-end checking, or tail chasing.

A dermatological workup should be performed for animals displaying overgrooming and excessive self-directed licking behaviors. A workup would include some or all of the following: evaluation and treatment for presumptive external parasites; cytologic examination of skin scrapings; fungal culture; evaluation of response to an exclusion diet; and assessment for atopy and endocrinopathies. Skin biopsies should also be considered. While not a diagnostic tool, one can also evaluate the pet's response to steroids, to help determine a potential role of pruritis.

Behavior or Medical?

Behavioral and medical pathologies are not mutually exclusive. While making a distinction is a common way to categorize the diagnoses, they should be considered synergistically. If you diagnose an underlying medical problem seemingly the cause of the repetitive behavior, you must still investigate the role, if any, behavior plays in the problem, and vice versa. Such inciting physical causes can be something like a physical irritation or lesion from fleas or a shaved area for a catheter. A compulsive drive to ingest non-food items can lead to needing surgery to remove the object. That said, gastrointestinal discomfort can contribute to the drive to ingest non-food items, as can gastrointestinal surgery to remove the items, creating a complicated "chicken or the egg" conundrum.

Common physiological differentials are listed in Table 18.2.

Neurological Disease

Seizures due to any number of underlying conditions, including neoplastic, should be considered if a behavior cannot be interrupted. There generally is a postictal phase, and other neurological deficits are usually present on a physical exam. Sensory neuropathies or cauda equina should be considered for those conditions that present as self-directed repetitive behaviors, such as tail chasing. Developmental neurological diseases can include hydrocephalus, syringomyelia, and lissencephaly. Interestingly, structural brain abnormalities were found in Doberman Pinschers diagnosed with compulsive disorders (Ogata et al. 2013).

Dermatological Disease

As cited above, medical causes of pruritis were found in 90% of cats presenting with presumptive psychogenic alopecia (Waisglass et al. 2006). Such causes include ectoparasites, food allergies, atopy, and bacterial or fungal disease such as dermatophytosis.

Infectious, Inflammatory, and Traumatic Causes

Infectious diseases or inflammatory processes, including those causing pain, that affect any organ system should also be considered if appropriate (Mills et al. 2020). Referred pain can present as a self-directed behavior. An example is painful nephroliths causing a cat to self-direct licking to the dorsal aspect over the kidneys. Infectious diseases can include rabies, feline infectious peritonitis (FIP), and feline immunodeficiency virus (FIV), and inflammatory diseases can include granulomatous meningioencephalitis. An example of how an inflammatory disease can play a role in a repetitive behavior is a case report of a Bull Terrier diagnosed with compulsive disorder, where

Table 18.2 Physiological differentials for repetitive behaviors.

Repetitive behavior	Possible medical causes
Psychogenic alopecia/ overgrooming	Inflammatory, infectious, abnormal nerve sensation, orthopedic problem or pain
Pica	Gastrointestinal problem (inflammatory, malabsorption), toxin
Light chasing	Ophthalmological problem (vitreous degeneration, retinal detachment), neurological problem (seizures, neoplastic)
Tail chasing	Neurological problem (spinal nerve problem), inflamed anal sacs, inflammatory, pain/injury to tail
Excessive licking of objects or air	Gastrointestinal problem (inflammatory, malabsorption, foreign body)
Circling (walking in circles)	Neurologic problem (seizures, neoplastic), ophthalmological problem (vitreous degeneration, retinal detachment)
Pacing	Pain or discomfort that decreases time spent lying down
Hind-end checking	Neurological problem (spinal nerve problem, neuromas), inflamed anal sacs, inflammatory, pain/injury to tail, pelvis, or stifles

one of the precipitating factors in the development of the behavior was anal sacculitis (Bain and Fan 2012).

If an animal presents for shadow, light, or "fly" chasing, a complete ophthalmological examination should be performed. Vitreous degeneration has been found as an inciting cause of this behavior in a Border Collie, who was also diagnosed with having displacement behaviors (Bain and Good 2015).

Excessive licking has been associated with underlying gastrointestinal pathologies, including inflammatory changes, foreign bodies, and neoplasia (Bécuwe-Bonnet et al. 2012).

Nutritional or Toxin

A nutritional cause of repetitive behaviors is unlikely to be seen unless there is an absorption or storage disease. Animals on an excessively low-protein diet may display unusual behaviors, as can animals with a thiamine deficiency. While not a nutritional disease per se, a pet with a liver shunt presenting with hepatic encephalopathy and head pressing may be misinterpreted as having a repetitive behavior. There is some evidence that gluten-sensitive Border Terriers may be predisposed to unusual movements (Lowrie et al. 2018).

Potential Genetic Predispositions

Species, breed, and family line dispositions for certain repetitive behaviors suggest a genetic predisposition for these behaviors. Of note, specific genetic links have been implicated in compulsive disorders in dogs (Dodman et al. 2010; Tang et al. 2014). Aside from specific genetic loci, there are some breeds that are seemingly more likely to develop these problems, as outlined in Table 18.3.

Table 18.3 Breed predispositions toward repetitive behaviors.

Repetitive behavior	Breeds
Acral lick granulomas/ dermatitis	Large breed dogs (retrievers)
Light or shadow chasing	Herding-type breeds
Spinning or tail chasing	Bull Terriers, German Shepherd Dogs
Freezing/trancing	Bull Terriers
Flank sucking	Doberman Pinschers
Checking hind end	Miniature Schnauzer
Pica	Siamese and other related breeds, Labrador Retrievers
Fabric chewing/eating	Siamese and other related breeds

Gathering a History

As with all aspects of veterinary medicine, history-taking is an important part of behavioral medicine (Horwitz 2000; Seibert and Landsberg 2008). It should be noted that client-reports and videorecorded evidence are more central for behavioral diagnoses than for physiological diagnoses (Nibblett et al. 2015; Palestrini et al. 2010).

Information on the pet's behavior during the incident includes the duration and description of the behavior, ease of distraction, and the frequency of such incidents. Once the incident has ended, how long does it take for the pet to return to its typical behavior? If other animals or people were involved, how did they respond during and after the fact?

An important technique to help diagnose the problem is videos of the pet when people are present, when the pet is completely alone, a demonstration of the behavior if it can be safely done, and a walkthrough of the environment in which the pet resides. Often, things can be seen on video that cannot be adequately described by clients (Scaglia et al. 2013).

Videos can also help identify environmental factors playing a role in the pet's behavior, especially if the appointment is in-clinic. Such factors that can be investigated are particular locations in which the pet performs the behavior (e.g. by the door in the kitchen), potential stressors (e.g. inappropriate locations for litterboxes, pet feeding locations next to one another), and perhaps family engagement with the pet. There could be subtle signs that the veterinarian may notice, especially if the behavior is caught on video. A subtle body movement, a specific direction in which the pet moves, and/or other physiological signs may be more apparent in a video compared to in-clinic.

Inform clients that, in many cases, repetitive behaviors may take weeks to months to decrease in frequency and intensity, and relapses may occur. These behaviors often require lifelong treatment to manage. If no improvement is seen after a few weeks, the diagnosis, treatment plan, medications, and client adherence to the plan should be reevaluated. Treatment plans should consider a client's ability and willingness to address the animal's behaviors. Clear communication about expectations should start with the initial diagnosis and prognosis. One should support the client through this journey with their pet, understanding that many things affect their ability to follow through with a treatment plan.

Have clients keep daily and/or weekly logs of the occurrence of the behavior, including duration and frequency of bouts. This will allow for accurate assessment of behavioral change and make it more objective for them. They may focus on "my dog still spins"; however, when reviewing logs, they can identify that the intensity has decreased, as has the frequency. Regular (semiannual to annual) monitoring is necessary for pets on long-term drug therapy; examination and laboratory evaluations (CBC, chemistry panel, urinalysis) should be conducted.

Treatment

Treatment comprises management, eliminating stressors in the environment, providing the animal with opportunities for choice of substitutive behaviors, providing structure and relationship-building exercises, desensitizing and counterconditioning to identifiable triggers that cause or exacerbate these behaviors, and utilizing medications to help alleviate underlying anxiety. While presented as distinct parts of a plan, there is considerable overlap. Of course, any contributing physiological problems should be acknowledged and treated appropriately. A summary of treatment is outlined in Table 18.4.

Table 18.4 Overview of treatment for repetitive behaviors in pets.

Physical health	**Rule out and treat any underlying and concurrent physiological condition**
Management	Avoid triggers that can cause stress, anxiety, or those that instigate or perpetuate behaviors Avoid purposeful or inadvertent reinforcement of the behavior Avoid aversive attempts at control Provide environmental enrichment to improve overall welfare
Tools	Tools for management (vinyl window cling, white noise, bandages) Tools for enrichment Avoid use of laser pointers
Training/behavior modification	Systematic desensitization and counterconditioning to triggers that can instigate repetitive behaviors, or those that cause stress or anxiety
Medications and alternative therapies *See Chapter* 21	Antidepressants: • To address an underlying compulsive disorder • To help ameliorate signs of stress and anxiety Other immediate-acting anxiolytics, nutraceuticals, or pheromones to help ameliorate signs of stress and anxiety Treatments for underlying physiological conditions

Management and Tools

Counsel clients on the importance of managing the environment so that the pet is less likely to continue to perform the behavior. An example is avoidance of potentially dangerous items that pets can ingest, should they have pica, wool, or fabric sucking. If a dog has acral lick dermatitis, you should medically manage the problem, including using bandages to help prevent self-mutilation.

Once identified, triggers causing anxiety or overarousal, should be eliminated and/or avoided. This can be very difficult, as some animals are very driven to perform repetitive behaviors in response to a fleeting exposure to the trigger. If these triggers cannot be avoided, then clients can perform desensitization and counterconditioning to these triggers, and/or utilize medications to help ameliorate the anxiety associated with the triggers.

In homes with multiple pets, make sure each has safe access to what it needs (food, water, and resting areas), along with the opportunity to eat, rest, and move around its environment undisturbed. This may mean separating pets during feeding times, providing multiple hiding places, and even rotating animals between rooms. If outside animals trigger the pet to display displacement behaviors, clients can discourage animals from entering the yard by removing bird feeders and can block the sight of outside animals with something like vinyl window film. If an animal is reactive to sounds, owners can play either classical music or white noise near the windows and doors to help block out environmental sound triggers.

Punishment for unwanted behaviors should be avoided, whether they are repetitive behaviors or others. Not only does this not address the underlying cause of a behavior, it also can cause an increase in anxiety and aggression and lead to diminished welfare (Herron et al. 2009). Yelling, swatting, hitting, and spraying with water are commonly thought of as punishing; however, punishment is in the eye of the beholder. What one animal considers tolerable, such as a pet's name uttered in a low voice, another finds aversive.

Not only should clients avoid items or triggers that can be dangerous or cause anxiety, but they should also provide appropriate alternatives that afford an animal sufficient mental and physical exercise. The perception of control is essential for well-being, and vital in helping to decrease stress in animals. It is important to provide foundations for animals to maintain their quality of life. These include: a stable, consistent environment that enhances learning; a safe environment free from fearful stimuli that allows exploration without harm; and satisfactory nutrition delivered in a way that the cat chooses to ingest it (Buffington and Bain 2020).

Increasing mental and physical stimulation, especially for indoor pets, is one way in which clients can positively affect their pets' well-being. There are many ways that this can be done, ranging from visual to olfactory enrichment, to interactive play, to food-dispensing and foraging "toys" (Figure 18.5).

Family involvement and interaction with their pet is important (Figure 18.6). This can range from something simple like petting and brushing, to interactive play sessions, walks and training classes. Playing with laser pointers should be discouraged, but if a client is going to utilize one, they should take care to ensure the game does not induce frustration or agitation (see Chapter 7 on Kitten behavior and development). A recent study demonstrated that laser light play was the largest predictor of "abnormal repetitive behaviors" in cats (Kogan and Grigg 2021).

Food-dispensing toys help to motivate the cat to engage with its environment in a meaningful manner, allowing a cat to display more species-typical behaviors of eating multiple times per day. There are many examples of food-dispensing toys, either purchased or homemade, many of which are discussed in Chapter 7. The website www.foodpuzzlesforcats.com presents a multitude of ideas.

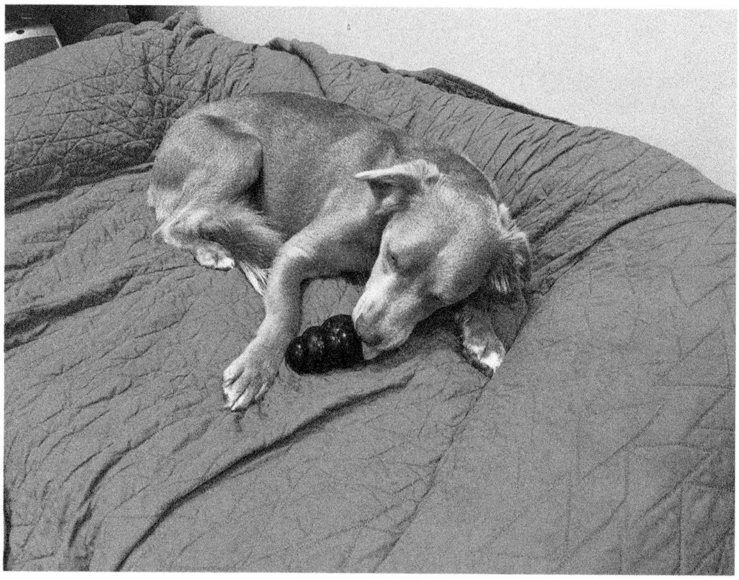

Figure 18.5 Food-dispensing puzzle toys, such as this Kong® (KONG Company, Golden, CO), provide long-lasting entertainment and can be especially helpful for dogs with repetitive oral behaviors. Keep in mind that black Kongs, such as the one shown here, are the most durable, and dogs should be supervised when first introduced, particularly if pica is a concern. *Source:* Meghan E. Herron.

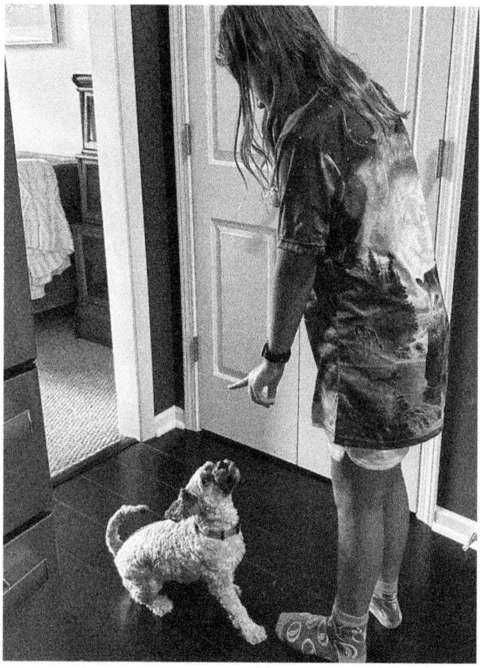

Figure 18.6 A child in the family works with her dog on positive reinforcement training for basic skills and manners. These skills will come in handy when she needs to distract her pet from unwanted repetitive behaviors. *Source:* Carrie Reyes.

Behavior Modification

If there is an underlying or concurrent behavior problem, that must also be treated. This is especially important when an animal is displaying displacement behaviors. Providing consistent manners in which to interact with the pet is a hallmark of any treatment plan. Utilizing positive reinforcement-based training, while giving the animal a perception of choice, provides a consistent and predictable manner of relating to one another.

Response substitution (differential reinforcement of an alternate behavior) is when an animal is positively reinforced for an alternate behavior, ideally one that is incompatible with the behavior you are attempting to change. Once the pet solidly learns the new behavior, the client can cue that behavior to redirect the pet away from the repetitive behavior. It is important that the cue for the new behavior be taught and rehearsed at times when the animal is calm and not already in the midst of a repetitive behavior episode. Gradually, the cue can be introduced and practiced during gradually more challenging situations.

When a trigger is identifiable, the client can work on **systematic desensitization** and **counterconditioning** (DS/CC) to change the animal's response to it. As discussed in Chapter 5, systematic desensitization is the process of reintroducing an animal to a triggering stimulus, ranging from sounds to sights of other pets, to flashing lights, in gradual increments. Counterconditioning is the process of changing the emotional state regarding the stimulus, usually from fear to a state of relaxation, utilizing something that the animal finds rewarding, such as a tasty treat.

The DS/CC exercises should be carried out in such small steps that the animal never crosses into a state of anxiety or fear (stays below threshold). Emphasize the importance of monitoring the pet's body language for signs of fear, anxiety, stress, and/or frustration (see Chapter 11). If the client attempts desensitization and counterconditioning when the animal is already anxious or aroused, the process will likely fail. They should start in a quiet, neutral setting and only gradually build up to the situation where the problem occurs. If the steps are too large, or occur too quickly, these techniques will not be effective. The client should not progress faster than what the pet can accept, and each session should end with a reward for desirable behavior before the pet is anxious or overaroused. Since the unwanted behavior took time to develop, look for small, incremental improvements rather than instant results. Ideally, sessions are kept short (just a minute or two) and repeated frequently. Since progress is often slow, the client should maintain a journal of the behavior to track the pet's progress more objectively, including information on the stimulus, intensity, distance, situation, and the pet's response.

Medications

Medications can help facilitate the behavioral modification program, and, in many cases, may be necessary for improvement. No drugs are labeled for use in dogs or cats for repetitive behaviors, and appropriate baseline screenings are indicated. The effects from the medications are not immediate and may take up to eight weeks to be fully appreciated. Clients often ask when the pet can be weaned off the medication, and the answer depends on the individual animal in the specific environment.

Aside from a purely physiological cause, different neurotransmitter systems have been implicated in the problems due to an underlying behavior, including and have included the opioid-mediated, dopaminergic, glutaminergic, and serotonergic (Brown et al. 1987). Clinical treatment is currently focused on the serotonergic system, and serotonergic medications are currently the first line of pharmacological intervention.

Fluoxetine has been the most extensively studied medications for the treatment of repetitive behaviors. While true stereotypic behavior is rarely, if ever found, in our companion animals, fluoxetine has been utilized to treat stereotypies in laboratory animals and captive wildlife (Arora et al. 2013; Poulsen et al. 1996; Woods et al. 1993; Yalcin and Aytug 2007). One study demonstrated effectiveness in the treatment of compulsive disorders in dogs, compared to placebo, albeit in the global evaluation, not in the daily diaries (Irimajiri et al. 2009).

Clomipramine, a tricyclic antidepressant, has been repeatedly studied as a treatment for compulsive disorders. One study determined that 75% of terriers diagnosed with tail chasing had a decrease of the behavior by 75% with clomipramine treatment, although there was no control group (Moon-Fanelli and Dodman 1998). However, another study did demonstrate effectiveness of clomipramine over a control group (Hewson et al. 1998). Another study demonstrated no effectiveness in treating cats with psychogenic alopecia with clomipramine (Mertens et al. 2006); however, it should be noted that, in another study, most cats with "psychogenic alopecia" had an underlying dermatological condition (Waisglass et al. 2006).

Current research in humans, and some limited documentation in dogs, has demonstrated that the glutaminergic system may play a role in some repetitive behaviors (Pittenger et al. 2011; Rodriguez et al. 2013). There is recent research on the potential efficacy of memantine in the treatment of canine compulsive disorders – both when used as a monotherapy and when combined with fluoxetine treatment (Schneider et al. 2009; Wald et al. 2009).

See Chapter 21 for specific psychopharmacological details, doses, and recommendations.

Nutraceuticals and Pheromones

While not directly treating repetitive behaviors, there are nutraceutical and pheromone products on the market labeled to help alleviate anxiety and promote relaxation. Nutraceutical ingredients L-theanine and alpha-casozepine have shown some limited evidence in published papers, albeit none specifically looking at repetitive behaviors, and few with a control group (Araujo et al. 2010; Beata et al. 2007; Pike et al. 2015; Stillo et al. 2021). Synthetic pheromone products, such as those that mimic what is produced by a lactating dog, have been shown to alleviate anxiety in some dogs; like the research in nutraceuticals, no studies have been done specifically looking at their use for repetitive behaviors (Frank et al. 2010).

Conclusion

There has been much written about repetitive behaviors in animals and humans, yet the underlying pathology is still not clear. Historically, papers published on this subject have lumped many of these behaviors erroneously under "compulsive" or "stereotypic," when in fact there is more evidence that other anxiety-related disorders can be found as the root cause of a repetitive behavior, such as with displacement behaviors. Further investigation has also led us to understand that many of these repetitive behaviors have an underlying physiological etiology. With the ever-changing information, it is important that you, as the veterinary clinician, gather a full history and do due diligence in ruling out pain or other physiological causes of repetitive behaviors. Treatment revolves around identifying the underlying reason for the behavior, be it behavioral and/or physiological, managing the environment, undertaking behavioral modification techniques, and medically managing the patient for all potential underlying causes.

References

Amat, M., de la Torre, J.L.R., Fatjó, J. et al. (2009). Potential risk factors associated with feline behaviour problems. *Appl. Anim. Behav. Sci. 121* (2): 134–139.

Amengual Batle, P., Rusbridge, C., Nuttall, T. et al. (2019). Feline hyperaesthesia syndrome with self-trauma to the tail: retrospective study of seven cases and proposal for an integrated multidisciplinary diagnostic approach. *J. Feline Med. Surg.* 21 (2): 178–185.

Araujo, J.A., de Rivera, C., Ethier, J.L. et al. (2010). ANXITANE® tablets reduce fear of human beings in a laboratory model of anxiety-related behavior. *J. Vet. Behav. 5* (5): 268–275. https://doi.org/10.1016/j.jveb.2010.02.003.

Arora, T., Bhowmik, M., Khanam, R., and Vohora, D. (2013). Oxcarbazepine and fluoxetine protect against mouse models of obsessive compulsive disorder through modulation of cortical serotonin and CREB pathway. *Behav. Brain Res. 247*: 146–152.

Bain, M.J. and Fan, C.M. (2012). Animal behavior case of the month. *J. Am. Vet. Med. Assoc. 240* (6): 673–675. https://doi.org/10.2460/javma.240.6.673.

Bain, M.J. and Good, K.L. (2015). Animal behavior case of the month. *J. Am. Vet. Med. Assoc. 247* (4): 352–355. https://doi.org/10.2460/javma.247.4.352.

Bamberger, M. and Houpt, K.A. (2006). Signalment factors, comorbidity, and trends in behavior diagnoses in cats: 736 cases (1991-2001). *J. Am. Vet. Med. Assoc. 229* (10): 1602–1606. https://doi.org/10.2460/javma.229.10.1602.

Beata, C., Beaumont-Graff, E., Diaz, C. et al. (2007). Effects of alpha-casozepine (Zylkene) versus selegiline hydrochloride (Selgian, Anipryl) on anxiety disorders in dogs. *J. Vet. Behav. 2* (5): 175–183. https://doi.org/10.1016/j.jveb.2007.08.001.

Beaver, B. (1994). *The Veterinarian's Encyclopedia of Animal Behavior*. Iowa State University Press.

Bécuwe-Bonnet, V., Bélanger, M.-C., Frank, D. et al. (2012). Gastrointestinal disorders in dogs with excessive licking of surfaces. *J. Vet. Behav.* 7 (4): 194–204.

Bradshaw, J.W.S., Neville, P.F., and Sawyer, D. (1997). Factors affecting pica in the domestic cat. *Appl. Anim. Behav. Sci. 52* (3-4): 373–379. http://www.sciencedirect.com/science/article/B6T48-3RH0C3B-J/2/eacc8602ebaecdd4a43f21fccd6bd59a.

Brown, S.A., Crowell-Davis, S., Malcolm, T., and Edwards, P. (1987). Naloxone-responsive compulsive tail chasing in a dog. *J. Am. Vet. Med. Assoc. 190* (7): 884–886.

Buffington, C.A.T. and Bain, M. (2020). Stress and feline health. *Vet. Clin.: Small Anim. Pract. 50* (4): 653–662. https://doi.org/10.1016/j.cvsm.2020.03.001.

Demontigny-Bédard, I., Beauchamp, G., Bélanger, M.-C., and Frank, D. (2016). Characterization of pica and chewing behaviors in privately owned cats: a case-control study. *J. Feline Med. Surg. 18* (8): 652–657.

Denerolle, P., White, S.D., Taylor, T.S., and Vandenabeele, S.I.J. (2007). Organic diseases mimicking acral lick dermatitis in six dogs. *J. Am. Anim. Hosp. Assoc. 43* (4): 215–220. http://www.jaaha.org/content/43/4/215.abstract.

Dodman, N., Bronson, R., and Gliatto, J. (1993). Tail chasing in a bull terrier. *J. Am. Vet. Med. Assoc. 202* (5): 758–760; 724 ref.

Dodman, N.H., Karlsson, E.K., Moon-Fanelli, A. et al. (2010). A canine chromosome 7 locus confers compulsive disorder susceptibility. *Mol. Psychiatry 15* (1): 8–10. https://doi.org/http://www.nature.com/mp/journal/v15/n1/suppinfo/mp2009111s1.html.

Frank, D., Beauchamp, G., and Palestrini, C. (2010). Systematic review of the use of pheromones for treatment of undesirable behavior in cats and dogs. *J. Am. Vet. Med. Assoc. 236* (12): 1308–1316.

Frank, D., Bélanger, M.C., Bécuwe-Bonnet, V., and Parent, J. (2012). Prospective medical evaluation of 7 dogs presented with fly biting. *Can. Vet. J.* 53 (12): 1279.

Hall, N.J., Protopopova, A., and Wynne, C.D. (2015). The role of environmental and owner-provided consequences in canine stereotypy and compulsive behavior. *J. Vet. Behav. 10* (1): 24–35.

Hart, B.L., Hart, L.A., and Thigpen, A.P. (2019). Characterization of plant eating in cats. *Proceedings of the 53rd Congress of the ISAE (International Society of Applied Ethology)*, Bergen, Norway: ISAE, *106*, 334–340.

Herron, M.E., Shofer, F.S., and Reisner, I.R. (2009). Survey of the use and outcome of confrontational and non-confrontational training methods in client-owned dogs showing undesired behaviors. *Appl. Anim. Behav. Sci. 117* (1-2): 47–54. http://www.sciencedirect.com/science/article/B6T48-4VFJS1D-2/2/aa7825255db8bf7960a78d845a183881.

Hewson, C., Luescher, U.A., Parent, J.M. et al. (1998). Efficacy of clomipramine in the treatment of canine compulsive disorder. *J. Am. Vet. Med. Assoc. 213* (12): 1760–1766.

Hewson, C.J., Luescher, U.A., and Ball, R.O. (1999). The use of chance-corrected agreement to diagnose canine compulsive disorder: an approach to behavioral diagnosis in the absence of a 'Gold Standard'. *Can. J. Vet. Res. 63* (3): 201–206. http://www.ncbi.nlm.nih.gov/pmc/articles/PMC1189548/pdf/cjvetres00011%2D0043.pdf/?tool=pmcentrez.

Horwitz, D.F. (2000). Differences and similarities between behavioral and internal medicine. *J. Am. Vet. Med. Assoc. 217* (9): 1372–1376.

Irimajiri, M., Luescher, A.U., Douglass, G. et al. (2009). Randomized, controlled clinical trial of the efficacy of fluoxetine for treatment of compulsive disorders in dogs. *J. Am. Vet. Med. Assoc. 235* (6): 705–709. https://doi.org/10.2460/javma.235.6.705.

Johnson, P.M. and Kenny, P.J. (2010). Dopamine D2 receptors in addiction-like reward dysfunction and compulsive eating in obese rats. *Nat. Neurosci.* 13 (5): 635–641.

Kogan, L.R. and Grigg, E.K. (2021). Laser light pointers for use in companion cat play: association with guardian-reported abnormal repetitive behaviors. *Animals 11* (8): 2178. https://www.mdpi.com/2076-2615/11/8/2178.

Longoni, R., Spina, L., Mulas, A. et al. (1991). (D-Ala2) deltorphin II: D1-dependent stereotypies and stimulation of dopamine release in the nucleus accumbens. *J. Neurosci. 11* (6): 1565–1576.

Lowrie, M., Smith, P., De Keuster, T., and Garosi, L. (2015). Trance-like syndrome in bull terriers. *Mol. Psychiatry* 15: 8–10.

Lowrie, M., Garden, O.A., Hadjivassiliou, M., et al. Characterization of paroxysmal gluten-sensitive dyskinesia in Border Terriers using serological markers. (2018) *Journal of Veterinary Internal Medicine. 32* (2) 775–781. https://doi.org/10.1111/jvim.15038

Mason, G. (2006). Stereotypic behaviour in captive animals: fundamentals and implications for welfare and beyond. In: *Stereotypic Animal Behaviour: Fundamentals and Applications to Welfare*, 2e (ed. G. Mason and J. Rushen), 325–356. CABI.

Mertens, P.A., Torres, S., and Jessen, C. (2006). The effects of clomipramine hydrochloride in cats with psychogenic alopecia: a prospective study. *J. Am. Anim. Hosp. Assoc. 42* (5): 336–343.

Mills, D.S., Demontigny-Bédard, I., Gruen, M., et al. (2020). Pain and problem behaviors in dogs and cats. *Animals*. 10(2) 318. https://doi.org/10.3390/ani10020318

Moon-Fanelli, A.A. and Dodman, N.H. (1998). Description and development of compulsive tail chasing in terriers and response to clomipramine treatment. *J. Am. Vet. Med. Assoc. 21* (8): 1252–1257.

Moon-Fanelli, A.A., Dodman, N.H., and Cottam, N. (2007). Blanket and flank sucking in Doberman Pinschers. *J. Am. Vet. Med. Assoc. 231* (6): 907–912.

Moon-Fanelli, A.A., Dodman, N.H., Famula, T.R., and Cottam, N. (2011). Characteristics of compulsive tail chasing and associated risk factors in Bull Terriers. *J. Am. Vet. Med. Assoc. 238* (7): 883–889. https://doi.org/10.2460/javma.238.7.883.

Nibblett, B.M., Ketzis, J.K., and Grigg, E.K. (2015). Comparison of stress exhibited by cats examined in a clinic versus a home setting. *Appl. Anim. Behav. Sci. 173*: 68–75. https://doi.org/10.1016/j.applanim.2014.10.005.

Ogata, N., Gillis, T.E., Liu, X. et al. (2013). Brain structural abnormalities in Doberman pinschers with canine compulsive disorder. *Prog. Neuro-Psychopharmacol. Biol. Psychiatry 45*: 1–6. https://doi.org/10.1016/j.pnpbp.2013.04.002.

Overall, K.L. and Dunham, A.E. (2002). Clinical features and outcome in dogs and cats with obsessive-compulsive disorder: 126 cases (1989–2000). *J. Am. Vet. Med. Assoc. 221* (10): 1445–1452. https://doi.org/10.2460/javma.2002.221.1445.

Palestrini, C., Minero, M., Cannas, S. et al. (2010). Video analysis of dogs with separation-related behaviors. *Appl. Anim. Behav. Sci. 124* (1-2): 61–67. https://doi.org/10.1016/j.applanim.2010.01.014.

Pike, A.L., Horwitz, D.F., and Lobprise, H. (2015). An open-label prospective study of the use of l-theanine (Anxitane) in storm-sensitive client-owned dogs. *J. Vet. Behav. 10* (4): 324–331. https://doi.org/10.1016/j.jveb.2015.04.001.

Pittenger, C., Bloch, M.H., and Williams, K. (2011). Glutamate abnormalities in obsessive compulsive disorder: neurobiology, pathophysiology, and treatment. *Pharmacol. Ther. 132* (3): 314–332.

Poulsen, E.M., Honeyman, V., Valentine, P., and Teskey, G. (1996). Use of fluoxetine for the treatment of stereotypical pacing behavior in a captive polar bear. *J. Am. Vet. Med. Assoc. 209*: 1470–1474.

Protopopova, A. (2016). Effects of sheltering on physiology, immune function, behavior, and the welfare of dogs. *Physiol. Behav.* 159: 95–103. https://doi.org/10.1016/j.physbeh.2016.03.020.

Rodriguez, C.I., Kegeles, L.S., Levinson, A. et al. (2013). Randomized controlled crossover trial of ketamine in obsessive-compulsive disorder: proof-of-concept. *Neuropsychopharmacology 38* (12): 2475–2483. https://doi.org/10.1038/npp.2013.150.

Santoro, D., Pucheu-Haston, C.M., Prost, C., et al. (2021). Clinical signs and diagnosis of feline atopic syndrome: detailed guidelines for a correct diagnosis. *Veterinary Dermatology 32* (1). 26–e6. https://doi.org/10.1111/vde.12935

Scaglia, E., Cannas, S., Minero, M. et al. (2013). Video analysis of adult dogs when left home alone. *J. Vet. Behav. 8* (6): 412–417.

Schneider, B.M., Dodman, N.H., and Maranda, L. (2009). Use of memantine in treatment of canine compulsive disorders. *J. Vet. Behav. 4* (3): 118–126. https://doi.org/10.1016/j.jveb.2008.10.008.

Seibert, L.M. and Landsberg, G.M. (2008). Diagnosis and management of patients presenting with behavior problems. *Vet. Clin. N. Am. Small Anim. Pract. 38* (5): 937–950. https://doi.org/10.1016/j.cvsm.2008.04.001.

Seksel, K. and Lindeman, M. (1998). Use of clomipramine in the treatment of anxiety-related and obsessive-compulsive disorders in cats. *Aust. Vet. J. 76* (5): 317–321.

Shumaker, A.K. (2019). Diagnosis and treatment of canine acral lick dermatitis. *Vet. Clin.: Small Anim. Pract.* 49 (1): 105–123.

Stillo, T., Norgard, R.J., Stefanovski, D. et al. (2021). The effects of Solliquin administration on the activity and fecal cortisol production of shelter dogs. *J. Vet. Behav. 45*: 10–15. https://doi.org/10.1016/j.jveb.2021.05.001.

Sueda, K.L.C., Hart, B.L., and Cliff, K.D. (2008). Characterisation of plant eating in dogs. *Appl. Anim. Behav. Sci. 111* (1–2): 120–132. https://doi.org/10.1016/j.applanim.2007.05.018.

Sulkama, S., Salonen, M., Mikkola, S., et al. (2022). Aggressiveness, ADHD-like behaviour, and environment influence repetitive behaviour in dogs. Scientific Reports, 12(12), 3520. https://doi.org/10.1038/s41598-022-07443-6

Tang, R., Noh, H.J., Wang, D. et al. (2014). Candidate genes and functional noncoding variants identified in a canine model of obsessive-compulsive disorder. *Genome Biol. 15* (3): R25. https://doi.org/10.1186/gb-2014-15-3-r25.

Tiira, K., Hakosalo, O., Kareinen, L. et al. (2012). Environmental effects on compulsive tail chasing in dogs. *PLoS One 7* (7): e41684. https://doi.org/10.1371/journal.pone.0041684.

Waisglass, S.E., Landsberg, G.M., Yager, J.A., and Hall, J.A. (2006). Underlying medical conditions in cats with presumptive psychogenic alopecia. *J. Am. Vet. Med. Assoc. 228* (11): 1705–1709. 10.2460/javma.228.11.1705.

Wald, R., Dodman, N., and Shuster, L. (2009). The combined effects of memantine and fluoxetine on an animal model of obsessive compulsive disorder. *Exp. Clin. Psychopharmacol. 17* (3): 191–197. https://doi.org/10.1037/a0016402.

Walsh, B.R. (2020). A critical review of the evidence for the equivalence of canine and human compulsions. *Appl. Anim. Behav. Sci. 234*: 105166.

Wassink-van der Schot, A.A., Day, C., Morton, J.M. et al. (2016). Risk factors for behavior problems in cats presented to an Australian companion animal behavior clinic. *J. Vet. Behav.* 14: 34–40. https://doi.org/10.1016/j.jveb.2016.06.010.

Woods, A., Smith, C., Szewczak, M. et al. (1993). Selective serotonin re-uptake inhibitors decrease schedule-induced polydipsia in rats: a potential model for obsessive compulsive disorder. *Psychopharmacology 112* (2): 195–198.

Yalcin, E. and Aytug, N. (2007). Use of fluoxetine to treat stereotypical pacing behavior in a brown bear (*Ursus arctos*). *J. Vet. Behav. 2* (3): 73–76.

Young, M.S. and Manning, T.O. (1984). Psychogenic dermatoses [dog and cat]. *Dermatology Rep. 3* (2): 1–8.

19

Repetitive and Other Abnormal Behaviors in Wild Animals Under Human Care

Mark Flint[1] *and Randall E. Junge*[2]

[1] *One Welfare and Sustainability Center, College of Veterinary Medicine, The Ohio State University, Columbus, OH, USA*
[2] *Columbus Zoo and Aquarium, Powell, OH, USA*

Introduction

The phrase *wild animals under human care* typically evoke thoughts of zoological parks, rehabilitation centers, or open-range conservation facilities that care for wild species under the auspice of education, conservation, and repatriation into the wild. Facilities like these have contributed to saving endangered species, offered sanctuaries to disused and misused animals, and increased our global awareness of the plight of many of the species found within. In contrast, unsuccessful attempts to keep wild animals under human care conjure images of pacing lions at zoos, malnourished polar bears performing stereotypes in stark exhibits, and mismatched species in the same pen, resulting in aggressive interactions.

Throughout history, wild animals have been held in private collections for a myriad of reasons, including entertainment, education, conservation, defense, and production, and these purposes persist to present day. Although some practices, such as circuses and the use of exotic animals as status symbols and beasts of war, are no longer socially acceptable nor common, many wild animals are still held publicly and privately under a range of health and welfare standards.

Some of these poorer conditions have given rise to repetitive and other abnormal behaviors, which have resulted in suffering of the animal. However, if good is to come from any of these practices that cause negative behaviors, it is to use them to learn and to improve the welfare and our understanding of the wild species being held.

In this chapter, we will first discuss behavior and other domains as a welfare indicator, associated challenges to using this tool in wildlife, and what constitutes a repetitive or aberrant behavior in wild animals. We will summarize where we have learned our lessons so that we may now apply this knowledge. We will then briefly review the negative behaviors seen in wild animals under human care in zoos and later explore in greater detail the non-zoo settings of free-ranging wildlife used in research. This final topic is discussed because it is important and largely absent in the literature. All of these settings provide a range of practices from which we can learn the spectrum of repetitive and aberrant behaviors seen. We will suggest how these clinical presentations may be diagnosed medically and used as indicators to result in positive outcomes. As with any health and well-being challenge, we will present prevention, management, and treatment strategies

Introduction to Animal Behavior and Veterinary Behavioral Medicine, First Edition. Edited by Meghan E. Herron.

Companion website: www.wiley.com/go/introductiontoanimalbehavior

based on known causative syndromes and environments.

The standard definition of **stereotypy** is a behavior that is repetitive and unvarying in its pattern, with a purpose of relieving stress related to underlying husbandry conditions, where an animal is unable to perform species-typical behaviors. However, this term may not completely define these behaviors in wildlife species; in part at least as wild animals may not be subject to direct husbandry. A more appropriate term, "abnormal repetitive behaviors" is defined as behaviors that are heavily repeated, invariant, and apparently functionless or maladaptive (Turner 1997).

Behavior and Other Domains as a Welfare Indicator

All animals interact with and respond to their environment — the habitat and its stressors. The degree of their engagement is dependent on the environment in which they are contained. Mimicking natural environments is believed to cause less stress by allowing the animal to conduct activities consistent with their "natural" behaviors. Seeing these behaviors in appropriate proportions and circumstances suggests to caregivers and ethologists that the basic behavioral needs of the animals are being met. However, seeing these behaviors in out-of-place instances or above or below the frequency expected to be "normal" can be indicative of a welfare problem. Therefore, knowing what is normal becomes an essential key to assessing welfare.

Starting with the Brambell report in 1965 that resulted in the Five Freedoms, basic needs and expressions were recognized in production animals to ensure they had a "life worth living" (Brambell 1965, FAWC 2009). As a result of an improved understanding of what domesticated animals need to have good welfare, these freedoms have since evolved into the Five Domains (Table 19.1), currently the most widely accepted approach to assessing the welfare of animals (Mellor et al. 2020). It uses not only behavior but also nutrition, environment, and health to predict a mental domain (that is, is the animal having a life worth living?). Based on production animals, can the Five Domains be directly applied to wild animals under human care to identify aberrant behaviors?

Unlike their domestic counterparts, there is often surprisingly little known about the specific health and welfare needs of wild animals (Flint and Bonde 2017). Using the

Table 19.1 The five freedoms, established in 1965 as part of the Brambell report are now more widely applied as the five domains.

Five freedoms	Five domains
1) Freedom from hunger and thirst	1) Nutrition — factors that involve the animal's access to sufficient, balanced, varied, and clean food and water.
2) Freedom from discomfort	2) Environment — factors that enable comfort through temperature, substrate, space, air, odor, noise, and predictability.
3) Freedom from pain, injury or disease	3) Health — factors that enable good health through the absence of disease, injury, impairment with a good fitness level.
4) Freedom to express normal behavior	4) Behavior — factors that provide varied, novel, and engaging environmental challenges through sensory inputs, exploration, foraging, bonding, playing, retreating, and others.
5) Freedom from fear or distress	5) Mental state — the mental state of the animal should benefit from predominantly positive states, such as pleasure, comfort, or vitality while reducing negative states such as fear, frustration, hunger, pain, or boredom.

Five Domains framework to determine mental wellbeing raises the following questions: what should the normal ethogram for this wild species be; what does this species eat long-term; how does this animal use the environment it is in; and what is the normal baseline for health? Sampling wild animals in their natural environment to get these answers almost certainly skews these findings. They do not behave normally when they are being watched, we seldom understand their ongoing year-round nutritional demands, they live in complex environments, but they do not necessarily interact with all parts of them, and clinical health profiles are largely limited to captured (stressed) or dead (usually not healthy) animals. As such, comparisons of "normal" can be difficult and many subtle aberrant deviations in each domain may be missed or even misinterpreted and challenging to use to gain a holistic impression.

Challenges and Using What We Know

On the surface, it appears the best tool we currently have to determine "normal" or "positive" to identify "aberrant" or "negative" — the Five Domains— may not directly be applicable to wild animals under human care due to the unknowns. Subsequently, subtle repetitive or abnormal behaviors may be difficult to confidently elucidate. However, this does not make application of the Five Domains untenable for wild animals under human care. Instead, it highlights the importance of using any setting as a learning opportunity and laterally applying lessons from the past or from other species to grow in knowledge. We will discuss these factors in this chapter.

As non-domesticated species, wild animals require specialized facilities and care to maintain their health and welfare. When successful, this can allow wild animals to thrive. This strategy has been commonly used to support survival of a species through reproduction. For example, *headstart programs* for reintroduction into the wild (Mortimer 1995). Conversely, when unsuccessful, this can force animals to suffer either overtly or subtly. Failure to meet the natural and behavioral needs of wild species can result in overt mortalities and morbidities or more subtle chronic stress that may eventually manifest as repetitive or other abnormal behaviors.

One of the primary challenges for wild animals under human care is that they exhibit a species-specific stress-susceptibility (Fischer and Romero 2018), often more than their domesticated counterparts. This is due, at least in part, to genetic selection. As discussed in Chapter 2, many of the domestic species we commonly see have been bred for purpose, be it high milk yields, meat production, companionship, or specific tasks like pulling a cart or catching a mouse. A big component of that genetic selection is being bred for domesticity— an ability to cope with man-made structures and practices (Ericcson and Jensen 2016). This has been refined over many generations. Wild animals, by definition, are not under human husbandry, or if they are, it is indirect management (such as preserving habitats) or recently (within a generation or two). Therefore, they have not had the selection of traits that necessarily allow them to cope with man-made structures or practices.

Compounding this issue is that many wild animal species do have a key behavioral adaptation for survival- the ability to mask any subtle signs of stress or injury (Dwyer 2004). This trait has been perfected to avoid appearing weak in the wild and susceptible to predation. When under human care and with species we are not as familiar with, this stoicism may result in missing subtle clues that something is not right. By the time it manifests as either a morbidity or aberrant behavior we do detect, it may be advanced state of disease or stress that is challenging to reverse. In the case of stress, a common example of an advanced manifestation is what we have traditionally known as **stereotypical behaviors**, like the conjured image we suggested at the start of this chapter of pacing lions in unenriched zoos in the old days.

However, with our increased knowledge of caring for wild species under human care, we know the early signs of stress and compromised welfare can be subtle. Further, as veterinarians, we can employ the behavioral nuances and cumulative knowledge briefly outlined so far with the Five Domains to combine clinical and physiological aspects to determine what is an aberrant behavior for the species of interest.

Allostatic Loads

One attempt to calculate the cumulative stressors on an animal that may result in aberrant behaviors is through determining its **allostatic load**. Established in humans, the concept of determining allostatic loads to estimate the cumulative health and welfare state of animals is now being applied to several wild and domesticated species — Western Lowland Gorillas, lemurs, and dairy cattle (Hartigan 2005, Edes et al. 2018, Seeley et al. 2021) (Figure 19.1). Allostatic load is the "wear and tear" on the body which accumulates as an individual is exposed to repeated or chronic stress. This strategy is showing great promise as a comprehensive diagnostic tool in welfare assessments and providing a potential quantitative measure for the "tipping point" of development of aberrant behaviors. It has been postulated that when in an adverse environment, animals undergo allostasis and alter their behavior to regain homeostasis. Measured using a myriad of biomarkers that vary for each situation and species, determining allostatic load can also employ other indicators such as clinical health, growth, reproductive capacity, and behavior. This suite of measures potentially provides a holistic overview of the welfare of the animal and can be used to measure the link between behavior and management.

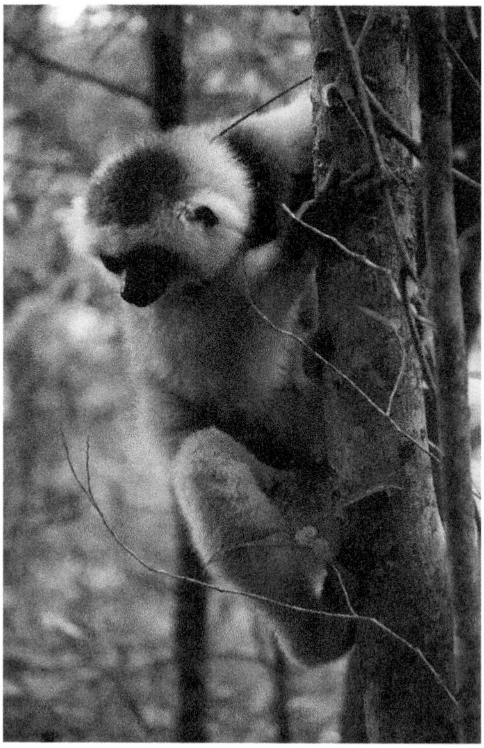

Figure 19.1 Diademed sifaka (*Propithecus diadema*), Madagascar. Allostatic load evaluation has been used to measure effects of anthropogenic stress (mining operations) on this species in the wild. *Source:* With permission from Randy Junge/Columbus Zoo and Aquarium.

Common Abnormal Repetitive Behaviors

Even with diagnostic advancements, observing and understanding fundamental behavior remains a key component of any welfare determination strategy. A behavior assessment, despite its limitations when applied to wild species, is a critical, non-invasive, and rapid tool we can and should routinely employ to determine the welfare of wild animals under human care. To facilitate this, and despite our gaps in knowledge, we do not have to keep reinventing the wheel. We can learn from the past, from similar species, and from what we know about farming and caring for non-domesticated species, as has been a trend in recent decades.

Lessons from the Past – Beasts of War

There is a long history of using exotic animals on the frontlines of war. For example, as early as the 4th Century BC, elephantry (military troops mounted on elephants) was used across

India and Asia to instill terror in the enemy (Nossov 2012). They are still used in Myanmar by the rebel Kachin Independence Army. During World War I, camels and donkeys carried troops and supplies in Sinai and Palestine's desert campaigns; and during both World Wars monkeys, bears, and lions were kept as mascots throughout Europe (Winn 2017).

Even in present day, exotic animals continue to be employed by the military. In the early days of the War on Terror, the flight response of herds of desert animals was used to detect camouflaged soldiers holding positions amongst rocks and outcrops. Navy dolphins, seals, and sea lions have been trained by the United States and the Russian Federation since the Vietnam War era, predominantly for mine detection and diver rescue. The United States still has an active U.S. Navy Marine Mammal Program. Russia reduced its Navy Dolphin program in the 1990's, although reports as recently as 2014 show dolphins on military records (Anon 2021).

Less gloriously, species such as monkeys in ancient China and pigeons and Mexican free-tailed bats in the United States were reportedly tested or used as living "suicide" bombers that infiltrated camps and sites to detonate explosives (Lyons 2016).

Given the difficulty and time required to breed many of these species of animals in captivity, exotics were (and are) captured from the wild, tamed and trained by handlers for specific uses, and then deployed in combat. Without the time needed to breed specific traits over several generations to select for a particular propensity to undertake these high-level tasks, the suitability and ability of the animal to cope with the assignment was/is unknown, and deleterious behavior reportedly resulted.

Not surprisingly, it is difficult to find details on the health and well-being of these animals, both as they have been lost in the annals of time before welfare and behavioral issues were identified as issues in animals and due to the classified status of many military activities. However, what information is available suggests that the sights, smells, and fear of war could send war elephants into a panic, causing them to run amok and indiscriminately cause injury. Similarly, the killing of their driver (tamer), with whom they bond, could result in the same fate. Also, the trauma of war can result in post-traumatic stress disorder (PTSD), as has been seen in numerous military working dogs returning from the Middle East in the last two decades. In several species, manifestations can include aggression in the form of biting, kicking, self-harm, or acral licking, and stereotypical repetitive pacing behaviors.

All is not lost in this history. For example, lessons learned have resulted in modern era military animals such as Navy dolphins having high level care and expertise to ensure their health and well-being; with ongoing and detailed monitoring. While controversy exists over their release back into the wild due to the loss of natural survival instincts, there are also reports that alternative human-care facilities can be employed. These tamed animals are well socialized and can be harmoniously retired to sanctuaries. The Ukraine used their retired Navy dolphins in 1997 as therapy animals for autistic and emotionally disturbed children (PBS 2014). Consequently, in the 20th and 21st Centuries, retirement in naturalistic environments or repatriation to the wild has become the objective of war animals.

Lesson from Recent Enterprises – Exotics in Production

Revolving around the leather, meat, or fiber trade, exotic animals in production have been in vogue for the better part of a century. Pythons, emus, ostriches, alligators, crocodiles, buffalo, llamas, alpacas, mink, deer, and rabbits are farmed around the globe. Each with their own production challenges, many of these species are raised for niche markets based on ever evolving production practices as we learn more about the species-specific needs and requirements. Centuries behind their domesticated counterparts in genetic selection and accumulated husbandry knowledge on what provides good welfare, they may be susceptible to accidental poor management that compromises their welfare and results in the manifestation of abnormal behaviors. And, as already noted, these undomesticated species pose the greatest risk of having subtle aberrant behaviors missed due to our lack of overall understanding of what is a normal behavior and what is required to satisfy their behavioral drives.

In the 1980s ostrich and emu farming for oil, meat, and leather became popular in many countries around the world. Enterprises ranged from "Mom and Pop" set-ups with a breeding pair of birds to farms comprised of hundreds of animals. Protracted abnormal behaviors in smaller holdings of emus have been recorded to include animals continuously pacing along the fences without eating or foraging if separated from conspecifics. Also reported, and although gregarious animals, immediately after changing pens, emus huddle (stay in groups in one corner) away from the emus already present in the pen. After regrouping, repetitive pecking at the fences can occur. Finally for small holdings, animals who were infrequently handled or stressed were prone to running into fences, jumping, kicking, slipping, stopping (balking), falling, and sitting (disinclination to move) when handled (Menon et al. 2014). Larger scale farms have similar aberrant behaviors, but they also face more serious aggression issues and pacing behaviors. Pacing behaviors are more apt to develop depending on pen design, where round or square pens without fence break resulted in circling around and around the fence line. Anecdotally, providing shiny objects as enrichment reduces aggression, presumably by creating displacement activities or allowing multiple hierarchies to form. In turn, breaking up fences by adding barriers that increase the complexity of the fence line reduces circling.

In the 1960s and 1970s in Africa, Australia, and the United States, wild crocodile and alligator hunting transitioned into farming. Direct harvest of wild crocodilians in all these regions had slowed down due to hunting pressures, reducing populations to near critically low levels (with Nile crocodiles and American alligators being listed as endangered). In response to the increasing demand for skins to supply the high-end fashion market, a sustainable ranching system was developed where eggs were harvested from the wild or breeding populations of animals were established on-farm with eggs collected and incubated through to hatch. The hatchlings were grown out to desired hide sizes to meet specific buyer demands. Today, these three species of crocodilian are farmed in state-of-the-art facilities that focus on developing welfare-oriented husbandry practices (Webb 2021). With 70 years of knowledge in place, noted aberrant behaviors these new facilities strive to reduce include caretaker avoidance preventing feeding, aggression among cohorts causing injury and isolation, cannibalism exacerbated by mixing size classes, and repetitive actions such as incessant "zombie" like swimming (either around the pen or with the snout pressed against the wall). To help achieve this, behavioral and morphometric measures are being combined with clinical parameters across the farmed species in comparison to wild counterpart behavior to develop the first allostatic load in non-mammalian species. Preliminary findings suggest that pen design, ambient light and temperature, appropriate nutrition, and careful husbandry can eliminate aberrant behaviors while achieving market requirements.

The alternatives to these production systems for some of these species are direct harvesting from the wild, where the animal is allowed to live a natural life until it is caught. For example, crocodiles and alligators are still routinely hunted in the wild for their skins and meat in the United States, Africa, and Australia; albeit in much smaller quantities than pre-1960s efforts (Webb 2021). Similarly, there are places like the Everglades in Florida where Burmese pythons have become established as invasive species and a burgeoning industry of making saleable products from wild harvested snakes has developed.

One argument for wild harvest of these species is that there are few to no reports of stereotypic behaviors in wild animals who are able to engage and live in natural environments unimpeded by anthropogenic activities. However, there is a general public distaste for wild harvesting as, like all species, overharvesting has been shown to decimate populations, with many being pushed to extinction, and contribute to ecological disturbances. Further, product quality may not be the same as their farmed counterparts. Finally, capture and harvest techniques may be below acceptable standards for humane euthanasia.

Applying What We have Learned in Zoos and Wildlife Sanctuaries

Stereotypic or repetitive behaviors are well-documented in wild animals when housed in unsatisfactory conditions. These behaviors are often redirected natural behaviors such as pacing or excessive grooming (Table 19.2). Such behaviors may be related to inappropriate housing, including small exhibit size, lack of security, proximity to threatening species, or noise and activity levels. They may also be related to the social environment, especially for social primates, herding or schooling species, or territorial individuals. The social environment includes not only the number of animals in a group, but also the sex ratios, age structure, and relatedness of individuals. Ideally, the social environment should match the natural social group structure (e.g. bonded pair, multigenerational, natal band, family group – see Chapter 4).

Stereotypies in ungulate species are most often oral or feeding behaviors such as inappropriate or functionless licking or chewing, or tongue-rolling. This is presumed to be related to significant differences in the captive diet, which often does not mimic the natural diet appropriately (Figure 19.2). Zoo ungulates spend less time foraging than their wild counterparts and may consume diets with varying levels of nutrient content, both of which can contribute to these abnormal behaviors. Low-fiber feed sources are believed to result in less feeling of satiety (less gut fill) which can contribute to abnormal feeding behaviors (Bergeron et al. 2006). See Chapter 20 for more details on abnormal repetitive behaviors in equine and livestock species.

Repetitive behaviors in captive carnivores are most often locomotive in nature, possibly related to hunting or ranging motivations. In human care this is often manifested as pacing. With ample supply of ready to eat food items, opportunity for an important carnivore behavior is absent. Additionally, some enclosures or husbandry practices remove exploratory and ranging activities, behaviors common to wild

Table 19.2 Example of abnormal repetitive behaviors in zoo and wildlife sanctuary animals.

Species	Behavior	Common root causes
Gorillas	Regurgitation and re-ingestion	Stress adaptation to give control/choice and to extend feeding time to natural duration in wild
Polar bears	Pacing	Displacement behavior for walking long distances for hunting, or an anticipatory behavior for routines
Elephants	Head bobbing	Anticipatory behavior to routines
Tigers	Pen circle/pacing	Displacement behavior for walking long distances for hunting, or an anticipatory behavior to routines
Snakes	Glass rubbing or "glass surfing"	Attempts to explore, poor husbandry, or stress
Ungulates	Bar biting or licking	Displacement of foraging behavior
Big cats	Over-grooming	Displacement activity for stress (Figure 19.3)

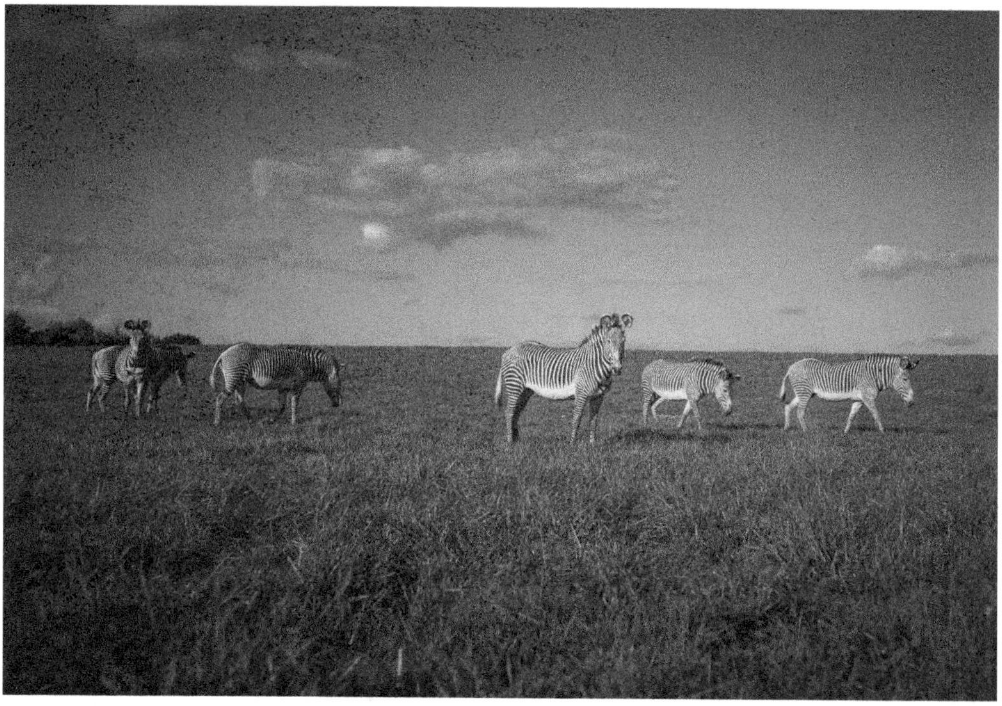

Figure 19.2 Grevy's zebra (*Equus grevyi*). Grazing animals in the wild spend a significant amount of time foraging. Feeding concentrated diets (pellets) or restricting feeding times when kept under human care can result in stereotypic behaviors. *Source:* With permission from G. Jones/Columbus Zoo and Aquarium.

carnivore species (Clubb and Vickery 2006). Captive carnivores may also engage in overgrooming, putting them at risk for skin lesions and infections (Figure 19.3).

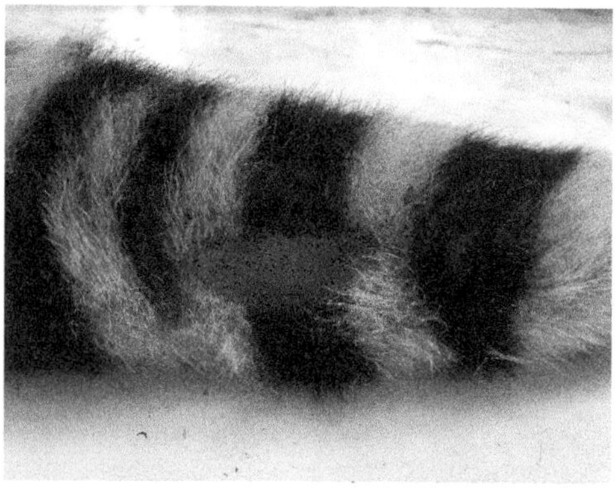

Figure 19.3 Tiger (*Panthera tigris*) with superficial trauma secondary to over-grooming. This abnormal repetitive behavior can be the result displacement activity due to stress. *Source:* With permission from Columbus Zoo and Aquarium.

Applying What We have Learned in Non-Zoo Settings

Wild Animals in our Changing World

Stereotypes or repetitive behaviors are postulated to arise in animals in artificial environments that do not meet their behavioral needs. However, it is possible for similar aberrant behaviors, even if not true stereotypies, to manifest in natural environments that have been either directly or indirectly manipulated by humans. With our changing environment, increasing global populations, and exploding human-wildlife interactions, even wild animals within their natural environment can demonstrate abnormal and aberrant mannerisms that are ultimately disruptive to their functioning and survival.

When we think of human induced stressors for wild animals, we think of the well-documented human–animal interactions that suggest these encounters are acutely impacting individuals and subtly deleterious for the species impacted over time. Examples include animal–motor vehicle encounters (e.g. deer or kangaroos; Figure 19.4) that typically result in the death of the animal, or local deforestation that displaces cohorts of high site fidelity species (e.g. koalas), causing stress-induced pathologies to enter the population and weaken the species' overall fitness. Some human-based changes may not be as obvious, yet they can still negatively impact a wild species. They do so by changing the environment sufficiently so as to alter the long-term learned behavior of individuals living within it, giving rise to abnormal behaviors.

Examples of this type of abnormal behavior in wild animals under human influences are not well-documented in the literature. However, known occurrences include populations of manatees and sea turtles near large infrastructures and individuals "rogue" elephants near villages.

The Florida manatee is a threatened species with fewer than 10,000 remaining individuals. Threats to survival include entanglement, watercraft interactions, harmful algal blooms, and loss of warm water refuges. The former two are caused by humans increased activity in waterways used by manatees, but the latter two are a result of larger scale environmental changes: agricultural activities causing nutrient run-off into waterways, which then fuels deadly algal blooms; and the retirement of artificial warm water refuges inhabited by manatees during the colder winter months, which cause a generational shift in behavior that results in seasonal spikes in morbidity and mortality. Manatees cannot tolerate waters below 20°C/68°F and are subject to cold stress syndrome. During the coldest part of winter, they seek warm water refuges from thermal upwellings, natural springs, and the discharge canals of powerplants. Since the advent of artificial warm water refuges in the 1960s, manatees have learned to preferentially use these sites over natural springs and thermals due to location and have altered their annual migration patterns to these discharge canals. As modern power stations replace these power plants and their associated warm water refuges, the abnormal behavior that has been conditioned over several generations to go to these refuges each winter no longer leads them to safety. As these plants shut down, generations of manatees are left not knowing the

(a) (b)

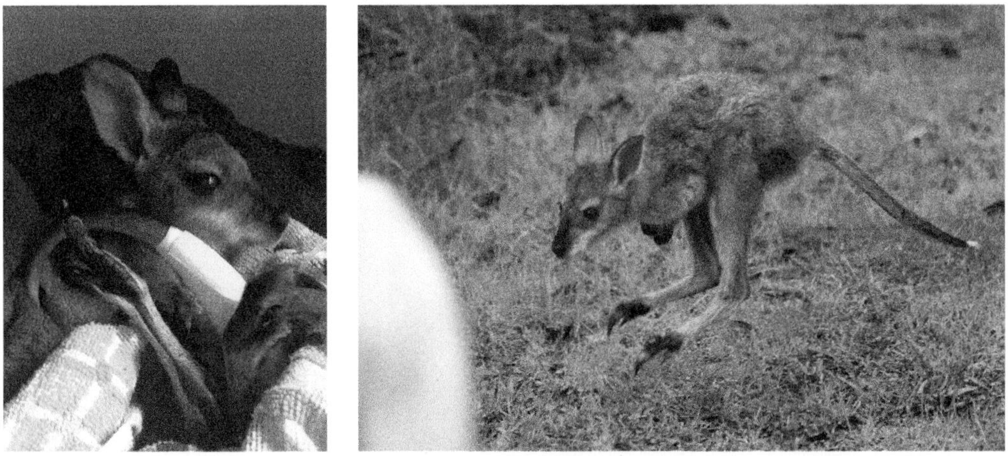

Figure 19.4 A baby eastern-grey kangaroo (*Macropus giganteus*) who received a fractured pelvis and tail when in the pouch of his mother who was hit and killed by a car in an area of heavy urbanization and wildlife displacement at (a) time of treatment and (b) after healing during fostering. *Source:* With permission from Mark Flint.

alternative historic natural sites to utilize and are susceptible to cold stress as winter water temperatures drop with no known refuge to annually migrate to (Bonde and Flint 2017).

Similar generational negative effects on behaviors have been seen in sea turtles returning to nest on natal beaches. It is believed they imprint on these beaches as hatchlings, but significant changes to the skyline (e.g. buildings) or wave current from altered water courses prevent their ability to identify their natal beach. The females ultimately resorb their clutches and fail to lay that season (Patrício et al. 2021).

Further, sea turtles are subject to an even greater anthropogenic induced change altering their innate behavior – climate change causing beach sand temperatures to become suboptimal for incubating eggs (Patrício et al. 2021). Turtles are changing their natal beach nesting behavior and finding beaches with cooler sand temperatures in novel areas. This generation shift will likely influence future generations as they imprint on these new beaches. Coupled with the rapid elevation in global temperatures, today's hatchlings may not be able to use their natal beach for nesting. The behavioral drivers that navigated turtles to their traditional natal beaches for thousands of years will be lost and subsequently replaced by abnormal nomadic nesting adaptations as a means of coping with the human-induced stressors. Nomadic lifestyles are postulated to lead to higher likelihoods of misadventure, detrimentally impacting sea turtle populations (Figure 19.5).

Finally, it has been reported that villages in Indian and African regional areas have increasingly been subject to "rogue" elephant attacks (Huggler 2006). These attacks are postulated to be caused by a myriad of reasons. In some cases, there are social herd dynamics displacing an individual elephant in a local village. While in other cases, it is the village activities that encroach on traditional elephant territory and then lead to "revenge" attacks by elephants on people for doing them harm. The latter two reasons are stressors caused by people resulting in abnormal behavior of animals in the wild.

Wildlife Used in Research

When one thinks of wild animals in laboratory research settings, negative images of monkeys in cages or rats in metabolic chambers spring to mind. These have been well covered in the literature on the repetitive and negative behaviors that can be caused and the welfare implications for the individual under such conditions (Bayne et al. 2014).

What is not as well-documented but is equally important is the influence on behavior and welfare of free-ranging wild animals used in research. Both authors of this chapter research wild animals in their natural habitats. Doing so, we interact with arboreal and aquatic

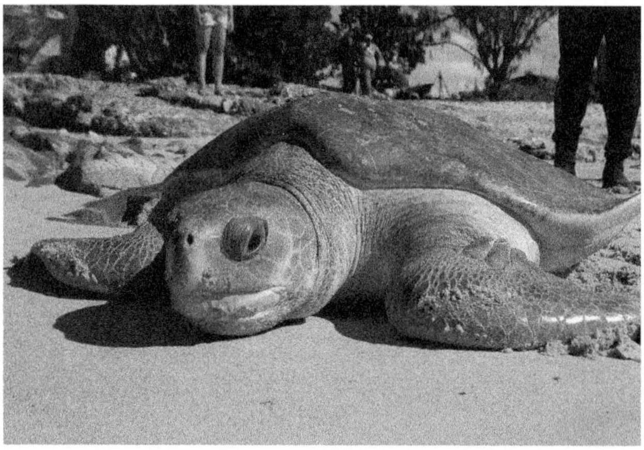

Figure 19.5 A flatback turtle (*Natator depressus*) found in waters at the cusp of its normal habitat range in central Queensland in 2008. There is growing evidence that nesting female turtles in Australia are starting to nest further south, using cooler sands to combat increased climate change-induced sand temperatures. Higher sand temperatures are feminizing populations in these temperature-related sex-determined species and are not compatible with successful incubation. *Source:* With permission from Mark Flint.

species in ways that could negatively impact the individual and the population if care was not taken. For example, if we were to capture an animal and use sedation without allowing full recovery in a safe place before release, the animal may be subject to misadventure or exposed to attack by their cohorts for smelling (of anesthesia) or behaving oddly. Similarly, some of the activities we undertake, such as placing radio transmitters, may impede movement or create a trapping hazard. This can draw attention to predators by causing an odd gait or swimming pattern or reduce the ability to swim/climb/run to keep up with its cohorts. This may result in isolation and dissociation from the group. Finally, examinations inducing capture-stress may disrupt natural cycles, like suppressing follicular development by catching at the start of breeding season or causing muscle damage (capture-stress myopathy) that reduces fitness (Figure 19.6).

To overcome these issues, all research conducted on free-ranging wildlife should include considerations including the types of drugs used to secure the animal; the size, weight, and placement of any monitoring devices (e.g. radiocollars); and the seasonality of any studies and capture-duration that may cause stress. All animals should be monitored not only for clinical signs of health prior to release, but also behaviorally as a function of their immediate and long-term welfare of the animal.

Prevention, Management, and Treatment

The best approach to control any disease is to prevent it from occurring in the first place. This is also true for abnormal behaviors. Ideally, regardless of whether the species is displayed, worked, farmed or in the wild, strategies to prevent the development of abnormal behaviors should be employed from the outset. However, the incorporation of welfare into human care endeavors involving animals is a relatively new concept borne from Ruth Harrison's *Animal Machines* in 1964. This groundbreaking book potentiated the Brambell Report in 1965, which first outlined the Five Freedoms (evolving into the Five Domains by 1994) (Harrison 1964; Brambell 1965; Mellor et al. 2020). So, it can be forgiven that preventive measures to stop poor behaviors and welfare developing in any animals, especially wild animals, under human care is only a recent concept. With that, managers of wild animals under human care are playing catch up to first understand what a normal, often subtle, behavior in a wild species is, and then how to weigh and incorporate that understanding into everyday management. Ethograms, comparative natural environment studies, health, allostatic loads, and anecdotal learnings can all be employed to quantify a preventive medicine regime. These regimes are often

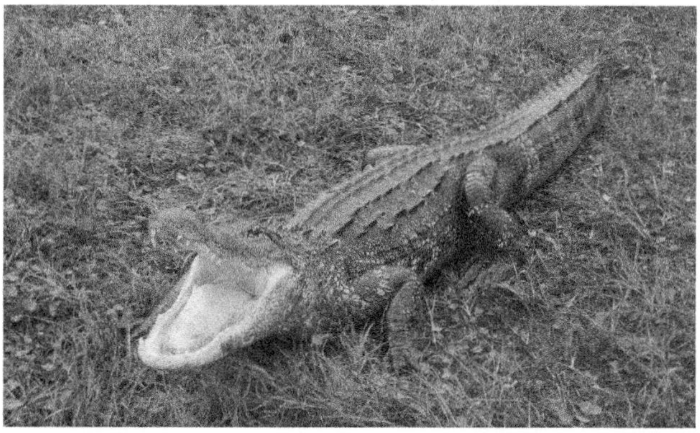

Figure 19.6 Free-ranging adult female American alligator at the start of breeding season showing defensive behaviors after being released from veterinary examination to determine reproductive status. Without care, this disturbance could disrupt her annual breeding cycle. *Source:* With permission from Jeffrey D. Miller/Biological Research and Education Consultants.

dynamic and should be adjusted as needed to refine and respond to changes as we learn more along the continuum of our gained knowledge. All regimes should include input from animal handlers, nutritionists, researchers, and animal health staff to be as holistic as practical.

Clinical veterinarians may be asked to assist in the management and/or elimination of repetitive behaviors in animals. These behaviors may be injurious (over-grooming, self-mutilation), objectionable (pacing), or interfere with normal behaviors or activities (inappropriate chewing or licking).

Attempts to eliminate or modify repetitive behaviors require a fundamental understanding of the origins (cause) of the behaviors. Attempts to eliminate behaviors without addressing the root cause will almost universally fail. Is an animal pacing because it is bored, or is it fearful and trying to escape the discomfort? Is the animal fearful of the environment, such as threatening animals nearby, loud noises, or large crowds?

Zoo animals' repetitive behaviors are likely related to factors in their environment. These include frustrated motivations to perform specific behaviors, paucity of behavioral opportunities, lack of sensory stimulation, and stress (Swaisgood and Shepherdson 2006). Regardless of the origin, addressing the concern begins with a thorough behavioral analysis (as described in Chapter 12). With a little creativity, the ABC's of a behavioral history may be applied to nondomestic animals. It is important to identify the Antecedent (A), or trigger, that initiates the behavior. Observant staff members will be able to identify an event (feeding, shifting, other animals, and crowds) that triggers the behavior. The behavior (B) should be described accurately by identifying verifiable facts (“**phenotypic description**”) rather than opinion or interpretation. For instance, “he paces when there are crowds” rather than “he hates people”. The final component is consequence (C). Some consequences are reinforcing (e.g. given extra food), which may further encourage the behavior.

Ideally, a complete medical evaluation should be performed at the onset. This examination should be designed to eliminate any underlying health concerns, as well as establish the animals health in case pharmacologic intervention is needed. Systemic illness may create debility or compromise that is distressful to an animal, resulting in repetitive behaviors as a coping mechanism. Specific etiologies, such as dental disease or fractures, or arthritis of limbs or spine, may alter normal behaviors, potentially resulting in misinterpretation.

Once underlying health issues are eliminated the repetitive behaviors can be addressed directly. Removal of the initiating cause is ideal but not always possible, either because it cannot be identified or cannot be reasonably eliminated. Modifications of the environment may mitigate or reduce stereotypies by increasing exploratory behavior, providing security, or reducing boredom (Figure 19.7). For zoo exhibited animals, providing seclusion or shelter may provide the feeling of security that is lacking.

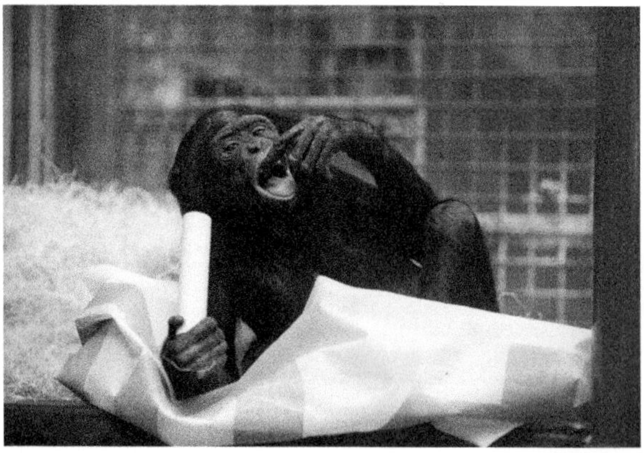

Figure 19.7 Bonobo (*Pan paniscus*). Enrichment activities such as puzzle feeders stimulate problem-solving behaviors in animals in human care. This activity can also mimic natural foraging behaviors. *Source:* With permission from A. Carberry / Columbus Zoo and Aquarium.

Environmental enrichment and training are valuable tools for reducing stress in animals under human care. When placed into limited environments and provided access to adequate food and access to (or elimination of) breeding partners, much of the stimulus for normal behaviors is eliminated. Enrichment and training may prevent those from being replaced by stereotypies. Enrichment consists of anything that engages an animal in something resembling natural behaviors, such as feeder puzzles or exhibit furniture. Training provides mental stimulation to animals and allows bonding with caretakers. Training also provides management opportunities by utilizing behaviors to perform exams, take weight measurements, or allow injections or blood collection opportunities (Figure 19.8). Enrichment strategies have been classified into the following categories (from Swaisgood and Shepherdson 2006):

- Mimicking nature – efforts to mimic the natural environmental factors to stimulate natural behaviors.
- Increasing physical complexity of the environment – efforts to promote exploration and sensory stimulation to encourage appropriate behaviors.
- Increasing sensory stimulation – to stimulate exploration, investigation, and increased natural behaviors.
- Meeting specific frustrated motivation – for example, increasing foraging for animals that appear to have repetitive behaviors related to lack of foraging.
- Removing sources of stress – changing exhibits or routines to minimize or remove a stressful situation (crowds, competition, and proximity).
- Giving the animal control – Puzzles or rewards for specific behaviors.

Pharmacologic intervention may be necessary and should be considered an appropriate tool if used properly. Psychopharmacology should not be the first or only management step for modifying behaviors but certainly have a place. In some instances, the calming effects

(a) (b)

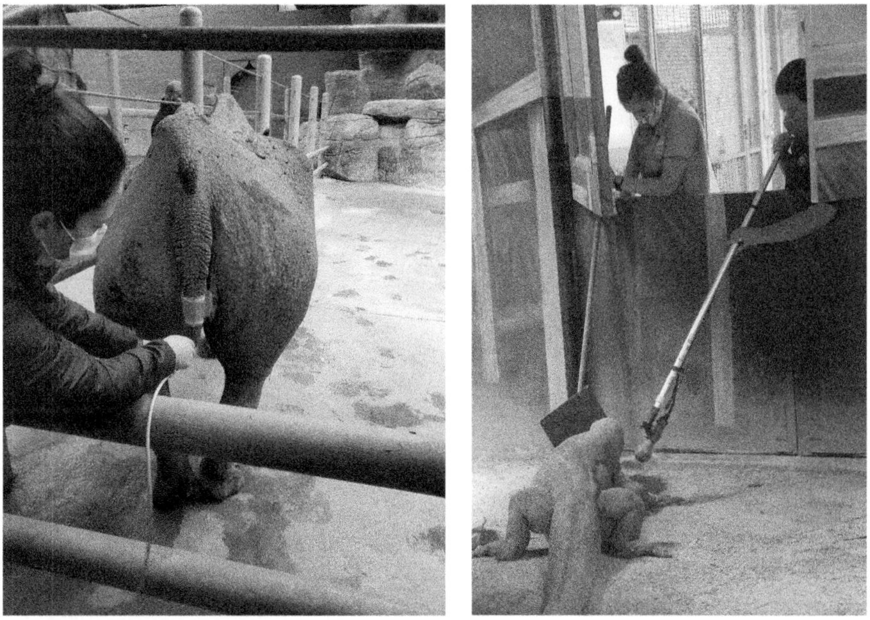

Figure 19.8 Conditioned behaviors allow medical procedures to be completed without additional stress of restraint or anesthesia. The black rhinoceros (a) (*Diceros bicornis*) is cooperating with voluntary blood pressure monitoring to manage hypertension. The Komodo dragon (b) (*Varanus komodoensis*) is conditioned to target the green square, allowing the veterinarian to apply laser therapy to an arthritic elbow. *Source:* Randy Junge/Columbus Zoo and Aquarium.

of tranquilizing agents can eliminate early or mild behaviors. Such medications may be given prophylactically in situations likely to cause stress for animals known to develop stereotypies. In some instances, repetitive behaviors may be long-established and deeply entrenched and continue beyond the elimination of stressors. In these cases, medication may be required to break the repetitive cycle.

There are a variety of psychotropic drugs available in veterinary and human medical fields. These work by different mechanisms and are recommended for modifying specific types of behavior such as anxiety, nervousness, compulsive behavior, and fearfulness (see Chapter 21 for more details). It is often difficult to define animal behaviors into these categories, and often behaviors overlap in cause and origin. Types of drugs and potential applications to wild animal species under human care are discussed in depth elsewhere (Marder and Posage 2005; Mills and Luescher 2006). Evaluation of the efficacy of medical management can be challenging. Often, dosing adjustments are needed to achieve the desired effect. If a chosen medication is not effective, consider trying a different compound with a different mode of action or target behavior. Often, several medications or doses are trialed before the desired effect is reached.

Medical intervention is a useful adjunct used in parallel with environmental or management changes that eliminate or reduce repetitive behaviors. It should not be used in the place of other modifications to reduce or eliminate the stimulus of repetitive behaviors. They may be initiated early in the process in order to prevent the behaviors from getting deeply ingrained. In all cases, the eventual goal is for medication to be gradually eliminated or at least greatly reduced. See Figures 19.9 and 19.10 for a breakdown of how to approach abnormal repetitive behaviors in wild animals under human care.

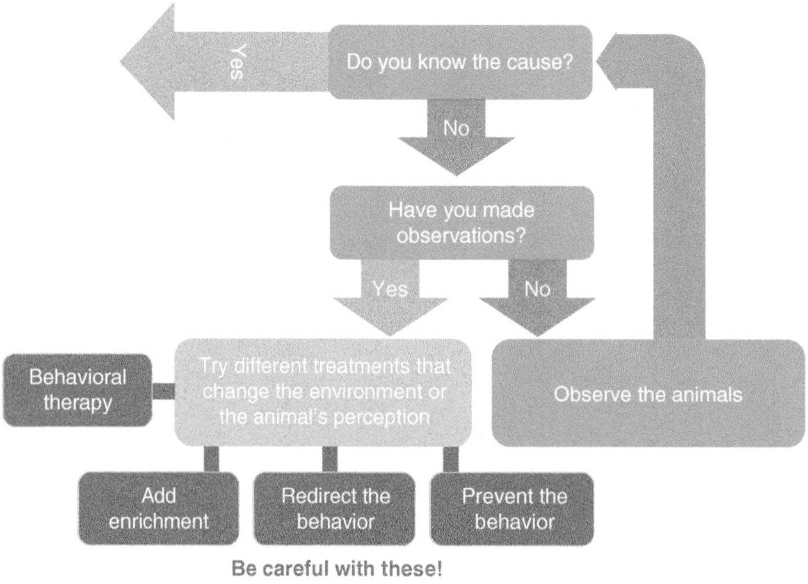

Figure 19.9 Diagram of how to proceed with a management and treatment plan for abnormal repetitive behaviors when you are not able to identify the root cause. Careful observation is required to determine which interventions may be most useful. When a cause cannot be identified, different treatments can be attempted to change the environment or the animal's perception. Be cautious with making major environmental changes abruptly or dramatically, as this can serve as an added stressor rather than an aide.

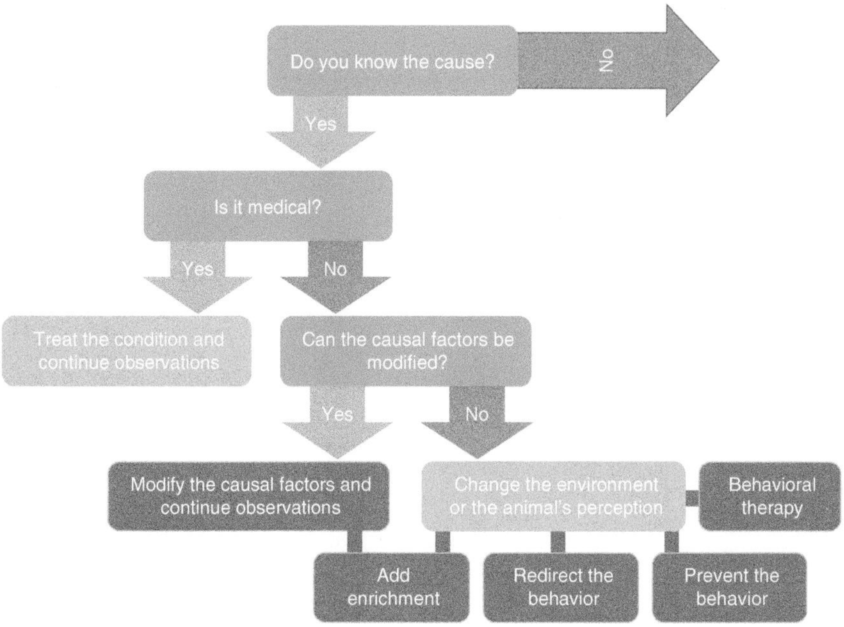

Figure 19.10 Diagram of how to proceed with a management and treatment plan for abnormal repetitive behaviors when you can identify the root cause. Differentiating and addressing medical etiologies is the first step toward addressing the cause before proceeding with behavioral intervention.

Conclusion

Repetitive or abnormal behaviors in wild animals under human care are undesirable occurrences as they signify an underlying stressor. Stress is often exacerbated by our limited detailed understanding of the exact social, behavioral, environmental, and physiological needs of the species under our charge. However, by carefully characterizing the behavior being observed in context of the holistic approach through frameworks such as the Five Domains, it is possible to try to understand the underlying cause and prevent or eliminate it. To best characterize, a suite of tools, including behavioral observation, clinical pathology, environmental assessment, and species-specific needs, can be employed. In this chapter, we defined how to identify aberrant behaviors and the associated limitations in wild animals, and identified several potential repetitive or abnormal behaviors that can occur under a range of circumstances where wild animals are under human influence, both direct and indirect. We suggested potential causes of these behaviors and clinical approaches to preventing and eliminating them. As with all species expressing abnormal behaviors, we cautioned our interpretation should be dynamic as we learn more about the animals under our care.

References

Anon (2021). Military marine mammals. https://en.wikipedia.org/wiki/Military_marine_mammal (accessed 01 May 2022).

Bayne, K.A.L., Turner, P.V., and American College of Laboratory Animal Medicine (2014). *Laboratory Animal Welfare*. Amsterdam; Boston: Elsevier/AP.

Bergeron, R., Badnell-Waters, A.J., Lambton, S., and Mason, G. (2006). Stereotypic oral behavior in captive ungulates: foraging, diet and gastrointestinal function. In: *Stereotypic Animal Behaviour- Fundamentals and Applications to Welfare*, 2e (ed. G. Mason and J. Rushen), 19–57. Wallingford UK: CABI.

Bonde, R.K. and Flint, M. (2017). Human interactions with sirenians. In: *Marine Mammal Welfare*, 299–314. Bristol: Springer International Publishing.

Brambell, R. (1965). Report of the Technical Committee to Enquire Into the Welfare of Animals Kept Under Intensive Livestock Husbandry Systems, Cmd. London, UK, Great Britain, Parliament: 1-84.

Clubb, R. and Vickery, S. (2006). Locomotory stereotypies in carnivores: does pacing stem from hunting, ranging or frustrated escape? In: *Stereotypic Animal Behaviour- Fundamentals and Applications to Welfare*, 2e (ed. G. Mason and J. Rushen), 58–85. Wallingford UK: CABI.

Dwyer, C.M. (2004). How has the risk of predation shaped the behavioural responses of sheep to fear and distress? *Anim. Welf.* 13 (3): 269–281.

Edes, A.N., Wolfe, B.A., and Crews, D.E. (2018). The first multi-zoo application of an allostatic load index to western lowland gorillas (*Gorilla gorilla gorilla*). *Gen. Comp. Endocrinol.* 266: 135–149.

Ericcson, M. and Jensen, P. (2016). Domestication and ontogeny effects on the stress response in young chickens (*Gallus gallus*). *Sci. Rep.* 6: https://doi.org/10.1038/srep35818.

FAWC (2009). *Farm Animal Welfare in Great Britain: Past, Present and Future*, 1–70. London: Farm Animal Welfare Council.

Fischer, C.P. and Romero, L.P. (2018). Chronic captivity stress in wild animals is highly species-specific. *Conser. Physiol.* 7 (1): https://doi.org/10.1093/conphys/coz1093.

Flint, M. and Bonde, R.K. (2017). Assessing welfare in individual sirenians in the wild and in captivity. In: *Marine Mammal Welfare* (ed. A. Butterworth), 381–393. Bristol: Springer.

Harrison, R. (1964). *Animal Machines.* London: FSC.

Hartigan, P. (2005). A primer on stress-related pathology 5. Allostatic load and the periparturient dairy cow. *Irish Vet. J.* 58 (4): 224–232.

Huggler, J. (2006). Animal behaviour: rogue elephants. https://www.independent.co.uk/climate-change/news/animal-behaviour-rogue-elephants-5330885.html (accessed 01 May 2022).

Lyons, C. (2016). Beasts of war. https://warfarehistorynetwork.com/2016/05/29/beasts-of-war/ (accessed 01 May 2022).

Marder, A. and Posage, J. (2005). Treatment of emotional distress and disorders – pharmacologic methods. In: *Mental Health and Well-being in Animals* (ed. F. McMillan), 159–166. Ames: Blackwell Publishing.

Mellor, D.J., Beausoleil, N.J., Littlewood, K.E. et al. (2020). The 2020 five domains model: including human–animal interactions in assessments of animal welfare. *Animals* 10 (10): 1870.

Menon, D.G., Bennett, D.C., and Cheng, K.M. (2014). Understanding the behavior of domestic emus: a means to improve their management and welfare—major behaviors and activity time budgets of adult emus. *J. Anim.* 2014: https://doi.org/10.1155/2014/938327.

Mills, D. and Luescher, A. (2006). Veterinary and pharmacological approaches to abnormal repetitive behavior. In: *Stereotypic Animal Behaviour- Fundamentals and Applications to Welfare*, 2e (ed. G. Mason and J. Rushen), 286–324. Wallingford UK: CABI.

Mortimer, J.A. (1995). Headstarting as a management tool. In: *Biology and Conservation of Sea Turtles* (ed. K.A. Bjorndal), 613–615. Washington, DC: Smithsonian Institution Press.

Nossov, K. (2012). *War Elephants.* Oxford: Osprey Publishing.

Patrício, A., Hawkes, L.A., Monsinjon, J.R. et al. (2021). Climate change and marine turtles: recent advances and future directions. *Endangered Species Research* 44: 363–395.

PBS (2014). The story of Navy dolphins. https://www.pbs.org/wgbh/pages/frontline/shows/whales/etc/navycron.html (accessed 01 May 2022).

Seeley, K.E., Proudfoot, K.L., Wolfe, B., and Crews, D.E. (2021). Assessing allostatic load in ring-tailed Lemurs (*Lemur catta*). *Animals (Basel)* 11 (11): 3074.

Swaisgood, R. and Shepherdson, D. (2006). Environmental enrichment as a strategy for mitigating stereotypies in zoo animals: a literature review and meta-analysis. In: *Stereotypic Animal Behaviour: Fundamentals and Applications to Welfare*, 256–285. CABI.

Turner, M. (1997). Towards an executive dysfunction account of repetitive behaviour in autism. In: *Autism as an Executive Disorder*, 57–100. Oxford University Press.

Webb, G.J.W. (2021). *Saltwater Crocodiles of the Northern Territory- Past, Present and Future*. Darwin: Colemans Printing.

Winn, P. (2017). War elephants still exist. But only in one forbidding place. https://theworld.org/stories/2017-02-27/war-elephants-still-exist-only-one-forbidding-place (accessed 01 May 2022).

20

Repetitive and Other Abnormal Behaviors in Livestock and Horses

Emily Miller-Cushon and Carissa Wickens

University of Florida, Department of Animal Sciences, Gainesville, FL, USA

Introduction

Behavior serves as an important tool for understanding an animal's health status and emotional state. Changes in natural behavior can provide early insight into developing disease or experiences of pain. Mindfulness of these behavioral changes can help identify clinical conditions (e.g. lameness scoring in dairy cattle). Behavior coinciding with painful procedures or disease is additionally observed in detail in research settings to establish a basis for understanding how animals experience pain, and how behavior may be incorporated in clinical examinations. Insufficient opportunity to engage in natural behavior for which animals are highly driven to perform can contribute to the development of abnormal repetitive behaviors, which have powerful implications for animal health. This section provides an overview of those behaviors, as well as behavioral indicators of sickness and pain, with examples drawn from horses and livestock species.

Behavioral Indicators of Sickness

Animals respond to developing illness with behavioral changes which function to conserve energy and mount an immune response (Hart 1988), and many behavioral changes coinciding with a febrile response, including lethargy and decreased appetite, are consistent across species.

Changes in rest and lying time may coincide with developing disease, although the nature of these changes may depend on the medical condition (Tucker et al. 2021). Lame dairy cows display increases in lying time, which suggests a greater motivation to lie down, whereas dairy cows with mastitis, an infection of the udder, decrease lying time, likely due to pain associated with pressure in this region. Therefore, duration of rest is not a straightforward indicator of welfare, although individual changes in behavior may be indicative of a problem.

Reduced feed intake is a widespread response to disease. Lame dairy cows exhibit decreases in feeding time as well as increases in feeding rate (Norring et al. 2014). Compared to healthy animals, morbid steers in feedlots will spend less time at the feed bunk, have fewer meals, and have a higher latency to begin feeding (Sowell et al. 1999). Sick dairy calves may reduce milk intake and consume milk more slowly (Borderas et al. 2009).

During subclinical and early stages of disease, animals will also reduce performance of behaviors that are less essential for survival, including play and social interactions. In a

Introduction to Animal Behavior and Veterinary Behavioral Medicine, First Edition. Edited by Meghan E. Herron.

Companion website: www.wiley.com/go/introductiontoanimalbehavior

more recent study, dairy calves subjected to an experimental respiratory disease challenge spent less time grooming and interacting socially, in addition to consuming less feed and spending more time resting (Hixson et al. 2018).

Behavioral Indicators of Pain

Behavioral changes can provide insight into the emotional experience of pain. They also provide important evidence to support provision of anesthetics and analgesics for routine painful procedures, including castration, disbudding/dehorning, and tail docking, which affect different livestock species. Painful procedures and conditions can result in spontaneous indicators of pain, such as changes in body posture and changes in normal behaviors, which may also resemble changes coinciding with disease. In addition, elicited indicators can provide insight into pain experienced in a particular region.

Some indicators of pain are elicited, including behavioral responses to palpation during examination and nociceptive responses when stimulated. It is common to examine animals with palpation during veterinary exams, and reactions to pressure can be a meaningful indicator of pain and sensitivity in a particular region. For example, Stojkov et al. (2015) found that when cows received rectal palpation, with and without uterine palpation, those with metritis (uterine infection post-calving) had a greater degree of back arch, suggesting that this may be an indicator of visceral pain. Pressure algometry is a useful tool used to assess sensitivity in specific regions. This involves quantifying the amount of pressure an animal will tolerate in a specific area, before moving away. For example, use of pressure algometry has revealed sensitivity in the area of a dairy calf's hornbud up to three weeks after disbudding (Adcock and Tucker 2018).

In addition to elicited indicators of pain, there is a wide range of spontaneous behavioral changes associated with pain, including changes in normal behavior and specific responses in the area of localized pain. For example, dairy calves reduce play behavior in response to pain following disbudding (Mintline et al. 2013; Špinka et al. 2001), an example of a change in duration of a normal behavior, and also increase ear flicks, a localized response to discomfort in a specific region. In horses, weight shifting, toe pointing, toe touching, biting at a limb, and excessive time spent recumbently indicate orthopedic pain. Horses experiencing abdominal pain can bite, paw, grind their teeth, flehmen, bite at their flank, stretch out, or roll. Ocular pain often manifests in squinting, excess tear production, rubbing of the eye(s) on a forelimb or nearby object, tilting of the head, or low head carriage. Horses in pain due to injury or illness may also become withdrawn and uninterested in their surroundings.

Understanding of these behavioral changes has been established through the use of continuous observation in research, but may also be assessed visually through brief observation of animals. For example, it may be quickly apparent that an animal seems uncomfortable, lethargic, or is moving in an unusual way. In some cases, behavior is a main diagnostic tool in the identification of injury. Lameness scoring in dairy cattle is used widely to identify animals with injuries and hoof problems. This scoring tool involves assessment of the evenness of the gait and animal posture, including back arch, as they walk.

In various species, **grimace scales** have been developed as an indicator of systemic pain. In cattle, Gleerup et al. (2015) describe a grimace scale based on ear posture, tension of muscles around eyes and evidence of "furrow lines," tension of facial muscles on the side of the head, and dilation of nostrils (Figure 20.1). Those authors found that grimace scale was affected by painful states, including lameness and post-surgical pain, and responded to analgesia.

Recently, the development and implementation of scoring systems to monitor and address pain in horses have received increased attention

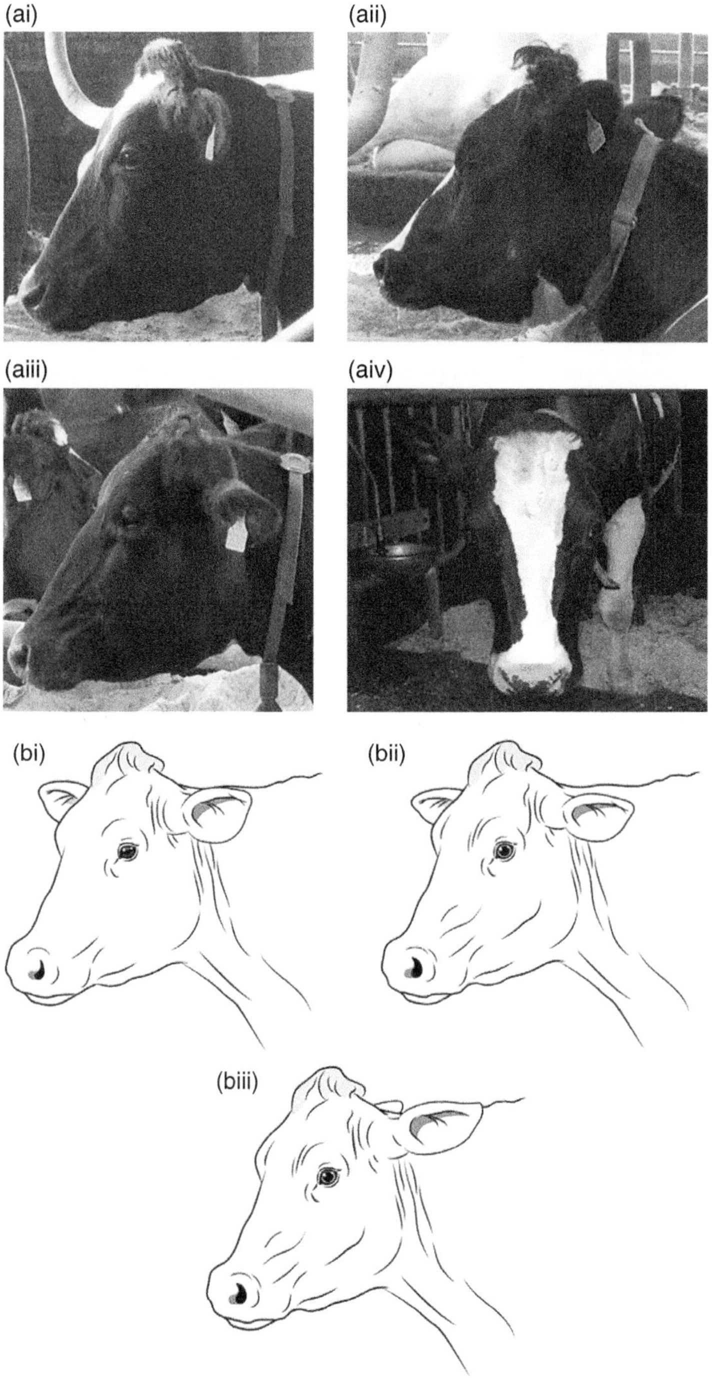

Figure 20.1 (a) Photos of a cow relaxing, not in pain (i), and three cows in pain: lameness (ii), compromised vascular system, udder sore, few and week peristaltic movements (iii), and post-surgical pain after rumen fistulation (iv). The features of the pain face of the cow comprise changes in four areas: (1) Ears: ears are tense and backwards (ii) or low/lambs ears (iii). (2) Eyes: eyes have a tense stare (ii + iv) or a withdrawn appearance (iii). Tension of the muscles above the eyes may be seen as "furrow lines" (iii + iv). (3) Facial muscles: tension of the facial muscles on the side of the head (ii + iii). (4) Muzzle: strained nostrils, the nostrils may be dilated, and there may be "lines" above the nostrils. There is increased tonus of the lips (ii + iii + iv). *Source:* Reproduced from Gleerup et al. (2015), with permission from Elsevier. (b) Illustrations of the Cow Pain Face. The scientific illustrations aim at accentuating the important changes in the facial expression without disturbances of the specific cow's individual expression. (i) Relaxed cow. (ii) Cow in pain with low ears/lambs ears. (iii) Cow in pain with ears tense and backwards. Illustrations Anders Rådén. *Source:* Reproduced with permission from Gleerup et al. (2015)/ELSEVIER.

in research and clinical settings. Specific methods and resources for identifying and monitoring pain include, but are not limited to, the Horse Grimace Scale (Dalla et al. 2014) (Figure 20.2), the Equine Discomfort Ethogram (Torcivia and McDonnell 2021 [https://www.mdpi.com/2076-2615/11/2/580]), and the Horse Chronic Pain Scale (HCPS; van Loon and Macri 2021). Horses may show reduced behavioral indicators of pain when people are present; thus the use of video recording and remote behavior monitoring can be helpful.

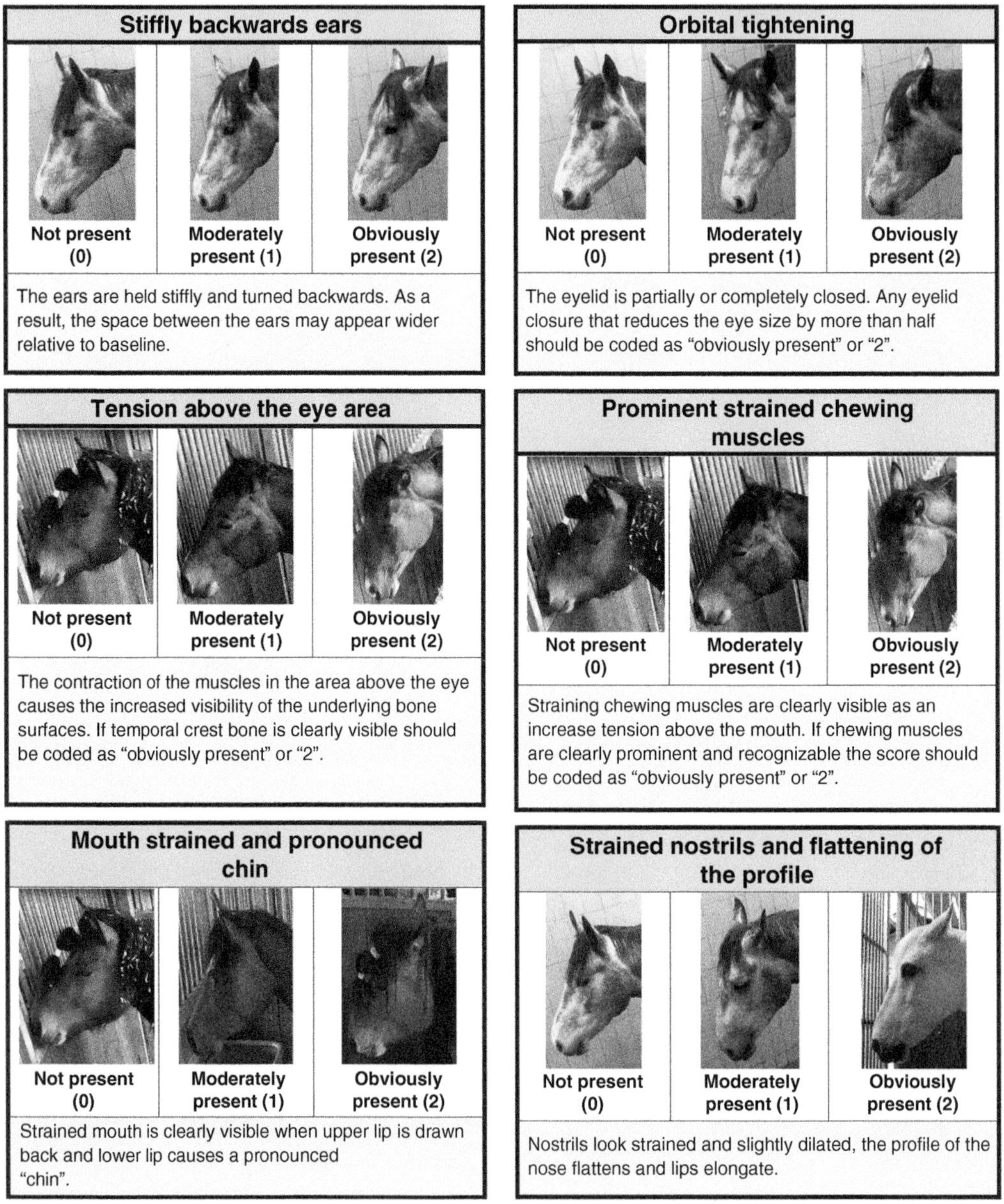
Stiffly backwards ears
Not present (0)
Moderately present (1)
Obviously present (2)
The ears are held stiffly and turned backwards. As a result, the space between the ears may appear wider relative to baseline.
Orbital tightening
Not present (0)
Moderately present (1)
Obviously present (2)
The eyelid is partially or completely closed. Any eyelid closure that reduces the eye size by more than half should be coded as "obviously present" or "2".
Tension above the eye area
Not present (0)
Moderately present (1)
Obviously present (2)
The contraction of the muscles in the area above the eye causes the increased visibility of the underlying bone surfaces. If temporal crest bone is clearly visible should be coded as "obviously present" or "2".
Prominent strained chewing muscles
Not present (0)
Moderately present (1)
Obviously present (2)
Straining chewing muscles are clearly visible as an increase tension above the mouth. If chewing muscles are clearly prominent and recognizable the score should be coded as "obviously present" or "2".
Mouth strained and pronounced chin
Not present (0)
Moderately present (1)
Obviously present (2)
Strained mouth is clearly visible when upper lip is drawn back and lower lip causes a pronounced "chin".
Strained nostrils and flattening of the profile
Not present (0)
Moderately present (1)
Obviously present (2)
Nostrils look strained and slightly dilated, the profile of the nose flattens and lips elongate.

Figure 20.2 Horse Grimace Pain Scale (HGS): The Horse Grimace Pain Scale with images and explanations for each of the six facial action units (FAUs). Each FAU is scored according to whether it is not present (score of 0), moderately present (score of 1) and obliviously present (score of 2). *Source:* Dalla et al. (2014)/ PLOS ONE / CC BY 4.0.

Cognitive Approaches to Understanding Emotional States

Considerable research effort in recent years has gone toward understanding emotional states in livestock, including pain as well as other negative states, such as fear. Cognitive approaches provide the most direct means to understanding pervasive mood states in animals. In a research setting, these cognitive tests provide convincing evidence that pain is a negative conscious experience and may have consequences for pervasive mood. The tests described in this section draw on methodology developed in the field of psychology and are generally practical to conduct only in a research setting, but these findings have important implications for how pain is understood and should be mitigated in a clinical setting.

Individual perceptions of pain, or other experiences, can be assessed through conditioned place preference tests. These tests involve two steps. First, through repeated exposure, animals acquire a learned association between different stimuli (differing in discriminative cues, such as color, pattern, and physical location) and an experience (such as the effects of a pain-mitigating drug). Second, preference for time spent near each stimulus is assessed. This provides a means to assess preference for an experience, such as pain relief. For example, in work described by Adcock and Tucker (2020), dairy calves learned that when they approached a colored panel (either white or black) in their home pen, they received a lidocaine cornual nerve block, whereas approaching the contrasting visual stimulus was associated with a control injection of saline. These authors then found that, following hot iron disbudding, calves were more likely to spend time near the visual stimulus associated with a lidocaine injection, compared to calves that received a sham disbudding procedure only. Findings like this provide convincing evidence that pain is a conscious experience that animals prefer to avoid.

There is also evidence that pain more generally causes negative judgment bias, or, in other words, pessimism. Pessimistic states are generally linked with negative moods, including depression in humans. Cognitive approaches to assessing judgment bias in animals can involve a go/no go task, where animals learn to approach a certain stimulus for a reward, and not approach the contrasting stimulus. Once this learning task is acquired, animals are presented with an ambiguous stimulus, and their response is recorded. For example, Neave et al. (2013) conducted a test where dairy calves learned to approach a colored screen (randomly assigned to be either red or white) in order to receive a reward of some milk, and they learned to not approach the contrasting cue (opposite color). Calves were then presented with screens that were shades in between red and white, which was an ambiguous cue. These authors found that, after calves were disbudded, they became less likely to approach the ambiguous cue. This suggests that those animals were more pessimistic, because they were less likely to interpret an ambiguous cue as being associated with a likely reward, suggesting that pain was associated with pessimism. This suggests that pain is not simply an unpleasant physical sensation, but an experience that has more general effects on mood. Similar work has been conducted with horses to evaluate affective state (Fureix et al. 2015) with results demonstrating a depression-like state characterized by withdrawn posture, lack of response to environmental stimuli, and reduced intake of sucrose (a measure of anhedonia).

Importance of Meeting Behavioral Needs

Good animal welfare depends on more than health and freedom from pain. Providing opportunities for motivated natural behaviors is critical for all animals. The basic concept of "behavioral needs" and indicators that they are not being met is described by Hughes and Duncan (1988). While behavioral needs are species-dependent, these involve some core elements, including opportunity for naturalistic foraging behavior and social interaction for naturally gregarious livestock species. Consequences of preventing expression of important behaviors are broad but can include increased fearfulness and frustration and development of abnormal behaviors.

Most species used for livestock production today are naturally gregarious, meaning that their evolutionary ancestors were social and that they would choose to reside in social groups under natural settings. However, livestock production occasionally involves periods of social isolation, for some specific procedure or phase of production, and some livestock species are routinely housed individually. In general, social isolation in livestock species is associated with a range of problematic behavioral outcomes, including fearfulness and development of abnormal behaviors. For example, dairy calves are reared in individual pens for the first weeks of life on some farms, and this practice can result in increased fearfulness, avoidance of novel objects and feeds, and even deficits in learning ability (reviewed by Costa et al. 2016). In the equine industry, stallions and performance horses are often housed singly in individual box stalls or small paddocks for extended periods of the day, under management conditions which limit social contact with other horses.

Livestock species are also motivated to perform aspects of natural foraging behavior, including searching for and manipulating feed. However, conventional livestock production often involves provision of high-quality and readily available feeds, which require no searching or exploration to acquire and less time to ingest. Prevention of opportunities for naturalistic foraging is also associated with a range of abnormal oral behaviors across various livestock species, which are described in detail later in this chapter. In general, it is well understood that provision of enrichments, resources that allow opportunity for natural behaviors and broader behavioral expression, is a means to improve animal welfare. This can involve access to social companions, opportunities for natural foraging or activities that mimic aspects of natural feeding behavior, and other opportunities to interact with objects or resources that facilitate any behavior – play, task completion, locomotor activities, grooming, and so on. Opportunity for broad behavioral expression can benefit emotional state. For example, sheep housed in an enriched environment, with greater space and more resources than sheep in standard housing, showed evidence of greater optimism when tested in a judgment bias task (Stephenson and Haskell 2020).

Common Abnormal Behaviors in Horses, Pigs, Cattle, and Poultry

Stereotypies are defined as repetitive, invariant behavior patterns with no obvious goal or function, and often arise in intensive housing environments which restrict expression of motivated natural behavior (Mason 1991). In ungulates, the most common **stereotypic behaviors** are oral stereotypies, such as tongue-rolling in cattle and cribbing in horses. In this section, common abnormal behaviors in livestock species are described, in terms of the appearance of the behavior and its typical prevalence. Management, feeding, and housing factors related to the development of these behaviors are addressed in "Prevention, Management, and Treatment Concepts."

Cattle

Cattle may perform tongue rolling (Figure 20.3) which is described as swinging of the tongue outside the mouth, from one side to the other, or repetitively rolling the tongue inside the mouth (Bergeron et al. 2006). Prevalence of tongue-rolling in a group of cattle depends greatly on feeding management and, specifically, foraging opportunities. In some research, as many as a third of the animals have been noted to perform this behavior, and this increases in response to certain nutritional factors like feed restriction (Redbo and Nordblad 1997). Frequency of oral

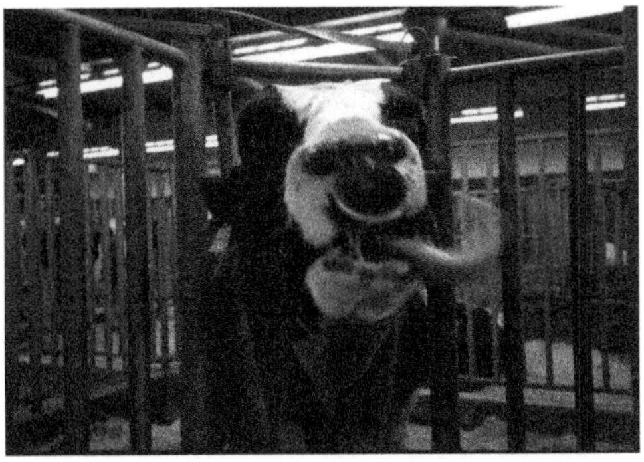

Figure 20.3 A bull rolls his tongue from one side to the other, repeatedly rolling his tongue inside of his mouth. This is a stereotypic behavior known as tongue rolling and is often related to feeding management and lack of foraging opportunities. *Source:* With permission from Katherine Houpt.

stereotypies is also variable between individuals and groups of animals. In one study, cattle spent between 1 and 9% of a 24 hour period performing oral stereotypies (primarily tongue-rolling) and had between 4 and 35 bouts of stereotypic behavior (Lindström and Redbo 2000). Most bouts of tongue-rolling occur primarily within 2–4 hours after feeding (Redbo 1990), and duration of bouts was reported to range between 10 and 320 seconds in one study (Seo et al. 1998).

While young dairy calves may perform tongue rolling, other oral behaviors are more common, including pen or self-directed non-nutritive sucking and licking (Figure 20.4), as well as cross-sucking (Figure 20.5) where suckling behavior is redirected to another calf's body (often the naval; see Table 20.1). These behaviors can occupy a large percentage of time in some cases. For example, individually housed milk-fed dairy calves were observed to spend over an hour during the day performing different types of abnormal oral behaviors in one study, including sucking on pen fixtures (Horvath et al. 2020).

Horses

Stereotypic behaviors in horses have often been referred to as "vices" or "stable vices," though behavior and welfare scientists

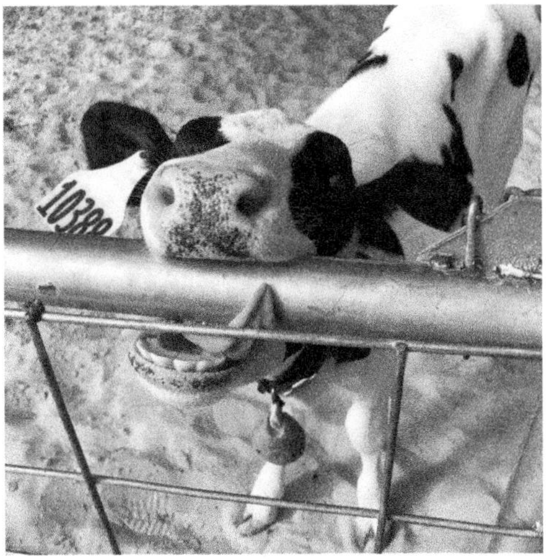

Figure 20.4 Image of a weaned heifer engaging in pen-directed sucking. *Source:* With permission from Katie Gingerich.

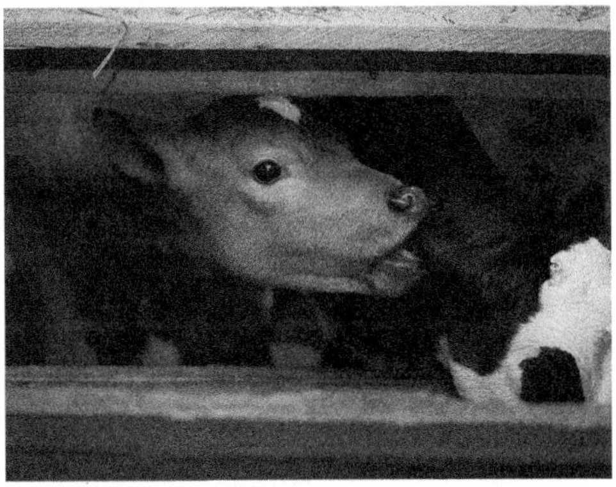

Figure 20.5 A calf engages in non-nutritive sucking of the ear of another calf who shares a pen. *Source:* victorass88/Adobe Stock.

Table 20.1 Stereotypic behaviors observed in cattle.

Behavior	Description
Tongue rolling	Affected animal flicks its tongue outside and rolls it back inside the mouth, followed by swallowing saliva
Cross-sucking	A calf will suck on other calves or the cow on any available appendage or skin tag, commonly the umbilical sheath of another calf
Pen sucking/ licking	A calf will suck or lick bars or other fixtures within their pen excessively

recommend moving away from this terminology. Use of the term "vice" implies blame on the horse, which can result in negative biases toward and reduced welfare of affected horses. Research studies conducted during the past two decades demonstrate stereotypic behaviors involve underlying psychological and physiological mechanisms, and there is some evidence for the combined influence of genetics and environment in the development and continued performance of these behaviors. A recent meta-analysis determined stereotypic behaviors occur in approximately 26% of the domestic horse population globally (Seabra et al. 2021). Stereotypic behaviors observed in horses are shown in Table 20.2 and include abnormal oral and locomotor behaviors, with cribbing, weaving, and stall walking being the most reported in the literature.

Pigs

Pigs commonly perform abnormal oral behaviors, including behaviors directed toward conspecifics, such as biting and chewing on the tail or ears, as well as solitary behaviors, such as sham chewing and bar biting (Brunberg et al. 2016). Tail-biting can lead to open wounds and severe injury to the recipient. These behaviors are reported frequently, with estimates of 30–70% of pig farms reporting some problems with tail-biting (Brunberg et al. 2016).

Poultry

Feather pecking occurs commonly in laying hens and involves pecking and pulling feathers from other birds, which can result in nude areas and skin damage. Different types of this behavior can occur, including gentle feather pecking which may relate to allopreening, and severe feather pecking (Figure 20.6). Evidence suggests that most birds perform or receive feather pecking at some point in their life; in one study, Daigle et al. (2015) found that approximately half of the population of birds both initiated and received feather pecking.

Table 20.2 Stereotypic behaviors observed in horses.

Behavior	Description
Cribbing or crib-biting	Horse places their incisor teeth on an object, pulls back while arching the neck, drawing air into the proximal esophagus, emitting an audible grunt
Weaving	Horse repeatedly shifts their weight back and forth between the right and left front legs, typically accompanied by swaying of the head, neck, and shoulders
Stall walking or box walking	Horse repetitiously walks part or all of their stall or paddock perimeter
Head bobbing or head shaking	Repetitive up and down motion of the head; head shaking is often accompanied by snorting, and horse attempts to rub the face and muzzle on a foreleg or other object (may not be considered a stereotypic behavior if causal factors involve neuropathic pain, allergies/photosensitivity)
Tongue rolling or tongue playing	Horse sticks out their tongue and twists it in the air
Self-mutilation behaviors	Flank biting where the horse bites at their own flank or stifle area causing wounds; can be accompanied by kicking out, squealing, striking, and self-directed biting of the legs, chest, and shoulder

Medical Considerations

In cattle, performance of abnormal oral behaviors may be associated with gut health. It has been speculated that tongue rolling may produce saliva, which acts as a buffer to increase rumen pH. In veal calves, performance of oral stereotypies was associated with reduced prevalence of abomasal ulcers at slaughter (Wiepkema et al. 1987), however, the nature of this relationship remains poorly understood, given complicated etiology of

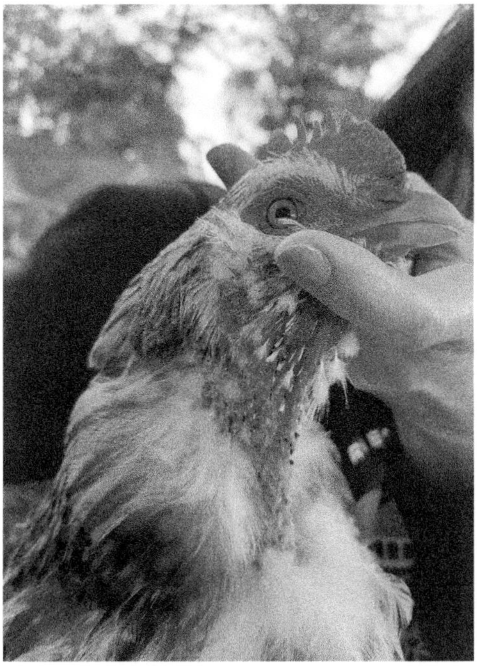

Figure 20.6 A hen has been the recipient of severe feather picking from another hen. *Source:* Dr. Sara Bennett.

abomasal ulcers. The relationship between performance of abnormal oral behaviors, diet, and gut health is described in more detail later in this chapter.

In horses, abnormal oral and locomotor behaviors can have deleterious health consequences. Cribbing behavior (Figure 20.7a) can lead to excessive wear of the incisor teeth (Figure 20.7b), and there is some evidence to suggest an association between cribbing behavior and epiploic foramen entrapment colic (van Bergen et al. 2021). Behaviors such as weaving and stall walking can be hard on hooves and legs, leading to musculoskeletal problems. Horses that perform stereotypic behaviors may also have difficulty maintaining body weight and body condition due to energy expenditure and reduced feed consumption during performance of the behavior(s).

Performance of abnormal behavior can be indicative of a health problem in the performing animal and can also cause injury to other animals. When abnormal oral behaviors are directed toward conspecifics, they can cause injury. Performance of self or cross-sucking behavior in calves can cause injury, as well as ingestion of urine (Figure 20.8). In particular, abnormal oral behavior in pigs and poultry directed toward other animals can cause severe injury. Tail-biting can lead to open wounds on recipients' tails. Feather-pecking in poultry can lead to areas of bare skin and bleeding.

(a) (b)

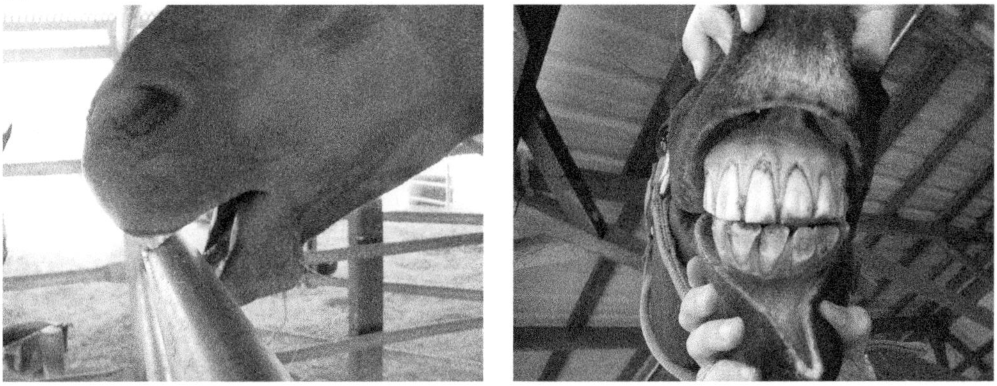

Figure 20.7 A horse engages in cribbing behavior by grasping stationary items, typically pen bars or the top rails of paddock fencing, and pulling with the incisors (a). Over time, the horse will cause substantial damage to the incisors (b), as well as fences and stalls. *Source:* Jeannine Berger.

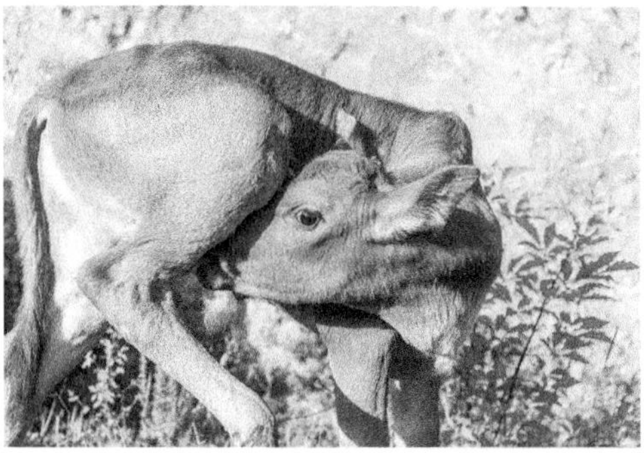

Figure 20.8 A calf engages in non-nutritive self-sucking behavior. This is an abnormal oral behavior that can lead to urine ingestion and damage to the prepuce. *Source:* Photo credit: THINK b / Adobe Stock

Both behaviors can develop into cannibalism, where recipient animals are badly injured and may die.

Prevention, Management, and Treatment Concepts

Foraging Opportunities, Feeding Behavior, and Nutritional Factors

The development of oral abnormal behaviors often relates to foraging opportunities. Provision of foraging material, where animals are provided hay or straw apart from their regular diet, reduces tongue rolling in cattle, non-nutritive oral behavior in calves, cribbing in horses, tail-biting in pigs, and feather pecking in poultry. Different theories have been proposed to explain the connection between feed restriction and forage provision and tongue-rolling, including that they result from frustrated feeding motivation (Lawrence et al. 1993) and may alleviate gastrointestinal dysfunction (Bergeron et al. 2006).

In cattle, tongue rolling is closely related to feeding time and feed restriction. For example, Redbo and Nordblad (1997) found that the prevalence of tongue rolling in a group of heifers fed ad libitum increased from 33% to 92% when they were fed restricted quantities of a high-energy, low-forage diet. The heifers that exhibited tongue-rolling prior to the period of feed restriction also increased the frequency of tongue-rolling bouts when roughage was restricted.

Provision of limited amounts of forage can both restrict feeding time, leaving animals motivated to perform foraging-related behavior, and reduce gut fill, leaving animals hungry. Research to date generally suggests that abnormal oral behaviors are mostly related to high motivation to perform foraging behavior, rather than hunger necessarily. In cattle, Lindström and Redbo (2000) attempted to experimentally decouple the effects of rumen fill and foraging time by manually adjusting rumen fill in cannulated dairy cows; they recorded occurrences of tongue-rolling in cattle that had long feeding time but low rumen fill, cattle that had short feeding time but high rumen fill, and cattle that had short feeding time or long feeding time and unmanipulated rumen fill. These researchers found that regardless of rumen fill, ability to forage decreased tongue-rolling. Cows with short feeding time but high rumen fill also had decreased stereotypies, possibly due to longer rumination time. There are also observations to suggest that tongue-rolling primarily occurs after a meal (Redbo 1990), suggesting that feeding motivation and resulting tongue-rolling are a result of frustrated foraging behavior, rather than lack of gut fill, which is greatest immediately after a meal. In pigs, there is also evidence that abnormal oral behaviors may be closely related to opportunities for oral manipulation rather than fiber ingestion and gut fill. For example, Fraser (1975) found that providing loose straw or straw bedding reduced oral stereotypies in sows, but that adding straw to the diet did not. Provision of straw accommodates motivation for oral manipulation and exploration in sows and reduces tail-biting behavior (reviewed by Brunberg et al. 2016).

Abnormal oral behaviors may also relate to gastrointestinal discomfort. In ruminants, diets that are high in concentrate and low in forage result in an excess of ruminal fermentation byproducts (particularly volatile fatty acids), resulting in low rumen pH (Forbes 2007). Consistently low rumen pH, or ruminal acidosis, may cause discomfort for the cow; there is evidence that cattle will choose to select long hay to attenuate this condition (Keunen et al. 2002). It is possible that tongue-rolling produces saliva that buffers the rumen, thereby reducing discomfort associated with low rumen pH. In sows, the addition of a bicarbonate buffer to the diet was also found to somewhat decrease oral stereotypies (Marchant-Forde and Pajor 2003), suggesting a relationship between gut acidity and abnormal oral behaviors. Similar relationships between gastrointestinal irritation, feeding of concentrates, and abnormal oral behaviors have been described in horses (Gillham et al. 1994; Nicol et al. 2002; Waters et al. 2002; Wickens et al. 2013).

Nutrition and ration formulation are important to consider in cases where abnormal oral behaviors are highly prevalent. Specific nutrient deficiencies can rapidly elicit severe feather pecking and cannibalism in poultry, although this problem is multi-factorial and also depends on environmental stressors (reviewed by Cronin and Glatz 2021; Kjaer and Bessei 2013). Inadequate nutrition may exacerbate tail-biting in pigs, including protein deficiencies (reviewed by Taylor et al. 2010).

In milk-fed calves, the development and prevalence of abnormal oral behaviors are closely related to milk feeding method, and specifically inadequate opportunity for suckling, but may also be affected by solid feed provision and enrichment. Dairy calves are conventionally reared apart from the dam and are fed milk, or milk replacer, for approximately the first seven to eight weeks of life. Provision of milk through a rubber artificial teat (Figure 20.9), which allows for natural suckling behavior, reduces performance of abnormal oral behaviors, compared to provision of milk from an open bucket, which requires that calves sip rather than suckle to ingest the milk. Calves are highly motivated to suck, and the action of suckling elicits the release of digestive hormones related to satiety, such as cholecystokinin and gastrin (De Passillé et al. 1993). This strong motivation to suckle exists apart from milk ingestion and may be redirected toward pen fixtures or other calves if there is inadequate opportunity for the calf to suckle during milk feeding. In addition to providing milk through a teat, suckling motivation may be redirected toward other outlets, such as provision of a dummy teat (Salter et al. 2021). As is the case for older cattle, abnormal oral behaviors in young calves are also reduced through provision of hay, perhaps due to opportunity to chew and orally manipulate feed.

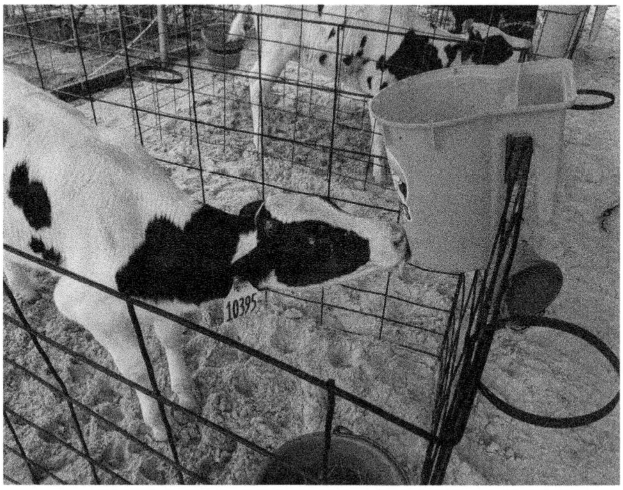

Figure 20.9 Image of a calf suckling milk from an artificial teat. *Source:* Photo by Emily Miller-Cushon, University of Florida.

Housing and Management

In general, housing animals in more restrictive spaces increases performance of abnormal behaviors. In cattle, isolated housing and limited space both increase performance of tongue rolling and other abnormal oral behaviors. For example, housing in tie stalls, which limit movement, increases oral abnormal behavior compared to housing that allows for more movement (Redbo 1992). Housing younger calves with social contact has also been found to reduce abnormal oral behavior, including stereotypic tongue rolling (Seo et al. 1998). In horses, multiple studies have consistently found insufficient or limited turnout time, which causes limited opportunities to socialize with other horses as well as limited grazing or foraging opportunities, is associated with increased risk of stereotypic behavior development (Waters et al. 2002; Wickens and Heleski 2010; Seabra et al. 2021). In laying hens, feather-pecking is greater in birds housed in cage systems (Figure 20.10a), compared to non-cage housing systems (Figure 20.10b) (van Staaveren et al. 2021).

Social dynamics in group-housed pigs and chickens may affect development of tail-biting and feather-pecking. Competition for access to feed is associated with increased tail-biting in sows (Brunberg et al. 2016). The relationship between group size or stocking density and abnormal oral behavior is less clear, although some evidence suggests that higher stocking densities may contribute to performance of abnormal behavior.

(a)

(b)

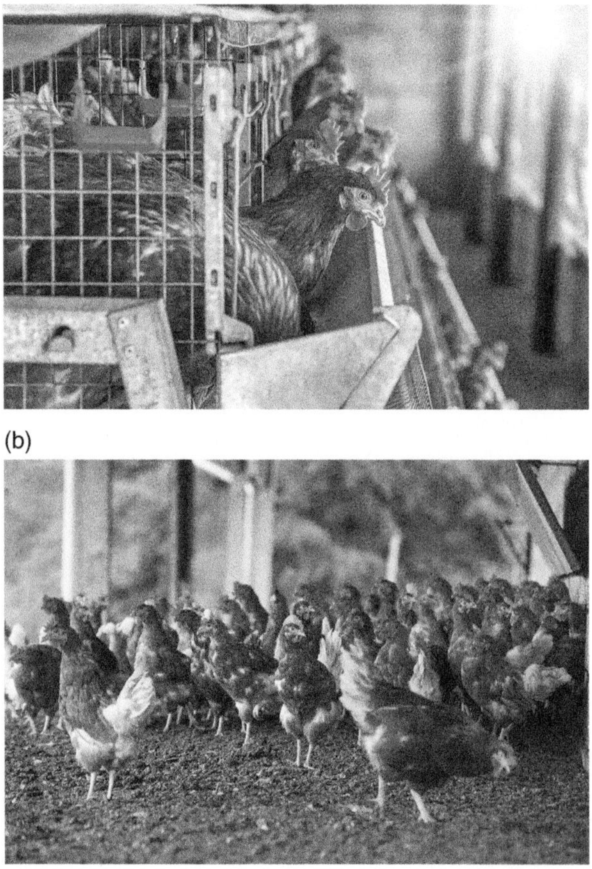

Figure 20.10 Traditional cage systems (a) for laying hens limit movement and are correlated with a higher incidence of feather picking, while those that allow for more free movement (b) tend to have lower feather picking rates (van Staaveren et al. 2021). *Source:* poco_bw/ Adobe Stock (a) and zlikovec/Adobe Stock (b).

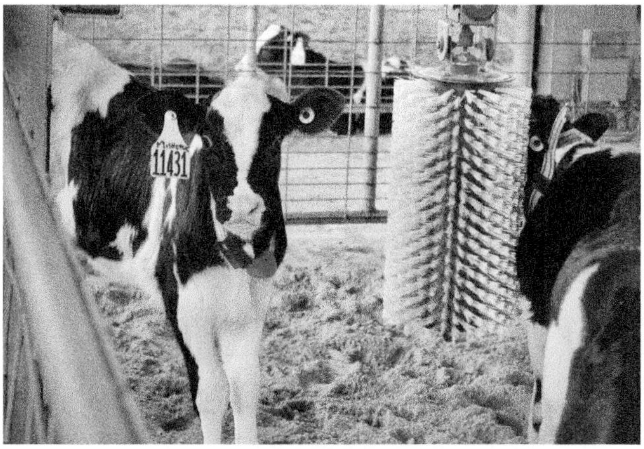

Figure 20.11 Image of a calf using a DeLaval swinging cow brush (DeLaval; Tumba, Sweden). *Source:* Photo by Samantha Doyle, University of Florida.

Environmental enrichment can be utilized to provide outlets for motivated natural behavior. Beyond provision of foraging material, social contact, and sufficient space, as discussed previously, additional enrichment items may provide opportunities for more complex behavior. In dairy calves, provision of brushes for grooming (either automated rotating brushes or manual brushes; see Figure 20.11) has been found to reduce duration of pen-directed sucking (Horvath et al. 2020). The addition of a horse-safe mirror in the stall has been shown to reduce weaving behavior and may also be effective in managing stall walking behavior. Providing horses with foraging devices (Figure 20.12) or objects such as a ball during stall confinement can help reduce the frequency or duration of the abnormal behavior. For sows, provision of enrichment items (Figure 20.13) which offer opportunities for oral manipulation (such as a ball or rope), can reduce tail-biting (reviewed by Henry et al. 2021). Enrichments are also effective in reducing feather-pecking in poultry, including material for dustbathing and foraging (van Staaveren et al. 2021).

Experts agree that environmental enrichment offers the most effective and welfare-friendly means to reduce abnormal behaviors. However, other means to thwart or prevent these behaviors are often adopted. Tail-docking in sows is a common and effective means to prevent tail-biting, and is often successful (reviewed by Henry et al. 2021). However, there are welfare concerns

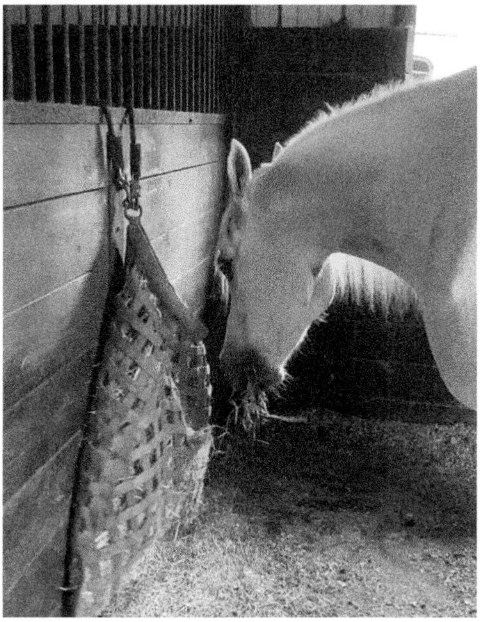

Figure 20.12 Image of a horse feeding from a slow feed, web hay bag to extend access to forage and feeding time while stalled. *Source:* Carissa Wickens.

surrounding tail-docking, including that it is painful and does not address the underlying cause of tail-biting, and it has been banned in the European Union. Similarly, beak trimming is used in laying hens to reduce damage caused through feather-pecking. Attempts to physically prevent stereotypic behaviors in horses (such as cribbing collars, application of distasteful substances to cribbing surfaces, and

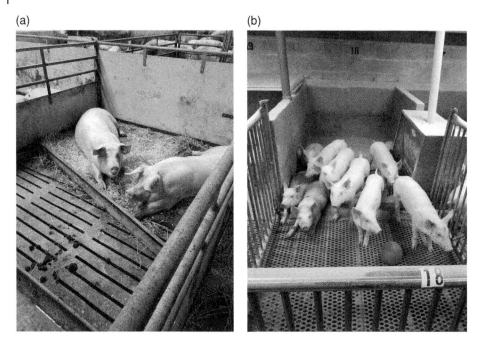

Figure 20.13 Provision of enrichment in the form of foraging material for sows (a) and rubber balls (b) used in nursery pens to reduce tail-biting and improve overall exploratory behavior. *Source:* With permission from Monique Pairis-Garcia.

anti-weave grills at the front of the stall) are only marginally successful in mitigating the behavior and may result in reduced welfare for the horse. Similarly, the use of nose flaps in dairy calves to prevent cross-sucking can prevent this behavior but does not address the underlying sucking motivation, and this problem is best addressed through milk feeding management and providing appropriate outlets for non-nutritive sucking. In general, strategies aimed at addressing the behavior should include consideration of potential causal factors and implementation of management practices that more closely mimic natural behaviors.

References

Adcock, S.J.J. and Tucker, C.B. (2018). The effect of disbudding age on healing and pain sensitivity in dairy calves. *J. Dairy Sci.* 101: 10361–10373.

Adcock, S.J.J. and Tucker, C.B. (2020). Conditioned place preference reveals ongoing pain in calves 3 weeks after disbudding. *Sci. Rep.* 10: 3849. https://doi.org/10.1038/s41598-020-60260-7.

Bergeron, R., Badnell-Waters, A.J., Lambton, S., and Mason, G. (2006). Stereotypic oral behaviour in captive ungulates: foraging, diet and gastrointestinal function. In: *Stereotypic Animal Behaviour: Fundamentals and Applications to Welfare*, 2e (ed. G. Mason and J. Rushen), 19–57. Cambridge, MA: CABI Publishing.

Borderas, T.F., Rushen, J., Von Keyserlingk, M.A.G., and De Passillé, A.M.B. (2009). Automated measurement of changes in feeding behavior of milk-fed calves associated with illness. *J. Dairy Sci.* 92 (9): 4549–4554.

Brunberg, E.I., Rodenburg, T.B., Rydhmer, L. et al. (2016). Omnivores going astray: a review and new synthesis of abnormal behavior in pigs and laying hens. *Front. Vet. Sci.* 3: 57. https://doi.org/10.3389/fvets.2016.00057.

Costa, J.H.C., von Keyserlingk, M.A.G., and Weary, D.M. (2016). Invited review: effects of group housing of dairy calves on behavior, cognition, performance, and health. *J. Dairy Sci.* 99: 2453–2467.

Cronin, G.M. and Glatz, P.C. (2021). Causes of feather pecking and subsequent welfare issues for the laying hen: a review. *Anim. Prod. Sci.* 61: 990–1005.

Daigle, C.L., Rodenburg, T.B., Bolhuis, J.E. et al. (2015). Individual consistency of feather pecking behavior in laying hens: once a feather pecker always a feather pecker? *Front. Vet. Sci.* 2: 6.

Dalla, C., E., Minero, M., Lebelt, D. et al. (2014). Development of the horse grimace scale (HGS) as a pain assessment tool in horses undergoing routine castration. *Plos One* 9 (3): e92281.

De Passillé, A.M.B., Christopherson, R., and Rushen, J. (1993). Nonnutritive sucking by the calf and postprandial secretion of insulin, CCK, and gastrin. *Physiol. Behav.* 54: 1069–1073.

Forbes, J.M. (2007). *Voluntary Food Intake and Diet Selection in Farm Animals*, 2e. Cambridge, MA: CABI.

Fraser, D. (1975). The effect of straw on the behaviour of sows in tether stalls. *Anim. Sci.* 21 (1): 59–68.

Fureix, C., Beauliey, C., Argaud, S. et al. (2015). Investigating anhedonia in a non-conventional species: do some riding horses *Equus caballus* display symptoms of depression? *Appl. Anim. Behav. Sci.* 162: 26–36.

Gillham, S.B., Dodman, N.H., Shuster, L. et al. (1994). The effect of diet on cribbing behavior and plasma β-endorphin in horses. *Appl. Anim. Behav. Sci.* 41: 147–153.

Gleerup, K.B., Andersen, P.H., Munksgaard, L., and Forkman, B. (2015). Pain evaluation in dairy cattle. *Appl. Anim. Behav. Sci.* 171: 25–32.

Hart, B.L. (1988). Biological basis of the behavior of sick animals. *Neurosci. Biobehav. Rev. 12* (2): 123–137.

Henry, M., Jansen, H., del Rocio Amezcua, M. et al. (2021). Tail-biting in pigs: a scoping review. *Animals* 11: 2002.

Hixson, C.L., Krawczel, P.D., Caldwell, J.M., and Miller-Cushon, E.K. (2018). Behavioral changes in group-housed dairy calves infected with Mannheimia haemolytica. *J. Dairy Sci.* 101 (11): 10351–10360.

Horvath, K.C., Allen, A.N., and Miller-Cushon, E.K. (2020). Effects of access to stationary brushes and chopped hay on behavior and performance of individually housed dairy calves. *J. Dairy Sci.* 103: 8421–8432.

Hughes, B.O. and Duncan, I.J.H. (1988). The notion of ethological 'need', models of motivation and animal welfare. *Anim. Behav.* 36: 1696–1707.

Keunen, J.E., Plaizier, J.C., Kyriazakis, L. et al. (2002). Effects of a subacute ruminal acidosis model on the diet selection of dairy cows. *J. Dairy Sci.* 85: 3304–3313.

Kjaer, J.B. and Bessei, W. (2013). The interrelationships of nutrition and feather pecking in the domestic fowl – a review. *Arch. Geflügelkd.* 77: 1–9.

Lawrence, A.B., Terlouw, E.C., and Kyriazakis, I. (1993). The behavioural effects of undernutrition in confined farm animals. *Proceed. Nutr. Soc.* 52 (1): 219–229.

Lindström, T. and Redbo, I. (2000). Effect of feeding duration and rumen fill on behaviour in dairy cows. *Appl. Anim. Behav. Sci.* 70: 83–97.

Marchant-Forde, J.N. and Pajor, E.A.2003). Dietary Sodium Bicarbonate and Stereotypic Behavior of Gestating Sows. Purdue University Swine Research Report. 72–75.

Mason, G.J. (1991). Stereotypies: a critical review. *Anim. Behav.* 41: 1015–1037.

Mintline, E.M., Stewart, M., Rogers, A.R. et al. (2013). Play behavior as an indicator of animal welfare: disbudding in dairy calves. *Appl. Anim. Behav. Sci.* 144 (1-2): 22–30.

Neave, H.W., Daros, R.R., Costa, J.H.C. et al. (2013). Pain and pessimism: dairy calves exhibit negative judgement bias following hot-iron disbudding. *Plos One* 9 (4): e96135.

Nicol, C.J., Davidson, H.P.D., Harris, P.A. et al. (2002). Study of crib-biting and gastric inflammation and ulceration in young horses. *Vet. Rec.* 151: 658–662.

Norring, M., Häggman, J., Simojoki, H. et al. (2014). Lameness impairs feeding behavior of dairy cows. *J. Dairy Sci.* 97 (7): 4317–4321.

Redbo, I. (1990). Changes in duration and frequency of stereotypies and their adjoining behaviours in heifers, before, during and after the grazing period. *Appl. Anim. Behav. Sci.* 26: 57–67.

Redbo, I. (1992). The influence of restraint on the occurrence of oral stereotypies in dairy cows. *Appl. Anim. Behav. Sci.* 35 (2): 115–123.

Redbo, I. and Nordblad, A. (1997). Stereotypies in heifers are affected by feeding regime. *Appl. Anim. Behav. Sci.* 53: 193–202.

Salter, R.S., Reuscher, K.J., and Van Os, J.M.C. (2021). Milk-and starter-feeding strategies to reduce cross sucking in pair-housed calves in outdoor hutches. *J. Dairy Sci.* 104: 6096–6112.

Seabra, J.C., Dittrich, J.R., and M.M. do Vale. (2021). Factors associated with the development and prevalence of abnormal behaviors in horses: systemic review with meta-analysis. *J. Equine Vet. Sci.* 106: 103750.

Seo, T., Sato, S., Kosaka, K. et al. (1998). Short communication: tongue-playing and heart rate in calves. *Appl. Anim. Behav. Sci.* 58: 179–182.

Sowell, B.F., Branine, M.E., Bowman, J.G.P. et al. (1999). Feeding and watering behavior of healthy and morbid steers in a commercial feedlot. *J. Anim. Sci.* 77 (5): 1105–1112.

Špinka, M., Newberry, R.C., and Bekoff, M. (2001). Mammalian play: training for the unexpected. *Quarterly Rev. Biology* 76 (2): 141–168.

Stephenson, E. and Haskell, M.J. (2020). The use of a "go/go" cognitive bias task and response to a novel object to assess the effect of housing enrichment in sheep (*Ovis aries*). *J. Appl. Anim. Welf. Sci.* 25: 6274.

Stojkov, J., von Keyserlingk, M.A.G., Marchant-Forde, J.N., and Weary, D.M. (2015). Assessment of visceral pain associated with metritis in dairy cows. *J. Dairy Sci.* 98: 5352–5361.

Taylor, N.R., Main, D.C.J., Mendl, M., and Edwards, S.A. (2010). Tail-biting: a new perspective. *The Vet. J.* 186: 137–147.

Torcivia, C. and McDonnell, S. (2021). Equine discomfort ethogram. *Animals* 11 (2): 580.

Tucker, C.B., Jensen, M.B., de Passille, A.M. et al. (2021). Invited review: lying time and the welfare of dairy cows. *J. Dairy Sci.* 104: 20–46.

Van Bergen, T., Wiemer, P., and Martens, A. (2021). Equine colic associated with small intestinal epiploic foramen entrapment. *Vet. J.* 269: 105608.

van Loon, J.P.A. and Macri, L. (2021). Objective assessment of chronic pain in horses using the horse chronic pain scale (HCPS): a scale-construction study. *Animals* 11 (6): 1826.

van Staaveren, N., Ellis, J., Baes, C.F., and Harlander-Matauschek, A. (2021). A meta-analysis on the effect of environmental enrichment on feather pecking and feather damage in laying hens. *Poultry Sci.* 100: 397–411.

Waters, A.J., Nicol, C.J., and French, N.P. (2002). Factors influencing the development of stereotypic and redirected behaviours in young horses: finding of a four year prospective epidemiological study. *Equine Vet. J.* 34: 572–579.

Wickens, C.L., McCall, C.A., Bursian, S. et al. (2013). Assessment of gastric ulceration and gastrin response in horses with history of crib-biting. *J. Equine Vet. Sci.* 33: 739–745.

Wickens, C.L. and Heleski, C.R. (2010). Crib-biting behavior in horses: a review. *Appl. Anim. Behav. Sci.* 128: 1–9.

Wiepkema, P., Vanhellemond, K., Roessingh, P., and Romberg, H. (1987). Behaviour and abomasal damage in individual veal calves. *Appl. Anim. Behav. Sci.* 18: 257–268.

21

Approach to Psychopharmacology in Companion Animals

M. Leanne Lilly

The Ohio State University, Veterinary Medical Center, Columbus, OH, USA

Introduction

Veterinary clinicians are reaching for psychosactive medications to combat fear, anxiety, and stress in pets, especially as the body of pet-related pharmacological literature expands (Crowell-Davis et al. 2019b; Sinn 2018). Anxiety-relieving medications facilitate learning and ease panic, allowing for more effective behavior modification and management. They also allow for tranquilization in situations where the pet is at risk for self-injury or escape. Psychopharmacology improves the lives of dogs, cats, and their families and may, in turn, be life-saving.

The choice to prescribe psychoactive medications is based on both the severity of the symptoms and the frequency and predictability of triggering events. Medications are also considered as an adjunct when appropriate behavior modification protocols have made insubstantial progress and the patient is still suffering, or when the patient is too stressed to eat or play at the lowest possible stimulus threshold, inhibiting effective counterconditioning. When there are underlying pathologies that make behavior modification alone unlikely to be successful, such as compulsive disorders, interstitial cystitis, or cognitive dysfunction, medications are also warranted as primary treatment modalities. Prescribing early in the treatment process may be appropriate when pet relinquishment or euthanasia is a risk if sufficient and rapid progress is not made, even if severity of the problem is only mild to moderate.

Keep in mind that, with few exceptions, most medications are not licensed or labeled for use in companion animals; doses are often extrapolated from human literature and use. Efficacy and safety studies in dogs and cats may be lacking to absent. While the goal of psychopharmacologic treatment is an improvement in behavior, all medications have a low risk of making things worse. In rare cases, you may see agitation, paradoxical excitement, and/or a general worsening of behavior problems. We can also occasionally see patients gain more confidence with treatment and, as a result, use more proactive distance increasing behaviors (aggression) rather than passive avoidance, an effect called disinhibition of aggression (Pineda et al. 2014; Simpson et al. 2007). This risk is low with most mediations, but clients should always be counseled to watch for them.

A physical examination and minimum database bloodwork (complete blood cell count, chemistry panel, urinalysis, and thyroid screen) are recommended prior to (Horwitz 2017) and within the first year of starting medications. The timing on that recommendation varies by

Introduction to Animal Behavior and Veterinary Behavioral Medicine, First Edition. Edited by Meghan E. Herron.

Companion website: www.wiley.com/go/introductiontoanimalbehavior

patient age, underlying medical conditions, ease of obtaining blood and urine samples, and clinician preference. When not approved by the Food and Drug Administration (FDA), disclosure of off-label usage is needed. Client education of potential side effects is always the clinician's responsibility.

Daily Medications

Often referred to as "baseline" or "long-lasting," daily psychotropic medications are those that are administered EVERY DAY, regardless of behavior or events, and take weeks to achieve therapeutic effects. These are not to be confused with immediate-acting medication that may start working the same day and may, thus, be used as often or as little as needed. Patients who experience fear in response to a host of non-predictable daily triggers (such as neighbors, other pets or children in the home, household appliances, car doors shutting, etc.) or are in a continual state of anticipation/anxiety are good candidates for 24/7 psychopharmacological support from a daily medication. This is achieved by using medications that make long lasting changes at the receptor level and are given every 12–24 hours.

The most prescribed and best studied medications in companion animals fall into five classes, three of which work primarily through serotonin reuptake inhibition. Serotonin reuptake inhibiting medications (SRIs) include the selective serotonin reuptake inhibitors (SSRIs), tricyclic antidepressants (TCAs), and serotonin and norepinephrine reuptake inhibitors (SNRIs). Other classes include the azapirones and monoamine oxidate inhibitors (MAOIs).

Serotonin Reuptake Inhibiting Drugs: SSRIs, TCAs, and SNRIs

Serotonin reuptake inhibitors (SRIs) are the most commonly used daily anti-anxiety medications in pets, though technically classified as antidepressants. These medications prevent the re-uptake of serotonin into the neuron that released it (presynaptic) by blocking the cell's serotonin reuptake pump (Ogata et al. 2019). Blocking this pump means that serotonin will linger for a longer time in the synaptic cleft, allowing it to bind more readily to 18+ postsynaptic serotonin receptors. That effect happens immediately, flooding all the serotonin receptors, even those which may not have desirable bodily effects. This is why we see side effects most commonly in the first two weeks of treatment. As the neurons re-acclimate to the flood of serotonin, the receptors are *down regulated* and side effects typically wane. The delays in therapeutic effect as well as the prolonged effect of SRIs are thought to stem from the down regulation of presynaptic serotonin **autoreceptors**, ultimately leading to increased serotonin production and release (Stahl 2008) (Figure 21.1). Because this mechanism takes several weeks, SRIs must be given regularly to achieve effect, and are not useful on an "as needed" basis.

All SRIs are metabolized by the liver (hepatic metabolism) and, to varying degrees, excreted by the kidneys (renal excretion), which is why pre-medication organ-screening lab testing is strongly recommended (Ogata et al. 2019). Follow-up blood and urine testing in 6–12 months is also recommended. SRIs may alter blood glucose (Meng et al. 2019; Ogata et al. 2019), and careful dosing and monitoring are warranted in diabetic patients. Platelet inhibition is possible with the use of SRIs, as platelets utilize serotonin surface receptors as part of the coagulation cascade (Milne and Cohn 1957). While it is not typically necessary or beneficial to stop SRIs prior to most surgical procedures, caution should be used when combining with other platelet-effecting medications (nonsteroidal anti-inflammatories [NSAIDs], steroids, and primary anti-coagulants) due to increased risk of gastrointestinal (GI) hemorrhage at least in humans (de Abajo et al. 1999; de Jong et al. 2003; Helin-Salmivaara et al. 2007; Meijer et al. 2004). For this reason, many clinicians recommend using GI protectants, such as proton-pump inhibitors, when combining SRIs

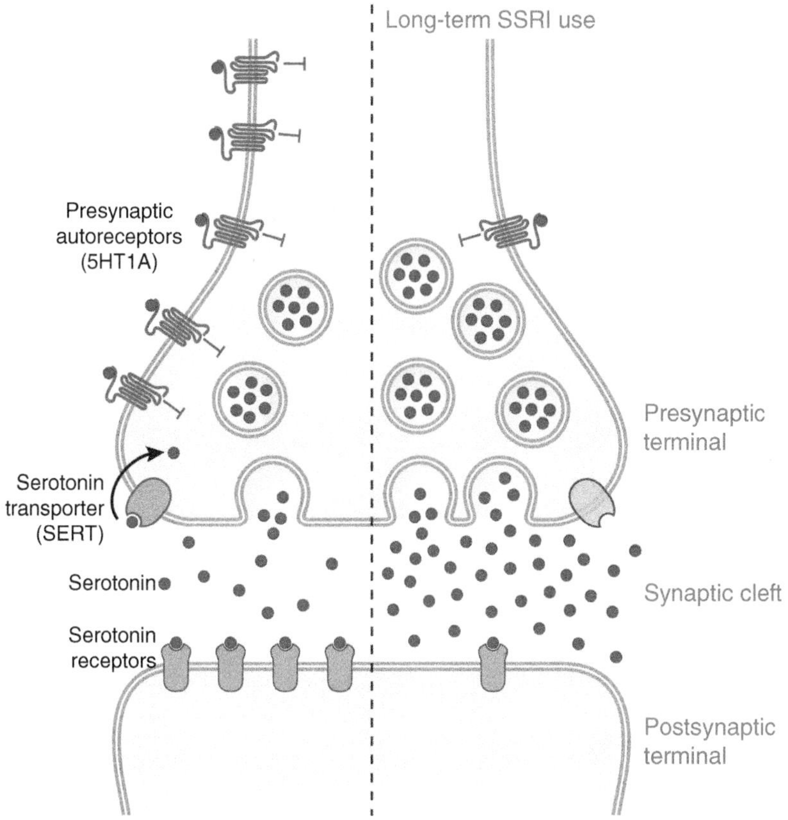

Figure 21.1 Effects of long-term SSRI use on the synapse of serotonin-releasing neurons. Note the decrease in number of pre-synaptic auto receptors (5HT1A) between the left and right (after long term SSRI use). This down regulation of 5HT1A is thought to cause the increase in serotonin released into the synaptic cleft (red dots). *Source:* Image credit: Tim Vojt, reproduced with permission from The Ohio State University.

and NSAIDs (de Abajo et al. 1999). Cats may develop functional urine retention *on any SRI*, presumably due to specific serotonin receptor subtypes in the bladder wall or sphincter (Ogata et al. 2019) that vary not only by species but by individual. Follow-up within two to three days of starting a SRI to confirm that a feline patient on fluoxetine is urinating normally is best practice. Dose reductions should be considered for patients with mild hepatic or renal compromise, though data on companion animal species is lacking and is typically derived from human literature (Ogata et al. 2019). Plasma levels of the drug, serotonin, or metabolites do not correlate with clinical response – response to treatment is judged purely on appreciable changes in behavior (Hiemke and Härtter 2000; van Harten 1993).

Selective serotonin reuptake inhibitors (SSRIs) are highly selective for serotonin reuptake inhibition and have little to no effect on other neurotransmitters, compared to other SRI classes. Commonly prescribed SSRIs include fluoxetine, paroxetine, and sertraline. This class may be preferred over others due to its lower side effect profile and affordable generic options. Depending on the medication and species being treated, SSRIs may be given once daily or twice daily. If patients have been taking SSRIs for several months, it is generally recommended to wean pets off gradually if discontinuation is desired (Dantas et al. 2019).

Tricyclic anti-depressants (TCAs) are also SRIs, with their name stemming from their three-ringed molecular structure. In addition to inhibiting serotonin reuptake, they also inhibit norepinephrine reuptake and have strong antihistamine and anticholinergic effects. Re-regulating norepinephrine may be involved in the fight/flight/freeze/fidget aspects of anxiety (Stahl 2008), making this a useful drug class for anxious pets. Commonly prescribed TCAs for dogs and cats include clomipramine and amitriptyline. Due to shorter half-lives, these medications are dosed every 12 hours in dogs and may have a slightly faster onset of therapeutic effect (3–5 weeks) compared to SSRIs (4–6 weeks) (Crowell-Davis 2019b). Due to their strong anticholinergic effects, they can be arrhythmogenic and may lower the seizure threshold more than SSRIs (Crowell-Davis 2019b). The immediate calming provided by the antihistamine effects makes them a reasonable first choice for patients who manifest their anxiety through frenetic behaviors (overactive, struggling to settle, rest, or be still). It is generally recommended to wean pets off gradually if they have been taking TCA for several months (Crowell-Davis 2019b).

Other Daily Medication Classes

Serotonin Norepinephrine reuptake inhibitors (SNRIs) have recently gained favor among human patients for depression and, following that, renewed interest in veterinary medicine. While theoretically they have a lower side effect profile than TCAs due to no primary antihistamine or anticholinergic effects, the literature on them in cats and dogs is sparse, with no placebo-controlled trials.

Azapirones are considered serotonin agonists. This means they stimulate postsynaptic serotonin autoreceptors in a way that mimics the binding of a serotonin molecule. They are commonly used in human psychiatry as add-ons to other antidepressants, such as selective serotonin reuptake inhibitors. While veterinary behavior specialists may utilize this combination, the practice is less common.

Monoamine oxidase inhibitors (MAOIs) are one of the older psychoactive medications. Originally anti-tuberculosis medications, MOAIs were found to have "mood elevating" effects on people, resulting in increased appetite, better sleep, sociability, and sometimes "dancing in the hall" (Ramachandraih et al. 2011). Monoamine Oxidase is the enzyme that breaks down any leftover serotonin, norepinephrine, and dopamine (monoamines) in the synaptic cleft (Stahl 2008). Inhibition of this breakdown causes all three neurotransmitters to be present in the synapse for longer. Unlike many of the other daily medications, MAOIs cannot be combined with other serotonin enhancing medications due to the increased risk of serotonin syndrome (Zoetis, Inc. 2014).

Specific Medications

Fluoxetine (Reconcile®, Prozac®); SSRI

The most well-known SSRI in humans as brand name Prozac®, fluoxetine has a canine counter-part, Reconcile®, which is labeled for the treatment of separation anxiety (Simpson et al. 2007). While most helpful in conjunction with a counterconditioning plan, it has also been shown to help without these steps (Landsberg et al. 2008) and to decrease negative cognitive bias or "pessimism" in dogs with separation anxiety (Karagiannis et al. 2015).

Though not labeled for this use in the United States, fluoxetine is often effective at decreasing urine marking in cats, with studies showing >90% reduction of urine marking in treated cats (Pryor et al. 2001). It has been tested for transdermal use, but roughly only 10% of transdermal fluoxetine makes it to a cat's bloodstream, making oral administration ideal (Ciribassi et al. 2003). The brand name product (Reconcile®) is flavored and comes in smaller mgs (8, 16, 32, 64), which may facilitate patient ingestion over the generic product (10 mg and 20 mg tablets and 10 mg, 20 mg, and 40 mg capsules).

Reports exist demonstrating a beneficial effect of fluoxetine in treating "owner" directed aggression (Dodman et al. 1996). Other studies show that fluoxetine decreases serum cortisol, the primary stress hormone, in dogs with aggression (Rosado et al. 2011). There is also a case series reporting beneficial impacts in treating acral lick dermatitis in dogs (Wynchank and Berk 1998).

Fluoxetine's two most common side effects are sedation and appetite suppression (Pryor et al. 2001; Simpson et al. 2007). Other forms of GI upset, including nausea and diarrhea, are uncommon but possible.

Fluoxetine inhibits several liver enzymes involved in drug metabolism, and this should be taken into account when combining with other medications ("Drug Bank: Fluoxetine," 2021; Law et al. 2014; Ogata et al. 2019). It also has long lasting metabolites with half-lives of 33–64 hours (*Reconcile - FDA initially published by Elanco 2007*, Drugs.com 2021). Consequently, it requires a five week washout period between discontinuation and starting an MAOI.

Sertraline (Zoloft®); SSRI

Sertraline (Zoloft®) is a less commonly utilized SSRI than fluoxetine, as it is a comparatively newer medication. There are no placebo-controlled trials for sertraline in dogs or cats, and there are only a handful of case reports for its use in treating acral lick granuloma (Rapoport et al. 1992), fear related aggression (Ballantyne 2017), and canine house soiling (Pryor 2003). Despite the limited literature, there are some benefits in selecting sertraline over fluoxetine: (1) Sertraline tends to be less sedating and less likely to suppress appetite (Garattini 1992; Sansone et al. 2000), (2) It is metabolized primarily in the liver, and much of it is cleared in feces rather than via the kidneys (Hiemke and Härtter 2000), and (3) In humans, sertraline is the least likely of the SSRIs to decrease seizure threshold (Hill et al. 2015).

Paroxetine (Paxil®); SSRI

Paroxetine (Paxil®) is another SSRI alternative to fluoxetine that is commonly prescribed to treat social and other anxiety disorders in people and may be used to treat various anxiety disorders in pets. Due to short half-life and lack of active metabolites, it is best to dose this medication every 12 hours, at least in dogs (Catterson and Preskorn 1996; Luescher 2003). It is particularly useful for picky eaters as it tends to enhance appetite, though decreases are possible (Ogata et al. 2019). Due to moderate anticholinergic side effects (dry eye, dry mouth, urine retention, constipation), caution should be used in patients with pre-existing conditions that would worsen with these effects (keratoconjunctivitis sicca, constipation/obstipation, urine retention or blocking) (Ogata et al. 2019); cats in particular seem to be sensitive to constipation effects (Frank and Dehasse 2003). While there are no placebo-controlled clinical trials for pets on paroxetine, there are published, peer-reviewed a case reports/series for generalized anxiety (Reisner 2003), territorial aggression and separation related problems in dogs (Herron 2010; Moesta 2014), and urine marking in cats (Pachel 2011; Pryor 2003).

Clomicalm® (Caniquell®/Clomipramine); TCA

Clomicalm® is the most serotonin-enhancing of the TCAs. It is FDA approved for the treatment separation anxiety in dogs (King et al. 2000; Podberscek et al. 1999). The label was approved at once daily or divided dosing, however, studies on metabolism support twice daily dosing due to rapid metabolism (King et al. 2000). Side effects of this medication may include GI upset (nausea, vomiting, or constipation), changes in appetite, sedation, increased anxiety or aggression, prolongation of the p-wave

(Reich et al. 2000), and anticholinergic side effects. Clomicalm may be prohibitively expensive for larger dogs, but recently a generic for dogs has been approved (CaniQuell®) based on equivalent absorption of the 20 mg tablets only.

Clomicalm® has been utilized in the treatment of many behavior disorders in dogs, such as conflict related aggression (see Chapter 15) (White et al. 1999), travel anxiety (Frank et al. 2006), tail chasing in bull terriers (Moon-Fanelli and Dodman 1998), and other compulsive behaviors (Overall and Dunham 2002). It has been used in cats to treat urine marking (Hart et al. 2005; Landsberg and Wilson 2005), though less effectively than fluoxetine, and has had some success in treating a variety of other behavior disorders in cats (Litster 2000), including psychogenic alopecia (Mertens et al. 2006) and compulsive behaviors (Seksel and Lindeman 1998).

Clomipramine may affect thyroid laboratory values and may lead to an artificially decreased total T4 but not free T4, T3, or TSH in dogs (Gulikers and Panciera 2003), and a 16–25% decrease in total T4, T3, and free T4 in cats (Martin 2010). Functionally, this means that a full thyroid function panel is particularly important when screening for hypothyroidism in dogs or hyperthyroidism in cats on clomipramine. A two-week wash-out period is needed between a TCA and an MAOI. Avoid use in patients with cardiac arrhythmias, constipation, seizures, or glaucoma (Crowell-Davis 2019a). Testicular hypoplasia may occur in intact males, especially at higher doses (Covetrus North America 2000; Elanco Inc. (US) 1999).

Amitriptyline; TCA

Amitriptyline is less **serotonergic**, more **antihistaminic**, more **anticholinergic**, and, thus, more sedating than Clomicalm® (Crowell-Davis 2019b). Essentially it has a side effect profile similar to Clomicalm®, with slight differences in cardiac rhythm changes. Amitriptyline may shorten the p-wave and Q-T intervals, having minimal arrhythmogenic potential at typical clinical doses (Reich et al. 2000). There are no placebo-controlled trials for amitriptyline in companion animals. Studies found little efficacy in the treatment of fear-related or conflict-related aggression (Virga et al. 2001), and it was less effective than Clomicalm® in reducing clinical signs associated with compulsive disorders in dogs. In an open treatment trial for separation anxiety, 60% of dogs given amitriptyline in combination with a behavior modification plan improved, though only 56% of these clients thought their success was due to the medication (Takeuchi et al. 2000).

Treatment with amitriptyline had no impact on acute, nonobstructive idiopathic lower urinary tract signs when given for 7 days (Kruger et al. 2003), but it did prevent recurrence of clinical signs at 6 and 12 months in roughly 60% of cats – a quarter of whom developed cystic calculi in the first 6 months (Chew et al. 1998). Studies suggest it may be useful in the treatment of psychogenic alopecia (Sawyer et al. 1999) as well as other compulsive behaviors in cats (Overall and Dunham 2002). Systemic absorption of amitriptyline after transdermal ear application in cats was below the level of quantification, making oral administration a must (Mealey et al. 2004).

Venlafaxine (Effexor®); SNRI

Venlafaxine is the first SNRI to be used in dogs and cats. There are no published placebo-controlled clinical trials, but several case series on its use in cats exist (Hopfensperger 2016; Katofiasc et al. 2002; Pflaum and Bennett 2021). The doses in dogs have been extrapolated from case series on cataplexy and early pharmacokinetic studies (Delucchi et al. 2010; Howell et al. 1994; Paul Wang et al. 1992). Recent retrospective studies in dogs suggest that venlafaxine may be more effective when used in conjunction with other adjunct behavior medications than when used alone and that it can be used to treat aggressive behavior without major adverse effects (Maffeo et al. 2023; Petroff 2022). In homes with cats, medication should be stored in a secure area as Effexor® prescribed for humans is the top reported unintentional drug ingestion by cats reported to poison control hotlines ("10 Poison Pills for Pets," 2021; Merola and Dunayer 2006).

Buspirone; Azapirone

The only azapirone commercially available in the United States is buspirone (Dantas and Crowell-Davis 2019a). Buspirone is unique among the daily medications in that it has direct agonist activity on 5HT1A receptors. Of particular clinical interest are its low side effect profile and rapid onset of therapeutic effects (2–7 days) (Dantas and Crowell-Davis 2019a). Considered the "bravery drug," buspirone is most useful in boosting confidence and social boldness in shy and fearful pets. An increase in friendly and affectionate behavior is a known and reported side effect (Hart et al. 1993). Caution should be exercised with aggressive patients, though, as there are reports of buspirone enhancing aggression in cats (Hart et al. 1993). For both cats and dogs, the increase in social boldness may prompt a more proactive aggressive response, therefore, this drug should be strictly avoided in pets with known aggression issues.

Studies have demonstrated some efficacy in treating urine marking behaviors in cats. That said, one published study showed that only 55% of treated cats had substantial reduction in urine marking frequency (Hart et al. 1993), which falls well below the efficacy reported for fluoxetine in the treatment of urine marking in cats (Pryor et al. 2001). Reports suggest a lack of efficacy in the treatment of feline **psychogenic alopecia** (Sawyer et al. 1999). It should be noted that buspirone was not detectable in plasma after transdermal application in cats, making oral administration a must (Mealey et al. 2004). In short, buspirone is a great first-line treatment for shy and fearful pets without known aggression problems, but there may be better options for pets with other behavioral pathologies and/or aggression issues.

Selegiline (Anipryl®); MAOI

The main MAOI used in behavioral medicine is selegiline which, under the brand name Anipryl®, is labeled for the treatment of Canine Cognitive Dysfunction (CCD) in the US (Zoetis, Inc. 2014) and as Selgian® for CCD and anxiety in the UK (Ceva 2021). While its primary effects are a result of slowed breakdown of dopamine, its increase in anti-oxidant activity through superoxide dismutase and catalase may also decrease the cellular changes (tangles and neuronal death) associated with CCD (Landsberg et al. 2013). Due to dangerous drug interactions and the risk of serotonin syndrome, selegiline requires at least a two-week washout period between its discontinuation and the start of another serotonin enhancing medication, such as fluoxetine, and requires a 5-week washout period between the discontinuation of fluoxetine and the start of selegiline (Zoetis, Inc. 2014). Caution must be used with several opioids (Dodam et al. 2004), metronidazole, prednisone, some antibiotics, and sympathomimetic and sympatholytic medications (Dodam et al. 2004; Fuller and Sajatovic 2009; Dantas and Crowell-Davis 2019b). Unlike in humans, the dietary impacts of tyramine found in aged foods like cheese and yogurt do not create a risk for life-threatening hypertension (Dantas and Crowell-Davis 2019b). Phenylpropanolamine, a common treatment for urinary incontinence in older dogs, is safe in combination with selegiline, though blood pressure evaluation before and after combining is recommended (Cohn et al. 2002). Though selegiline is often used to treat cognitive changes in cats, its use is off-label, and there is no placebo-controlled trial in cats (Landsberg et al. 2010; Sordo and Gunn-Moore 2021).

Selecting a Daily Medication

Specific drug selection and dose (Table 21.1) are based on individual pet and client needs, taking therapeutic needs, side effect profiles,

Table 21.1 Daily medication doses.

Daily medication generic name	Canine oral dose	Feline oral dose
Fluoxetine	1.0–4 mg/kg Q24 h	0.5–1.5 mg/kg Q24 h
Sertraline	1–5 mg/kg Q24 h or divided	0.5–1.5 mg/kg Q24 h
Paroxetine	0.5–2 mg/kg Q12[a]–24 h	0.5–1.5 mg/kg Q24 h
Clomipramine	2–4 mg/kg Q12 h	0.25–1 mg/kg Q24 h
Amitriptyline	2–6 mg/kg Q12 h	0.5–2 mg/kg Q24 h
Venlafaxine	2–4 mg/kg Q12 h	0.6–1.7 mg/kg Q24[b] h
Buspirone	0.5–2 mg/kg Q8–12 h	0.5–1 mg/kg Q12 h
Selegiline	0.5–1mg/kg Q24 h	0.25–0.5 mg/kg Q24 h

Daily medications commonly used in veterinary medicine (Crowell-Davis, Sharron L., and Lansberg, Gary M. 2009; Crowell-Davis et al. 2019b; Landsberg et al. 2013).

[a] Based on (Luescher 2003).

[b] Based on (Pflaum and Bennett 2021 and Hopfensperger 2016).

and financial constraints into consideration. Rarely is there a "go to" medication for each specific condition, rather the selection should be based on the needs unique to each patient. For example, in the treatment of canine separation anxiety, many options exist. If you have more comfort prescribing a medication with strong literature support, your best selection is likely Reconcile® (fluoxetine) or Clomicalm® (clomipramine), as each carries specific FDA labels for the treatment of separation anxiety. If more substantial and immediate calming effects are needed, such as those provided by drugs that have strong antihistamine effects, then Clomicalm® may be your better option of the two. That said, if cost is a major concern, clients may find the generic fluoxetine to be more affordable than Clomicalm® or clomipramine in many pharmacies. If your patient also historically has a finicky appetite, then fluoxetine may not actually be an appropriate first choice. Instead, you might opt for paroxetine (Paxil®) for its appetite enhancing effects, despite its lack of FDA labeling and fewer placebo-controlled trials. If your patient is also an epileptic, then paroxetine would not be the best first choice (Hill et al. 2015). In this case, sertraline (Zoloft®) would be a safer choice and should also have neutral effects on appetite. In summary, your first recommendation is to attempt to follow medications with FDA labels for specific indications in dogs and cats. When that is not readily available for the syndrome or species you are treating, or if the side effect profile or cost makes those drugs contraindicated or unfeasible, you can examine the side effect profile and costs of other options within the same or similar classes of drugs. Keep in mind that trial and error is commonplace with psychotropic medications, and your first choice may not yield the desired effect. If you are not seeing the results you had hoped for after six to eight weeks, you can attempt a dose increase. If you are seeing no results or adverse effects, then you will need to discontinue that medication and move onto another. Some patients take three, four, or even five attempts at daily drug establishment. You are wise to counsel clients and provide realistic expectations as they begin this journey with their pet.

Event Medications

Patients who experience extreme fear or **phobia** of a predictable and unavoidable trigger, such as fireworks, veterinary visits, thunderstorms, or being home alone, may benefit from immediate, as-needed pre-"event" psychopharmacologic support. Patients who qualify for daily medications may also have conditions that fall into this category. If daily medication is not sufficient or if immediate daily control is needed while waiting the four to six weeks for daily medications to reach therapeutic effects, *event* medications may be warranted *daily*. Apart from combinations from inside the same class, event medications can be mixed and matched together as well as with daily medications, vastly expanding your pharmacologic toolkit.

Clonidine; α-2 Agonist

Clonidine is an α-2 agonist used to treat hypertension, Attention Deficit Hyperactivity Disorder (ADHD), and Post Traumatic Stress Disorder (PTSD) in humans (Fuller and Sajatovic 2009; Ming et al. 2011). The most likely side effects in pets include sedation, GI upset, and a drop in blood pressure. In obese dogs, it may decrease both hypertension and insulin resistance, though these effects are not seen in dogs with normal body condition (Rocchini et al. 1999). Onset to effect is about 30–60 minutes, and duration of effect can vary between patients (4–8 hours). Clonidine is hepatically metabolized and renally excreted (Ogata and Dodman 2011). Polytherapy is common with clonidine, and it has been used in combination with SSRIs, TCAs, or buspirone for the management of noise phobia, separation related problems, and aggression in dogs (Ogata and Dodman 2011). There are a variety of studies in rats (Brusberg et al. 2008; Li et al. 2007; Romero-Sandoval and Eisenach 2007) and humans (Nitta et al. 2013; Reuben et al. 1998; Wahi et al. 2016), that suggest clonidine may have analgesic properties in spinal tissues, but this has not been assessed in companion animals. Clonidine may also be useful in the treatment of inflammatory bowel disease (IBD) in both dogs and cats (Washabu 2013).

Sileo® (Dexmedetomidine Gel 0.25 ml per dot, 0.09 mg/ml); α-2 Agonist

Sileo® oral transmucosal gel is FDA approved for noise and storm fear in dogs, dosed on dots per weight, applied directly to the gums. Doses can be repeated every 2 hours, up to five times in a 24-hour period. An opened tube loses its potency after four weeks and will lose it within two weeks if not stored in the dark at room temperature. Vomiting is the most common side effect (Zoetis 2016). Unlike the powerful sedative effects seen in injectable alpha-2 agonists, the oral transmucosal gel seems to elicit minimal sedation in dogs. In fact, in an at home clinical trial treating dogs with phobias related to fireworks from 6 p.m. to 2 a.m., >85% of dogs whose fear improved were still noted to be awake and alert (Korpivaara et al. 2017). Note that clients must wear gloves when administering this medication, and it may not be safe to administer it to dogs with family-directed aggression due to close contact with the dog's mouth during drug administration.

Trazodone; SARI

Trazodone is a serotonin antagonist reuptake inhibitor (SARI). It antagonizes serotonin auto-receptors, giving it the same overall effect as an SSRI without the four- to six-week lag time. The onset of effect takes 90–120 minutes, and effects typically last 7–8 hours. It also has an antihistamine property that provides immediate calming effects in most dogs. Like most other serotonin enhancing drugs, it is metabolized by the liver and cleared by the kidneys (Dantas and Crowell-Davis 2019a). Side effects include GI upset, worsening of pre-existing incontinence, and lowering of the seizure threshold (Hill et al. 2015). Less likely is agitation, and even rarer is priapism (reported in humans) and liver enzyme elevation (Arnold et al. 2021; Gilbert-Gregory et al. 2016; Gruen et al. 2017; Gruen and Sherman 2008).

In dogs, trazodone has been shown to facilitate calm behavior after orthopedic surgery (Gruen et al. 2017), to reduce anxiety-related behaviors during hospitalization (Gilbert-Gregory et al. 2016), and as an adjunct medication for a range of anxiety related disorders: separation anxiety, storm phobia, generalized anxiety, noise phobia, compulsive disorder, and travel phobia, with or without concurrent aggression diagnoses (Gruen and Sherman 2008). It reduces isoflurane levels needed to maintain anesthesia (Hoffman et al. 2018) and may also decrease transitional stress and, thus, upper respiratory infections in dogs acclimating to shelters (Abrams et al. 2020).

Primary literature on the use of trazodone in cats is sparse but has been useful for veterinary visits (Orlando et al. 2016; Stevens et al. 2016). It decreased blood pressure when given to cats, with no echocardiographic or heart rate changes (Fries et al. 2019).

Gabapentin and Pregabalin

Gabapentin is named because it was synthesized to be an analogue of the inhibitory neurotransmitter γ-amino-butyric acid, or GABA (Crowell-Davis et al. 2019a). Interestingly, neither gabapentin nor pregabalin interact with GABA receptors at all and instead act diffusely by blocking α2–δ subunits of voltage-gated Ca2+ channels, earning the term **neuromodulator** (Plumb 2015). Both medications take 30–60 minutes to reach therapeutic effects, and effects last about 8 hours. Gabapentin has dose-dependent sedative and minimal anticonvulsant effects (Stahl 2008; Battistin et al. 1984) and was shown to be effective in managing storm fears in a placebo-controlled trial (Bleuer-Elsner et al. 2001). Side effects may include excess sedation, ataxia, agitation, increased vocalization, or decreased appetite (Crowell-Davis et al. 2019a); cats may be more prone to vomiting (van Haaften et al. 2017). Because gabapentin is predominantly cleared by the kidneys (Vollmer et al. 1986; Adrian et al. 2018; Siao et al. 2010), screening for renal insufficiency is recommended prior to daily use.

Like trazodone, gabapentin decreases the amount of isoflurane needed to keep dogs anesthetized (Johnson et al. 2019). In cats, gabapentin has been a game changer in the treatment of veterinary clinic FAS. Multiple placebo-controlled trials show it to be effective at decreasing travel and veterinary exam-related anxiety (Pankratz et al. 2017; van Haaften et al. 2017). Be aware that liquid gabapentin for humans (Neurontin®) contains xylitol, and veterinarians need to exercise caution when prescribing liquid formulations for dogs and cats (American Veterinary Medical Association 2017). A recent study in cats, using a liquid formulation of pregabalin (Bonqat®), demonstrated substantial reduction in signs of FAS associated with travel to and experiences during veterinary visits (Lamminen et al. 2023).

Neurologists may recommend gabapentin to manage parasethesias and neuropathic and chronic pain in cats (Guedes et al. 2018) and dogs (Giudice et al. 2019; Mitton et al. 2019; Plessas et al. 2015). Recently, though, pregabalin has demonstrated greater efficacy in the treatment of neuropathic pain (Sanchis-Mora et al. 2019; Schmierer et al. 2020; Thoefner et al. 2020). Trials with pregabalin in the treatment of anxiety are lacking in dogs, though promising in humans and cats (Generoso et al. 2017).

Benzodiazepines

Benzodiazepines are classified as **anxiolytic** and are the primary anti-**panic** medications. Specific medications in this class include alprazolam, diazepam, lorazepam, clonazepam, clorazepate, and chlordiazepoxide. They facilitate the activity of the main inhibitory neurotransmitter, GABA, with their panic-alleviating effects stemming from this activity in the amygdala (Stahl 2008). Clients often remark that after administering a benzodiazepine, their pet seems "happy" or "playful" for the first time in situations that would normally trigger crippling fear and panic. One advantage of using a benzodiazepine over another medication is that they start working as soon as they are absorbed – as quickly as 30 minutes for many patients (Landsberg et al. 2013). They are selected based on duration of time needed for relief and hepatic metabolism pathways. See Table 21.2 for specific benzodiazepine doses and durations of effect.

Benzodiazepines are all metabolized by the liver using various cytochrome pathways, with the exception of lorazepam, which is glucuronidated (Gerkens et al. 1981; Crowell-Davis 2019a). This makes lorazepam a

Table 21.2 Event medication doses.

Medication	Dogs	Cats
Clonidine	0.01–0.05 mg/kg PO q6–12 h	0.005–0.01 mg/kg PO Q12 h
Sileo® gel	125 mcg/m^2 as number of dots/lb of body weight, oral transmucosal may be repeated every 2 h up to 5 times per 24 h period	
Trazodone	4–18 g/kg PO Q8 h, not exceeding 300 mg/dose	50–100 mg/cat PO Q12 h
Gabapentin	5–50 mg/kg PO Q8–12 h	2–30 mg/kg PO Q8 h Up to 49.6 mg/kg situationally
Bonqat®		5 mg/kg PO 90 min before the start of transportation
Alprazolam	0.02–0.1 mg/kg PO Q4–12 h	0.125–0.25 mg/cat PO Q8–12 h or 0.02–0.1 mg/kg PO Q8–12 h
Diazepam	0.5–2.2 mg/kg PO Q4–6 h	Avoid
Clorazepate	0.5–2.2 mg/kg PO Q4–24 h	Avoid
Clonazepam	0.1–0.5 mg/kg Q8–12 h	0.015–0.25 mg/kg Q12–24 h
Chlordiazepoxide	2–6.6 mg/kg Q8–12 h	Avoid
Lorazepam	0.02–0.2 mg/kg Q8–24 h	0.125–0.25 mg/cat PO Q12–24 h or 0.03–0.08 mg/kg PO Q12 h

Crowell-Davis and Lansberg 2009; Crowell-Davis et al. 2019b; Landsberg et al. 2013; Lilly 2020; Pankratz et al. 2017; Zoetis 2016 and 2023.

potentially safer option for dogs with liver damage and for cats. Diazepam is associated with fulminant and fatal hepatic necrosis in cats (Center et al. 1996; Hughs et al. 1996); both clorazepate and chlordiazepoxide share the entire metabolic pathway with diazepam (Crowell-Davis 2019a) so all three drugs are best avoided in cats.

Benzodiazepines may increase appetite. This is a desirable side effect as it may increase interest in positive reinforcement training and counterconditioning efforts (Brown et al. 1976; Herron et al. 2008; Landsberg et al. 2013). While this class of drugs may work wonders for some patients, they also come with a high likelihood of undesirable side effects. In one retrospective study, approximately one out of three dogs prescribed diazepam were reported to have paradoxical excitation or profound agitation. Due to their muscle relaxing effects, ataxia is a common side effect which tends to wane with repeated dosing. Clients should be cautioned about blocking off stairs and monitoring pets' jumping on and off of furniture to prevent injurious falls during initial dosing. Other adverse side effects include disinhibition of aggression, vomiting, and sedation (Crowell-Davis and Lansberg 2009; Crowell-Davis 2019b; Herron et al. 2008). After prolonged, regular use, the dose should be tapered rather than stopped suddenly, as physical dependence is possible and has been demonstrated in dogs and other species (Crowell-Davis 2019a). Careful patient selection for benzodiazepines is warranted as there is a potential for human abuse.

Acepromazine

Acepromazine is a phenothiazine neuroleptic (anti-psychotic). It works by blocking dopamine in the muscle motor pathway, causing stillness. This stillness should not be mistaken for anxiolysis or "calmness". There is anecdotal evidence that startle reactions and noise phobias may worsen with the use of this medication, and there are documented reports of acute aggression (Seibert and Crowell-Davis 2019). Common side effects include profound sedation. Less common effects include hyperthermia, ataxia, hyperglycemia, hypotension, and paradoxical excitation (Posner 2017; Seibert and Crowell-Davis 2019). Acepromazine also has **antiemetic** properties, making it a potentially useful adjunct to anxiolytic medications for pets with comorbid motion sickness (Valverde et al. 2004). Keep in mind that dogs who are homozygous for the p-glycoprotein defect commonly found in collies, Australian shepherds, Shetland and Old English sheep dogs may require decreased dosing (Deshpande et al. 2016; Geyer et al. 2005; Mealey and Meurs 2008; Neff et al. 2004). Acepromazine is best used in combination with anxiety-relieving medications when more profound tranquilization is desired. We typically do not dose acepromazine with alpha-2 agonists due to their opposing effects on blood pressure.

Polytherapy

As mentioned above, *event* medications can be combined with longer lasting *daily* medications. This expands treatment options substantially, but the decision-making process can be intimidating, especially considering the literature on polytherapy in animals is sparse. So, when is polytherapy warranted, and how should you approach it?

Indications for polytherapy:

1) Immediate relief of symptoms is needed:
   Some patients' behavior is concerning enough that immediate alleviation of clinical signs is needed – whether for their welfare, safety, or ability to stay in their current home and/or to avoid euthanasia. In Chapter 12, we referred to the use of "crisis buster" medications for this reason. Those patients are in a crisis state and cannot afford to wait four to six weeks for an SSRI or TCA to start working. If that is the case, then starting one of the *event* medications on a *daily* basis, every 8–12 hours BEFORE starting your *daily*, longer-lasting medications can give your patient (and client) some immediate benefit. The *event* medication can then be maintained daily while onboarding a *daily* medication. When we do this, we refer to the initial rapid acting *event* medication as a **bridge medication**. In some cases, you can wean the patient off of the bridge medication once your *daily* medication reaches therapeutic levels. Choosing what medication to use as a bridge follows the same process as if you were using it on its own: what side effects may be useful? (Think – antihistamine effects of trazodone in a dog with concurrent pruritus), Which side effects may not be tolerated (Think – worsening of aggression with a benzodiazepine) or medically contraindicated? (Think – clonidine in a patient with congestive heart failure).
2) The daily medication is not sufficient for certain anticipated stressful events:
   Some patients have known and anticipated events that trigger panic and stress that are likely to override the effects of their daily medication. Consider storms, vet visits, visitors, or neighboring construction, for example. In those situations, you typically have time to start a daily medication first and to test an event medication later. Once you have confirmed there are no major side effects from the daily medication (give it for at least 5–10 days), you can have the client administer a test dose of an event medication on a day when no stressful events are anticipated. That way, they have a dose plan in place prior to the stressful event, whether it occurs during daily medication onboarding, or after.
3) The daily medication is helpful, but not quite enough, even at maximum dose:
   Often, when patients struggle with severe behavioral disorders, even the maximum

dose of a daily medication may not be enough to adequately control their symptoms. Many clients may not want to risk regression by weaning their pet off a medication that has been at least moderately helpful in order to try a new daily medication. In these cases, it is reasonable to add an *event* medication every 8–24 hours on a *daily* basis. For some patients, there is a specific time of day when symptoms are at their worst, such as early evening hours when the family is starting to settle but the patient is spiraling with anxiety. For these patients, a once daily mid-afternoon dose of an event medication may be indicated. In other cases, the need is full-time and *event* medications can be given every 8–12 hours, every day.

In some advanced cases, polytherapy that involves two or more drugs that fall into the *daily* category may be warranted. For example, buspirone is sometimes used in careful combination with SSRIs as a means of boosting serotonin production in serotonin releasing neurons (Dantas et al., 2019). Occasionally, amitriptyline may be added to an SSRI, such as fluoxetine, for greater therapeutic effect. These cases are best managed by a board-certified veterinary behaviorist, when possible, due to the risk of **serotonin syndrome** (Box 21.1) and drug interaction potential. The combination of more than one drug within the same class (i.e. fluoxetine and sertraline) or the use of a SRI with a MAOI is typically contraindicated due to the high risk of serotonin syndrome (Ogata et al. 2019) (See Box 21.1). Judicious use of *daily* medications with *event* medications that modulate serotonin is safer and more common, but clients should still be informed of the drug interaction risks.

Administering Medications

Pets who are highly food-motivated may readily take pills covered in anything that smells and tastes delicious, but others are far pickier. There are several different approaches to getting medications into pets in a non-stressful manner. In general, "pilling" a pet is not recommended, as it can cause fear, and in some cases aggression, toward the person administering the drug. Alternatives to pilling include:

1) Teaching the patient to take pills as a pattern hidden in the second treat in a 3-treat series ("treat-pill-treat" method)
   This method is best accomplished using soft food with a crunchy texture added. For example, you can make a treat ball from canned dog food or commercially available pill disguising treats by mixing the treats with crushed crackers or potato chips (Figure 21.2). This gives added texture to disguise the hard texture of the pill. Many pets will reject a treat ball once a harder texture is detected. By offering treat balls with

Box 21.1 Serotonin Syndrome

Definition: A syndrome that occurs when too much serotonin floods the synaptic cleft, typically a result of overdose or a combination of serotonin-enhancing drugs, such as MAOIs and SSRIs.

Signs:

- Hyperthermia
- Tachycardia
- Tremors
- Profound agitation
- Seizures
- Collapse

Treatment: Cyproheptadine 1.1 mg/kg PO or rectally Q8 h (Mensching 2012)

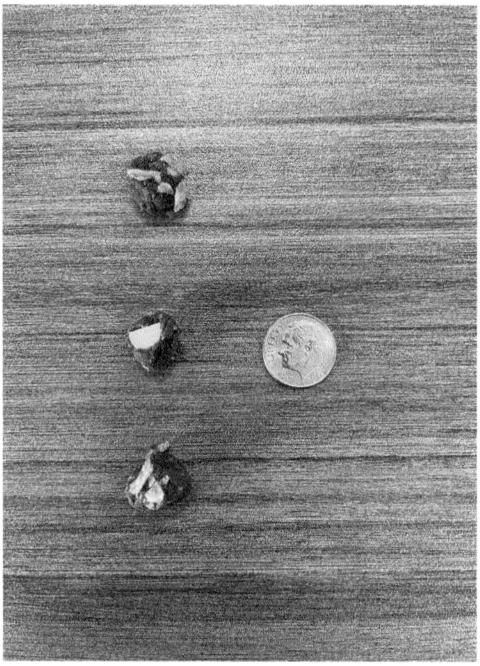

Figure 21.2 Pills can be disguised and more readily consumed when coated with a highly palatable and sticky food substance and given in a "treat-pill-treat" method. The addition of a crunchy texture to the treat balls, such as the potato chip crumbs shown here, prevents pets from immediately rejecting the hard texture of the tablet. *Source:* Meghan E. Herron.

crunchy food textures several times prior to attempting to hide a pill inside, we can teach our pets to be more trusting of harder textures. By hiding the pill in the second of a three-treat series, we can typically count on them to have swallowed the second treat as the third one is presented before realizing there was a pill inside.

2) Compounding medication into a flavored liquid or treat that can be given alone or added to food

   Many online pharmacies offer compounding, but quality assurance varies widely. Best practice is to utilize online pharmacies which are accredited by the National Association of Board of Pharmacy (NABP). These pharmacies will have a *pharmacy* domain name or can be found on the NABP registry. Pharmacies registered with the F8/9/2022DA as 503B with online portals are known as "outsourcing facilities" and also meet all NABP standards. You may still need to disguise flavored medications in palatable food and/or utilize the "treat-pill-treat" method. For liquid medications, the "parfait" or "sandwich" method of putting palatable liquid food (poultry flavored baby food, Churu® paste, etc.) in a syringe before and after the medication so that the pet can voluntarily lick palatable food from the syringe before and after licking flavored liquid medication (Figure 21.3). Liquid medications should not be forcefully squirted into a pet's mouth, as syringe avoidance will likely result, making future administration difficult.

3) Transdermal application of a compounded medication

   This last option comes with some caveats. There are more systems and options available than there are data; for example, many medications can be purchased from a variety of vendors as transdermal. However, we only have data for effective absorption of transdermal mirtazapine (Mirataz®) and methimazole (Boretti et al. 2014; Hoffman et al. 2002; Sartor et al. 2004). Altering the pH and binding agents of medications for compounded options may alter their bioavailability.

See the online materials for a special handout on conditioning pets to take medication readily in food.

Weaning

There is a common misconception that once you start a psychotropic medication, the treatment must be life-long. While indeed there are pets whose behavioral pathologies warrant long-term psychotropic medication therapy,

(a) (b)

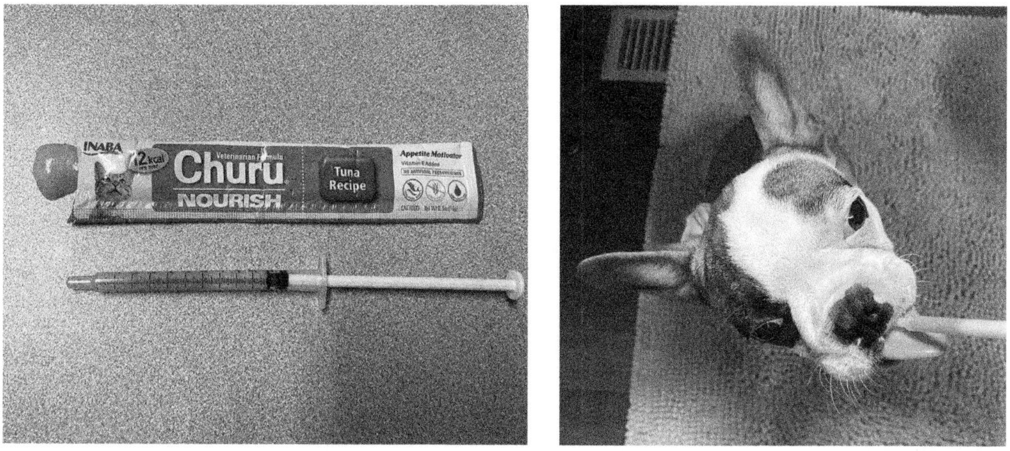

Figure 21.3 Medication "parfait." Liquid medications can be sandwiched in a syringe between palatable liquid foods, such as the Churu paste shown here (a). This allows the pet to readily consume (b) and have an enjoyable experience before and after taking the medication, making future administration easier.

many pets can and should eventually be weaned off their medications. Much depends on the severity of the illness, the ability of the client to manage triggers, and/or the progress that can be made through behavior modification and training. Separation anxiety is one condition where weaning is often possible. In the initial Clomicalm® trials for separation anxiety, only 5% of dogs worsened when therapy was discontinued after 30 weeks (King et al. 2004). In one trial where urine marking cats were treated with fluoxetine for 8 weeks, a very short time, 11% remained marking free after fluoxetine was discontinued (Pryor et al. 2001). The choice to wean involves a continued balancing act between the benefits and the costs. A typical approach for patients responding well to behavior modification is to maintain the support of medication until clinical signs resolve and all behavioral goals are met. At that point, medications should be maintained for a minimum of 90 additional days, at which point weaning, rather than abrupt discontinuation, can be attempted (Crowell-Davis, et al., 2019). Weaning is typically accomplished by decreasing the dose by 25% every 2–4 weeks. If there is a return of undesirable behaviors, therapy is resumed at the lowest effective dose and the plan is re-evaluated.

When weaning for the purpose of changing a medication that is not providing adequate relief for the patient, the process can be much faster. This is especially true for patients who have been on therapy for only a few weeks or months. In these cases, you could consider cutting the dose in thirds or halves every few days, then providing a washout period without medication to make sure the initial drug is eliminated prior to starting the new medication. Washout periods depend on the half-life of the individual drug being discontinued. Most SSRIs, SNRIs, and TCAs have a half-life of 24 hours or less, except for fluoxetine and its active metabolites, which have half-lives of several days. When changing from fluoxetine to another drug with SRI properties, a washout period of 6 days is recommended. As stated previously, a washout of 5 weeks is recommended when changing from fluoxetine to a MAOI. See Box 21.2 for weaning plan examples.

Box 21.2 Sample weaning plans for patients on psychotropic medications

Scenario 1: Patient is a 30 kg dog with separation anxiety who has been receiving Reconcile® (fluoxetine) 32 mg once daily for 2 months with no noticeable change in behavior. You are electing to change to Clomicalm® (clomipramine) to see if greater relief is possible with a new medication.

Plan: Because the client reports minimal relief from the current medication and the pet has only been on this medication for a short period, you may make this change quickly: Decrease Reconcile® to 16 mg once daily for 6 days, then discontinue and wait 6 days before starting Clomicalm®.

Scenario 2: Patient is a 30 kg dog who has been receiving Reconcile® (fluoxetine) 32 mg for the past 2 years for separation anxiety and has had a complete resolution of clinical signs for the past 4 months.

Plan: Because we have resolved clinical signs for more than 3 months, an attempt to wean off Reconcile is warranted. Since we want to assess carefully how well the patient can succeed off medication and because therapy has been longer term, we will wean much more slowly: Decrease Reconcile to 24 mg once daily for 4 weeks. Record home alone behavior each week and as long as there is no worsening of behavior after 4 weeks, decrease to 16 mg once daily. If video monitoring of home alone behavior confirms there is still no worsening of behavior after 4 additional weeks, decrease again to 8 mg once daily. If the patient is still successful 4 weeks later, you may discontinue Reconcile entirely and check in with the patient in one week to ensure there is no return of symptoms and that video monitoring confirms the resolution of clinical signs.

References

10 Poison Pills for Pets (2021). American Veterinary Medical Association. https://www.avma.org/resources/pet-owners/petcare/10-poison-pills-pets (accessed 21 December 2021).

Abrams, J., Brennen, R., and Byosiere, S.-E. (2020). Trazodone as a mediator of transitional stress in a shelter: effects on illness, length of stay, and outcome. *J. Vet. Behav.* 36: 13–18. https://doi.org/10.1016/j.jveb.2020.01.001.

Adrian, D., Papich, M.G., Baynes, R. et al. (2018). The pharmacokinetics of gabapentin in cats. *J. Vet. Intern. Med.* 32: 1996–2002. https://doi.org/10.1111/jvim.15313.

American Veterinary Medical Association (2017). *Eliminate Xylitol from Canine Prescriptions*. American Veterinary Medical Association https://www.avma.org/blog/eliminate-xylitol-canine-prescriptions (accessed 25 August 2021).

Arnold, A., Davis, A., Wismer, T., and Lee, J.A. (2021). Suspected hepatotoxicity secondary to trazodone therapy in a dog. *J. Vet. Emerg. Crit. Care* 31: 112–116. https://doi.org/10.1111/vec.13028.

Ballantyne, K.C. (2017). Animal behavior case of the month. *J. Am. Vet. Med. Assoc.* 251: 296–298. https://doi.org/10.2460/javma.251.3.296.

Battistin, L., Varotto, M., Berlese, G., and Roman, G. (1984). Effects of some anticonvulsant drugs on brain GABA level and GAD and GABA-T activities. *Neurochem. Res.* 9: 225–231. https://doi.org/10.1007/BF00964170.

Bleuer-Elsner, S., Medam, T., and Masson, S. (2001). Effects of a single oral dose of gabapentin on storm phobia in dogs: a double-blind, placebo-controlled crossover trial. *Vet. Rec.* e453: https://doi.org/10.1002/vetr.453.

Boretti, F.S., Sieber-Ruckstuhl, N.S., Schäfer, S. et al. (2014). Transdermal application of methimazole in hyperthyroid cats: a long-term follow-up study. *J. Feline Med. Surg.* 16: 453–459. https://doi.org/10.1177/1098612X13509808.

Brown, R.F., Houpt, K.A., and Schryver, H.F. (1976). Stimulation of food intake in horses by diazepam and promazine. *Pharmacol. Biochem. Behav.* 5: 495–497.

Brusberg, M., Ravnefjord, A., Lindgreen, M. et al. (2008). Oral clonidine inhibits visceral pain-related viscerosomatic and cardiovascular responses to colorectal distension in rats. *Eur. J. Pharm.* 591: 243–251. https://doi.org/10.1016/j.ejphar.2008.06.056.

Catterson, M.L. and Preskorn, S.H. (1996). Pharmacokinetics of selective serotonin reuptake inhibitors: clinical relevance. *Pharmacol. Toxicol.* 78: 203–208. https://doi.org/10.1111/j.1600-0773.1996.tb00206.x.

Center, S.A., Elston, T.H., Rowland, P.H. et al. (1996). Fulminant hepatic failure associated with oral administration of diazepam in 11 cats. *J. Am. Vet. Med. Assoc.* 209: 618–625.

Ceva (2021). SELGIAN®Package Insert.

Chew, D.J., Buffington, C.A., Kendall, M.S. et al. (1998). Amitriptyline treatment for severe recurrent idiopathic cystitis in cats. *J. Am. Vet. Med. Assoc.* 213: 1282–1286.

Ciribassi, J., Luescher, A., Pasloske, K.S. et al. (2003). Comparative bioavailability of fluoxetine after transdermal and oral administration to healthy cats. *Am. J. Vet. Res.* 64: 994–998. https://doi.org/10.2460/ajvr.2003.64.994.

Cohn, L.A., Dodam, J.R., and Szladovits, B. (2002). Effects of selegiline, phenylpropanolamine, or a combination of both on physiologic and behavioral variables in healthy dogs. *Am. J. Vet. Res.* 63: 827–832. https://doi.org/10.2460/ajvr.2002.63.827.

Covetrus North America, 2000. Clomipramine Hydrochloride - Covetrus North America: Veterinary Package Insert.

Crowell-Davis, S.L. and Lansberg, G.M. (2009). Pharmacology and pheromone therapy. In: *BSAVA Manual of Canine and Feline Behavioural Medicine*, 2e, 245–258. British Small Animal Veterinary Association.

Crowell-Davis, S.L. (2019a). Tricyclic antidepressants. In: *Veterinary Psychopharmacology*, 231–256. Hoboken, NJ: Wiley-Blackwell.

Crowell-Davis, S.L. (2019b). Benzodiazepines. In: *Veterinary Psychopharmacology*, 67–102. Hoboken, NJ: Wiley-Blackwell.

Crowell-Davis, S.L., Iriajiri, M., and Dantas, L.M.d.S. (2019a). Anticonvulsants and mood stabilizers. In: *Veterinary Psychopharmacology*. Hoboken, NJ: Wiley-Blackwell.

Crowell-Davis, S.L., Murray, T., and Dantas, L.M.d.S. (2019b). *Veterinary psychopharmacology*, 2e. Hoboken, NJ: Wiley-Blackwell.

Dantas, L.M.d.S. and Crowell-Davis, S.L. (2019a). Miscellaneous serotonergic agents. In: *Veterinary Psychopharmacology*, 129–146. Hoboken, NJ: Wiley-Blackwell.

Dantas, L.M.d.S. and Crowell-Davis, S.L. (2019b). Monoamine oxidase inhibitors. In: *Veterinary Psychopharmacology*, 185–190. Hoboken, NJ: Wiley-Blackwell.

Dantas, L.M.d.S., Crowell-Davis, S.L., and Ogata, N. (2019). Combinations. In: *Veterinary Psychopharmacology*, 281–290. Hoboken, NJ: Wiley-Blackwell.

de Abajo, F.J., Rodríguez, L.A.G., and Montero, D. (1999). Association between selective serotonin reuptake inhibitors and upper gastrointestinal bleeding: population based case-control study. *BMJ* 319: 1106–1109.

de Jong, J.C.F., van den Berg, P.B., Tobi, H., and de Jong-van den Berg, L.T.W. (2003). Combined use of SSRIs and NSAIDs increases the risk of gastrointestinal adverse effects. *Br. J. Clin. Pharmacol.* 55: 591–595. https://doi.org/10.1046/j.0306-5251.2002.01770.x.

Delucchi, L., Martino, P., Baldovino, A. et al. (2010). Use of venlafaxine in the treatment of a canine narcolepsy-cataplexy case. *J. Small Anim. Pract.* 51: 132–132. https://doi.org/10.1111/j.1748-5827.2009.00908.x.

Deshpande, D., Hill, K.E., Mealey, K.L. et al. (2016). The effect of the canine ABCB1-1Δ mutation on sedation after intravenous administration of acepromazine. *J. Vet. Intern. Med.* 30: 636–641. https://doi.org/10.1111/jvim.13827.

Dodam, J.R., Cohn, L.A., Durham, H.E., and Szladovits, B. (2004). Cardiopulmonary effects of medetomidine, oxymorphone, or butorphanol in selegiline-treated dogs. *Vet. Anaesth. Analg.* 31: 129–137. https://doi.org/10.1111/j.1467-2987.2004.00164.x.

Dodman, N.H., Donnelly, R., Shuster, L. et al. (1996). Use of fluoxetine to treat dominance aggression in dogs. *J. Am. Vet. Med. Assoc.* 209: 1585–1587.

Plumb, D.C. (2015). *Plumb's Veterinary Drug Handbook*, 7e. Stockholm, Wisconsin: PharmaVet.

Drug Bank: Fluoxetine (2021). Drug bank. https://go.drugbank.com/drugs/DB00472 (accessed 23 June 2021).

Elanco Inc. (US) (1999). Clomicalm. Elanco US Inc.: Veterinary Package Insert.

Frank, D. and Dehasse, J. (2003). Differential diagnosis and management of human-directed aggression in cats. *Vet. Clin. N. Am. Small Anim. Pract.* 33: 269–286. https://doi.org/10.1016/S0195-5616(02)00131-6.

Frank, D., Gauthier, A., and Bergeron, R. (2006). Placebo-controlled double-blind clomipramine trial for the treatment of anxiety or fear in beagles during ground transport. *Can. Vet. J.* 47: 1102–1108.

Fries, R.C., Kadotani, S., Vitt, J.P., and Schaeffer, D.J. (2019). Effects of oral trazodone on echocardiographic and hemodynamic variables in healthy cats. *J. Feline Med. Surg.* 21: 1080–1085. https://doi.org/10.1177/1098612X18814565.

Fuller, M.A. and Sajatovic, M. (ed.) (2009). *Drug Information Handbook for Psychiatry: Including Psychotropic, Nonpsychotropic, and Herbal Agents*, 7e. Lexi-Comp Inc.

Garattini, S. (1992). An update on the pharmacology of serotoninergic appetite-suppressive drugs. *Int. J. Obes. Relat. Metab. Disord.* 16 (Suppl 4): S41–S48.

Generoso, M.B., Trevizol, A.P., Kasper, S. et al. (2017). Pregabalin for generalized anxiety disorder: an updated systematic review and meta-analysis. *Int. Clin. Psychopharmacol.* 32: 49–55. https://doi.org/10.1097/YIC.0000000000000147.

Gerkens, J.F., Desmond, P.V., Schenker, S., and Branch, R.A. (1981). Hepatic and extrahepatic glucuronidation of lorazepam in the dog. *Hepatology* 1: 329–335. https://doi.org/10.1002/hep.1840010409.

Geyer, J., Döring, B., Godoy, J.R. et al. (2005). Frequency of the nt230 (del4) MDR1 mutation in Collies and related dog breeds in Germany. *J. Vet. Pharmacol. Ther.* 28: 545–551. https://doi.org/10.1111/j.1365-2885.2005.00692.x.

Gilbert-Gregory, S.E., Stull, J.W., Rice, M.R., and Herron, M.E. (2016). Effects of trazodone on behavioral signs of stress in hospitalized dogs. *J. Am. Vet. Med. Assoc.* 249: 1281–1291. https://doi.org/10.2460/javma.249.11.1281.

Giudice, E., Crinò, C., Barillaro, G. et al. (2019). Clinical findings in degenerative lumbosacral stenosis in ten dogs—a pilot study on the analgesic activity of tramadol and gabapentin. *J. Vet. Behav.* 33: 7–15. https://doi.org/10.1016/j.jveb.2019.05.004.

Gruen, M.E., Roe, S.C., Griffith, E.H., and Sherman, B.L. (2017). The use of trazodone to facilitate calm behavior after elective orthopedic surgery in dogs: results and lessons learned from a clinical trial. *J. Vet. Behav.* 22: 41–45. https://doi.org/10.1016/j.jveb.2017.09.008.

Gruen, M.E. and Sherman, B.L. (2008). Use of trazodone as an adjunctive agent in the treatment of canine anxiety disorders: 56 cases (1995–2007). *J. Am. Vet. Med. Assoc.* 233: 1902–1907. https://doi.org/10.2460/javma.233.12.1902.

Guedes, A.G.P., Meadows, J.M., Pypendop, B.H. et al. (2018). Assessment of the effects of gabapentin on activity levels and owner-perceived mobility impairment and quality of life in osteoarthritic geriatric cats. *J. Am. Vet. Med. Assoc.* 253: 579–585. https://doi.org/10.2460/javma.253.5.579.

Gulikers, K.P. and Panciera, D.L. (2003). Evaluation of the effects of clomipramine on canine thyroid function tests. *J. Vet. Intern. Med.*

17: 44–49. https://doi.org/10.1111/j.1939-1676.2003.tb01322.x.

Hart, B.L., Cliff, K.D., Tynes, V.V., and Bergman, L. (2005). Control of urine marking by use of long-term treatment with fluoxetine or clomipramine in cats. *J. Am. Vet. Med. Assoc.* 226: 378–382. https://doi.org/10.2460/javma.2005.226.378.

Hart, B.L., Eckstein, R.A., Powell, K.L., and Dodman, N.H. (1993). Effectiveness of buspirone on urine spraying and inappropriate urination in cats. *J. Am. Vet. Med. Assoc.* 203: 254–258.

Helin-Salmivaara, A., Huttunen, T., Grönroos, J.M. et al. (2007). Risk of serious upper gastrointestinal events with concurrent use of NSAIDs and SSRIs: a case-control study in the general population. *Eur. J. Clin. Pharmacol.* 63: 403–408. https://doi.org/10.1007/s00228-007-0263-y.

Herron, M. (2010). Animal behavior case of the month. *J. Am. Vet. Med. Assoc.* 237: 916–918. https://doi.org/10.2460/javma.237.8.916.

Herron, M.E., Shofer, F.S., and Reisner, I.R. (2008). Retrospective evaluation of the effects of diazepam in dogs with anxiety-related behavior problems. *J. Am. Vet. Med. Assoc.* 233: 1420–1424. https://doi.org/10.2460/javma.233.9.1420.

Hiemke, C. and Härtter, S. (2000). Pharmacokinetics of selective serotonin reuptake inhibitors. *Pharmacol. Ther.* 85: 11–28. https://doi.org/10.1016/S0163-7258(99)00048-0.

Hill, T., Coupland, C., Morriss, R. et al. (2015). Antidepressant use and risk of epilepsy and seizures in people aged 20 to 64 years: cohort study using a primary care database. *BMC Psychiatry* 15: https://doi.org/10.1186/s12888-015-0701-9.

Hoffman, E.A., Aarnes, T.K., Ricco Pereira, C.H. et al. (2018). Effect of oral trazodone on the minimum alveolar concentration of isoflurane in dogs. *Vet. Anaesth. Analg.* 45: 754–759. https://doi.org/10.1016/j.vaa.2018.08.002.

Hoffman, S.B., Yoder, A.R., and Trepanier, L.A. (2002). Bioavailability of transdermal methimazole in a pluronic lecithin organogel (PLO) in healthy cats. *J. Vet. Pharmacol. Ther.* 25: 189–193. https://doi.org/10.1046/j.1365-2885.2002.00405.x.

Hopfensperger, M. J. (2016). Use of oral venlafaxine in cats with feline idiopathic cystitis or behavioral causes of periuria. *Proceedings of the American College of Veterinary Behaviorists (ACVB) Annual Symposium*. ACVB: 13–17. Horwitz, D.F. (2017). *Blackwell's Five-Minute Veterinary Consult Clinical Companion: Canine and Feline Behavior*. Hobokon, NJ: Wiley.

Howell, S.R., Hicks, D.R., Scatina, J.A., and Sisenwine, S.F. (1994). Pharmacokinetics of venlafaxine and O-desmethylvenlafaxine in laboratory animals. *Xenobiotica* 24: 315–327. https://doi.org/10.3109/00498259409045895.

Hughs, D., Moreau, R.E., Overall, K.L., and Winkle, T.J.V. (1996). Acute hepatic necrosis and liver failure associated with benzodiazepine therapy in six cats, 1986–1995. *J. Vet. Emerg. Crit. Care* 6: 13–20. https://doi.org/10.1111/j.1476-4431.1996.tb00030.x.

Johnson, B.A., Aarnes, T.K., Wanstrath, A.W. et al. (2019). Effect of oral administration of gabapentin on the minimum alveolar concentration of isoflurane in dogs. *Am. J. Vet. Res.* 80: 1007–1009. https://doi.org/10.2460/ajvr.80.11.1007.

Karagiannis, C.I., Burman, O.H., and Mills, D.S. (2015). Dogs with separation-related problems show a "less pessimistic" cognitive bias during treatment with fluoxetine (Reconcile™) and a behaviour modification plan. *BMC Vet. Res.* 11: https://doi.org/10.1186/s12917-015-0373-1.

Katofiasc, M.A., Nissen, J., Audia, J.E., and Thor, K.B. (2002). Comparison of the effects of serotonin selective, norepinephrine selective, and dual serotonin and norepinephrine reuptake inhibitors on lower urinary tract function in cats. *Life Sci.* 71: 1227–1236. https://doi.org/10.1016/S0024-3205(02)01848-9.

King, J.N., Overall, K.L., Appleby, D. et al. (2004). Results of a follow-up investigation to a clinical trial testing the efficacy of clomipramine in the treatment of separation anxiety in dogs. *Appl. Anim. Behav. Sci.* 89: 233–242. https://doi.org/10.1016/j.applanim.2004.06.003.

King, J.N., Simpson, B.S., Overall, K.L. et al. (2000). Treatment of separation anxiety in dogs with clomipramine: results from a prospective, randomized, double-blind, placebo-controlled, parallel-group, multicenter clinical trial. *Appl. Anim. Behav. Sci.* 67: 255–275. https://doi.org/10.1016/S0168-1591(99)00127-6.

Korpivaara, M., Laapas, K., Huhtinen, M. et al. (2017). Dexmedetomidine oromucosal gel for noise-associated acute anxiety and fear in dogs—a randomised, double-blind, placebo-controlled clinical study. *Vet. Rec.* 180: 356–356. https://doi.org/10.1136/vr.104045.

Kruger, J.M., Conway, T.S., Kaneene, J.B. et al. (2003). Randomized controlled trial of the efficacy of short-term amitriptyline administration for treatment of acute, nonobstructive, idiopathic lower urinary tract disease in cats. *J. Am. Vet. Med. Assoc.* 222: 749–758. https://doi.org/10.2460/javma.2003.222.749.

Lamminen, T., Korpivaara, M., Aspegrén, J., Palestrini, C., & Overall, K. L. (2023). Pregabalin alleviates anxiety and fear in cats during transportation and veterinary visits—A clinical field study. *Animals*, 13(3): 371.

Landsberg, G.M., Denenberg, S., and Araujo, J.A. (2010). Cognitive dysfunction in cats: a syndrome we used to dismiss as 'old age.'. *J. Feline Med. Surg.* 12: 837–848. https://doi.org/10.1016/j.jfms.2010.09.004.

Landsberg, G.M., Hunthausen, W.L., Ackerman, L.J., and Fatjó, J. (2013). Pharmacologic intervention in behavior therapy. In: *Behavior Problems of the Dog and Cat*, 113–138. Edinburgh: Saunders Elsevier.

Landsberg, G.M., Melese, P., Sherman, B.L. et al. (2008). Effectiveness of fluoxetine chewable tablets in the treatment of canine separation anxiety. *J. Vet. Behav.: Clin. Appl. Res.* 3: 12–19. https://doi.org/10.1016/j.jveb.2007.09.001.

Landsberg, G.M. and Wilson, A.L. (2005). Effects of clomipramine on cats presented for urine marking. *J. Am. Anim. Hosp. Assoc.* 41: 3–11. https://doi.org/10.5326/0410003.

Law, V., Knox, C., Djoumbou, Y. et al. (2014). DrugBank 4.0: shedding new light on drug metabolism. *Nucleic Acids Res.* 42: D1091–D1097. https://doi.org/10.1093/nar/gkt1068.

Li, C., Sekiyama, H., Hayashida, M. et al. (2007). Effects of topical application of clonidine cream on pain behaviors and spinal fos protein expression in rat models of neuropathic pain, postoperative pain, and inflammatory pain. *Anesthesiology* 107: 486–494. https://doi.org/10.1097/01.anes.0000278874.78715.1d.

Lilly, M. L. (2020). General psychopharmacology: meds for now and later. *Proceedings from the Midwest Veterinary Conference (MVC)*, Columbus, OH: MVC.

Litster, A. (2000). Use of clomipramine for treatment of behavioural disorders in 14 cats – efficacy and side-effects [WWW Document]. URL /paper/Use-of-Clomipramine-for-treatment-of-behavioural-in-Litster/9a52c84711832c3024c513c03a8fa11 2ef2d0a7a (accessed 2 March 2021).

Luescher, A.U. (2003). Diagnosis and management of compulsive disorders in dogs and cats. *Vet. Clin. N. Am. Small Anim. Pract.* 33: 253–267. https://doi.org/10.1016/S0195-5616(02)00100-6.

Maffeo, N.N., Springer, C.M., and Albright, J.D. (2023). A retrospective study on the clinical use and owner perception of venlafaxine efficacy as part of a multimodal treatment for canine fear, anxiety, and aggression. *J. Vet. Behav.* 64-65: 54–59.

Martin, K.M. (2010). Effect of clomipramine on the electrocardiogram and serum thyroid concentrations of healthy cats. *J. Vet. Behav.* 5: 123–129. https://doi.org/10.1016/j.jveb.2009.12.019.

Mealey, K.L. and Meurs, K.M. (2008). Breed distribution of the ABCB1-1Δ (multidrug sensitivity) polymorphism among dogs undergoing ABCB1 genotyping. *J. Am. Vet. Med. Assoc.* 233: 921–924. https://doi.org/10.2460/javma.233.6.921.

Mealey, K.L., Peck, K.E., Bennett, B.S. et al. (2004). Systemic absorption of amitriptyline and buspirone after oral and transdermal administration to healthy cats. *J. Vet. Intern. Med.* 18: 43–46. https://doi.org/10.1111/j.1939-1676.2004.tb00133.x.

Meijer, W.E.E., Heerdink, E.R., Nolen, W.A. et al. (2004). Association of risk of abnormal bleeding with degree of serotonin reuptake inhibition by antidepressants. *Arch. Intern. Med.* 164: 2367. https://doi.org/10.1001/archinte.164.21.2367.

Meng, H., Lu, J., and Zhang, X. (2019). Metabolic influences of commonly used antidepressants on blood glucose homeostasis. *Indian J. Pharm. Sci.* 81: 188–189. https://doi.org/10.36468/pharmaceutical-sciences.498.

Mensching, D. (2012). Chapter 14 - Nervous system toxicity. In: *Veterinary Toxicology*, 2e (ed. R.C. Gupta), 207–222. Boston: Academic Press https://doi.org/10.1016/B978-0-12-385926-6.00014-4.

Merola, V. and Dunayer, E. (2006). The 10 most common toxicoses in cats. *DVM* 360: 330–342.

Mertens, P.A., Torres, S., and Jessen, C. (2006). The effects of clomipramine hydrochloride in cats with psychogenic alopecia: a prospective study. *J. Am. Anim. Hosp. Assoc.* 42: 336–343. https://doi.org/10.5326/0420336.

Milne, W.L. and Cohn, S.H. (1957). Role of serotonin in blood coagulation. *Am. J. Physiol. Legacy Cont.* 189: 470–474. https://doi.org/10.1152/ajplegacy.1957.189.3.470.

Ming, X., Mulvey, M., Mohanty, S., and Patel, V. (2011). Safety and efficacy of clonidine and clonidine extended-release in the treatment of children and adolescents with attention deficit and hyperactivity disorders. *Adolesc. Health Med. Ther.* 2: 105–112. https://doi.org/10.2147/AHMT.S15672.

Mitton, L.F., Sanchis-Mora, S., Pelligand, L. et al. (2019). Clinical usage of gabapentin in dogs under primary veterinary care in the UK. In: *BSAVA Congress Proceedings 2019*, 478. BSAVA Library https://doi.org/10.22233/9781910443699.74.2.

Moesta, A. (2014). Animal behavior case of the month. *J. Am. Vet. Med. Assoc.* 244: 1149–1152. https://doi.org/10.2460/javma.244.10.1149.

Moon-Fanelli, A.A. and Dodman, N.H. (1998). Description and development of compulsive tail chasing in terriers and response to clomipramine treatment. *J. Am. Vet. Med. Assoc.* 212: 1252–1257.

Neff, M.W., Robertson, K.R., Wong, A.K. et al. (2004). Breed distribution and history of canine mdr1-1Δ, a pharmacogenetic mutation that marks the emergence of breeds from the collie lineage. *PNAS* 101: 11725–11730. https://doi.org/10.1073/pnas.0402374101.

Nitta, R., Goyagi, T., and Nishikawa, T. (2013). Combination of oral clonidine and intravenous low-dose ketamine reduces the consumption of postoperative patient-controlled analgesia morphine after spine surgery. *Acta Anaesthesiol. Taiwanica* 51: 14–17. https://doi.org/10.1016/j.aat.2013.03.003.

Ogata, N., Dantas, L.M.d.S., and Crowell-Davis, S.L. (2019). Selective serotonin reuptake inhibitors. In: *Veterinary Psychopharmacology*, 103–128. Hoboken, NJ: Wiley-Blackwell.

Ogata, N. and Dodman, N.H. (2011). The use of clonidine in the treatment of fear-based behavior problems in dogs: an open trial. *J. Vet. Behav.: Clin. Appl. Res.* 6: 130–137. https://doi.org/10.1016/j.jveb.2010.10.004.

Orlando, J.M., Case, B.C., Thomson, A.E. et al. (2016). Use of oral trazodone for sedation in cats: a pilot study. *J. Feline Med. Surg.* 18: 476–482. https://doi.org/10.1177/1098612X15587956.

Overall, K.L. and Dunham, A.E. (2002). Clinical features and outcome in dogs and cats with obsessive-compulsive disorder: 126 cases (1989-2000). *J. Am. Vet. Med. Assoc.* 221: 1445–1452. https://doi.org/10.2460/javma.2002.221.1445.

Pachel, C.L. (2011). Animal behavior case of the month. *J. Am. Vet. Med. Assoc.* 239: 1433–1434. https://doi.org/10.2460/javma.239.11.1433.

Pankratz, K.E., Ferris, K.K., Griffith, E.H., and Sherman, B.L. (2017). Use of single-dose oral gabapentin to attenuate fear responses in cage-trap confined community cats: a double-blind, placebo-controlled field trial. *J. Feline Med. Surg.* 20 (6): 535–543. https://doi.org/10.1177/1098612X17719399.

Paul Wang, C., Howell, S.R., Scatina, J., and Sisenwine, S.F. (1992). The disposition of venlafaxine enantiomers in dogs, rats, and humans receiving venlafaxine. *Chirality* 4: 84–90. https://doi.org/10.1002/chir.530040204.

Petroff, M. (2022). A retrospective study of the efficacy of venlafaxine in 130 dogs with aggression disorders. 2022 Veterinary Behavior Symposium Proceedings. American College of Veterinary Behaviorists.

Pflaum, K. and Bennett, S. (2021). Investigation of the use of venlafaxine for treatment of refractory misdirected play and impulse-control aggression in a cat: a case report. *J. Vet. Behav.* 42: 22–25. https://doi.org/10.1016/j.jveb.2020.10.008.

Pineda, S., Anzola, B., Olivares, A., and Ibáñez, M. (2014). Fluoxetine combined with clorazepate dipotassium and behaviour modification for treatment of anxiety-related disorders in dogs. *Vet. J.* 199: 387–391. https://doi.org/10.1016/j.tvjl.2013.11.021.

Plessas, I.N., Volk, H.A., Rusbridge, C. et al. (2015). Comparison of gabapentin versus topiramate on clinically affected dogs with Chiari-like malformation and syringomyelia. *Vet. Rec.* 177: 288–288. https://doi.org/10.1136/vr.103234.

Podberscek, L., Hsu, Y., and Serpell, J.A. (1999). Evaluation of clomipramine as an adjunct to behavioural therapy in the treatment of separation-related problems in dogs. *Vet. Rec.* 145: 365–369. https://doi.org/10.1136/vr.145.13.365.

Posner, L.P. (2017). Sedatives and traquilizers. In: *Veterinary Pharmacology and Therapeutics* (ed. J.E. Riviere and M.G. Papich), 324–369. Ames, Iowa: Wiley-Blackwell.

Pryor, P. (2003). Animal behavior case of the month. *J. Am. Vet. Med. Assoc.* 223: 1117–1119. https://doi.org/10.2460/javma.2003.223.1117.

Pryor, P.A., Hart, B.L., Cliff, K.D., and Bain, M.J. (2001). Effects of a selective serotonin reuptake inhibitor on urine spraying behavior in cats. *J. Am. Vet. Med. Assoc.* 219: 1557–1561. https://doi.org/10.2460/javma.2001.219.1557.

Ramachandraih, C.T., Subramanyam, N., Bar, K.J. et al. (2011). Antidepressants: from MAOIs to SSRIs and more. *Indian J. Psychiatry* 53: 180–182. https://doi.org/10.4103/0019-5545.82567.

Rapoport, J.L., Ryland, D.H., and Kriete, M. (1992). Drug treatment of canine acral lick. An animal model of obsessive-compulsive disorder. *Arch. Gen. Psychiatry* 49: 517–521. https://doi.org/10.1001/archpsyc.1992.01820070011002.

Drugs.com (2021). Reconcile - FDA prescribing information, side effects and uses. Initially published by Elanco 2007 [WWW Document]. Drugs.com. https://www.drugs.com/pro/reconcile.html (accessed 23 June 2021).

Reich, M.R., Ohad, D.G., Overall, K.L., and Dunham, A.E. (2000). Electrocardiographic assessment of antianxiety medication in dogs and correlation with serum drug concentration. *J. Am. Vet. Med. Assoc.* 216: 1571–1575. https://doi.org/10.2460/javma.2000.216.1571.

Reisner, I.R. (2003). American college of veterinary behaviorists 2003 scientific session abstracts. *J. Am. Anim. Hosp. Assoc.* 39 (5): 509–512. Diagnosis of canine generalized anxiety disorder and its management with behavioral modification and fluoxetine or paroxetine: a retrospective summary of clinical experience (2001-2003). https://doi.org/10.5326/0390509.

Reuben, S.S., Steinberg, R.B., Madabhushi, L., and Rosenthal, E. (1998). Intravenous regional clonidine in the management of sympathetically maintained pain. *Anesthesiology* 89: 527–530.

Rocchini, A.P., Mao, H.Z., Babu, K. et al. (1999). Clonidine prevents insulin resistance and hypertension in obese dogs. *Hypertension* 33: 548–553.

Romero-Sandoval, A. and Eisenach, J.C. (2007). Clonidine reduces hypersensitivity and alters the balance of pro- and anti-inflammatory leukocytes after local injection at the site of inflammatory neuritis. *Brain, Behav. Immun., Neuropathic Pain, Glia and Cytokines* 21: 569–580. https://doi.org/10.1016/j.bbi.2006.09.001.

Rosado, B., García-Belenguer, S., León, M. et al. (2011). Effect of fluoxetine on blood concentrations of serotonin, cortisol and dehydroepiandrosterone in canine aggression. *J. Vet. Pharmacol. Ther.* 34: 430–436. https://doi.org/10.1111/j.1365-2885.2010.01254.x.

Sanchis-Mora, S., Chang, Y.M., Abeyesinghe, S.M. et al. (2019). Pregabalin for the treatment of syringomyelia-associated neuropathic pain in dogs: a randomised, placebo-controlled, double-masked clinical trial. *Vet. J.* 250: 55–62. https://doi.org/10.1016/j.tvjl.2019.06.006.

Sansone, R.A., Wiederman, M.W., and Shrader, J.A. (2000). Naturalistic study of the weight effects of amitriptyline, fluoxetine, and sertraline in an outpatient medical setting. *J. Clin. Psychopharmacol.* 20: 272–273.

Sartor, L.L., Trepanier, L.A., Kroll, M.M. et al. (2004). Efficacy and safety of transdermal methimazole in the treatment of cats with hyperthyroidism. *J. Vet. Intern. Med.* 18: 651–655. https://doi.org/10.1111/j.1939-1676.2004.tb02601.x.

Sawyer, L.S., Moon-Fanelli, A.A., and Dodman, N.H. (1999). Psychogenic alopecia in cats: 11 cases (1993-1996). *J. Am. Vet. Med. Assoc.* 214: 71–74.

Schmierer, P.A., Tünsmeyer, J., Tipold, A. et al. (2020). Randomized controlled trial of pregabalin for analgesia after surgical treatment of intervertebral disc disease in dogs. *Vet. Surg.* 49: 905–913. https://doi.org/10.1111/vsu.13411.

Seibert, L. and Crowell-Davis, S.L. (2019). Antipsychotics. In: *Veterinary Psychopharmacology*, 201–215. Hoboken, NJ: Wiley-Blackwell.

Seksel, K. and Lindeman, M. (1998). Use of clomipramine in the treatment of anxiety-related and obsessive-compulsive disorders in cats. *Aust. Vet. J.* 76: 317–321. https://doi.org/10.1111/j.1751-0813.1998.tb12353.x.

Siao, K.T., Pypendop, B.H., and Ilkiw, J.E. (2010). Pharmacokinetics of gabapentin in cats. *Am. J. Vet. Res.* 71: 817–821. https://doi.org/10.2460/ajvr.71.7.817.

Simpson, B.S., Landsberg, G.M., Reisner, I.R. et al. (2007). Effects of reconcile (fluoxetine) chewable tablets plus behavior management for canine separation anxiety. *Vet. Ther.* 8: 18–31.

Sinn, L. (2018). Advances in behavioral psychopharmacology. *Vet. Clin.: Small Anim. Pract.* 48: 457–471. https://doi.org/10.1016/j.cvsm.2017.12.011.

Sordo, L. and Gunn-Moore, D.A. (2021). Cognitive dysfunction in cats: update on neuropathological and behavioural changes plus clinical management. *Vet. Rec.* 188: 30–41. https://doi.org/10.1002/vetr.3.

Stahl, S.M. (2008). *Stahl's Essential Psychopharmacology: Neuroscientific Basis and Practical Applications*. Cambridge University Press.

Stevens, B.J., Frantz, E.M., Orlando, J.M. et al. (2016). Efficacy of a single dose of trazodone hydrochloride given to cats prior to veterinary visits to reduce signs of transport- and examination-related anxiety. *J. Am. Vet. Med. Assoc.* 249: 202–207. https://doi.org/10.2460/javma.249.2.202.

Takeuchi, Y., Houpt, K.A., and Scarlett, J.M. (2000). Evaluation of treatments for separation anxiety in dogs. *J. Am. Vet. Med. Assoc.* 217: 342–345.

Thoefner, M.S., Skovgaard, L.T., McEvoy, F.J. et al. (2020). Pregabalin alleviates clinical signs of syringomyelia-related central neuropathic pain in Cavalier King Charles Spaniel dogs: a randomized controlled trial. *Vet. Anaesth. Analg.* 47: 238–248. https://doi.org/10.1016/j.vaa.2019.09.007.

Valverde, A., Cantwell, S., Hernández, J., and Brotherson, C. (2004). Effects of acepromazine on the incidence of vomiting associated with opioid administration in dogs. *Vet. Anaesth. Analg.* 31: 40–45. https://doi.org/10.1111/j.1467-2995.2004.00128.x.

van Haaften, K.A., Forsythe, L.R.E., Stelow, E.A., and Bain, M.J. (2017). Effects of a single preappointment dose of gabapentin on signs of stress in cats during transportation and veterinary examination. *J. Am. Vet. Med. Assoc.* 251: 1175–1181. https://doi.org/10.2460/javma.251.10.1175.

van Harten, J. (1993). Clinical pharmacokinetics of selective serotonin reuptake inhibitors. *Clin. Pharmacokinet.* 24: 203–220. https://doi.org/10.2165/00003088-199324030-00003.

Virga, V., Houpt, K., and Scarlett, J. (2001). Efficacy of amitriptyline as a pharmacological adjunct to behavioral modification in the management of aggressive behaviors in dogs. *J. Am. Anim. Hosp. Assoc.* 37: 325–330. https://doi.org/10.5326/15473317-37-4-325.

Vollmer, K.O., von Hodenberg, A., and Kölle, E.U. (1986). Pharmacokinetics and metabolism of gabapentin in rat, dog and man. *Arzneimittelforschung* 36: 830–839.

Wahi, A., Singh, A.K., Syal, K. et al. (2016). Comparative efficacy of intrathecal bupivacaine alone and combination of bupivacaine with clonidine in spinal anaesthesia. *J. Clin. Diagn. Res.* 10: UC06–UC08. https://doi.org/10.7860/JCDR/2016/16343.7565.

Washabu, R.J. (2013). Antispasmodic agents. In: *Canine and Feline Gastroenterology*, 481–485. St Louis, MO: Saunders.

White, M.M., Neilson, J.C., Hart, B.L., and Cliff, K.D. (1999). Effects of clomipramine hydrochloride on dominance-related aggression in dogs. *J. Am. Vet. Med. Assoc.* 215: 1288–1291.

Wynchank, D. and Berk, M. (1998). Fluoxetine treatment of acral lick dermatitis in dogs: a placebo-controlled randomized double blind trial. *Depress. Anxiety* 8: 21–23.

Zoetis (2023). Bonqat Package Insert.

Zoetis (2016). Sileo Package Insert.

Zoetis, Inc. (2014). ANIPRYL® selegiline HCl (L-deprenyl HCl) Tablets.

22

Chemical Restraint and Sedation in Small Animals

M. Leanne Lilly

The Ohio State University, Veterinary Medical Center, Columbus, OH, USA

Introduction

What is Chemical Restraint?

Chemical restraint is the use of medications classically referred to as "sedatives" or "tranquilizers" to facilitate veterinary procedures, examinations, diagnostic testing, and treatment. However, this definition and the lump terms "sedative and tranquilizer" leave out critical understanding of these medications: (1) the dose, route, and patient status can all result in differing levels of sedation from the same substance; (2) medications that decrease anxiety may or may not result in sedation but can facilitate handling; (3) analgesia can improve handling even without impairing patient mentation or motor functions; and (4) medications that solely inhibit motor function without addressing underlying pain, fear, or anxiety, are rarely appropriate as solo agents.

When is Chemical Restraint Indicated?

Veterinarians "should provide the least restraint required to allow the specific procedure(s) to be performed properly, should minimize fear, pain, stress, and suffering for the animal, and should protect both the animal and personnel from harm. Every effort should be made to ensure adequate and ongoing training in animal handling and behavior by all parties involved, so that distress and physical restraint are minimized." (American Veterinary Medical Association n.d.)

Chemical restraint and sedation (CRS) are suggested for *any* patient undergoing a socially invasive or painful procedure. For a patient with pre-existing behavioral concerns, CRS may be necessary even for benign procedures such as vaccines and venipuncture. In these cases, chemical restraint is indicated not just for everyone's safety but also to prevent sensitization to handling and resultant fear, anxiety, stress, and aggression at subsequent visits. Remember that fear is the number one cause of aggressive behavior. Appropriate CRS plans decrease fear, which then decreases aggressive behavior, which then allows for safe and effective handling. In reducing patient emotional pain and distress, we decrease potential for aggression during future visits, improve patient welfare, and increase client perceptions of compassion. CRS is warranted in the following situations (Yin 2009a, 2009b, 2009c; Herron and Shreyer 2014):

- *Marked or moderate fear due to minimal handling*: "alligator rolling", flinching and vocalizing in response to minimal touch,

Introduction to Animal Behavior and Veterinary Behavioral Medicine, First Edition. Edited by Meghan E. Herron.

Companion website: www.wiley.com/go/introductiontoanimalbehavior

releasing anal glands, urinating, flailing, panicked attempts to flee, in addition to moderate fear signs.

- *Moderate fear during handling and more extensive handling/procedures are needed*: crouching, cowering, urinating, trembling, tail tucking, head turned away, avoiding eye contact, lip-licking, yawning, lip smacking, teeth chattering; felines hiding in corners, "meatloaf" position, flat ears, hissing.
- *Moderate fear-related aggression in handling history or with handling currently*: growling, barking while backing up, "whale eye" stiff staring.
- *Aggressive behavior at any point in history for handling or before handling*: barking, lunging, hackles up, snarling, snapping, tail up stiff, ears forward, showing just the front teeth; felines who are hissing, yowling, swatting, lunging, attempting to bite.
- *A particularly painful or socially invasive procedure for any pet*: ruptured anal glands, lancing an abscess, cast placement, most radiographs, abdominal ultrasound, wound debridement, esophageal tube placement, etc.

Medications and Routes

Oral Medications

Oral **psychotropic medications** are extensively discussed as *event* medications in Chapter 21. When these medications are given specifically for the event of a veterinary clinic visit, we refer to them as **pre-visit pharmaceuticals** (PVPs). These medications alone may be sufficient for mildly invasive procedures in some patients. They can be combined with most CRS injectable medications (see below), and we recommend using both PVPs and CRS for aggressive patients, more invasive procedures, or as part of an anesthetic plan. *Note: Behavior patients who are taking medications daily should* ***continue*** *to take them for planned sedation or anesthesia.*

Oral medications should:

- always be tested at home *before* the appointment *with time for adjustment* (set this expectation for the client; is that a week before or three days before?)
- be administered well before their anticipated onset of effect (typically 90–120 minutes before the patient *gets into the car* for the appointment, as well as the evening prior).

With few exceptions, waiting until the patient arrives at the hospital to give PVPs runs an increased risk of effect failure due to continued stress, heightened arousal, and trigger stacking from the various hospital stimuli (Albright et al. 2017). This is especially true for aggressive patients. As discussed in Chapter 21, immediate-acting oral medications are best given when the pet is in a calm state. If PVPs are given during a time of high stress, patient arousal is likely to override most, if not all, of the therapeutic effects. For this reason, most clinicians recommend giving a dose of the PVPs the night prior to the anticipated veterinary visit as well as the morning of the visit, allowing at least two hours for effect. Sileo® is the only exception – with its rapid 20-minute onset of action, it should be administered 2–3 minutes before the patient leaves the house and can be readministered upon arrival if needed (Box 22.1).

Choosing a Pre-Visit Pharmaceutical

Key aspects of appropriate PVPs include (1) fast onset of action, (2) predictable duration of action, and (3) adequate fear and/or anxiety-relieving effects. We have many immediate acting *event* medications at our disposal – see Chapter 21 for doses, duration of action, and other details. The most frequently used PVP in dogs is likely trazodone, due to its low side effect profile, wide dosing range, and published safety and efficacy as an event medication (Gilbert-Gregory et al. 2016, Gruen et al. 2014). Many clinics have a standard dosing plan for trazodone, given to ALL surgical patients both the evening prior and morning of scheduled surgery days (see Table 22.1).

Box 22.1 Spotlight on Sileo®

Sileo (Zoetis, Inc. [Parsippany-Troy, NJ]) is one of the few PVPs that works quickly enough for the client to give upon arrival in the hospital with an onset time of 20 minutes. This use is off-label as it is FDA approved only for the treatment of noise fears in dogs. The labeled doses are anxiolytic, and are unlikely to cause sedation- 87% of patients who saw improvement in noise fear-related signs were not noted to be sedate (Korpivaara et al. 2017). Consequently, judicious patient selection, use with other medications, or at doses similar to other OTM protocols (see below) can help this be a useful tool in your behavior tool box.

Table 22.1 Sample pre-surgical dose chart for trazodone in dogs, based on body weight. This dose should be given the evening prior to and the morning of (two hours prior to leaving the home) scheduled surgery days. Note that dogs with known fear, anxiety, and stress during veterinary visits often require higher doses of trazodone and/or a combination of trazodone with other PVPs.

Weight (lbs)	Dose of trazodone
Up to 10	25 mg (50 mg: ½ tablet)
10–20	50 mg
20–40	75 mg (50 mg: 1.5 tablets)
40–60	100 mg
60–80	150 mg (100 mg: 1 tablet + 50 mg: 1 tablet)
Over 80	200–300 mg (100 mg: 2–3 tablets)

Source: Adapted from Gigi's, Canal Winchester, OH.

When trazodone is not a good fit for a dog, due to adverse effects (e.g. agitation, urinary incontinence, gastrointestinal (GI) upset, tremors/seizures), either clonidine or gabapentin are appropriate alternatives. Clonidine, an alpha-2 agonist, typically has a rapid onset of action (30–60 minutes) and has both sedative and anxiety-relieving properties (Ogata and Dodman 2011). Gabapentin, a neuromodulator, also has a rapid onset of action (30–60 minutes), as well as sedative and anxiety-relieving properties. Due to its potential analgesic effects against spinal pain and paresthesias (Giudice et al. 2019; Mitton et al. 2019), gabapentin may be a better first choice for dogs with known spinal or other neuropathic pain or those who may undergo vertebral or amputation surgeries. Both trazodone and gabapentin have been shown to lower the mean alveolar concentration of isoflurane needed to keep dogs anesthetized (Hoffman et al. 2018; Johnson et al. 2019), making them potentially beneficial additions to all surgical anesthetic plans.

Gabapentin is typically the PVP of choice for cats, as multiple placebo-controlled trials show it to be effective at decreasing travel and veterinary exam-related anxiety in this species (Pankratz et al. 2018; van Haaften et al. 2017). Another reason gabapentin is a good first choice PVP for cats is that it lacks the bitter flavor present in most other immediate-acting medications. The capsules can be opened and their contents mixed with palatable food, such as poultry-flavored baby food or canned tuna fish. For unsocialized feral cats, gabapentin can be compounded into a liquid and squirted into the mouth through the trap cage bars (Figure 22.1). A recent study in cats, using a liquid formulation of pregabalin (Bonqat®), demonstrated substantial reduction in signs of FAS associated with travel to and experiences during veterinary visits

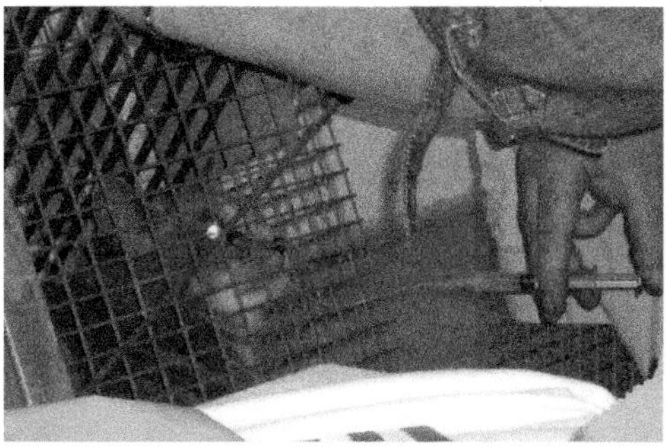

Figure 22.1 Many oral pre-visit pharmaceuticals are available in or can be compounded into liquid form and safely administered to cats through the cage bars when they open their mouths. In some cases, injectable medications can be given transmucosally in this manner. *Source:* Photo credit: Kat Pankratz.

(Lamminen et al. 2023). Regardless of which medication, avoid mixing PVPs with cats' regular canned food diets, as food aversions can result in taste-sensitive cats.

Creating a Combination Oral Plan

Patients with high levels of fear, anxiety, and stress (FAS) during veterinary visits often require a cocktail of medications as part of the PVP plan. Furthermore, if trials of a monotherapy PVP have been attempted at home and even the maximum doses have not provided adequate relief, it may be necessary to add in a second or third medication. For pets who require more substantial tranquilization, acepromazine can be *added* to the PVP plan. Since it has no fear or anxiety-reducing properties, acepromazine should *not* be used as a sole agent PVP. See Tables 22.2 and 22.3 for examples of oral medication combinations in dogs and cats.

Table 22.2 Example combination PVPs for dogs.

Trazodone and gabapentin	Trazodone and clonidine
• Trazodone and acepromazine	• Gabapentin and clonidine
• Gabapentin and Sileo®	• Gabapentin and acepromazine
• Trazodone, gabapentin, and clonidine	
• Trazodone, gabapentin, and acepromazine	
• Trazodone and Sileo®	
• Trazodone, Sileo®, gabapentin	

For non-aggressive patients, a benzodiazepine such as lorazepam, diazepam, or alprazolam can be added to any of the above combinations.

Table 22.3 Example combination PVPs for cats.

Trazodone and gabapentin	Trazodone and lorazepam
• Trazodone and acepromazine	• Gabapentin and acepromazine
• Lorazepam and acepromazine	• Gabapentin and lorazepam

For the behavior patient who is already on a *daily* medication (see Chapter 21), these combinations are still safe with the following caveats:

- Trazodone may increase the risk of serotonin syndrome, though this is less common in dogs than humans, and frequently, maximum doses of both are used in aggressive patients, provided they are not on additional serotonin enhancing medications (Cerenia, tramadol, and mirtazapine etc.).
- TCAs may decrease the hypotensive effects of clonidine and increase sedative effects.

Injectable Medications

When used for the purpose of eliciting rapid onset anxiolysis and sedation in a patient with behavioral concerns, injectable medications are almost always given intramuscularly (IM). Few patients with FAS will tolerate the careful restraint needed for an intravenous (IV) injection, and, therefore, only medications that are safe to give IM are highlighted in this chapter. Note that some of these medications are safe and effective when given via the oral transmucosal route (absorbs through the patient's gums, sublingual area, or cheek mucosa). Those doses are specified by the letters "OTM" when mentioned below.

Analgesics

Pain can worsen existing anxiety, fear, and/or aggression or cause aggression on its own as a defensive strategy when tolerance for physical handling is limited (as discussed in Chapter 15). Pain is often under-appreciated in behavior patients. Often, these patients are only examined under sedation, where an accurate pain assessment is not possible, and/or their fear, aggression, and reactivity upon entering the hospital cause a flood of stress hormones (cortisol and adrenaline) that attenuate pain responses. They may also be more inhibited from showing voluntary signs of pain (pulling away, whimpering, guarding an area) because they are already afraid. As discussed in Chapter 11, freezing is a common coping strategy for profoundly fearful patients. When in doubt, it is safest to assume and treat pain rather than not. While the use of polypharmacy for analgesia has become the gold standard, things can get complicated when the patient is already on other daily medications, and special attention should be paid to daily psychotropic medications.

A note on non-steroidal anti-inflammatories (NSAIDs)

Platelets have serotonin reuptake transporters and utilize serotonin as part of the coagulation cascade. In humans, the combination of an NSAID and an SSRI may increase the risk of GI bleeds, or lead to poor clotting after surgery (de Jong et al. 2003; Helin-Salmivaara et al. 2007). In some human cases, they share cytochrome-P450 (CYP450) substrates (meaning they affect the liver metabolism of each other's parent compounds or metabolites), but this has not been extensively evaluated in canines or felines compared to humans. NSAIDS are not sedatives and provide no anxiolytic effects.

Opioids

This class includes drugs that block pain signals by binding to opioid receptors on nerve cells in the brain, spinal cord, GI tract, and other organs in the body, such as the heart and lungs. The major receptor types include mu, delta, and kappa, with full (pure) receptor agonists having the greatest **analgesic effects** (compared to partial receptor agonists). Pure agonists also have more potential for cardiovascular and respiratory depression and should be used with caution and close supervision. Opioid drugs may affect the metabolism and concentration of other medications when they share, inhibit, or induce CY450 substrates. For example, some opioids have a range of cardiovascular effects that may interact negatively with psychotropic medications (Behzadi et al. 2018). Methadone has the highest capacity to prolong the Q-T interval portion of the cardiac electrical rhythm compared to other opioids in humans, and oxycodone has dose-dependent prolongation of Q-T interval. This risk is relatively low with morphine and buprenorphine and is not reported with hydromorphone (Behzadi et al., 2018). While these risks seem lower in dogs overall, amitriptyline may also prolong the Q-T interval and its combination with certain opioids should be weighed carefully (Reich et al. 2000; Borer-Weir 2014).

Butorphanol: 0.1–0.4 mg/kg IM, IV, SC, or OTM – dogs and cats (Plumb 2015).

This is a mixed agonist (kappa agonist, and partial antagonist at mu receptors). This may explain, why experientially it provides more sedation but less analgesia, and its propensity for being far less emetic than morphine and, in some reports, buprenorphine. It is cleared from the bloodstream far more slowly by cats than dogs, giving it a half-life roughly equivalent to buprenorphine, with analgesia lasting ~2.5–3 hours (KuKanich and Papich 2017).

Buprenorphine: 0.01–0.04 mg/kg IM, IV, SC dogs and cats; 0.02–0.04 mg/kg OTM dogs and cats (Steagall et al. 2014; Abbo et al. 2008); Simbadol® 0.24 mg/kg SC in cats (labeled dose); 0.03 mg/kg IN in dogs (Enomoto et al. 2022).

This is a mixed agonist (partial mu agonist with high affinity, and a full kappa antagonist). This mixed action gives it a better safety profile than a pure mu agonist, and in cats produces less dysphoria, excitement, vomiting, or nausea. In dogs, buprenorphine is relatively well absorbed when given IN with an average bioavailability of 57.5%, while OTM has an average bioavailability of 41.41%. Sedative effects may last for 2–6+ hours and the analgesic effects of formulations other than Simbadol® last around 4 hours, but metabolites may have analgesic effects. Buprenorphine has excellent bioavailability through the mucous membranes in cats (Robertson et al. 2003), but has poor oral bioavailability (~10–20%) so direct gum or buccal pouch contact is key for at home or in hospital administration (Bullingham et al. 1983).

Morphine: 0.2–1 mg/kg IM, 0.5 mg/kg IV, 1 mg/kg OTM dogs; 0.05–0.25 mg/kg IM, IV cats.

Morphine is a pure mu agonist making it a powerful analgesic. Onset is 3 minutes IV, 15 minutes IM, SQ, (Donald C. Plumb 2015), and 45–60 minutes OTM (Herron 2016), and duration is 1–4 hours. Side effects include mild bradycardia, respiratory suppression, ataxia, vomiting, and histamine release (Donald C. Plumb 2015).

Hydromorphone: 0.05–0.1 mg/kg IM, IV dogs and cats.

This is a full mu agonist, but also has activity for delta and kappa receptors, though very low affinity for these receptors comparatively (Gharagozlou et al. 2006; *Hydromorphone* 2022). Onset is 3 minutes when given IV and 15 minutes when given IM (Donald C. Plumb 2015). Its use is contraindicated in patients with severe renal insufficiency or those who are severely debilitated. Side effects include sedation, mild bradycardia, respiratory suppression, mild ataxia, and vomiting. Hydromorphone has not been reported to have any Q-T interval prolongation (Behzadi et al., 2018) and histamine release risks are low (KuKanich and Papich 2017).

Alpha-2 Agonists

Alpha-2 agonists are drugs that stimulate alpha-2 receptors in the central and peripheral nervous system (CNS and PNS), resulting in a reduction in **sympathetic nervous system** output, anxiolysis, and analgesia. Sedative and anxiolytic effects are a result of receptor stimulation in the locus coeruleus, and analgesic effects are mediated by activation of alpha-2 receptors in the dorsal horn of the spinal cord. Alpha-2a receptors mediate sedation, analgesia, hypotension, and bradycardia, while alpha-2b receptors mediate the initial surge in vascular resistance and reflex bradycardia (Lemke 2004). The ability of a drug to cross the blood-brain barrier determines whether a drug has effects on the CNS, PNS, or both.

Dexmedetomidine (Dexdomitor®) 10–40 mcg/kg IM dogs and cats (Zoetis Inc. 2015) or 20–40 mcg/kg OTM dogs and cats (Cohen and Bennett 2015; Dent et al. 2019).

This drug is routinely used for sedation, due to its increased specificity for auto-receptors in the CNS, slowing the release of norepinephrine to decrease anxiety and motor activity. Cats seem to be particularly sensitive to its emetic effects and this is worse with OTM than injection, and as a solo agent (Slingsby et al. 2009; Santos et al. 2010; Porters et al. 2014). Because of the propensity for bradycardia and hypotension, dexmedetomidine should be avoided in pets with cardiovascular disease. It can be reversed with Antisedan® (atipamezole).

Detomidine 0.35 mg/m^2 2 mg/m^2 OTM dogs and cats, 0.35 mg/m^2 IV dogs and cats.

This drug is less routinely used for injectable sedation in cats and dogs, but has been through pharmacokinetic evaluation IV and OTM in dogs (Messenger et al. 2016; Kasten et al. 2018). The OTM route is less effective at sedating dogs, likely due to its ~30% bioavailability, and takes an average 60 minutes to reach maximum concentration. The most common side effect reported was vomiting. The use of the equine OTM Dormosedan® gel (Zoetis [Parsippany-Troy, NJ]) 7.6 mg/ml facilitates easier application than the injectable due to smaller volumes and has been used off-label in dogs at a dose of 224 mcg/kg, often as a pre-euthanasia PVP. (For Dormosedan® use in horses, see product insert by Zoetis). OTM has been reversed with 0.1 mg/kg Antisedan® (atipamezole) IM (Kasten et al. 2018).

Zenalpha® (medetomidine/vatinoxan) 1 mg/m^2 medetomidine IM, dogs only (Zenalpha® product insert).

Zenalpha® (Dechra Veterinary Products [Overland Park, KS]) is a combination alpha-2 agonist (medetomidine) and peripheral alpha-2 antagonist (vatinoxan). Medetomidine is responsible for sedative and analgesic effects, while vatinoxan selectively binds and blocks peripheral alpha-2 receptors and has limited penetration across the blood-brain barrier. Similar to other alpha-2 agonists, medetomidine as a sole agent leads to bradycardia and hypotension, due to peripheral alpha-2 agonism. The addition of vatinoxan blocks these effects, giving it a lower cardiovascular side effect profile, without hindering the central sedative effects (Rolfe et al. 2012). Zenalpha is approved only for IM administration in dogs and is not approved for any use in cats. In the editor's experience, the maintenance of normal blood pressure allows for better ease of venipuncture and catheter placement. Effects last about 35-40 minutes and most dogs wake up without the need for a reversal agent.

Benzodiazepines

Oral benzodiazepines are discussed in Chapter 21 and the effects of injectable benzodiazepines are similar, but have a more profound and immediate onset.

Midazolam (Versed®) 0.2–0.4 mg/kg IM, IV dogs and cats (Donald C. Plumb 2015).

Midazolam is an injectable benzodiazepine that is safe if injected outside of the vein (unlike diazepam). It can also be absorbed intranasally, though the efficacy of this route has only been studied for seizures in dogs versus sedation in birds (Sadegh 2013; Schwartz et al. 2013; Araghi et al. 2016; Charalambous et al. 2017). It can cause respiratory compromise and disinhibition of existing aggression. This is most common in already agitated or profoundly panicked patients and should consequently rarely if ever be used as a single agent especially for highly aroused patients. Increased appetite, muscle relaxation, and ataxia may also be seen (Posner 2017). Midazolam can be reversed with flumazenil though fewer practices carry this reversal agent in comparison to Atisedan® (Posner 2017).

NMDA Antagonists

Ketaset® (ketamine): 1–5 mg/kg IM, OTM (bitter); 1-2.5 mg/kg IV dogs and cats (Donald C. Plumb 2015).

Ketamine is an NMDA (N-methyl-D-aspartate amino acid) antagonist, dissociative, and general anesthetic. Most practitioners are familiar with ketamine as part of "kitty magic" (dexmedetomidine, ketamine, and an opioid); or in combination with diazepam (IV) for induction in a variety of species as it is one of the most commonly used anesthetics across veterinary medicine (Morgan et al. 2012). However, ketamine can also be utilized as part of an OTM protocol at similar doses but with lesser effect due to lower bioavailability (Grove and Ramsay 2000). This may be most useful in aggressive or unsocialized feral cats requiring urgent care, whose mouth we can access through a kennel door during hissing but who cannot be otherwise safely handled for an injection (Figure 22.1).

Telazol® (tiletamine/zolazepam) 5–10 mg/kg tiletamine IM dogs and cats, IV dogs only; 5–7.5 mg/kg OTM dogs and cats.

Telazol® is a combination of an NMDA antagonist dissociative anesthetic (tiletamine) with a benzodiazepine (zolazepam), (Zoetis Inc. 2019). The zolazepam will wear off first, leaving most patients in a dissociative state that lasts longer (2–4+ hours) than functional sedation (30–60 minutes). It may exacerbate pancreatitis and has the potential to cause respiratory depression, so it should be avoided or used with caution in patients with a history of pancreatic disease or respiratory compromise (Zoetis Inc. 2019). It can be combined with alpha-2 agonists or acepromazine for particularly aggressive patients or in end-of-life situations. Telazol® is FDA-approved for IV induction of anesthesia in dogs, but NOT in cats, though has been used off-label OTM for sedation in the buccal pouch of cats (Nejamkin et al. 2020). Using Telazol® OTM will decrease respiratory and heart rates as well as systolic pressure in the same manner it does when given IV or IM.

Other Injectable Options

Alfaxalone 0.2–4.5 mg/kg IM or IV dogs, 2.2–10.8 mg/kg IM or IV cats.

This is a neurosteroid injectable anesthetic, like propofol, but can be given either IV or IM. Its mechanism works by actively enhancing $GABA_A$ activity (Jurox Animal Health 2019). When used as a sole agent, the volume needed to induce adequate sedation in highly agitated patients can be higher than is feasible to administer IM. When used in combination with opioids or alpha-2 agonists, the volume needed is lower, but the overall volume of the injection may still be too high, particularly for a highly stressed or aggressive patient. Alfaxalone's use when given IM is, commonly restricted to smaller patients (<5 kg). The Multi-Dose product, Alfaxan®, is only labeled for IV use, is FDA approved in cats and dogs, and is legally marketed to, but not labeled for, use in minor, non-food producing species, including exotics (Medicine, C. for V 2020). Alfaxalone is hepatically metabolized and has linear kinetics so additional dosing or volume results in proportionally longer anesthesia. Apnea is the most common side effect (Jurox Animal Health 2019).

Quick dosing guide for commonly used *injectable* chemical restraint:

Drug	Dose	Route	Species
Butorphanol	0.1–0.4 mg/kg	IM, IV, SC	Dog, cat
Buprenorphine	0.01–0.04 mg/kg	IM, IV, SC	Dog, cat
Simbadol®	0.24 mg/kg	SC	Cat
Morphine	0.2–1.0 mg/kg	IM	Dog
	0.5 mg/kg	IV (slow)	Dog
	0.05–0.25 mg/kg	IV (slow), IM	Cat
Hydromorphone	0.05–0.1 mg/kg	IM, IV	Dog, cat
Dexmedetomidine	10–40 mcg/kg	IM, IV	Dog, cat
Midazolam	0.2–0.4 mg/kg	IM, IV, SC, IN	Dog, cat
Ketamine	1–5 mg/kg	IM	Dog, cat
	1–2.5 mg/kg	IV	Dog, cat
Telazol®	5–10 mg/kg	IM	Dog, cat
Alfaxalone	0.2–4.5 mg/kg	IM, IV	Dog
	2.2–10.8 mg/kg	IM, IV	Cat

Quick dosing guide for *OTM* chemical restraint:

Drug	Dose	Species
Butorphanol	0.2–0.4 mg/kg OTM	Dog, cat
Buprenorphine	0.02–0.04 mg/kg OTM	Dog, cat
Dexmedetomidine	20–40 mcg/kg OTM	Dog, cat
Telazol®	5–7.5 mg/kg OTM	Dog, cat

Protocols, Combinations, and Decision-Making

Overall, the plan for most patients with substantial behavioral needs coming into the hospital for pre-planned visits is:

1) Have client give oral PVPs the evening prior to and morning of the scheduled visit.
2) Have skilled staff provide injectable IM sedation upon arrival (in the parking lot, if needed).
3) Induce with IV anesthesia once patient sedates (if going to surgery or other procedure/diagnostics that require anesthesia).
4) Perform the procedure immediately.
5) Recover patient from anesthesia.
6) For aggressive patients, place a basket muzzle or Elizabethan collar on the dog once extubated.
7) Reverse sedation (when indicated).
8) Send patient home as soon as medically safe to do so.

On an urgent basis, or for initial patient visits where behavioral or analgesic needs arise unexpectedly, we may have to skip straight to step 2.

Injectable CRS Protocols

As mentioned above, patients with profound fear and/or aggressive behavior seldom tolerate the restraint necessary to give IV injections.

This means CRS is best given *quickly via IM routes*. Protocols for CRS combinations or "cocktails" vary based on health status, age, pain and invasiveness of the procedure, and clinician comfort. See Figure 22.2a–d for examples in dogs and Figure 22.3a–c for examples in cats.

Oral Transmucosal CRS Protocols

There are some patients for whom the IM injection is too traumatic, regardless of how quickly we can administer it. In these cases, it may be more reasonable for a client to administer the CRS through the OTM route (on the gums, inside the cheeks). See Box 22.2 for screening questions to ask clients before allowing them to administer OTM CRS to their own pets. If client involvement is not a safe or feasible option, you may combine the CRS liquid, mixed with something sticky, such as peanut butter (check for allergies) or squeeze cheese, over a large surface area and allow the patient to lick it up. When swallowed, CRS is not systemically absorbed, therefore, increased contact time is necessary. Hence, the use of sticky foods to prevent immediate swallowing (Figure 22.4). OTM requires higher doses (Figure 22.5) due to slower absorption and onset of effects, and some agents are bitter (Telazol®, ketamine). However, for a patient you cannot safely approach or approach without extreme fear, it is a valuable option.

Safely Getting Injections into Your Patients

Injections can be made safer through a variety of equipment: muzzles, cones, and/or blankets. If muzzling for an injection, ideally the muzzle should stay on until the patient is unconscious or through the entire procedure. The exception is the patient who can only tolerate the muzzle for the 30 seconds or so for injection, then their arousal escalates. Patients can be enticed into muzzles or tolerate muzzling with a small amount of sticky food. Avoid tenting or drawing back once the needle is in position for aggressive patients; plunge medications quickly and with purpose- these medications are all safe if accidentally given IV so you do not need to pull back to check for blood in the syringe before IM CRS injections.

Epaxial muscles may be easier to reach in cats and in taller dogs and provide a wider, broader target that does not require palpation to avoid peripheral nerves. The hamstrings (semimembranosus and tendinosus muscles) or the lateral muscles (biceps femoris or vastus lateralis) are alternative IM injection sites but can be more difficult to access quickly and can be more sensitive areas. Each clinician will develop their own preferences based on experience and physical abilities. Walking or "dive by" injections, where the patient is distracted in front, briefly restrained by leaning against the wall by their guardian, and injected from behind by a person they did not know was there (hiding around a corner or in a room) can facilitate the injection process itself in the short term. Alternatively, the patient can be walked by an experienced handler and kept moving during the injection process, while the clinician or technician follows and administers an injection through a butterfly catheter (Figure 22.6). See the online materials for video examples. Squeeze cages are not widely available and are often more stressful for patients, but can be used as a last resort for safety.

Long-term, teaching patients who are fearful in the veterinary setting to enthusiastically wear a muzzle, practice desensitization and counter conditioning to injections (walking or otherwise), or to take OTM medications directly will facilitate the future veterinary visits. The alternative is a patient that sensitizes over time, making each visit more challenging and stressful (Howell and Feyrecilde 2018).

Achieving and Maintaining Sedation

While injections have a rapid onset of action, the stress of the clinic environment can decrease CRS efficacy (Albright et al. 2017).

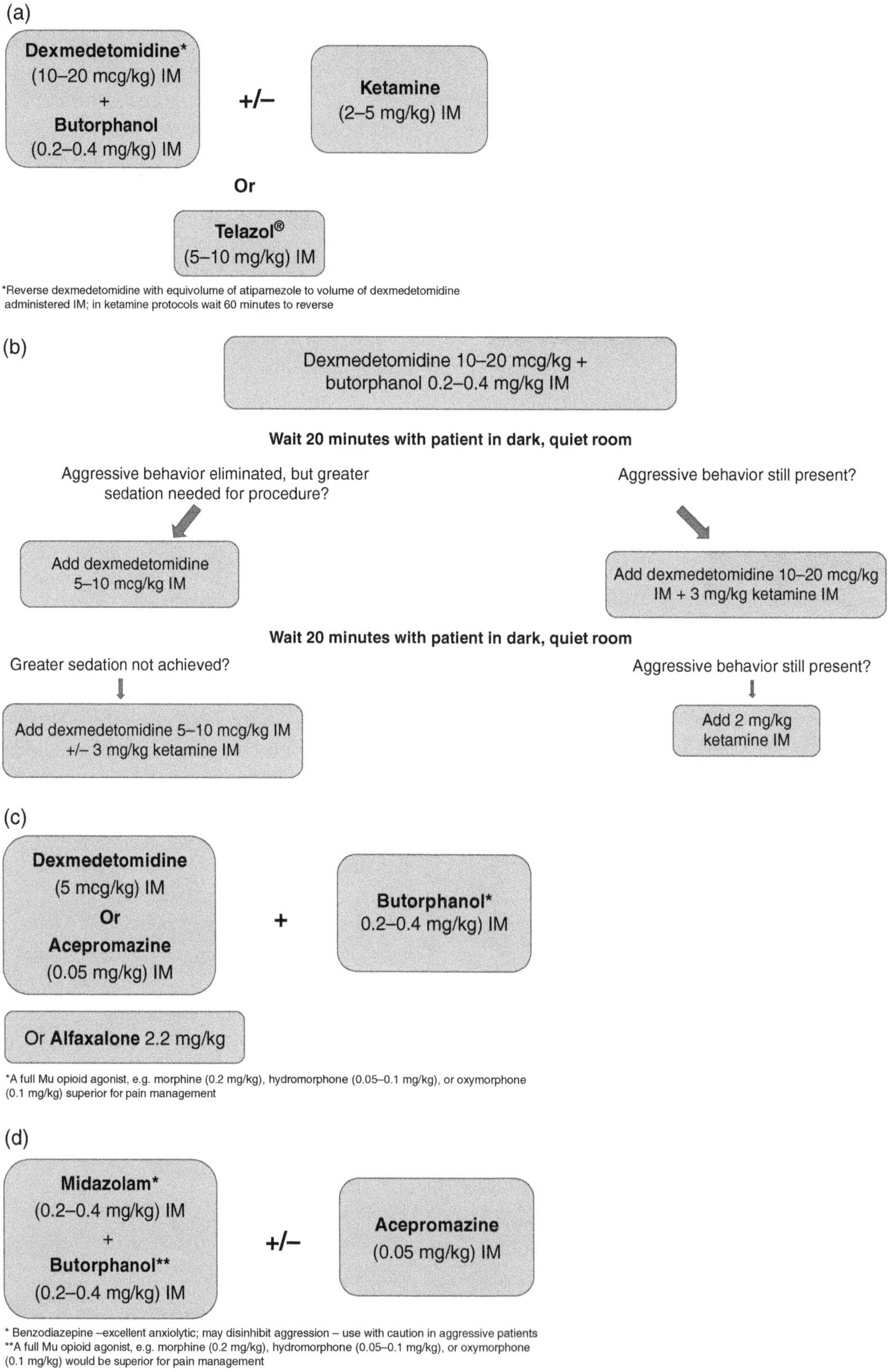
(a)
Dexmedetomidine* (10–20 mcg/kg) IM + Butorphanol (0.2–0.4 mg/kg) IM
+/–
Ketamine (2–5 mg/kg) IM
Or
Telazol® (5–10 mg/kg) IM
*Reverse dexmedetomidine with equivolume of atipamezole to volume of dexmedetomidine administered IM; in ketamine protocols wait 60 minutes to reverse
(b)
Dexmedetomidine 10–20 mcg/kg + butorphanol 0.2–0.4 mg/kg IM
Wait 20 minutes with patient in dark, quiet room
Aggressive behavior eliminated, but greater sedation needed for procedure?
Add dexmedetomidine 5–10 mcg/kg IM
Aggressive behavior still present?
Add dexmedetomidine 10–20 mcg/kg IM + 3 mg/kg ketamine IM
Wait 20 minutes with patient in dark, quiet room
Greater sedation not achieved?
Add dexmedetomidine 5–10 mcg/kg IM +/– 3 mg/kg ketamine IM
Aggressive behavior still present?
Add 2 mg/kg ketamine IM
(c)
Dexmedetomidine (5 mcg/kg) IM Or Acepromazine (0.05 mg/kg) IM
+
Butorphanol* 0.2–0.4 mg/kg) IM
Or Alfaxalone 2.2 mg/kg
*A full Mu opioid agonist, e.g. morphine (0.2 mg/kg), hydromorphone (0.05–0.1 mg/kg), or oxymorphone (0.1 mg/kg) superior for pain management
(d)
Midazolam* (0.2–0.4 mg/kg) IM + Butorphanol** (0.2–0.4 mg/kg) IM
+/–
Acepromazine (0.05 mg/kg) IM
* Benzodiazepine –excellent anxiolytic; may disinhibit aggression – use with caution in aggressive patients
**A full Mu opioid agonist, e.g. morphine (0.2 mg/kg), hydromorphone (0.05–0.1 mg/kg), or oxymorphone (0.1 mg/kg) would be superior for pain management

Ideally, the patient is kept separate from triggering stimuli before, during, and after CRS is administered. This may mean injections are given in the vehicle, parking lot, or outdoors if entering the clinic or hospital triggers high FAS. Once injected, the patient should be escorted to a quiet area where the lights can be dimmed and auditory stimuli minimized. Care should be taken to avoid loud or crowded areas when moving the patient to this quiet area. A single burst of reactivity can delay/inhibit onset of sedation and relaxation. As discussed in Chapter 11, white noise and classical music can provide a sound buffer as well as encourage relaxation for the patient. Cotton balls can be placed in the ears (be sure to count so that you know how many to remove), and the head can be lightly covered with a towel if the lights cannot be dimmed. Cats can be kept in their carriers, covered by a towel, until sedation is achieved. Minimize touch or keep a steady hand on the patient at all times so that they are not startled by petting or the repeated stopping and starting of touch. For dogs, if they are not already muzzled, one should be placed when safe to do so, prior to starting any procedure or treatment. If the dog is undergoing surgery, the muzzle can be removed after propofol induction in time for intubation.

Monitoring and Safety

The degree of close monitoring necessary for patients receiving CRS will vary based on the medications used and duration of sedation. At minimum, oxygen saturation and auscultation are necessary every five minutes with a starting and ending temperature to ensure cardiovascular stability. Best practices are to treat any fully unconscious patient more like an anesthetized one and monitor circulatory flow, oxygenation, and ventilation. Commonly, this is done through oxygen saturation, electrocardiogram, and blood pressure measurements, every 5–10 minutes, all of which should be documented in the medical record. Much like planning for the patient's arrival and necessary veterinary care, planning for/in case of adverse responses to CRS is required. Have reversal medications, oxygen, and endotracheal tubes and ties nearby (American College of Veterinary Anesthesiologists 2009).

Figure 22.2 (a) CRS plan for a young, healthy, but aggressove dog. An alpha-2 agonist is combined with an opioid, such as butorphanol. A full mu opioid agonist, e.g. morphine (0.2 mg/kg), hydromorphone (0.05–0.1 mg/kg), or oxymorphone (0.1 mg/kg) should be used in pre-surgical CRS plans or for patients in need of superior pain management. (b) Decision tree for a first time CRS plan for healthy, aggressive dogs. An alpha-2 agonist is combined with an opioid, such as butorphanol and given IM. A full mu opioid agonist, e.g. morphine (0.2 mg/kg), hydromorphone (0.05–0.1 mg/kg), or oxymorphone (0.1 mg/kg) should be used in pre-surgical CRS plans or for patients in need of superior pain management. If the aggressive behavior is still present after allowing the patient to settle in a dark quiet room for 20 minutes, give a second dose of dexmedetomidine (10–20 mcg/kg) AND ketamine 3 mg/kg IM. If after this initial 20 minutes the aggressive behavior has subsided, but greater sedation is still needed to accomplish the necessary tasks, give a second dose of dexmedetomidine at 5–10mcg/kg. In either case, additional dexmedetomidine and/or ketamine can be given, as long as you do not exceed 40 mcg/kg dexmedetomidine or 5 mg/kg ketamine. (c) CRS plan for a geriatric, aggressive dog. A low-dose of an alpha-2 agonist is combined with an opioid, such as butorphanol. When cardiac output may be compromised, an alpha-2 agonist should be avoided altogether and acepromazine can be given, instead, for added tranquilization. An alternative protocol for small dogs when cardiac disease or output is a concern is alfaxalone in combination with an opioid of choice. (d) CRS plan for a geriatric or debilitated dog who is fearful but not aggressive. The benzodiazepine, midazolam, is combined with an opioid, such as butorphanol. If additional tranquilization is needed, acepromazine can be added.

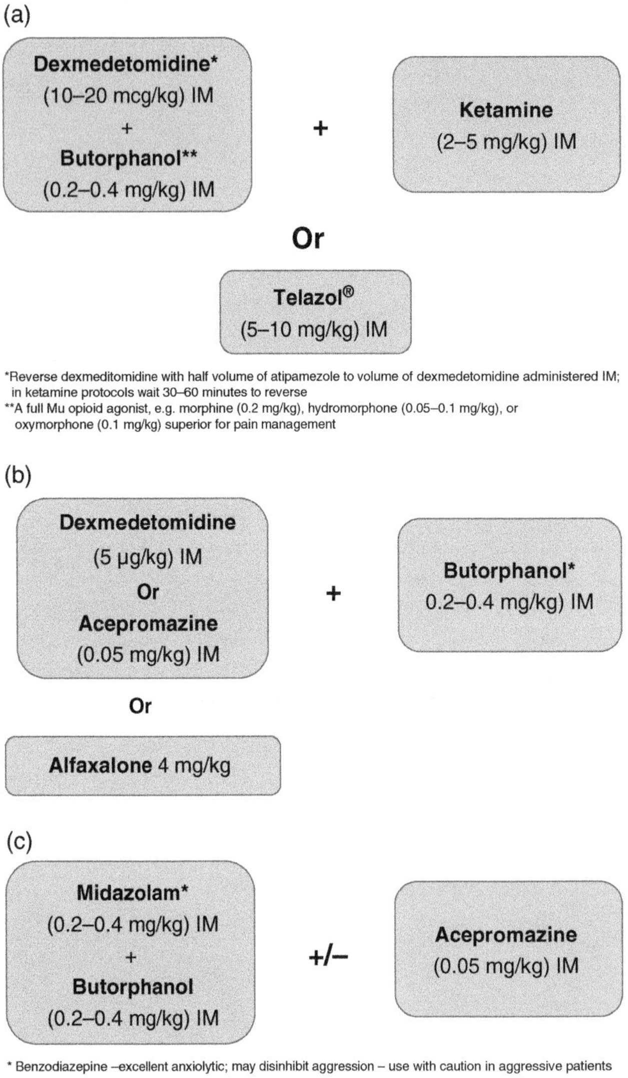
(a)
Dexmedetomidine* (10–20 mcg/kg) IM + Butorphanol** (0.2–0.4 mg/kg) IM
+
Ketamine (2–5 mg/kg) IM
Or
Telazol® (5–10 mg/kg) IM
*Reverse dexmeditomidine with half volume of atipamezole to volume of dexmedetomidine administered IM; in ketamine protocols wait 30–60 minutes to reverse
**A full Mu opioid agonist, e.g. morphine (0.2 mg/kg), hydromorphone (0.05–0.1 mg/kg), or oxymorphone (0.1 mg/kg) superior for pain management
(b)
Dexmedetomidine (5 µg/kg) IM Or Acepromazine (0.05 mg/kg) IM
+
Butorphanol* 0.2–0.4 mg/kg) IM
Or
Alfaxalone 4 mg/kg
(c)
Midazolam* (0.2–0.4 mg/kg) IM + Butorphanol (0.2–0.4 mg/kg) IM
+/−
Acepromazine (0.05 mg/kg) IM
* Benzodiazepine –excellent anxiolytic; may disinhibit aggression – use with caution in aggressive patients

Figure 22.3 (a) CRS plan for a young, healthy, but aggressive cat. The combination known as “kitty magic” included an alpha-2 agonist, combined with an opioid, such as butorphanol, and the dissociative anesthetic, ketamine. A full mu opioid agonist, e.g. morphine (0.2 mg/kg), hydromorphone (0.05–0.1 mg/kg), or oxymorphone (0.1 mg/kg) should be used in place of butorphanol in pre-surgical CRS plans or for patients in need of superior pain management. An alternative is Telazol. A separate opioid injection can be given once the pet is sedate if analgesic support is needed (e.g. the cat is having surgery). (b) CRS plan for a geriatric, aggressive cat. A low-dose of an alpha-2 agonist is combined with an opioid, such as butorphanol. A full mu opioid agonist, e.g. morphine (0.2 mg/kg), hydromorphone (0.05–0.1 mg/kg), or oxymorphone (0.1 mg/kg) should be used in pre-surgical CRS plans or for patients in need of superior pain management. When cardiac output may be compromised, alpha-2 agonists should be avoided altogether and acepromazine can be given, instead, for added tranquilization. An alternative protocol when cardiac disease or output is a concern is alfaxalone in combination with an opioid of choice. (c) CRS plan for a geriatric or debilitated cat who is fearful but not aggressive. The benzodiazepine, midazolam, is combined with an opioid, such as butorphanol. A full mu opioid agonist, e.g. morphine (0.2 mg/kg), hydromorphone (0.05–0.1 mg/kg), or oxymorphone (0.1 mg/kg) should be used in pre-surgical CRS plans or for patients in need of superior pain management. If additional tranquilization is needed, acepromazine can be added.

Box 22.2

Having the client administer OTM CRS: Due to inherent risks of having clients handle the mouths of their own pets during a veterinary visit, you need to screen for comfort and potential for aggression before proceeding. There are several questions you need to ask before allowing a client to administer OTM medications to their own pet:

1) Has your pet ever growled, snarled, stiffened, or bitten when you have touched or tried to open their mouth?
2) Is your pet head-shy or fearful when you pet or touch near the face or mouth?
3) Has your pet growled, snarled, stiffened, or bitten if you have touched them while eating or taking a treat?
4) Do you feel both physically and emotionally comfortable lifting up the side of your pet's mouth and applying medication to their gums?

If the client reveals any history of aggression or fear regarding the handling of the head, face, or mouth, or if you sense any hesitation in their words or non-verbal body language, do not involve the client in the process. You are liable for their injuries within the practice, even if it is a result of their own pet's behavior.

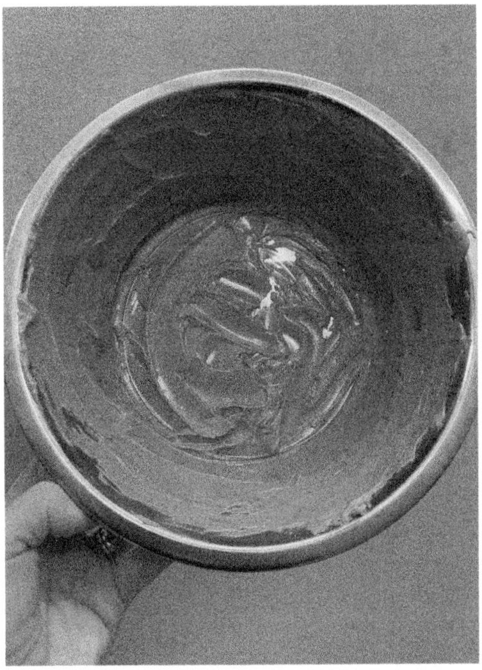

Figure 22.4 A CRS combination of dexmedetomidine and butorphanol has been mixed with peanut butter and smeared all around a large, metal water bowl. The patient can be given the bowl in a quiet room with the client and allowed to slowly lick and absorb the drugs. *Source:* Meghan E. Herron.

Pre-calculate reversal medications and/or cardiovascular event medications. In larger hospitals, where access to reversal agents may require logging in to dispensing systems such as Cubex®, pre-draw reversal for alpha-2 agonists (atipamezole).

Record Keeping and Communication

Documenting drug doses administered is a legal requirement for every practice. However, of equal importance to long-term success is documentation of *response* to used doses *and* restraint methods. For aggressive and fearful patients, this information needs to be exceptionally easy to find in case of urgent/emergent care needs, keeping in mind exposure to clinic activities may decrease efficacy of sedation (Albright et al. 2017). Consider using the same flag system used to denote significant allergies to denote sedation and restraint successes (Figure 22.7).

Additionally, flags such as "Caution"/ "Will Bite"/"Muzzle" often provide inadequate

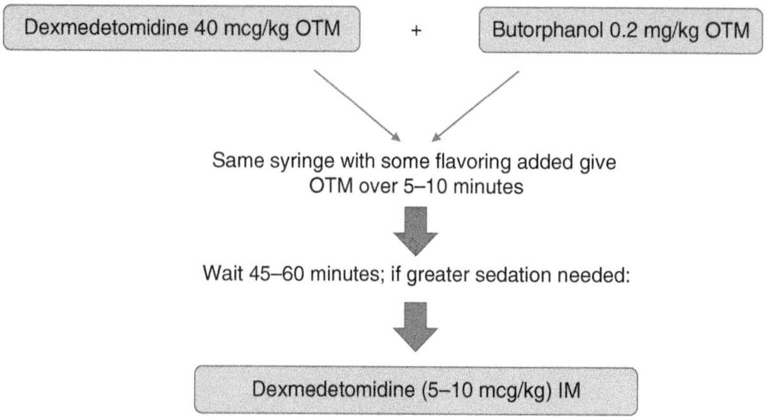
Dexmedetomidine 40 mcg/kg OTM
+
Butorphanol 0.2 mg/kg OTM
Same syringe with some flavoring added give OTM over 5–10 minutes
Wait 45–60 minutes; if greater sedation needed:
Dexmedetomidine (5–10 mcg/kg) IM

Figure 22.5 Oral transmucosal (OTM) CRS plan for dogs. A higher dose is required for the alpha-2 agonist, dexmedetomidine, due to anticipated spillage and swallowing. This dose is combined with an opioid, such as morphine, in an oral syringe. A viscous, flavored food, such as maple syrup or honey, is added for palatability and increased mucosal contact time. Be aware that morphine typically triggers vomiting once absorbed. These doses in large breed dogs can become cost prohibitive for some clients.

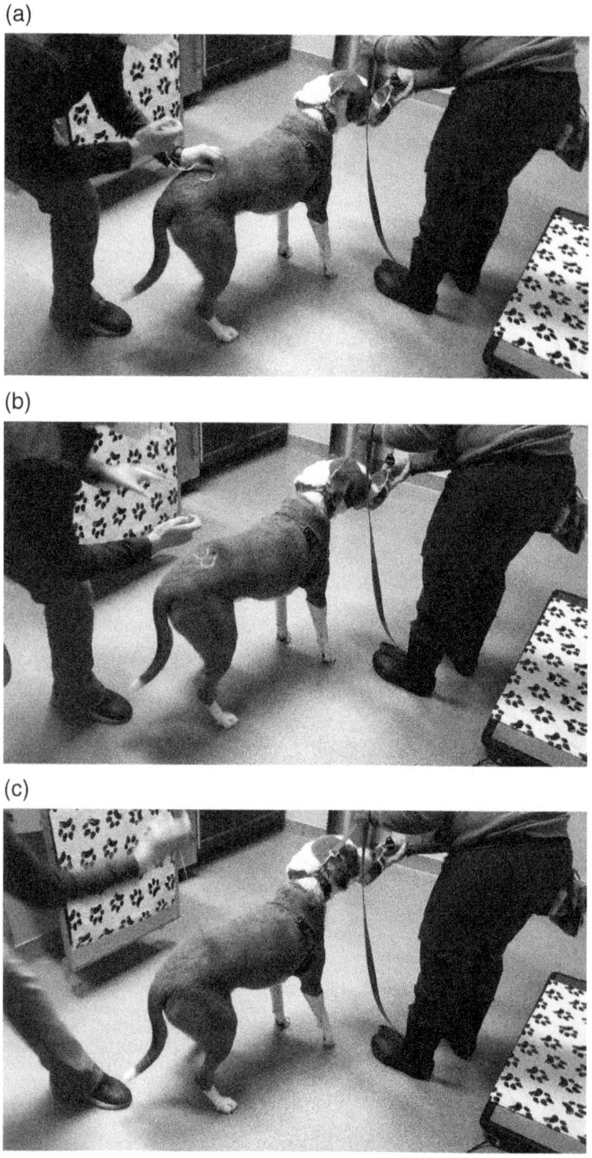
(a)
(b)
(c)

Figure 22.6 For patients who cannot be safely muzzled, injectable chemical restraint and sedation can be quickly injected through a butterfly catheter while the patient is fed and handled with a tight high collar held by an experienced handler (a). This injection should be quick and deliberate (b) and the person giving the injection should step back immediately after injecting (c). This takes practice! *Source:* Photo credit: Meghan E. Herron.

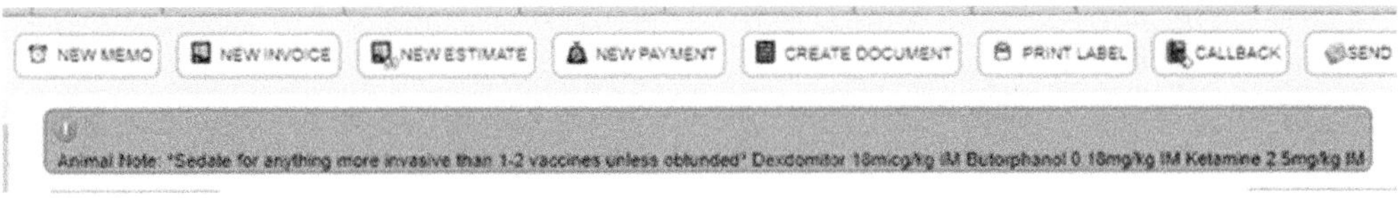

Figure 22.7 Example of a red flag alert system in an electronic medical record that alerts the clinician to the patient's tolerance for handling and need for sedation.

information especially when there are rotations or changes in personnel. Instead, flags like "Muzzle for nail trims, will eat distractedly for physical exams and vaccines" are far more informative about how to proceed for a specific patient. Additional details should be somewhere documented in the patient chart. Those details should describe the handling so that someone with no experience with that patient can recreate the situation and use objective, observable behaviors- much like a surgery report. See Box 22.3 for an example of handling details that can be included in a medical record.

Interpretations such as "dumb/mean/stubborn" are not reflective of the animal's true state or motivation (fear) and do not promote appropriate medical and evidence-based approaches to that patient (see Chapter 11). Detailed documentation with appropriate, observable body language increases the safety of future visits, increases appointment efficiency, increases practice communication, and increases perceived value to clients while improving patient welfare (Herron and Shreyer 2014). When you enter into the profession as a graduate, you will take an oath to protect animal health and welfare and to relieve suffering. Taking the time to create and document handling and sedation plans facilitates upholding that oath by maintaining welfare and alleviating suffering during or caused by the veterinary experience.

Box 22.3 Example of patient handling notes to facilitate ease of handling in future visits

"Patient stopped eating when approached near neck for attempt at jugular blood draw. Blood was drawn with her standing on the couch, owner at her head, scratching her head and neck, and Dr. X doing the same with her hand around the wing of atlas in case physically restraining her neck or head was needed. Patient was provided with spray cheese on a lick plate which she ate readily. Technician drew from her left lateral saphenous without any flinching, moving, or pause in eating."

References

Abbo, L.A., Ko, J.C.H., Maxwell, L.K. et al. (2008). Pharmacokinetics of buprenorphine following intravenous and oral transmucosal administration in dogs. *Vet. Ther.* 9 (2): 83–93.

Albright, J.D., Seddighi, R.M., Ng, Z. et al. (2017). Effect of environmental noise and music on dexmedetomidine-induced sedation in dogs. *PeerJ* 5: e3659. https://doi.org/10.7717/peerj.3659.

American College of Veterinary Anesthesiologists (2009). Recommendations for monitoring anesthetized veterinary patients- small animal. https://acvaa.org/wp-content/uploads/2019/05/Small-Animal-Monitoring-Guidlines.pdf (Accessed 29 June 2022).

American Veterinary Medical Association (n.d.) Physical restraint of animals. https://www.

avma.org/resources-tools/avma-policies/physical-restraint-animals (Accessed 17 May 2022).

Araghi, M., Azizi, S., Vesal, N. et al. (2016). Evaluation of the sedative effects of diazepam, midazolam, and xylazine after intranasal administration in juvenile ostriches (*Struthio camelus*). *J. Av. Med. Surg.* 30 (3): 221–226. https://doi.org/10.1647/2015-110.

Behzadi, M., Joukar, S., and Beik, A. (2018). Opioids and cardiac arrhythmia: a literature review. *Med. Prin. Pract.* 27 (5): 401–414. https://doi.org/10.1159/000492616.

Borer-Weir, K. (2014). Chapter 5 – Analgesia. In: *Veterinary Anaesthesia, 11e* (ed. K.W. Clarke, C.M. Trim, and L.W. Hall), 101–133. Oxford: W.B. Saunders https://doi.org/10.1016/B978-0-7020-2793-2.00005-0.

Bullingham, R.E.S., McQuay, H.J., and Moore, R.A. (1983). Clinical pharmacokinetics of narcotic agonist-antagonist drugs. *Clin. Pharmacokinet.* 8 (4): 332–343. https://doi.org/10.2165/00003088-198308040-00004.

Charalambous, M., Bhatti, S.F.M., Van Ham, L. et al. (2017). Intranasal midazolam versus rectal diazepam for the management of canine status epilepticus: a multicenter randomized parallel-group clinical trial. *J. Vet. Intern. Med.* 31 (4): 1149–1158. https://doi.org/10.1111/jvim.14734.

Cohen, A.E. and Bennett, S.L. (2015). Oral transmucosal administration of dexmedetomidine for sedation in 4 dogs. *Can. Vet. J.* 56 (11): 1144–1148.

Dent, B.T., Aarnes, T.K., Wavreille, V.A. et al. (2019). Pharmacokinetics and pharmacodynamic effects of oral transmucosal and intravenous administration of dexmedetomidine in dogs. *Am. J. Vet. Res.* 80 (10): 969–975. https://doi.org/10.2460/ajvr.80.10.969.

Enomoto, H., Love, L., Madsen, M. et al. (2022). Pharmacokinetics of intravenous, oral transmucosal, and intranasal buprenorphine in healthy male dogs. *J. Vet. Pharmacol. Ther.* 45 (4): 358–365. https://doi.org/10.1111/jvp.13056.

Federal Drug Administration. (2020) FDA adds alfaxan multidose IDX index of legally marketed unapproved new animal drugs for minor species', *FDA* [Preprint] https://www.fda.gov/animal-veterinary/cvm-updates/fda-adds-alfaxan-multidose-idx-index-legally-marketed-unapproved-new-animal-drugs-minor-species (accessed 25 June 2022).

Gharagozlou, P., Hashemi, E., DeLorey, T.M. et al. (2006). Pharmacological profiles of opioid ligands at Kappa opioid receptors. *BMC Pharmacol.* 6: 3. https://doi.org/10.1186/1471-2210-6-3.

Gilbert-Gregory, S.E., Stull, J.W., Rice, M.R., and Herron, M.E. (2016). Effects of trazodone on behavioral signs of stress in hospitalized dogs. *J. Am. Vet. Med. Assoc. 249* (11): 1281–1291.

Giudice, E., Crinò, C., Barillaro, G. et al. (2019). Clinical findings in degenerative lumbosacral stenosis in ten dogs—A pilot study on the analgesic activity of tramadol and gabapentin. *J. Vet. Behav.* 33: 7–15. https://doi.org/10.1016/j.jveb.2019.05.004.

Grove, D.M. and Ramsay, E.C. (2000). Sedative and physiologic effects of orally administered α2-adrenoceptor agonists and ketamine in cats. *J. Am. Vet. Med. Assoc.* 216 (12): 1929–1932. https://doi.org/10.2460/javma.2000.216.1929.

Gruen, M.E., Roe, S.C., Griffith, E. et al. (2014). Use of trazodone to facilitate postsurgical confinement in dogs. *J. Am. Vet. Med. Assoc. 245* (3): 296–301.

van Haaften, K.A., Forsythe, L.R.E., Stelow, E.A., and Bain, M.J. (2017). Effects of a single preappointment dose of gabapentin on signs of stress in cats during transportation and veterinary examination. *J. Am. Vet. Med. Assoc.* 251 (10): 1175–1181. https://doi.org/10.2460/javma.251.10.1175.

Helin-Salmivaara, A., Huttunen, T., Grönroos, J.M. et al. (2007). Risk of serious upper gastrointestinal events with concurrent use of NSAIDs and SSRIs: a case-control study in the general population. *Eur. J. Clin. Pharmacol.* 63 (4): 403–408. https://doi.org/10.1007/s00228-007-0263-y.

Herron, M.E. (2016). *Better Living Through Chemistry: Utilizing Chemical Restraint to Aid in Low Stress Handling in Small Animal Practice*. San Antonio, TX: *American Veterinary Medical Association Convention.*

Herron, M.E. and Shreyer, T. (2014). The pet-friendly veterinary practice: a guide for practitioners. *Vet. Clin. North America: Small Anim. Pract.* 44 (3): 451–481. https://doi.org/10.1016/j.cvsm.2014.01.010.

Hoffman, E.A., Aarnes, T.K., Ricco Pereira, C.H., Lerche, P., Bednarski, R.M., and McLoughlin, M. A. (2018). Effect of oral trazodone on the minimum alveolar concentration of isoflurane in dogs. *Vet. Anaesth. Analg.* 45(6): 754–759. https://doi.org/10.1016/j.vaa.2018.08.002

Howell, A. and Feyrecilde, M. (2018). *Cooperative Veterinary Care*. Wiley-Blackwell Available at: https://www.wiley.com/en-us/Cooperative+Veterinary+Care-p-9781119130543 (Accessed 25 June 2022).

Hydromorphone (2022). Drug bank. https://go.drugbank.com/drugs/DB00327 (Accessed 19 June 2022).

Johnson, B.A., Aarnes, T.K., Wanstrath, A.W. et al. (2019). Effect of oral administration of gabapentin on the minimum alveolar concentration of isoflurane in dogs. *Am. J. Vet. Res.* 80 (11): 1007–1009. https://doi.org/10.2460/ajvr.80.11.1007.

de Jong, J.C.F., van den Berg, P.B., Tobi, H., and de Jong-van den Berg, T.W. (2003). Combined use of SSRIs and NSAIDs increases the risk of gastrointestinal adverse effects. *British J. Clin. Pharmacol.* 55 (6): 591–595. https://doi.org/10.1046/j.0306 5251.2002.01770.x.

Jurox Animal Health (2019). Alfaxan multidose prescribing summary. St. Joseph MO. https://jurox.com/us/alfaxan/prescribing-summary (Accessed 22 January 2022).

Kasten, J.I., Messenger, K.M., and Campbell, N.B. (2018). Sedative and cardiopulmonary effects of buccally administered detomidine gel and reversal with atipamezole in dogs. *Am. J. Vet. Res.* 79 (12): 1253–1260. https://doi.org/10.2460/ajvr.79.12.1253.

Korpivaara, M., Laapas, K., Huhtinen, M. et al. (2017). Dexmedetomidine oromucosal gel for noise-associated acute anxiety and fear in dogs—a randomised, double-blind, placebo-controlled clinical study. *Vet. Rec.* 180 (14): 356. https://doi.org/10.1136/vr.104045.

KuKanich, B. and Papich, M.G. (2017). Opioid analgesic drugs. In: *Veterinary Pharmacology and Therapeutics*, 165–449. Hoboken, NJ: Wiley-Blackwell.

Lamminen, T., Korpivaara, M., Aspegrén, J., Palestrini, C., and Overall, K.L. (2023). Pregabalin alleviates anxiety and fear in cats during transportation and veterinary visits—A clinical field study. *Animals.* 13(3): 371.

Lemke, K.A. (2004) 'Perioperative use of selective alpha-2 agonists and antagonists in small animals', *Can. Vet. J.*, 45(6):475–80. PMID: 15283516; PMCID: PMC548630.

Messenger, K.M., Hopfensperger, M., Knych, H.K., and Papich, M.G. (2016). Pharmacokinetics of detomidine following intravenous or oral-transmucosal administration and sedative effects of the oral-transmucosal treatment in dogs. *Am. J. Vet. Res.* 77 (4): 413–420. https://doi.org/10.2460/ajvr.77.4.413.

Mitton, L.F., Sanchis-Mora, S., Pelligand, L. et al. (2019). Clinical usage of gabapentin in dogs under primary veterinary care in the UK. BSAVA Congress Proceedings 2019. BSAVA Library, pp. 478–478. Available at https://doi.org/10.22233/9781910443699.74.2.

Morgan, C.J.A., Curran, H.V., and the Independent Scientific Committee on Drugs (ISCD) (2012). Ketamine use: a review. *Addiction* 107 (1): 27–38. https://doi.org/10.1111/j.1360-0443.2011.03576.x.

Nejamkin, P., Cavilla, V., Clausse, M. et al. (2020). Sedative and physiologic effects of tiletamine–zolazepam following buccal administration in cats. *J. Feline Med. Surg.* 22 (2): 108–113. https://doi.org/10.1177/1098612X19827116.

Ogata, N. and Dodman, N.H. (2011). The use of clonidine in the treatment of fear-based behavior problems in dogs: an open trial.

J. Vet. Behav.: Clin. Appl. Res. 6 (2): 130–137. https://doi.org/10.1016/j.jveb.2010.10.004.

Pankratz, K.E., Ferris, K.K., Griffith, E.H., and Sherman, B.L. (2018). Use of single-dose oral gabapentin to attenuate fear responses in cage-trap confined community cats: a double-blind, placebo-controlled field trial. *J. Feline Med. Surg.* 20 (6): 535–543. https://doi.org/10.1177/1098612X17719399.

Porters, N., Bosmans, T., Debille, M. et al. (2014). Sedative and antinociceptive effects of dexmedetomidine and buprenorphine after oral transmucosal or intramuscular administration in cats. *Vet. Anaesth. Analg.* 41 (1): 90–96. https://doi.org/10.1111/vaa.12076.

Posner, L.P. (2017). Sedatives and traquilizers. In: *Veterinary Pharmacology and Therapeutics*, 9e (ed. J.E. Riviere and M.G. Papich), 324–369. Ames, Iowa: Wiley-Blackwell.

Plumb, D.C. (2015). *Plumb's Veterinary Drug Handbook*, 7e. Stockholm, Wisconsin: PharmaVet.

Reich, M.R., Ohad, D.G., Overall, K.L., and Dunham, A.E. (2000). Electrocardiographic assessment of antianxiety medication in dogs and correlation with serum drug concentration. *J. Am. Vet. Med. Assoc.* 216 (10): 1571–1575. https://doi.org/10.2460/javma.2000.216.1571.

Robertson, S.A., Taylor, P.M., and Sear, J.W. (2003). Systemic uptake of buprenorphine by cats after oral mucosal administration. *Vet. Rec.* 152 (22): 675–678. https://doi.org/10.1136/vr.152.22.675.

Rolfe, N., Kerr, C., and McDonell, W. (2012). Cardiopulmonary and sedative effects of the peripheral α2-adrenoceptor antagonist MK 0467 administered intravenously or intramuscularly concurrently with medetomidine in dogs. *Am. J. Vet. Res.* 73: 587–594.

Sadegh, A.B. (2013). Comparison of intranasal administration of xylazine, diazepam, and midazolam in budgerigars (*Melopsittacus undulatus*): clinical evaluation. *J. Zoo Wildlife Med.* 44 (2): 241–244. https://doi.org/10.1638/2009-0116R3.1.

Santos, L.C.P., Ludders, J.W., Erb, H.N. et al. (2010). Sedative and cardiorespiratory effects of dexmedetomidine and buprenorphine administered to cats via oral transmucosal or intramuscular routes. *Vet. Anaesth. Analg.* 37 (5): 417–424. https://doi.org/10.1111/j.1467-2995.2010.00555.x.

Schwartz, M., Muñana, K.R., Nettifee-Osborne, J.A. et al. (2013). The pharmacokinetics of midazolam after intravenous, intramuscular, and rectal administration in healthy dogs. *J. Vet. Pharmacol. Ther.* 36 (5): 471–477. https://doi.org/10.1111/jvp.12032.

Slingsby, L.S., Taylor, P.M., and Monroe, T. (2009). Thermal antinociception after dexmedetomidine administration in cats: a comparison between intramuscular and oral transmucosal administration. *J. Feline Med. Surg.* 11 (10): 829–834. https://doi.org/10.1016/j.jfms.2009.03.009.

Yin, S. (2009a). Chapter 11. General handling principles. In: *Low Stress Handling Restraint and Behavior Modification of Dogs & Cats: Techniques for Developing Patients Who Love Their Visits*, 191–233. Cattle Dog Publishing.

Yin, S. (2009b). Chapter 14. Dealing with difficult dogs. In: *Low Stress Handling Restraint and Behavior Modification of Dogs & Cats: Techniques for Developing Patients Who Love Their Visits*, 301–340. Cattle Dog Publishing.

Yin, S. (2009c). Chapter 16. Handling difficult cats. In: *Low Stress Handling Restraint and Behavior Modification of Dogs & Cats: Techniques for Developing Patients Who Love Their Visits*, 387–404. Cattle Dog Publishing.

Steagall, P.V.M., Monteiro-Steagall, B.P., and Taylor, P.M. (2014). A review of the studies using buprenorphine in cats. *J. Vet. Intern. Med.* 28 (3): 762–770. https://doi.org/10.1111/jvim.12346.

Zoetis Inc. (2015). Dexdomitor package insert. https://www2.zoetisus.com/content/_assets/docs/Petcare/dexdomitor05-pi.pdf (Accessed 22 January 2022).

Zoetis Inc. (2019). Telazol product insert. https://www2.zoetisus.com/content/_assets/docs/vmips/package-inserts/telazol.pdf (Accessed 22 January 2022).

23

Behavior Considerations for Aging Dogs and Cats

Margaret O'Brian

Southeast Animal Behavior and Training, Charlotte, NC, USA

Introduction

If we are lucky enough, our dogs and cats' lifespans extend into their senior years. From a client's perspective, this can be a time where behavioral changes are simply thought of as an unavoidable byproduct of age, arthritis, and other medical or sensory changes. From this lens, issues may go unaddressed – not for lack of worry or a desire to help their pets through these changes, but more so a lack of awareness regarding treatment options.

How many times have you heard a client say "ah doc, they are just getting old" when you note lameness in their 12-year-old dog. While we may perceive this as a lack of empathy for their pet's struggles, many clients do not recognize signs of pain or disease in pets. It is our job as the veterinarian to help families understand the importance of recognizing senior pet behavior changes to ensure the best quality of life possible through the end stage of their lives.

Sensory Changes

Sensory changes are to be expected in our senior dog and cat population. Although at times it feels like our pets get selective sensory loss (you cannot hear me say your name in the yard, but you can hear the treat bag opening from the floor below?), we know that these sensory changes can affect their perception of the environment and, subsequently, their behavior.

Vision loss may result in an animal that is more easily startled or concerned about sounds outside that they cannot identify or localize. The neighbor's new shrubbery may have been perceived as a great new sniff and pee spot previously, but now it is menacing and something to avoid. Pets with vision changes may also struggle more with alterations in the environmental layout, such as furniture rearrangements or replacements. For pets already bumping into objects in the house, these changes can be especially problematic. A dog may not explore or interact with toys or people the way they used to due to reluctance to navigate through the home. Similarly, cats may not feel confident enough to leap to their favorite high resting spot. Non-slip surfacing, ramps or step stools can help our pets navigate their environment with more confidence. Avoiding frequent or sudden big changes in the layout of the home can minimize stress in older pets, especially those with significant vision loss. If pets appear more nervous to approach an item, speak in a light-hearted manner to them and allow them to approach at their own pace.

Introduction to Animal Behavior and Veterinary Behavioral Medicine, First Edition. Edited by Meghan E. Herron.

Companion website: www.wiley.com/go/introductiontoanimalbehavior

Like vision deficits, hearing impairments can result in a heightened startle response. This is particularly true if animals are touched when they do not hear the person or other animal approach, which can result in a rapid fright response and even trigger aggression. It is never advisable to touch animals when they do not have awareness of your approach, i.e. let sleeping dogs lie, but this is especially true in our senior dogs. The one bright side of hearing loss in pets is that they may no longer be able to hear triggers that used to bother them, such as smoke detector beeps, thunderstorms, or fireworks. However, even dogs with hearing loss may feel vibrations of fireworks or thunderstorms despite this sensory change. Ongoing treatment of sound related fears should be based on the pet's clinical response, not the client's perception of whether the pet can hear adequately.

When we consider senior pets being more easily startled due to sensory loss, it is important to also consider the potential contribution of pain. Rapid muscle tension or movement that a pet would otherwise avoid can result in discomfort. This can contribute to nervous or aggressive behavior, as a pet will want to move away from this sudden, perceived threat quickly.

Olfaction is incredibly important for communication and feeding behaviors in animals. As social creatures who rely on odors and pheromones for intra-species communication, changes in olfaction can affect how pets interact with each other and with us (Bakker et al. 2022). Feeding behavior is also closely linked to olfactory perception, especially for cats. Cats will often smell their food exhaustively to assess its freshness and safety (Aldrich and Koppel 2015). An inability to smell food can, thus, affect taste secondarily, reducing the value and satisfaction of food. Fortunately, even into old age, many dogs and cats will still maintain a strong sense of smell, despite other sensory losses. As one of the strongest senses, we can use this as an avenue for enrichment and to aid in the management of other sensory losses. For example, allowing dogs to go for "sniff walks" – meandering adventures where each blade of grass and every flower and leaf can be investigated and introducing scent work training – teaching dogs to "hunt" for hidden scents around the home, can be highly stimulating. You can also advise clients to scent mark areas around the home so that they can be more easily identified. For example, resting areas can be marked with a vanilla scent, water bowls with lavender, and doors to the outside with peppermint.

Touch and taste changes are less clinically relevant, but individual pets may have medical concerns that lead to changes in this area that can correspond to behavioral concerns.

Musculoskeletal Pain

Imagine a distraught client calling you because her 10-year-old dog growled and snapped her for the first time in his entire life. She was petting him while he rested on the couch like she always does– this was not a new circumstance and he behaved in such an out of character way. She is convinced that the dog has a brain tumor or is mad at her for changing over to low-fat treats last week. What do you tell her?

Aggression is the most common behavioral concern presented to veterinary behaviorists. When aggression is first noted in the senior pet, especially under circumstances that a pet has experienced countless times before, pain-related aggression should be your top differential diagnosis. As discussed in Chapter 15, the initial onset of aggression in dogs typically occurs prior to or as a dog goes through social maturity (one to three years of age). Mature dogs with a sudden onset of aggression almost always have an underlying medical reason behind the behavior. In the case of the client who called you, the aggression was reported to be secondary to touch, making it likely the dog was physically uncomfortable. Often, musculoskeletal discomfort or pain can lower the threshold for aggression.

Other behavioral changes include the development or escalation of noise fears/phobias.

Interestingly, noise fears have been associated with musculoskeletal pain in dogs (Lopes Fagundes et al. 2018). The sudden muscle tension associated with startling can create a learned association between noises and physical pain. When noise fears are associated with musculoskeletal pain, they are more likely to present later in life and more likely to develop fear in general areas where they previously experienced the noises, whether a sound is currently present or not. For example, a painful dog who heard a car backfire on one street may avoid this street moving forward to avoid a repeat scary and, presumably, painful experience. Pain management is an important aspect of treating these patients, rather than being solely addressed from an anxiety standpoint (Mills et al. 2020).

Cats are not only predators, but their small stature makes them feel like prey animals in relation to larger carnivores, such as dogs. This means their outward signs of illness and musculoskeletal pain are often subtle. Cats with osteoarthritis may not solicit or tolerate physical affection as they have previously. They may also be less likely or less able to reach typical vertical resting or feeding spots. Elevation helps cats feel safe and secure, and if they are unable to comfortably access these areas, their quality of life can suffer.

When speaking with clients, you may find it helpful to create empathy for the changes their pet is experiencing. One might ask them to consider what they would do if their 85-year-old grandmother was resting on the couch. Would they shake her awake? Would you shove her off the furniture and expect her not to react? Likely not, so we need to offer our pets the same level of respect and patience.

Pain management is beyond the scope of this chapter, but an in-depth investigation of suspected physical discomfort is the first step in helping these animals. Other comfort-related recommendations for households with senior pets include non-slip flooring options, elevated food and water dishes (dogs), harnesses to avoid excessive neck pressure, and providing steps or ramps to higher resting spots (Figure 23.1).

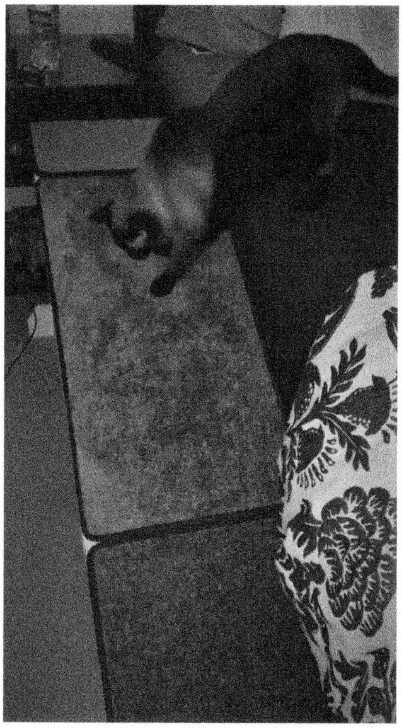

Figure 23.1 Sake, aged 16, has osteoarthritis. This carpeted ramp (CozyUp Bed Ramp [PetSafe®, Knoxville, TN]) gives him an easy, comfortable means of accessing his favorite resting spot on his human's bed. *Source:* With permission from Kristin Quisenberry.

Brain Changes

Rule Out Physical Disease

As pets age, they become more vulnerable to metabolic, neoplastic, and other degenerative disease processes. These can have broad ranging effects on behavior and make underlying etiology of certain behavioral changes challenging. For example, a senior cat starts urinating outside the litterbox. Is this a lower urinary tract concern? Is a musculoskeletal issue reducing the cat's willingness to walk up the stairs to access the litterbox? Could the cat have hyperthyroidism that is increasing urine production?

Or is the social upheaval of a recently added kitten triggering urine marking in this cat?

All behavior changes in senior pets should first be evaluated as a symptom of a medical problem. A minimum database of screening tests (full physical exam, a complete blood count, serum chemistry profile, total T4, and urinalysis), as well as additional testing, depending on the presentation (imaging, culture, and sensitivity), is indicated (Horwitz and Pike 2014).

Neurologic and behavior problems are another area that overlaps more commonly in senior years. Circling, pacing, and/or aggression with no discernible trigger should be worked up for primary neurologic etiologies.

The tricky aspect is that behavioral and medical issues do not occur in a vacuum and are rarely mutually exclusive. The diagnoses can be a combination of medical and behavioral concerns, and the treatment, likewise, needs to address the whole problem.

Cognitive Dysfunction Syndrome

Cognitive dysfunction syndrome (CDS) is a neurodegenerative disorder that results in gradual cognitive decline.

Prevalence of CDS

The prevalence of CDS in dogs varies from 14.2 to 73.0% depending on the study and the age group (Neilson et al. 2001; Osella et al. 2007; Salvin et al. 2010). However, consistent findings show that the older dogs get, the more likely they are to develop CDS (Fast et al. 2013; Osella et al. 2007; Salvin et al. 2010; O'Brian et al. 2021). One study found that only 1.9% of dogs identified as having signs consistent with CDS had received an actual diagnosis of CDS from their veterinarian, indicating that this is a markedly underdiagnosed condition (Salvin et al. 2010). In cats, the prevalence ranges from 13% of cats $\geq$8 years of age (MacQuiddy et al. 2022), 28% of cats 11–14 years of age, to >50% of cats 15 years of age or older (Gunn-Moore et al. 2007).

Human Correlation

Cognitive dysfunction syndrome has overlapping pathological and clinical markers as cognitive impairment, including Alzheimer's disease, in humans. Dogs have been used as a model for Alzheimer's disease in people due to these similarities (Cummings et al. 1996b).

CDS Pathophysiology

There are macro- and microscopic brain changes associated with CDS. Macroscopic changes include hippocampal atrophy, enlarged sulci, and enlarged ventricles (Pugliese et al. 2010). These changes can be seen with advanced imaging and support, but do not definitively diagnose CDS. Microscopic changes that confirm a CDS diagnosis include the presence of amyloid-beta plaques and hyperphosphorylated tau proteins in brain cells (Cummings et al. 1996a; Smolek et al. 2016; Schmidt et al. 2015). These can only be identified post-mortem, making them unhelpful in establishing a diagnosis in living pets. Amyloid-beta plaques accrue in the cells of the prefrontal cortex and hippocampus and can lead to memory and learning deficits, as well as decreased ability to voluntarily control elimination. Hyperphosphorylated tau protein changes disrupt transport mechanisms and lead to cell death. As cell pathology progresses to the parietal lobe, pets may display spatial disorientation, wandering, and reduced ability to process visual stimuli. Lastly, as the temporal and occipital lobe cells are damaged, auditory and visual deficits may be observed.

Because macroscopic changes do not definitively diagnose CDS, many clients are unlikely to pursue advanced imaging. Microscopic changes can only be identified post-mortem, making CDS a diagnosis of exclusion.

Making a Diagnosis

In most cases we rely primarily on client observed behavioral changes in pets to diagnose this disease (Landsberg et al. 2012). The first step is to evaluate, diagnose, and treat underlying medical issues that contribute to behavior changes in senior pets. This means completing the minimum database investigation and any additional testing that appears clinically relevant for that patient's problem list. Once you have ruled out a medical cause for the behavior changes, you can screen for symptoms of CDS. The acronym most commonly used to describe the clinical signs of CDS is DISHAA- *d*isorientation, changes in *i*nteractions with owners, *s*leep wake cycle alterations, *h*ouse soiling, and changes in *a*ctivity level or *a*nxiety (Landsberg et al. 2012).

There are multiple surveys available to assess and score these changes. The DISHAA Cognitive Dysfunction Evaluation Tool developed by Dr. Gary Landsberg and the Purina Institute is one of the most accessible and most convenient of these surveys (https://www.purinainstitute.com/centresquare/nutritional-and-clinical-assessment/dishaa-assessment-toolavailable in the online materials for Chapter 23). A high score on this survey is indicative of a high degree of CDS-related impairment.

Clients should begin filling out these surveys at routine exams every 6 months, starting when their dog turns eight years of age. Going through this survey may prompt them to bring up changes they have noticed at home that they otherwise may not have thought to bring to your attention. Remind them that they are scoring based on changes in behavior, not long-standing severity. For example, a dog that has severe, persistent separation anxiety should not score highly on the question evaluating separation anxiety if this behavior has not changed with time. Reassure your clients that a high score does not necessarily imply CDS unless underlying medical issues have been ruled out or adequately addressed.

Treatment

Enrichment and Training

Mental engagement is an important component of treating any behavior concern, and this is certainly the case with CDS. Studies show that regular training has a protective benefit against CDS. (Head et al. 2009). Encourage clients to sign their dogs up for mentally stimulating activities, such as "trick" training or scent work. They can also increase exposure to external stimuli by taking their time on walks. A senior dog may not want to go for their historical 60-minute brisk walk or jog, but they can still spend daily time going outside the home, moving at their pace around the neighborhood (Figure 23.2). Consider wagons or strollers to continue these adventures when dogs have reached their physical comfort limit (Figure 23.3).

One study showed that a once a week class specifically for senior dogs had a protective benefit against the progression of signs associated with CDS compared to dogs who did not attend classes (O'Brian et al. 2021). During the class, clients were educated on common changes seen in senior dogs and given recommendations for improving comfort and mobility. The dogs were taught two new "tricks" every week and encouraged to interact with puzzle toys. In this author's opinion, the only class cuter than Puppy Kindergarten is Senior Dog Class (Figure 23.4). If your clinic has the space, consider offering a similar course.

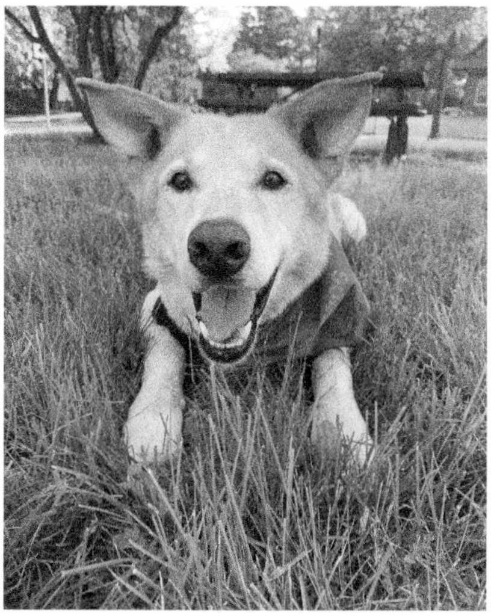

Figure 23.2 Balto, aged 12, enjoys time outdoors as part of his sensory enrichment routine. *Source:* Margaret O'Brian.

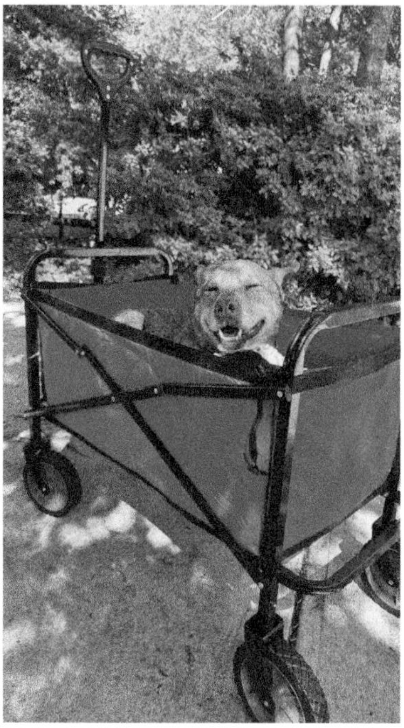

Figure 23.3 Dylan, aged 12, enjoys his daily walks with a little help from this wagon. Since he is unable to walk more than a few feet at a time, the wagon gives him the ability to explore the outdoor environment in comfort for extended periods of time. *Source:* Margaret O'Brian.

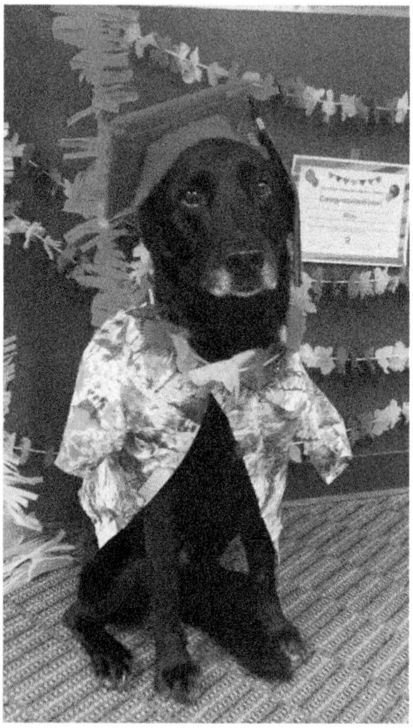

Figure 23.4 A graduate of Senior Dog Class displays his cap and gown proudly. *Source:* Margaret O'Brian.

Enrichment through food puzzles can encourage dogs to use cognitive skills during meals. Meals can be moved from bowls to food dispensing toys. Hidden treats in "snuffle mats" (Figure 23.5) can be placed on an elevated surface to reduce neck strain. Frozen food toys allow dogs to settle on the floor in a comfortable position.

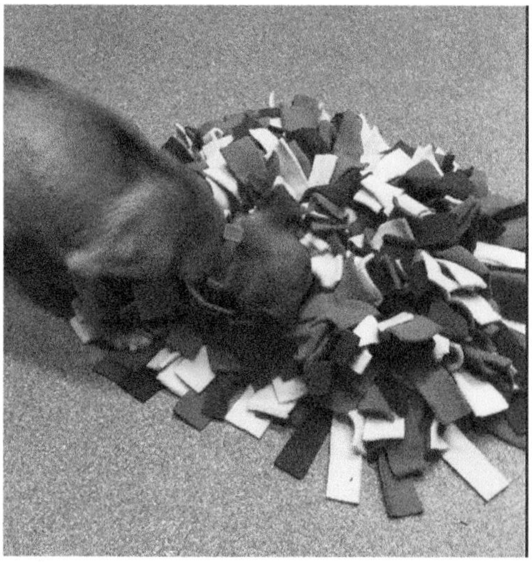

Figure 23.5 A snuffle mat serves as a food puzzle. Treats and dry kibble can be hidden in between the fleece flaps so that the dog must sniff and hunt for the goodies. This makes for great mental stimulation for aging pets. *Source:* Meghan E. Herron.

Diet

Unless there are medical concerns requiring a different diet, dogs and cats should be eating age-appropriate food. There are diets not only aimed at senior cats and dogs but aimed specifically to help with cognitive decline.

Hill's Prescription Diet – Brain Aging Care (b/d™) contains high levels of omega-3 fatty acids and antioxidants, L-carnitine to enhance mitochondrial function, and fruits and vegetables rich in flavonoids and carotenoids. Clinical trials demonstrated an improvement in learning in senior dogs with diet change alone (Dodd et al. 2003), and dogs treated with a combination of Hill's b/d and enrichment demonstrated even greater improvement in learning (Milgram et al. 2005).

Purina ProPlan® Veterinary Diets – Neurocare contains medium-chain triglyceride vegetable oils, antioxidants, and omedga-3 fatty acids and is high in protein to help maintain muscle mass. Research demonstrates improvement in clinical signs of CDS in dogs (Pan et al. 2018).

Nutraceuticals and Supplements

Pets may be on a different diet for medical reasons, and/or clients may be more hesitant to change their pets' diets in general. The good news is that there are many supplements available aimed at treating cognitive dysfunction that may be more feasible for clients to implement than a diet change. Targeted age recommendations may vary based on the supplement, but in general clients should be encouraged to start their pets on a cognition-supporting supplement starting around eight years of age. Signs of cognitive decline are often missed, and we are best to treat proactively as pets age.

Senilife® (Ceva Animal Health, Lenexa, KS) is available for both dogs and cats in the US. This supplement contains phosphatidylserine (which improves nerve-cell communication), pyridoxine (which plays a role in brain function and health), gingko biloba extract (which improves cerebral blood flow, increases glucose metabolism, and has an antioxidant effect), and resveratrol and D-alpha-tocopherol (antioxidants which have neuroprotective benefits). Two clinical trials demonstrated improvement in learning when compared to placebo (Osella et al. 2007; Araujo et al. 2008). Researchers also demonstrated that the earlier this supplement is started, the bigger the impact it can have on the pet's behavior.

Aktivait® (VetPlus, Lytham, Lancashire, UK) is available for dogs and cats in the UK. It contains phosphatidylserine, omega-3 fatty acids, L-carnitine (which plays a role in cellular metabolism and healthy mitochondrial function), vitamin E, vitamin C, and selenium (all of which have antioxidant effects).

Supplements containing SAM-e are available for dogs and cats globally. SAM-e is a free radical scavenger. SAM-e plays a role in the synthesis of serotonin - use caution when combining a SAM-e supplement with other serotonergic medications. Studies suggest SAM-e may improve some of the clinical signs associated with CDS, including a 50% reduction in mental impairment scores (Rème et al. 2008).

Canine Senior Vitality and Feline Senior Vitality supplements (VetriScience Laboratories, Williston, VT) are multivitamins available for dogs and cats in the US. They contain magtein (a synthesized form of magnesium, which is an important cofactor for many brain enzymes), DMG (which is a precursor for SAMe), medium chain triglycerides, omega-3 fatty acids, resveratrol, and choline (which support liver and nerve function).

Pharmacological Interventions

In addition to supplements, there are prescription medications available for use to treat cognitive decline and the associated clinical signs in dogs.

Selegiline [Anipryl® (Zoetis, Parsippany, NJ)] is a monoamine oxidase inhibitor (MAOI) that is FDA-approved for the treatment of CDS in dogs, and it is also used off-label in cats (Pan 2013). In an open-label trial, over 77% of dogs treated with selegiline showed improvement in the clinical signs associated with CDS (Campbell, Trettien, and Kozan 2001). It functions by inhibiting monoamine-oxidase B, an enzyme that breaks down dopamine, serotonin, and norepinephrine. This allows more dopamine, serotonin, and norepinephrine to circulate in the brain. MAOIs are also thought to reduce free radicals. Selegiline can take four to six weeks to reach therapeutic effect. Side effects are uncommon but may include sedation, decreased appetite, GI upset, and irritability. Selegiline may interact with other medications, especially those that increase dopamine, serotonin, or norepinephrine (SSRIs, TCAs, alpha-2 agonists, amphetamines, tramadol, opioids, and Amitraz).

Some senior pets with escalating anxiety may benefit from a daily anti-anxiety medication, such as an SSRI. SSRIs should be prioritized over TCAs in senior pets due to their comparatively fewer side effects and contraindications. Refer to Chapter 21 for more details on SSRI versus TCA therapies in dogs and cats.

Additionally, as-needed medications may be appropriate for a pet that has a predictable and specific area of concern. For example, one of the most common complaints from senior pet families is a change in sleep patterns. Many dogs suffering from sleep-wake cycle changes are up pacing and panting much of the night. This also means the humans in their household are getting little sleep. Benzodiazepines can be used prior to bedtime for dogs and cats, as they provide anxiolytic, sedative, and muscle-relaxing effects. Lorazepam is one benzodiazepine that does not have any active hepatic metabolites, making it a safe first option benzodiazepine for use in senior dogs and cats. Gabapentin may provide anxiolytic, sedative, and neuropathic pain reduction (see Chapter 21). It is another safe option to trial for improved nighttime sleep in both dogs and cats.

Addressing Specific Concerns Associated with CDS

House Soiling

Once you have ruled out and/or treated medical concerns related to inappropriate elimination in the home, guide clients on how to address CDS-related house soiling, as this is one of the most distressing and frustrating problems for pet households.

Advise clients to go back to basic puppy house training. This means taking the dog out on a leash, rewarding with a treat within one to three seconds of the pet eliminating outdoors, employing strict supervision while home with the dog, and considering management such as diapers or belly bands to prevent indoor elimination. Pets should never be scolded for soiling in the house, as this can lead to additional anxiety and behavior problems. Clients should clean soiled areas with an enzymatic cleaner and block access to these areas if and when possible. House soiling as a result of cognitive decline is thought to stem from a loss of previously learned behavior and the ability to voluntarily "hold it" until they are in an outdoor environment. However, consider the possibility that the increased anxiety component of cognitive decline is relevant and make plans to address the underlying anxiety issue along with the training.

Sleep/Wake Cycle Changes

Once you have ruled out and treated medical concerns related to changes in the sleep-wake cycle, particularly physical discomfort leading to a difficulty settling, advise clients on helping pets sleep through the night. Like house soiling, disruption in sleep can cause substantial client stress. Environmental interventions that may help include synthetic pheromone diffusers, white noise machines, night lights, or, for some pets, blackout curtains. Clients should try to keep dogs active throughout the day and implement enrichment and training as discussed previously. Clients can trial various sleep comfort options, including cooling mats, bolstered dog beds, and/or stairs that allow pets to more easily access the client's bed (if that is desired).

Prognosis

CDS is ultimately a progressive disease with no definitive cure. The main risk factor for cognitive decline is increasing age. One study demonstrated that without treatment, 48% of dogs aged 11–14 years already showing clinical signs of CDS in one behavioral category developed signs in two or more categories within 6–18 months (Neilson et al. 2001). The treatment options described here can help slow the progression of this disease and improve quality of life for our senior pets. As the primary care veterinarian, we can help clients recognize the clinical signs associated with CDS and understand that there are treatment options available.

References

Aldrich, G.C. and Koppel, K. (2015). Pet food palatability evaluation: a review of standard assay techniques and interpretation of results with a primary focus on limitations. *Animals* 5 (1): 43–55.

Araujo, J.A., Landsberg, G.M., Milgram, N.W. et al. (2008). Improvement of short-term memory performance in aged Beagles by a nutraceutical supplement containing phosphatidylserine, *Ginkgo biloba*, vitamin E, and pyridoxine. *Can. Vet. J.* 49: 379–385.

Bakker, J., Leinders-Zufall, T., and Chamero, P. (2022). The sense of smell: role of the olfactory system in social behavior. In: *Neuroscience in the 21st Century: From Basic to Clinical*, 1215–1243. Cham: Springer International Publishing.

Campbell, S., Trettien, A., and Kozan, B. (2001). A noncomparative open-label study evaluating the effect of selegiline hydrochloride in a clinical setting. *Vet. Ther.* 2 (1): 24–39.

Cummings, B.J., Head, E., Afagh, A.J. et al. (1996a). β-Amyloid accumulation correlates with cognitive dysfunction in the aged canine. *Neurobiol. Learn. Mem.* 66: 11–23.

Cummings, B.J., Head, E., Ruehl, W. et al. (1996b). The canine as an animal model of human aging and dementia. *Neurobiol. Aging* 17: 259–268.

Dodd, C.E., Zicker, S.C., Jewell, D.E. et al. (2003). Can a fortified food affect the behavioral manifestations of age-related cognitive decline in dogs? *Vet. Med.* 98 (5): 396–408.

Fast, R., Schütt, T., Toft, N. et al. (2013). An observational study with long-term follow-up of canine cognitive dysfunction: clinical characteristics, survival, and risk factors. *J. Vet. Intern Med.* 27: 822–829.

Gunn-Moore, D., Moffat, K., Christie, L.A., and Head, E. (2007). Cognitive dysfunction and the neurobiology of ageing in cats. *J. Small Anim. Prac.* 48 (10): 546–553.

Head, E., Nukala, V.N., Fenoglio, K.A. et al. (2009). Effects of age, dietary, and behavioral enrichment on brain mitochondria in a canine model of human aging. *Exp. Neurol.* 220: 171–176.

Horwitz, D.F. and Pike, A.L. (2014). Common sense behavior modification: a guide for practitioners. *Vet. Clin. North America, Small Anim. Pract.* 44 (3): 401–426.

Landsberg, G.M., Nichol, J., and Araujo, J.A. (2012). Cognitive dysfunction syndrome. A disease of canine and feline brain aging. *Vet. Clin. North America Small Anim. Pract.* 42: 749–768.

Lopes Fagundes, A.L., Hewison, L., McPeake, K.J. et al. (2018). Noise sensitivities in dogs: an exploration of signs in dogs with and without musculoskeletal pain using qualitative content analysis. *Front. Vet. Sci.* 5: 17.

MacQuiddy, B., Moreno, J., Frank, J., and McGrath, S. (2022). Survey of risk factors and frequency of clinical signs observed with feline cognitive dysfunction syndrome. *J. Feline Med. Surg.* 24 (6): e131–e137.

Milgram, N.W., Head, E., Zicker, S.C. et al. (2005). Learning ability in aged beagle dogs is preserved by behavioral enrichment and dietary fortification: a two-year longitudinal study. *Neurobiol. Aging* 26 (1): 77–90.

Mills, D.S., Demontigny-Bédard, I., Gruen, M. et al. (2020). Pain and problem behavior in cats and dogs. *Animals* 10 (2): 318.

Neilson, J.C., Hart, B.L., Cliff, K.D. et al. (2001). Prevalence of behavioral changes associated with age-related cognitive impairment in dogs. *J. Am. Vet. Med. Assoc.* 218: 1787–1791.

O'Brian, M.L., Herron, M.E., Smith, A.M., and Aarnes, T.K. (2021). Effects of a four-week group class created for dogs at least eight years of age on the development and progression of signs of cognitive dysfunction syndrome. *J. Am. Vet. Med. Assoc. 259* (6): 637–643.

Osella, M.C., Re, G., Odore, R. et al. (2007). Canine cognitive dysfunction syndrome: prevalence, clinical signs and treatment with a neuroprotective nutraceutical. *Appl. Anim. Behav. Sci. 105* (4): 297–310.

Pan, Y.L. (2013). Cognitive dysfunction syndrome in dogs and cats. *CABI Rev.* 2013: 1–10.

Pan, Y., Landsberg, G., Mougeot, I. et al. (2018). Efficacy of a therapeutic diet on dogs with signs of cognitive dysfunction syndrome (CDS): a prospective double blinded placebo controlled clinical study. *Front. Nutr.* 5: 127.

Pugliese, M., Carrasco, J.L., Gomez-Anson, B. et al. (2010). Magnetic resonance imaging of cerebral involutional changes in dogs as markers of aging: an innovative tool adapted from a human visual rating scale. *Vet. J.* 186: 166–171.

Rème, C.A., Dramard, V., Kern, L. et al. (2008). Effect of S-adenosylmethionine tablets on the reduction of age-related mental decline in dogs: a double-blinded, placebo-controlled trial. *Vet. Ther.: Res. Appl. Vet. Med. 9* (2): 69–82.

Salvin, H.E., McGreevy, P.D., Sachdev, P.S. et al. (2010). Under diagnosis of canine cognitive dysfunction: a cross-sectional survey of older companion dogs. *Vet. J.* 184: 277–281.

Schmidt, F., Boltze, J., Jäger, C. et al. (2015). Detection and quantification of β-amyloid, pyroglutamyl Aβ, and tau in aged canines. *J. Neuropathol. Exp. Neurol.* 74: 912–923.

Smolek, T., Madari, A., Farbakova, J. et al. (2016). Tau hyperphosphorylation in synaptosomes and neuroinflammation are associated with canine cognitive impairment. *J. Comp. Neurol.* 524: 874–895.

Appendix A

Books to Keep in Practice – Clinical Textbook Recommendations

General

Broom, D.M. (2021). *Broom and Fraser's domestic animal behaviour and welfare 6th edition*. CABI.

Crowell-Davis, S.L., Murray, T.F., and de Souza Dantas, L.M. (2019). *Veterinary psychopharmacology*. John Wiley & Sons.

Houpt, K.A. (2018). *Domestic animal behavior for veterinarians and animal scientists*. John Wiley & Sons.

Dogs and Cats

Denenberg, S. (ed.) (2020). *Small animal veterinary psychiatry*. CABI.

DiGangi, B.A., Cussen, V.A., Reid, P.J., and Collins, K.A. (ed.) (2022). *Animal behavior for shelter veterinarians and staff*. John Wiley & Sons.

Horwitz, D. and Mills, D., 2009. *BSAVA manual of canine and feline behavioural medicine*.

Horwitz, D.F. (ed.) (2018). *Blackwell's five-minute veterinary consult clinical companion: canine and feline behavior*. John Wiley & Sons.

Landsberg, G., Radosta, L., and Ackerman, L. (ed.) (2023). *Behavior problems of the dog and cat*. Elsevier Health Sciences.

Overall, K. (2013). *Manual of clinical behavioral medicine for dogs and cats*. Elsevier Health Sciences.

Stelow, E.A. (ed.) (2023). *Clinical handbook of feline behavior medicine*. John Wiley & Sons.

Yin, S.A. (2009). *Low stress handling, restraint and behavior modification of dogs & cats: techniques for developing patients who love their visits*. Cattle Dog Publishing.

Horses

Beaver, B.V. (2019). *Equine behavioral medicine*. Academic Press.

McDonnell, S.M. (2003). *The equid ethogram: a practical field guide to horse behavior*. Eclipse Press.

McGreevy, P. (2012). *Equine behavior: a guide for veterinarians and equine scientists*. Elsevier Health Sciences.

Introduction to Animal Behavior and Veterinary Behavioral Medicine, First Edition. Edited by Meghan E. Herron.

Companion website: www.wiley.com/go/introductiontoanimalbehavior

Farm Animals

Ekesbo, I. and Gunnarsson, S. (2018). *Farm animal behaviour: characteristics for assessment of health and welfare.* CABI.

Exotic Animals

Bays, T.B., Lightfoot, T., and Mayer, J. (2006). *Exotic pet behavior: birds, reptiles, and small mammals.* Elsevier Health Sciences.

Luescher, A. (ed.) (2006). *Manual of parrot behavior.* Wiley-Blackwell.

Tynes, V.V. (ed.) (2010). *Behavior of exotic pets.* John Wiley & Sons.

Appendix B

Teaching Your Cat to Like the Carrier

Lisa Radosta

Florida Veterinary Behavior Service, West Palm Beach, FL, USA

Most cats hate the carrier, and it is easy to understand why. Cats go into the carrier only when something bad is going to happen, like a long car ride or a trip to the veterinarian. It takes just one negative experience for your kitty to believe that the carrier is bad news. But you can change that perception.

The first thing is choosing the best carrier for your cat. In general, try to choose a sturdy carrier that comes apart in several places (such as a plastic carrier with a removable top section) so that your cat can be lifted out easily or examined by the veterinarian inside the carrier if necessary. Then follow these dos and don'ts to help your cat love the carrier.

Do:

- Get the carrier out of the garage, clean it up, and put it in the area where your cat usually hangs out.
- Take the carrier apart by taking the top off and removing the door for a couple of weeks to help your cat feel comfortable and perhaps rest in the bottom portion.
- Put your cat's bed in the carrier.
- Make the carrier positive and encourage discovery by placing special toys and treats inside or feeding your cat there.
- Consider placing the carrier in a safe elevated spot where your cat likes to spend time, such as a couch, a chair, or a wide windowsill.
- Teach your cat to get into the carrier with clicker training or luring.
- Use a synthetic pheromone spray inside the carrier for thirty minutes before calling your cat to the carrier.
- Give your cat palatable food treats while inside the carrier.
- When your cat is comfortable in the carrier, take them on short rides while encouraging a positive emotional state with delicious foods.
- Keep the carrier level in the car by using towels or bumpers.
- Clean the inside of the carrier with an unscented cleaner after each use.

Don't:

- Pull the carrier out and try to force your cat inside immediately before a veterinary visit.
- Bring the carrier out only when you have to take your cat somewhere.
- Dump your cat out onto the examination table at the veterinarian's office.

If your cat already has a negative conditioned emotional response to the carrier, desensitization and counterconditioning may be necessary to change their emotional state. Desensitization and classical counterconditioning (DS/CC) is a process by which the cat is slowly exposed to the stimulus (the carrier) while using a positive stimulus (food) to change the cat's emotional state.

Introduction to Animal Behavior and Veterinary Behavioral Medicine, First Edition. Edited by Meghan E. Herron.

Companion website: www.wiley.com/go/introductiontoanimalbehavior

Glossary

Acral lick dermatitis A self-inflicted skin irritation/infection, sometimes forming thick, firm granulomas, which results from excessive licking of the lower legs and feet.

Affective aggression Aggression with an underlying emotional basis, accompanied by a high degree of sympathetic nervous system activation, vocalizations, and threat displays, with the goal of threatening harm to the individual perceived as a potential danger.

Affiliative behaviors Behaviors that show friendly intent and a desire to get closer to another being.

Aggression An act or threat of an act by one individual that threatens to harm another.

Agonistic Any activity related to fighting, including threats, aggression, submission, and retreat.

Alloparenting Giving parental care to young that are not one's own direct offspring.

Allostatic load The "wear and tear" on the body which accumulates as an individual is exposed to repeated or chronic stress.

Altricial Being relatively immobile and underdeveloped at birth, requiring parental care for a period of time.

Analgesic effects Pain-relieving effects.

Anticholinergic Effects created when a substance blocks the action of the neurotransmitter acetylcholine at synapses in the central and peripheral nervous system. Common anticholinergic effects include dry eyes, dry mouth, urine retention, and constipation.

Antiemetic Having anti-nausea properties.

Antihistaminic Effects created when a substance blocks histamine receptors. The most common antihistaminic effect is sedation.

Anxiolytic Anxiety-relieving.

Artificial selection The process by which humans select physical and/or behavioral traits in animals and breed them based on their liking, rather than what might be fit for survival in a natural environment. Also known as "selective breeding."

Associative learning The process by which two distinct stimuli, events, or cues become associated with one another in the mind after being experienced together.

Attention seeking behavior Behavior displayed with the intent of gaining attention from another being. This is a learned behavior after certain behaviors have been reinforced with attention.

Autonomic nervous system A component of the peripheral nervous system that regulates involuntary physiological processes, including heart rate, blood pressure, respiration, and digestion. It comprises two antagonistic sets of nerves, the sympathetic and parasympathetic nervous systems.

Introduction to Animal Behavior and Veterinary Behavioral Medicine, First Edition. Edited by Meghan E. Herron.

Companion website: www.wiley.com/go/introductiontoanimalbehavior

Autoreceptor A receptor on a nerve cell that responds to a neurotransmitter released from the same nerve cell on which it is located.

Aversion tests Tests that measure negative motivations. Animals can learn to avoid an unpleasant stimulus by changing its behavior and/or location. These tests are used to determine what animals find to be aversive or unpleasant.

Bachelor herds A group of nonbreeding juvenile male animals of the same species that form their own herd away from the main herd that contains both males and females.

Binocular vision Vision obtained by seeing something simultaneously with both eyes. This requires coordination from both eyes to merge the image they each see into one. This allows for better three-dimensional visual perception. Front facing eyes that are close together have better binocular vision as there is more overlap between what each eye sees.

Breeders The term used to refer to the male and female in a pack of animals who mate and produce offspring. Most packs include only one breeding pair, unless their numbers and resources are high. This pair will suppress breeding of other animals within the pack.

Bridge medication An immediate-acting medication used to provide immediate relief of fear, anxiety, and/or stress while awaiting the full therapeutic effects of a longer-acting, more delayed onset psychotropic medication.

Chemical restraint The use of injectable medications to provide a quick-onset of sedation, anxiolysis, and relaxation.

Classical conditioning A learning process in which involuntary responses develop after repeated associations are made between an unconditioned stimulus and a neutral stimulus. When a stimulus becomes a cue or trigger for a reflex behavior and emotion (fear or pleasure), it is considered to be classically conditioned stimulus. This is an unconscious, automatic learning process.

Cognitive dysfunction syndrome A neurodegenerative disorder that results in gradual cognitive decline.

Colonies (feline) Groups of feral cats which linger and live around regular food sources, typically food set out by humans.

Complex dominance hierarchy A form of social hierarchy that includes linear, triangular, and dyad components.

Compulsive behaviors Abnormal, regularly repeated behaviors that occur even in the absence of their original context or trigger. There often is an underlying anxiety disorder in animals showing these behaviors.

Conditioned emotional response A learned emotional response to a previously neutral stimulus as a result of classical conditioning whereby the neutral stimulus was repeatedly paired with an unconditioned stimulus.

Conditioned reinforcer A stimulus that was once neutral now elicits a positive emotional response, after a period of training where it was paired repeatedly with something that triggered an unconditioned positive emotional response.

Conditioned stimulus A stimulus that was once neutral now elicits an emotional response, after a period of training where it was paired repeatedly with something that triggered an unconditioned emotional response.

Conspecifics Members of the same species.

Contiguity The principle that for learning to occur, the response must occur in the presence of or very soon after a stimulus is presented. This means that associations between two events or stimuli will only occur when they occur relatively close together in time.

Contingency The extent that a stimulus or cue predicts an event will follow.

Continuous reinforcement schedule A training schedule whereby a desired behavior is reinforced every single time it occurs.

Counterconditioning The process of changing a negative emotional response (fear) to a positive one (happy) by associating a previously conditioned fear-eliciting stimulus with one that naturally elicits a positive emotional response (often food). Over time, the triggering stimulus will change from triggering fear to triggering an animal to feel happy.

Desensitization The process of reducing a behavioral/fear response over time. This occurs by presenting fear-eliciting stimuli repeatedly at low intensities until the animal habituates to it. Over time the intensity is gradually increased. To be effective, the intensity of the stimulus must never go above the threshold of triggering fear.

Despotic dominance hierarchy A hierarchy in which one individual has a higher social rank or dominance over all other individuals who all share the same subordinate status.

Differential reinforcement The reinforcement of a new, desirable behavior while withholding or preventing reinforcement for an unwanted behavior.

Dilution effect The principle that a large group of animals has a better chance of eluding a predator than does one animal alone. The "safety in numbers" principle.

Displacement behaviors Behaviors performed out of context in relation to the situation. Often starts when an external stressful event occurs.

Docility A naïve openness to tameness and a willingness to interact with humans. One of the most important character traits to favor domestication.

Domesticated A term used to describe species of animals whose genotype and phenotype have been changed from their original wild ancestor through the process of artificial selection of traits that favor domestication.

Domestication See Domesticated.

Domestication syndrome Coined by Charles Darwin as a suite of modified characteristic traits involving physiology, morphology, and behavior that consistently occur together across species of domestic animals.

Dominance An achieved social status of having preferential access to resources over another social group member.

Dominance theory A scientifically inaccurate theory that humans and dogs exist within the same hierarchical structure and that humans must assert a dominant position in their relationship in order to maintain desirable behaviors.

Driving line An imaginary, approximate vertical line around the area of the shoulder of a horse. Directing your focus in front of this part of a horse's body will cause them to move back or away from you, while putting pressure behind this area will cause them to move forward or turn their rear end away from you. Your position in relation to this line will determine the direction a horse will move in front of, or behind, this line.

Epigenetics The study of how behavior and the environment can change gene activity without changing the DNA sequence.

Extinction The gradual weakening of a conditioned behavioral response when the reinforcement that had been maintaining that behavior is no longer provided.

Fear The emotional response of an animal to the perception of present danger.

Fear period A period of time in early development where dogs are particularly sensitive to frightening events. They may go unnoticed by human companions but may present as a sudden fearfulness or suspicion toward new things. Frightening experiences during this period may lead to long-lasting fears/phobias.

Feral A word used to describe an individual whose species has gone fully down the genetic path to domestication, perhaps having sustained selective breeding or even line breeding, but which has been living without direct human care since infancy, i.e. feral cats, feral pigs, feral Mustangs.

Fixed interval reinforcement schedule As part of positive reinforcement training, the animal is given reinforcement for a cued behavior after a fixed amount of time has elapsed, i.e. every 10 seconds, every 30 seconds, or every 2 minutes.

Fixed ratio reinforcement schedule As part of positive reinforcement training, the animal is given reinforcement after a specified number of responses, i.e. after taking two steps forward.

Flehmen A behavior in which an animal inhales deeply with the mouth open and the nostrils curled up as a means of detecting and moving pheromones through the ducts that connect the nares and the vomeronasal epithelium.

Flight zone/distance The distance around an animal within which a person can approach before the animal moves away.

Flooding A form of training that involves forced exposure to a stimulus that triggers a conditioned negative emotional response until the animal habituates and then no longer exhibits that response.

Food aversion A strong dislike for a particular food after experiencing nausea and/or gastrointestinal illness shortly after eating this food previously.

Gape A behavior in which an animal inhales with the mouth open, moving the head side-to-side as a means of detecting and moving pheromones through the ducts that connect the mouth and the vomeronasal epithelium. In dogs and cats, the ducts reside just caudal to the upper incisor teeth.

Grimace scale A scale used to evaluate facial expressions specifically related to pain as a means of objectively scoring pain based on the position of an animal's eyes, nose, and cheeks.

Habituation The diminishing of an emotional or behavioral response to a stimulus after repeated exposure to it. A form of nonassociative learning where animals no longer find something unpleasant or threatening because it has not caused them harm or discomfort.

Home range The area in which an animal lives and moves on a periodic basis but is not necessarily actively defended.

Horizontal streak An area within the retina, linear in shape, with a high concentration of ganglion cells, which allows for a linear streak of high visual acuity.

Hypothalamo-pituitary-adrenal (HPA) axis A complex set of direct influences and feedback interactions among the hypothalamus, the anterior pituitary gland, and the adrenal cortices. This axis controls the release and inhibition of the stress hormone, cortisol.

Imprinting A form of learning in newly hatched birds in which they fix their attention on the first moving object they see. This then triggers an immediate bond and, typically, a lifelong propensity to follow that object (typically their parent[s]).

Instrumental learning see Operant conditioning.

Juvenile period The developmental period following the socialization period where an animal is rapidly growing and gaining independence prior to becoming sexually mature.

Learned helplessness Failure of an animal to attempt to escape an aversive stimulus or situation which occurs after that animal has been repeatedly exposed to said aversive stimulus or situation and been unable to escape. Eventually, the animal stops attempting to escape and behaves as if it is helpless to change the situation. This state is a potential consequence of flooding and other aversive training methods.

Linear dominance hierarchy A linear form of social status ranking where each animal is dominant over the animals below it and submissive/deferential to those above it in the hierarchy in relation to access to valuable resources, such as food, shelter, and mates. Formerly and colloquially known as a "pecking order."

Local enhancement The enhancement in attractiveness of an area or object after one member of a group explored or investigated it. Individuals are attracted to areas where conspecifics have previously been but are not necessarily still present when the next animal explores the object or area.

Luring A form of positive reinforcement training where an animal's interest in enticements/rewards is used to create a behavior. As the animal sniffs/investigates/follows the enticement, its body is manipulated into the desired position, which can then be marked with a conditioned reinforcer and/or access to the enticement/reward.

Matriarchal A form of social organization in which the eldest females lead the family group. Matriarchal groups often include several related females who may help cooperatively rear their young.

Middening An animal's deposition of feces for the purpose of marking.

Misdirected play A phenomenon common in kittens and young cats where normal play-related behaviors, including stalking, chasing, grabbing, and biting are directed onto undesirable targets. Sometimes referred to as "play-related aggression."

Mobbing A group of animals surround and attack a threat or predatory in order to drive it off.

Monocular vision Occurs in animals with laterally placed eyes, allowing them to process two separate images at one time. This allows for a wide peripheral field of vision, but poor depth perception and poor visual acuity on what is directly in front of them.

Natal bands A social structure whereby animals form a group, consisting of one or two dominant males, multiple females, and their offspring. The dominant male drives off other males and has the highest social ranking of the group. Multiple natal bands may be present in a herd of animals.

Natural selection Terms coined by Charles Darwin that describe the process whereby organisms better adapted to their environment tend to survive and produce more offspring. These terms encompass the "survival of the fittest" concept.

Neonatal period The period in early development just after birth when newborn animals are highly dependent on their dam for nourishment and safety. Neonatal dogs and cats have limited sensory limitations and are dependent on the dam for elimination and warmth.

Neuromodulator A substance that potentiates or inhibits the transmission of a nerve impulse but is not the actual means of transmission itself.

Nonassociative learning A process in which an animal's behavior toward a specific stimulus changes over time in the absence of any evident link to (association with) consequences or other stimuli that would lead to such change. There are two major forms of nonassociative learning: habituation and sensitization.

Operant conditioning The process by which voluntary behaviors are trained in response to a given cue, either through reinforcement or punishment.

Pairing territorial A social organization characterized by a male and female pair occupying and defending a territory.

Pandora syndrome A term coined by Dr. C. A. Buffington that refers to a pathologic condition resulting from anxiety associated with chronic perception of threat.

Panic Sudden, uncontrollable fear or anxiety, which may lead to erratic, fleeing, or aggressive behavior.

Parallel dominance hierarchy A social ranking system seen in groups where animals of different ages coexist. In these groups, there is a linear hierarchy among adults and a similar linear hierarchy in the juveniles within the group.

Pavlovian conditioning See Classical conditioning.

Peri-domestic Animals who have become adapted to human settlements and environments through natural selection. They provide no utility to humans and their traits are not selected for based on human preference.

Phenotypic description Objective descriptions of physical characteristics or behaviors that include statements of verifiable fact, not opinion or subjective judgment.

Pheromones Natural, nonvolatile, chemical substances that an animal releases into the environment that affect the behavior or physiology of others of its species, including themselves.

Phobia Excessive, extreme, irrational, fear or panic about a situation, living creature, place, or thing.

Pica The ingestion of nonfood items.

Pinnal distance The distance on an animal's head between the two pinnae, allowing the brain to localize sound based on the differences in the time arrival of hearing impulses.

Point of balance An area located near the point of the shoulder of cattle that determines which way an animal will move based on where the handler approaches. If the handler approaches the pressure zone behind the point of balance, the animal gets the signal to move forward. If the handler moves in front of the point of balance, the animals gets the signal to move backward.

Polyestrous A female reproductive pattern that includes more than one estrus cycle in a one-year period.

Precocial/Precocious Being relatively mobile and having close to full sensory abilities at birth. Precocial species can stand, walk, and follow their dam within hours of birth.

Preferred associates Two individuals who form a bond and prefer to be within proximity to each other and to engage in mutual affiliative behaviors.

Prenatal period The period that encompasses the time an animal spends in utero and/or the time between conception and birth.

Pressure zone The zone just outside of the flight zone of an animal where a handler can slowly move into, in order to guide the animal to move, not flee, away from you.

Pre-visit pharmaceuticals (PVPs) Immediate-acting medications given to a pet prior to a veterinary visit for the purpose of easing fear, anxiety, and stress in the veterinary setting.

Primary reinforcers Stimuli that serve as rewards for a behavior because they are naturally reinforcing. The animal does not need to be taught to enjoy them because they naturally elicit a positive emotion or sensation.

Problem Oriented Veterinary Behavior Record Behavioral health documentation based on observed behavior, assessment of the behavior, and a plan for modification.

Psychogenic alopecia Excessive self-directed licking which results in areas of hair loss that cannot be connected to an underlying medical etiology.

Psychotropic medication Drugs that affect mood and emotional states, and, therefore behavior, by altering or enhancing neurotransmitter release and/or uptake in the brain.

Punishment A type of operant conditioning where an undesirable consequence occurs after a behavior that then reduces the likelihood that behavior will happen again in the future.

Redirection and distraction The process of reorienting an animal to another behavior or stimulus to decrease the focus on the original stimulus.

Reinforcement A type of operant conditioning where a desirable consequence occurs after a behavior that then increases the likelihood that behavior will happen again in the future.

Repetitive disorder A broad term that refers to multiple abnormal or problematic behaviors with repetitive natures.

Resource holding potential The ability of an animal to win in an all-out fight or contest, mostly based on their size, strength, endurance, and weapons.

Response substitution See Differential reinforcement.

Ritualized behaviors Behaviors that feign attack without the intent of causing harm. The intention is to showcase one's fighting ability.

Secondary reinforcers Rewards that were once neutral stimuli that come to gain value of their own by being paired with primary reinforcers. A form of conditioned reinforcers.

Semi-domestic Species who are part of and derived from human-occupied environments but have not been subjected to conscious selective breeding. They are still capable of living independent of humans.

Sensitization A process in which an animal has a more pronounced reaction to a stimulus than it did the first time it was exposed to that stimulus.

Serotonergic Anything that potentiates and/or involves the neurotransmitter, serotonin.

Serotonin syndrome A condition resulting from accumulation of excessively high levels of serotonin in the body, often due to the overdose or combination of serotonergic drugs.

Sexual maturity The age at which animals develop the physical capability to reproduce. Sexually dimorphic physical and behavioral traits become apparent during this time in sexually intact animals.

Sexual selection A form of natural selection where traits evolve through preference by one sex for certain characteristics in individuals of the other sex.

Shaping A method of reinforcement training where successive approximations of the final, full desired behavior are reinforced until the final behavior is achieved.

Snapping (in foals) The act of opening and closing of the mouth with retracted lips in response to another horse, often as a result of being fearful of the other horse, but mostly signals that they are socially immature.

Social buffering The concept that the presence of a social support system helps buffer or shield an individual from the negative impacts of a stressful event.

Social facilitation Animals in groups engaging in behaviors that appear to have been elicited by seeing the same behavior in other group members.

Social maturity The age at which animals demonstrate their full repertoire of adult behaviors. This period ends the transition between adolescence and adulthood.

Social referencing The process by which one individual's emotional state is affected by the emotional state of another group member.

Socialization The process of providing animals with exposure (neutral or positive) to various people, animals, places, and objects during a defined sensitive period early in life so that they do not grow up being afraid of these stimuli later in life.

Socialization period A developmental period in animals whereby they can make broad generalizations based on a few experiences. Social and emotional experiences during this time may have a greater and longer-lasting impact in comparison to similar or more extensive experiences later in life. Lack of exposure to social and nonsocial stimuli during this period often leads to the development of adult problem behaviors.

Solitary territorial A social organization where adults occupy and defend their own territories males typically solitary and females with young.

Stereotypic behavior See Stereotypy.

Stereotypy A behavior that is repetitive and unvarying in its pattern, with a purpose of relieving stress related to underlying husbandry conditions, where an animal is unable to perform species-typical behaviors.

Submissive behaviors Gestures that signal retreat and the intention to cause no harm, in an attempt to end an interaction.

Sympathetic nervous system Part of the autonomic nervous system that regulates an animal's involuntary/automatic response to threat or excitement. Adrenaline released from the adrenal glands prepares the body for survival by increasing heart and respiratory rates, mobilizing glucose from the liver, dilating the pupils, increasing circulation to the muscles and skin, and ceasing nonessential functions such as digestion.

Systematic desensitization See Desensitization.

Tame An acquired loss of fear of humans. This can occur among various wild animal species when individual animals have had early contact with humans.

Tapetum lucidum The reflective portion of the retina that allows light to be reflected and, therefore, enhanced. This reflection allows for better vision in low light settings and can be visualized by a green or yellow reflection when direct light hits the eyes.

Territorial Social organization where an animal or animals works to gain and/or maintain exclusive access to the resources in a fixed area.

Touch gradient The concept of keeping in constant physical contact with an animal in order to prevent startle during an exam or procedure.

Transitional period The developmental period between the neonatal and socialization periods in puppies and kittens. It is a time of rapid motor and behavior changes.

Triangular dominance hierarchy A social hierarchy between three individuals where the relationship between these individuals may vary relative to each other, forming a triangle. Animal A has a higher rank over B, B has a higher rank over C, but C has a higher rank over A.

Trigger stacking Occurs when multiple stressful events occur in a short period of time, causing an exaggerated behavioral response compared to what might typically be elicited from a single stressful event.

Unconditioned stimulus A stimulus that automatically triggers an unconditioned emotional or reflex response without any learning or previous exposure.

Urine marking Deposition of urine for the purpose of leaving a social message or signal.

Variable interval reinforcement schedule A schedule of reinforcement whereby an animal is reinforced based on an interval of time, but the time varies between reinforcement, regardless of how many times the correct behavior is performed.

Variable ratio reinforcement schedule A schedule of reinforcement whereby an animal is reinforced after a varying number of times the behavior is correctly performed.

Vomeronasal organ A group of sensory receptors located in the soft tissue of the nasal septum, in the nasal cavity, just above the hard palate responsible for detecting nonvolatile compounds (pheromones).

Wild Species of animals whose phenotype has not undergone artificial selection.

Winner–loser effect The effect whereby an outcome of a contest is influenced by the individual's previous contest results.

Index

a

Abandonment 54
ABCs of behavioral history 249, 250
Abnormal repetitive behaviors 408
 in cattle 408–409
 feeding behavior 412
 foraging opportunities 412
 gastrointestinal discomfort 412–413
 in horses 409–410
 medical considerations 410–412
 nutritional factors 413
 in pigs 410
 in poultry 410, 411
 in wild animals
  allostatic load 388
  behavior assessment 388
  captive carnivores 391–392
  defined 386
  environmental enrichment and training 397
  Five Domains framework 386–387
  human-induced stressors. 392–394
  management and treatment plan 396–399
  in non-zoo settings 392–395
  oral/feeding behaviors 391, 392
  pharmacologic intervention 397–398
  preventive measures 395
  skin infections 392
  in zoos and wildlife sanctuaries 391
Academically trained behaviorists 259–260
Acepromazine 201–202, 429–430
Acral lick dermatitis (ALD) 372, 373
ADAPTIL® 211, 232, 257
Affective aggression 289
Affiliative behaviors 32, 47–50, 290, 291
Aggression 47
 affective 289
 canine (*see* Dog aggression)
 dominance ranks 47
 fear-based 43
 feline (*see* Cat aggression)
 horses (*see* Equine aggression)
 neurophysiology of 289–290
 predatory (*see* Predatory behavior)
 protective 43, 53
 RHP 46–47
Aging dogs and cats
 brain changes 463–464
 cognitive dysfunction syndrome
  definition of 464
  diagnosis 464–465
  diet 466–467
  enrichment and training 465–466
  house soiling 468
  nutraceuticals and supplements 467
  pathophysiology 464
  pharmacological interventions 467–468
  prevalence of 464
  prognosis 468–469
  sleep/wake cycle changes 468
 musculoskeletal pain 462–463
 sensory changes
  hearing 462
  olfaction 462
  taste 462
  visual 461
Agonistic behavior 39–43
Agonistic interactions 291, 292
Aktivait® 467
Alfaxalone 449–450
Allogrooming 48, 304
Alloparenting 54
Allorubbing 48
Allostatic loads 388
Alpha-2 agonists 427, 448–449
Alprazolam 429
Amitriptyline 424, 426
Analgesics 446–447
Anipryl® 425
Antecedents 249
Antianxiety medications 284
Antiemetic properties 430

Introduction to Animal Behavior and Veterinary Behavioral Medicine, First Edition. Edited by Meghan E. Herron.

Companion website: www.wiley.com/go/introductiontoanimalbehavior

Anti-panic medication 428
Anxiety 315–316
Anxiolytic medication. *See* Antianxiety medications
Anxitane 283
Applied animal behaviorists 260
Artificial selection 11
Asocial 37
Associative learning 96–99, 101
Assortative mating 15
Audition
- auditory signal 73
- cats 76
- dogs 75–76
- hearing range 73
- horses 74–75
- pinnal distance 74
- ruminants 76–77

Autonomic nervous system 80
Autoreceptors 420
Aversion 168
Aversion (learning) tests 168, 171
Azapirone 422, 425

b

Bachelor herds 37
Behavioral wellness assessment 247–248
Behavior consultants 259
Behavior-focused visit 262
Behavior professionals
- certifications 263–264
- finding 260–261
- red flags 261
- types of 259–260

Behavior triage 244–249
- phenotypic descriptions 250
- red flags 252
- medical rule outs 252–253
- minimum diagnostic database 254
- recommended referral 258–259
- safety advice 253–255
- stress reduction 255–258

Belyaev, Dimitry 22
Benzodiazepines 428–429, 449, 468
Beta-blocking drugs 201
Bifidobacterium longum 284
Binocular vision 66, 67
Bird vision 72, 73
Bite threat 352
Botai 20
Brambell report (1965) 386
Breeders 46
Bridge medication 430
Bullmastiff 43, 44
Buprenorphine 447
Buspirone 425, 426
Butorphanol 447

c

Canine. *See* Dogs
Canine Behavior Assessment and Research Questionnaire (C-BARQ) scores 118
Canine cognitive dysfunction (CCD) 425
Caniquel® 424
Canis familiaris 46
Capture myopathy 17
Cat aggression
- abnormal 292–293
- aggression between cats 303–306
- behavior modification 298–299
- defensive/fear-related aggression 295, 300, 304
- environmental modification 296–298
- frustration-related 300
- irritable 296
- misdirected play behaviors 303
- normal 290–292
- offensive 295–296
- pain and 294
- pathological 301–303
- to people 300–303
- petting-induced 300–301
- physical disease and 293–295
- physiological 301
- psychoactive medications 299–300
- redirected 296, 304
- safety and management 296–297, 305–306
- territorial 295, 300, 304
- treatment of 296–299, 304–306

Cats
- agonistic interactions 291, 292
- allogrooming and allorubbing 48, 304
- altricial 135
- behavioral needs 144–149
- behavioral wellness assessment 248
- breeds 16–17
- chewing 145–147
- colonies 290
- countertops 147, 149
- developmental periods in 136–137
  - juvenile 141, 142
  - neonatal 137–138
  - prenatal 137
  - seniors 142
  - sexual maturity 142
  - socialization 136, 139–142
  - social maturity 142
  - transitional 138–139
- domestication 15–17
- elimination disorders 269
  - anxiety 277, 278
  - diets, supplements, and medications 283–284
  - FIC 274, 278
  - history taking 272–275
  - litter box aversion 276
  - litter box management and hygiene 279–281
  - location aversion 277
  - location preference 277
  - LUTD 274, 275
  - management of soiled areas 281
  - multimodal environmental modification 281–282
  - substrate aversion 276–277
  - substrate preference 277, 278
  - synthetic pheromones 282–283
  - treatment principles 279
  - undesirable toileting 271–272
- excessive licking 372
- food aversion 82
- gape 140, 141

habituation 97
handling (*see* Croney's assessment and plan system)
handling tools
carrier 234–235
EZ Nabber 237–238
FELIWAY Classic and Optimum 237
muzzles 238, 298
towel wrapping and restraint 225–227, 235–236
hearing 76
hunting 144
hyperthyroidism in 253
indoor *vs.* outdoors 148, 149
kitten socialization classes 141, 142
laser pointer games 145
latrine 143–144
living with multiples 149–150
non-threatening approach 219
normal elimination behavior 269
middening 271
sniffing 270
toileting 270
urine marking 270–271
olfactory system 81
osteoarthritis 276
play 256, 292
psychogenic alopecia 373, 425
red flag kittens 150–151, 252
scratching 146–148
taste 81
thermal comfort 213
toys for 144–146
veterinary visits 150
vision 70, 71
wild-crossed breeds 145
Cattle
abnormal oral behaviors
artificial teat 413
cross-sucking 409
environmental enrichment 414
gastrointestinal discomfort 410–413
management 412–416
non-nutritive sucking/licking 409, 412
nose flaps 416
tongue-rolling 408–410, 412
aversion tests 168, 171
fear 168
following behavior 172–173
green, yellow and red zones 169–170
handling
handler skills, attitude, and personality 175
negative 171
positive 171–172
training handlers 175–176
headlocks 174
hearing 76–77, 166–167
high arousal negative emotional state 167–168
movement
flight zone 173
point of balance 173–174
pressure zone 173
negative affective states 168–169
pain in 406
play behavior 169
positive affective states 169
restraining 174
rumen fill 412
signals of affect 167
stress 167–168
swinging cow brush 414
tactile sensation 167
understanding emotional states 407
vision 71–72, 165–166
vocalization 77
Chemical restraint and sedation (CRS) 228–229, 443
achieving and maintaining sedation 451–453
alpha-2 agonists 448–449
analgesics 446–447
benzodiazepines 449
documentation 455, 457
indications for 443–444
injectable CRS protocols 450–451
for cats 451, 454
for dogs 451–453
injectable medications 446, 449–450
monitoring and safety 453, 455
NMDA antagonists 449
opioids 447–448
oral medications 444–449
oral transmucosal (OTM) 451, 455, 456
pre-visit pharmaceuticals (PVPs)
choosing 444–446
combination 446
red flag alert system 455, 457
safe injection practices 451, 456
Chewing
cats 145–147
dogs 123
Chickens
imprinting 52
social facilitation 49
Classical conditioning 96–98, 162, 294, 298, 302
Clomicalm® 423–424, 426, 433
Clomipramine 379, 424, 426
Clonidine 427, 429, 445
Cognitive dysfunction syndrome (CDS) 344, 345
definition of 464
diagnosis 464–465
diet 466–467
enrichment and training 465–466
house soiling 468
nutraceuticals and supplements 467
pathophysiology 464
pharmacological interventions 467–468
prevalence of 464
prognosis 468–469
sleep/wake cycle changes 468
Colonies, feline 290
Commercial breeding operations (CBO) 112

Communication skills 245
Competition
 reproductive 35, 36
 resource 35, 36
Competitive agonistic interactions 39–41
Complex hierarchy 45–46
Compulsive disorder 343–344
Conditioned emotional response (CER) 97
Conditioned reinforcers 94, 98, 157
Conditioned response (CR) 97, 98
Conditioned stimulus (CS) 97, 98
Conditioned taste aversion (CTA) 81
Conflict aggression, in dogs 323
Conflict in social groups 39. *See also* Social group(ing)
 aggression 43–44
 competitive agonistic interactions 39–41
 determinants of contest outcomes 41
 owner *vs.* intruder 43
 perceived resource value 41–42
 resolution 39
 resource holding potential 41, 42
 ritualized behavior 40
 submissive behavior 40
 winner–loser effects 42
Conspecifics 31, 65
Context-specific aggression 44
Contingency 93–94
Continuous reinforcement schedule 104
Cooperative hunting 34
Coprophagia 154–156
Corticotropin-releasing hormone (CRH) 92
Cortisol 92, 112
Counterconditioning (CC) 107, 215, 223–225, 329–330
Crisis buster medication 258
Croney's assessment and plan system 206–207
 assess the environment 207–214
 assess the patient's comfort level and intent 214–215
 assess yourself
  inaccurate patient descriptors 220
  language and attitude 219–220
  non-threatening body language 215, 218–219
 make a handling plan 220–221
  canine handling tools 229–234
  chemical restraint 228–229
  counterconditioning 223–225
  feline handling tools 234–238
  needs *vs.* wants algorithm 221–223
  PVPs 228
  safe and effective restraint 225–226

d

Dachshunds 317
DAMNIT-B scheme 253
Darwin, C., 11, 16
Defensive aggression
 in cats 295, 300, 304
 in dogs 314
Desensitization. *See* Systematic desensitization and counterconditioning
Despotic hierarchy 45
Detomidine 448
Detomidine hydrochloride 202
Developmental periods, in cats 136–137
 juvenile 141, 142
 neonatal 137–138
 personality 143
 prenatal 137
 seniors 142
 sexual maturity 142
 socialization 136, 139–142
 social maturity 142
 transitional 138–139
Developmental periods, in dogs 111
 fear 116
 juvenile 117
 neonatal 112–113
 prenatal 111–112
 sexual maturity 117–118
 socialization 114–116
 social maturity 118
 summary of 112, 118–119
 transitional 113–114
Developmental periods, in horses 153
 mare–foal communication 156
 neonatal period
  coprophagia 154–156
  lateral recumbency 154, 155
  licking 153, 154
  precocious 153
Dexmedetomidine 427, 448
Diazepam 429
Dichromats 66, 67
Diet 466–467
Differential reinforcement 105
Diffusers 211, 232, 283
Dilution effect 33
Distraction 105
Doberman Pinscher 371–372, 374
Docility 11
Dog aggression
 aggression between dogs in same household 326
 aggression secondary to high arousal 324
 bite assessment scale 332
 body language 313–315
 conflict-related aggression 323
 defensive 314
 definition of 311
 diagnosis 320
  aggression screen 320–322
  history taking 320–322
  medical assessment and rule outs 320, 323–325
  observation 320

dominance hierarchy 325
episodic dyscontrol 324
euthanasia 334
fear-related 313, 323
human-directed 325
influencing factors
  age 318
  arousal 316
  breed differences 316–318
  environmental factors 318–319
  fear, anxiety, and pain 315–316
  impact of learning 319–320
  sex 318
intraspecific 325–326
irritable aggression 324
leash reactivity 319, 328
management 326–327
  avoidance of triggers 327
  behavior modification 328–331
  counterconditioning 329–330
  positive punishment 330–331
  psychotropic medications 331
  safety and management tools 327–328
  systematic desensitization 330
  teaching alternative behaviors 329
maternal aggression 324
mixed 314, 315
as normal behavior 311
offensive 314, 315
pain-related aggression 324
predatory behavior 311–313
prognosis 331–333
redirected aggression 324
rehoming 333–334
resource guarding 323
socially facilitated aggression 324–325
social status aggression 324
territorial aggression 323–324
Dog appeasing pheromones (DAP) 232
Dog crates 327
Dogs
  agonistic behavior 42–43
  barking 124–125
  behavioral wellness assessment 247
  chewing 123
  deafness in 75
  developmental periods in 111
    fear 116
    juvenile 117
    neonatal 112–113
    prenatal 111–112
    sexual maturity 117–118
    socialization 114–116
    social maturity 118
    transitional 113–114
  domestication 14–15
  elimination behaviors 125–126
  emotional contagion 49
  excitable behaviors 124–125
  fear of loud noises 343
  flank-sucking 371–372
  food aversion 81
  handling (*see* Croney's assessment and plan system)
  handling tools
    DAP 232
    Elizabethan collar restraint 234
    muzzle 229–231
    ThunderCap 232–233
    Thundershirt 233
    towel restraint 233
  head collars 328
  hearing 75–76
  housetraining 125–126
  jumping 124
  lateral recumbency 226
  mounting 124
  mouthing 123
  muzzles 327–328
  negative reinforcement 100
  non-threatening approach 215, 218–219
  olfactory system 80–81
  oral behaviors 123–124
  OTM CRS plan 456
  pack 46
  play behavior 50, 256
  puppy classes 121–122
  red flag puppies 127–128, 252
  resource guarding 123–124
  sensitization 96–97
  separation-related behaviors 126–127
  social buffering 49
  SRD in (*see* Separation-related disorders (SRD))
  taste 81
  ThunderCap 207, 229
  towel wraps 225, 227
  vaccination 122
  venipuncture 226
  vision 70–71
Domestication
  behavioral adaptation 12
  cats 15–17
  centers of 8, 10
  defined 7
  dogs 14–15
  donkey 20
  entrained beasts 22
  farm animals 17–19
  farm-fox experiment 22–23
  feral animal 13
  Fertile Crescent 10
  horses 19–21
  origin of 8–10
  pathways to 13–14
  peri-domestic animals 13
  semi-domestic animals 13
  tameness 12–13
  traits of
    climate adaptability 11
    docility 11
    fast growth rate 11
    flexible diet 10–11
    group living 10
    limited ability 11
    parental-offspring bonding 10
    promiscuous mating 10
    short flight distance 10
  wild animals 13
  wolves 14–15

Domestication syndrome 11–12
Dominance 47
  hierarchies 45–46
  theory 47
Driving line of horses 193
Ducks
  abandonment of young 54
  imprinting 52

e

Electronic fencing 102
Elimination disorders of cats 269
  anxiety 277, 278
  feline interstitial cystitis 274, 278
  history taking 272–275
  litter box aversion 276
  location aversion 277
  location preference 277
  lower urinary tract diseases 274, 275
  substrate aversion 276–277
  substrate preference 277, 278
  treatment principles 278–279
    diets, supplements, and medications 283–284
    litter box management and hygiene 279–281
    management of soiled areas 281
    multimodal environmental modification 281–282
    synthetic pheromones 282–283
  undesirable toileting 271–272
Elizabethan collar restraint 234
Endocrine system 5
Entrained beasts 22
Environmental enrichment 255–256
Epigenetics 135
Equine. *See* Horses
Equine aggression 351
  assessment 361–363
  bite threat 352
  fear-induced 356–357
  foal rejection 357–359
  human-directed 360, 361
  intermale aggression 360, 361
  learning 359–360
  mares in breeding shed 360
  maternal 357
  medication 363
  pain-induced 353–354
  play 359
  social/dominance-related/competitive 354–355
  stallions in breeding shed 360
  territorial 355–356
  tips to manage 363
  treatment strategies 354–360
Equine appeasing pheromone (EAP) 80
Essential oils 211
Ethological approach 4
Euthanasia 334
Exercise 256, 346
Experiential approach 4–5
Extinction 104
Ezee-Visit Pet Vet Mat® 211
EZ Nabber 237–238

f

Fabric sucking 371
Farm animals 17–19
Farm-fox experiment 22–23
Fear
  in cattle 168
  definition 168
  of loud noises 343
Fear, anxiety, and stress (FAS) 214–215
Fear, anxiety, stress, conflict, and panic (FAS-CP) 91–93
Fear Free 215–217, 265
Fear period 116
Fear-related aggression 43
  in cats 295, 300, 304
  in dogs 313, 315–316, 323
  in horses 356–357
Feline. *See* Cats
Feline hyperesthesia syndrome 371
Feline inappropriate elimination (FIE) 269
Feline interstitial cystitis (FIC) 274, 278, 294
Feline undesirable elimination (FUE) 269
Felis silvestris 16, 17
FELIWAY® Classic 237, 257, 282–283
FELIWAY Multi-cat 257, 283
FELIWAY Optimum 237, 257, 283
Feral animal 13, 17
Fertile Crescent 10, 16
Fitness 32
Five Domains 386–387
Five Freedoms 386
Fixed interval reinforcement schedule 104
Fixed ratio reinforcement schedule 104
Flank-sucking 371–372
Flehmen 79, 158
Flight distance 169
Flight zone 173
Flooding 105, 157
Fluconazole 81
Fluoxetine 379, 422–423, 426
Fluralaner 81
Foal rejection 160, 357–359
Followers 53
Food aversion (FA) 81–82
Foraging efficiency 34, 36
Four habits model 246, 247
Frustration-related aggression 300

g

Gabapentin 202, 428, 429, 445–446, 468
Gamma-aminobutyric-acid (GABA) 201, 202
Gape, in cats 140, 141
Gastrointestinal (GI) upset 82
Generalized anxiety disorder (GAD) 343
Gonadectomy 117–118
Grandin, Temple 172
Great Pyrenees 43, 44
Grimace scales 404
Group hunting 34
Gustatory comfort 212–213

h

Habituation 97
Halter training 157, 158
Handlers
  skills, attitude, and personality 175
  training 175–176
Handling animals
  cats and dogs (*see* Croney's assessment and plan system)
  cattle
    affective emotional states 167–169
    following behavior 172–173
    green, yellow and red zones 169–170
    handler skills, attitude, and personality 175
    movement 173–174
    negative handling 171
    positive handling 171–172
    positive reinforcement 174–175
    training handlers 175–176
  horses 189
    approach and haltering 190–192
    approach and retreat 190
    approaching the client horse 189–190
    body language and emotional states 181–186
    drug administration 200–203
    halting 194
    injections 196, 198
    leading 191, 193–195
    lunging 195
    picking up hooves 195–198
    sending 194–195
    temperature measurement 196, 199
    turning 194
  low-stress 206
Handling tools
  cats
    carrier 234–235
    EZ Nabber 237–238
    FELIWAY Classic and Optimum 237
    muzzles 238
    towel wrapping and restraint 225–227, 235–236
  dogs
    DAP 232
    Elizabethan collar restraint 234
    muzzle 229–231
    ThunderCap 232–233
    Thundershirt 233
    towel restraint 233
  horses
    gloves 186
    halters and ropes 186–188
    treat holder 187–189
    treats 186, 187
Hearing, cattle 166–167
Heifers 48
Hens 32
  conflict in social groups 39
  management of abnormal behavior 414, 415
  stereotypic behaviors in 410, 411
Hiders 53
Hind-end checking 370, 374
Home range 37
Horizontal streak 68
Horse Grimace Scale (HGS) 406
Horses
  adult behavior 162
  aggression in (*see* Equine aggression)
  classical conditioning 162
  cribbing behavior 410, 411
  domestication 19–21
  driving line 193
  drugs effects 201
    acepromazine 201–202
    beta-blocking drugs 201
    detomidine hydrochloride 202
    gabapentin 202
    trazodone 202
  EAP 80
  emotional states
    green zone 182–183
    red zone 185–186
    yellow zone 183–185
  examination 194
  flehmen 79, 158
  foal rejection 160
  food aversion 81
  grazing 158, 159
  halter training 157, 158
  handling skills 189
    approach and haltering 190–192
    approach and retreat 190
    approaching the client horse 189–190
    drug administration 200–203
    halting 194
    injections 196, 198
    leading 191, 193–195
    lunging 195
    picking up hooves 195–198
    sending 194–195
    temperature measurement 196, 199
    turning 194
  handling tools
    gloves 186
    halters and ropes 186–188
    treats 186–188
  hearing 74–75
  imprint training 157
  management of abnormal behavior 414
  mare–foal communication 156
  medications 200–201
  neonatal period
    coprophagia 154–156
    lateral recumbency 154, 155
    licking 153, 154
    precocious 153
  nickering 156
  olfactory system 79–80
  orphan foal 160
  pain in 406
  play 158
  positive reinforcement 157–159

Horses (*cont'd*)
  problem prevention
    Tips 162
  procedures aversion
    198, 200
  sickness 159–160
  snapping 156
  social preference
    development 158, 159
  stereotypic behaviors in
    409–411
  touch gradient 194
  understanding emotional
    states 407
  vision 66, 68–69
  vital signs 183
  weaning 160–162
Housing 414–416
Human color vision 66, 68–69
Human-directed
    aggression 325
Hydromorphone 448
Hypothalamic-pituitary-adrenal
    (HPA) axis 92, 112, 167
Hypothalamus 92

i

Imprinting 52–53
Imprint training 157
Information transfer 34, 36
Injections
  for horses 196, 198
  intramuscular 198
  intravenous 196, 198
Instrumental learning 97–99
Intermale aggression 360, 361
Intermittent separation-related
    disorders 339–340, 348

j

Juvenile period
  in cats 141, 142
  in dogs 117, 119

k

Ketamine 449
Ketaset™ 449
Kitten socialization classes
    141, 142
Kungas 20–21

l

Laser pointer games 145
Lateral recumbency 226
Learned helplessness 105
Learning 91
  associative 96–99
  choosing the right training
    method 101–103
  consistency 94
  contingency 93–94
  dealing with changing/
    unwanted behaviors 103
    counterconditioning 107
    desensitization and
      counterconditioning
      107
    differential
      reinforcement 105
    extinction 104
    flooding 105
    luring 106
    redirection and
      distraction 105
    reinforcement
      schedule 104
    shaping 106
    systematic desensitization
      106
  extrinsic factors 93
  impact on aggression
    319–320
  intrinsic factors 91
  non-associative 96–97
  pain 93
  punishment 95–96
  reinforcement 94–95
  responses 96
  saliency 94
Levamisole 81
Licking, excessive
    372, 374, 375
Light chasing 370, 374
Linear hierarchy 45, 291
Litter box
  aversion 276
  management and
    hygiene 279–281
Local enhancement 34
Location aversion 277
Locoweed 81, 82
Lorazepam 468
Lower urinary tract diseases
    (LUTD) 274, 275
Low Stress Handling® 206,
    221. *See also* Croney's
    assessment and
    plan system
Lunging 195
Luring 106

m

Main olfactory epithelium
    (MOE) 80, 81
Manatees 393–394
"Many Eyes hypothesis" 34
Mare–foal
    communication 156
Maternal aggression
  in dogs 324
  in horses 357
Matriarchal 37
Medium chain triglycerides
    (MCT) 82
Methadone 447
Methodical selection 11
Midazolam 449
Middening 271
Military working dogs,
    reinforcement 95
Misdirected play 136, 303
Mobbing 33–34
Modern horse 21
Monoamine oxidase inhibitors
    (MAOIs) 422, 425,
    467–468
Monocular vision 66, 67
Morphine 447–448
Mother–offspring bonds
    50–54
Mouthing, dogs 123
Mules 21
Multi-cat environment 149–150
Multimodal environmental
    modification (MEMO)
    281, 282
Musculoskeletal pain 462–463
Music exposure 76, 77, 209
Muzzle 227–228
  for cats 238, 298
  for dogs 327–328
    basket style 229, 230,
      231, 328
    client's comfortness
      231–232
    "drive-by" muzzling
      method 230–231
    goals of 230
    proper placement of 230
    sleeve-style 229
    training advice 230
  safe injection practices 451

n

Natal bands 38
National Association of Board of Pharmacy (NABP) 432
Natufians 10
Natural selection 11, 32
Needs *vs.* wants algorithm 221–223
Negative punishment 100–101
Negative reinforcement 100, 101
Neonatal period
  in cats 137–138
  in dogs 112–113, 118
Neoteny 12
Neuromodulator 428
Neutral stimulus (NS) 97, 98
NMDA antagonists 449
Non-associative learning 96–97
Non-steroidal anti-inflammatories (NSAIDs) 447
Nonverbal communication 245
Nutraceuticals 380, 467

o

Odor
  emotional 79
  identifier 79
  response
    dogs 81
    horses 79–80
Offensive aggression
  in cats 295–296
  in dogs 314, 315
Olfaction 77–78
  cats 81
  dogs 80–81
  horses 79–80
  pheromones 79
  scents/odors 78–79
  VNO 78
Olfactory comfort 209–211
Operant conditioning 97–99, 101, 224, 298, 302
Opioids 447–448
Oral transmucosal (OTM) CRS plan 451, 455, 456
Orphan foal 160
Oxytocin 51

p

Pacing 370, 374
Pack 46
Pain
  analgesics 446–447
  animal learning 93
  behavioral indicators of 404–406
  in cattle 167
  in cow 405
  in horses 406
  musculoskeletal 462–463
Pain-induced aggression
  in cats 294
  in dogs 315–316
  equine 353–354
Pairing-territorial grouping 37
Palatable food 212, 223–225
Pandora syndrome 278
Parallel hierarchy 45
Parent–offspring relationships 50–54
Paroxetine 423, 426
Pathogen transmission 35, 36
Pavlovian conditioning 97
Paxil® 423
Pecking order 44
Perceived resource value 41–42
Peri-domestic animals 13
Persistent separation-related disorders 338, 347–348
Personality
  in cats 143
  handler's 175
Pessimistic states 406
Pet Professional Guild 265
Petting-induced aggression 300–301
Phenotypic description 396
Pheromones 79, 146, 209, 211, 256–257, 282–283, 380
Phobia 426
Physical activity 256, 346
Physiological approach 5
Pica 371, 374
Pigs
  aggressiveness of 44, 46
  emotional contagion 49
  environmental enrichment 415, 416
  music exposure 77
  sound localization 77
  stereotypic behaviors in 410
  taste 81
  vision 71
  winner–loser effects 42
Pinnal distance 74
Plant-eating, excessive 371
Play 49–50
  cats 144–146, 256, 292
  cattle 169
  dogs 256
  equine 158, 359
  misdirected 303
Point of balance 173–174
Polyestrous animal 17
Polytherapy 430–431
Porcine reproductive and respiratory syndrome (PRRS) 35
Positive punishment 100, 101
Positive reinforcement 99–101, 174–175
Post-traumatic stress disorder (PTSD) 389
Predator defense 33–34, 36
Predatory behavior 289, 311–313
Preferred associates 48, 291, 355
Prenatal period
  in cats 137
  in dogs 111–112
Pressure algometry 404
Pre-visit pharmaceuticals (PVPs) 223, 228, 444–446
Primary reinforcers 94
Problem oriented veterinary behavior record (POVBR) 361–362
Professional trainers 259
Pro-social behaviors 47–48. *See also* Affiliative behaviors
Protective aggression 43, 53
Prozac® 422
Przewalski's horse 21
Psychoactive medications 299–300
Psychogenic alopecia 372–374, 425

Psychopharmacology, in companion animals 419
administering medications 431–432
daily medications 423–426
SNRIs 422
SRIs 420–422
SSRIs 421
TCAs 422
event medications 426–430
polytherapy 430–431
weaning 432–434
Psychotropic medications 200, 331, 444. *See also* Antianxiety medication and Anxiolytic medications
Punishment 95–96, 99, 220, 299
negative 100–101
positive 100, 101, 330–331
timing of 96
Puppy classes 121–122
Puppy visit checklist 120–121
Purina Veterinary ProPlan Calming Care 284

r

Reconcile® 422
Red flags 252
behavior professional 261
kittens 150–151
puppies 127–128
Redirected aggression 296, 304
Redirection 105
Reflective listening 245
Reinforcement 93, 99
differential 105
negative 100, 101
positive 99–101
timing of 96
Reinforcement schedule 104
continuous 104
fixed interval 104
fixed ratio 104
variable interval 104
variable ratio 104
Reinforcers 94–95
Rejection 54
Repetitive behaviors, in companion animals. *See also* Abnormal repetitive behaviors
attention-seeking behaviors 368, 369
behavior modification 378–379
breed predispositions 375
compulsive behaviors 368–369
definition of 367
differential diagnoses 367, 368
displacement behaviors 368
family involvement and interaction 377, 378
hallucinatory
fly snapping 371
light/shadow chasing 370
reflection fixation 371
skin rippling 371
history-taking 375–376
locomotory
freezing/trancing 370
hind-end checking 370
pacing 370
spinning and tail chasing 370
management and tools 377–378
medications 379–380
nutraceuticals 380
oral
acral lick dermatitis 372, 373
excessive licking 372
excessive plant-eating 371
fabric/wool sucking 371
flank-sucking 371–372
pica 371
psychogenic alopecia 372, 373
pheromones 380
physiological differentials 373–375
stereotypic behaviors 368–370
treatment for 376
Reproduction, benefits of group living 34, 36
Reproductive competition 35, 36
Resource competition 35, 36
Resource guarding, dogs 123–124
Resource holding potential (RHP) 41, 42, 46–47
Response substitution 378
Restraint
chemical 228–229
Elizabethan collar 234
guidelines for 226
for longer period 226–228
safe and effective 225–226
towel 233
Rhinoceros 397
Ritualized behavior 40
Rope halters, for horses 188
Royal Canin Calm diet 284
Rumen fill 412
Ruminants
hearing 76–77
vision 71–72

s

SAM-e 467
Scratching, horses 157–159
Sea turtles 394
Secondary reinforcers 94
Sedation 228. *See also* Chemical restraint
Selective serotonin reuptake inhibitors (SSRIs) 299–300, 306, 363, 421–423, 468
Selegiline 425, 426, 467–468
Semi-domestic animals 13
Senilife® 467
Sensitization 96–97
Sensory perception 65
audition
auditory signal 73
cats 76
dogs 75–76
hearing range 73
horses 74–75
pinnal distance 74
ruminants 76–77

olfaction 77–78
cats 81
dogs 80–81
horses 79–80
pheromones 79
scents/odors 78–79
VNO 78
taste 81–82
vision
binocular 66, 67
birds 72, 73
cats 70, 71
dichromatic 66, 67
dogs 70–71
electromagnetic spectrum of visible light 66
horses 66, 68–69
monocular 66, 67
ruminants/cattle 71–72
trichromatic 66, 67
Separation-related disorders (SRD)
age of onset 340
associated with human sleep times 340, 348
breed and sex factors 340
CDS 345
contexts of incidents 345
diagnoses 343–345
distress surrounding departures and arrivals 342
hyper/insecure attachment 342
incidence of 337
independence training 346
intermittent 339–340, 348
normal 338
persistent 338
juvenile onset 339
medication 347
pharmacological intervention 347
secondary 339
shelter/rescue dog 338–339
risk factors 340
secondary 339
signs of 340–341
treatment 345–348
underlying diseases 345
video recording 342, 345
Serotonin 290, 299, 363
Serotonin antagonist reuptake inhibitor (SARI) 427–428
Serotonin norepinephrine reuptake inhibitors (SNRIs) 422, 424–425
Serotonin reuptake inhibitors (SRIs) 420–422
Serotonin syndrome 431
Sertraline 423, 426
Sexual maturity
in cats 142
in dogs 117–119
Sexual selection 11
Shaping, behavior 106
Sheep, selection of birth sites 32
Shock collars 102
Sickness, behavioral indicators of 403–404
Sileo® 427, 429, 444, 445
Skin rippling 371
Snakes 66
Snapping 156
Snuffle mats 466
Social buffering 48–49, 213
Social facilitation 34, 49
Social group(ing). *See also* Conflict in social groups
affiliative behaviors 47–50
aggressiveness, RHP and dominance rank 46–47
dominance hierarchies 45–46
female grouping 37
multi-male and multi-female 38, 45
pairing-territorial 37
pecking order 44
pro-social behaviors 47–48
single male-multiple female 38
solitary-territorial 36–37
sows 38
Sociality 31
benefits of
examples of 36
foraging efficiency 34
information transfer 34
predator defense 33–34
reproductive benefits 34
costs of
examples of 36
parasites and disease 35
predation risk 34–35
reproductive competition 35
resource competition 35
evolution and environmental constraints 31
Socialization classes, for kittens 141, 142
Socialization period
in cats 136, 139–141
in dogs 114–116, 119
tips 115
Socially facilitated aggression 324–325
Social maturity
in cats 142
in dogs 118, 119
Social referencing 214
Solitary-territorial grouping 36–37
Sows 38
Spinning 370, 375
Stereotypic(al) behaviors 387, 408. *See also* Abnormal repetitive behaviors
Stereotypy 386
Stress 92, 167–168
Submissive behavior 40
Substrate aversion 276–277
Sympathetic nervous system (SNS) 92, 448
Sympathoadrenal medullary (SAM) pathway 167
Systematic desensitization 106, 330
Systematic desensitization and counterconditioning 107, 198, 200, 305, 379

t

Tactile comfort 211–212
Tail-biting 410
Tail chasing 370, 374
Taming 12–13
Tapetum lucidum 70
Telazol® 449

Territorial aggression (TA) 343
in cats 295, 300, 304
in dogs 323–324
equine 355–356
Territoriality 36
Thermal comfort 213
Thiabendazole 81
Thiram 81
ThunderCap 207, 229, 232–233
ThunderEase 211, 257
Thundershirt 233
Topical analgesics 212
Touch gradient (TG) 194, 212
Towel wrapping and restraint
cats 225–227, 235–236
dogs 233
half-burrito 236
Toys 144–146, 377–378
Transitional period
in cats 138–139
in dogs 113–114, 119
Trazodone 202, 427–429, 444–446
Triangular hierarchy 45–46
Trichromatic vision 66, 67
Tricyclic antidepressants (TCAs) 299–300, 306, 422–424
Trigger stacking 251, 253

u

Unconditioned response (UCR) 97, 98
Unconditioned stimulus (UCS) 97–99
Unconscious selection 11
Urine marking 270–271, 343

v

Vaccination 122
Variable interval reinforcement schedule 104
Variable ratio reinforcement schedule 104
Venipuncture 226
Venlafaxine 424–426
Veterinary behaviorists 260
Veterinary visits
cats 150
dogs
checklist 120–121
first veterinary visit 119–120
future visits 121
happy visit 227
presence of familiar members 213, 214
Vision
binocular 66, 67
birds 72, 73
cats 70, 71
cattle 165–166
dichromatic 66, 67
dogs 70–71
electromagnetic spectrum of visible light 66
horses 66, 68–69
monocular 66, 67
ruminants/cattle 71–72
trichromatic 66, 67
Visual comfort 207–209
Vomeronasal organ (VNO) 78, 80, 81

w

Weaning
gradual 161, 162
horses 160–162
Wild animals
abnormal repetitive behaviors in
allostatic load 388
behavior assessment 388
captive carnivores 391–392
defined 386
environmental enrichment and training 397
Five Domains framework 386–387
human-induced stressors. 392–394
management and treatment plan 396–399
manatees 393–394
non-zoo settings 392–395
oral/feeding behaviors 391, 392
pharmacologic intervention 397–398
preventive measures 395
sea turtles 394
skin infections 392
stereotypical behaviors 387
zoos and wildlife sanctuaries 391
beasts of war 388–389
in changing world 392–394
domestication 13
under human care 387–388
in production 389–391
Wildcats 16, 17
Winner–loser effects 42
Wolves
domestication 14–15
fights 41

y

Y-maze 168

z

Zenalpha® 448–449
Zenidog® 257
Zoloft® 423, 426
Zylkene® 284